Hearing Loss: Neural Consequences

Hearing Loss: Neural Consequences

Editor: David Crow

AMERICAN
MEDICAL PUBLISHERS
www.americanmedicalpublishers.com

AMERICAN
MEDICAL PUBLISHERS
www.americanmedicalpublishers.com

Cataloging-in-Publication Data

Hearing loss : neural consequences / edited by David Crow.
p. cm.
Includes bibliographical references and index.
ISBN 979-8-88740-173-7
1. Deafness. 2. Hearing disorders. 3. Nervous system--Diseases. 4. Neurology. I. Crow, David.
RF290 .H433 2023
617.8--dc23

American Medical Publishers,
41 Flatbush Avenue,
1st Floor, New York,
NY 11217, USA

ISBN 979-8-88740-173-7 (Hardback)

Contents

Preface

Hearing loss refers to a partial or complete inability to hear. It can be present at birth or it may develop later in life. It can affect one or both ears. Hearing problems in children may impair their ability to acquire spoken language, while social and occupational challenges are created for adults. Hearing loss can be permanent or temporary. When it occurs due to age, it often affects both ears and is caused by the loss of cochlear hair cell. There are various causes of hearing loss such as birth complications, certain medications or toxins, genetics, exposure to noise, trauma to the ear, some infections and ageing. Neural consequences of hearing loss can be seen in the structure of auditory cortex in humans. This book unravels the recent studies on hearing loss. It also strives to provide a fair idea about its neural consequences. This book will serve as a reference to a broad spectrum of readers.

This book has been the outcome of endless efforts put in by authors and researchers on various issues and topics within the field. The book is a comprehensive collection of significant researches that are addressed in a variety of chapters. It will surely enhance the knowledge of the field among readers across the globe.

It gives us an immense pleasure to thank our researchers and authors for their efforts to submit their piece of writing before the deadlines. Finally in the end, I would like to thank my family and colleagues who have been a great source of inspiration and support.

Editor

Preface

1

Unilateral hearing during development: hemispheric specificity in plastic reorganizations

Andrej Kral[1]*, Silvia Heid[1,2], Peter Hubka[1] and Jochen Tillein[1,2]

[1] *Cluster of Excellence, Department of Experimental Otology, Institute of Audioneurotechnology, ENT Clinics, Hannover Medical School, Hannover, Germany*
[2] *Department of Physiology and Otolaryngology, J. W. Goethe University, Frankfurt am Main, Germany*

***Correspondence:**
Andrej Kral, Institute of Audioneurotechnology, Hannover School of Medicine, Feodor-Lynen-Str. 35, D-30625 Hannover, Germany
e-mail: kral.andrej@mh-hannover.de

The present study investigates the hemispheric contributions of neuronal reorganization following early single-sided hearing (unilateral deafness). The experiments were performed on ten cats from our colony of deaf white cats. Two were identified in early hearing screening as unilaterally congenitally deaf. The remaining eight were bilaterally congenitally deaf, unilaterally implanted at different ages with a cochlear implant. Implanted animals were chronically stimulated using a single-channel portable signal processor for two to five months. Microelectrode recordings were performed at the primary auditory cortex under stimulation at the hearing and deaf ear with bilateral cochlear implants. Local field potentials (LFPs) were compared at the cortex ipsilateral and contralateral to the hearing ear. The focus of the study was on the morphology and the onset latency of the LFPs. With respect to morphology of LFPs, pronounced hemisphere-specific effects were observed. Morphology of amplitude-normalized LFPs for stimulation of the deaf and the hearing ear was similar for responses recorded at the same hemisphere. However, when comparisons were performed between the hemispheres, the morphology was more dissimilar even though the same ear was stimulated. This demonstrates hemispheric specificity of some cortical adaptations irrespective of the ear stimulated. The results suggest a specific adaptation process at the hemisphere ipsilateral to the hearing ear, involving specific (down-regulated inhibitory) mechanisms not found in the contralateral hemisphere. Finally, onset latencies revealed that the sensitive period for the cortex ipsilateral to the hearing ear is shorter than that for the contralateral cortex. Unilateral hearing experience leads to a functionally-asymmetric brain with different neuronal reorganizations and different sensitive periods involved.

Keywords: cochlear implant, plasticity, single-sided deafness, critical periods, development

INTRODUCTION

In developmental manipulations of the symmetry of auditory input, as occurs with unilateral deafness (Reale et al., 1987; Vale et al., 2004; Langers et al., 2005; Burton et al., 2012; Kral et al., 2013) or asymmetric moderate hearing loss (King et al., 2001; Popescu and Polley, 2010), the hemispheres can be differentiated in respect of the anatomical relationship to the (better) hearing ear. Plastic reorganizations are often reported in the hemisphere contralateral to the hearing ear. However, the ipsilateral cortex also receives asymmetric input and likely participates in behavioral consequences of unilateral hearing. The present study investigates whether the function of the primary field A1 of the ipsilateral and the contralateral cortex differs in unilateral deafness.

The primary auditory cortex contains mainly binaural neurons—neurons responsive to stimulation of only one ear are virtually absent (Zhang et al., 2004). Many different aural interaction patterns have been described in neuronal recordings, even in the same neurons, depending on the exact binaural temporal and intensity relations (Zhang et al., 2004). The majority of auditory neurons has receptive fields covering large portions of the contralateral hemifield (Middlebrooks et al., 1994). Stimulation of one ear most frequently leads to excitation in the neurons of the contralateral cortex but may cause excitation or inhibition in the ipsilateral cortex (Imig and Adrián, 1977). Because of the stronger responses at the contralateral cortex, and because of the shorter latency of the responses at the contralateral cortex, the term "aural dominance" (Imig and Adrián, 1977) or aural preference (Kral et al., 2013) has been introduced. Contralateral "dominance" is the consequence of the cortical representation of the contralateral acoustic hemifield.

Recently, effects of unilateral deafness have attracted clinical interest owing to the predominantly monaural therapy of prelingual deafness with one cochlear implant (Graham et al., 2009; Gordon et al., 2013) and the relatively high incidence of unilateral deafness (Eiserman et al., 2008; Watkin and Baldwin, 2012). Unilateral deafness is now considered an indication for cochlear implantation of the deaf ear, but so far mainly in cases of postlingual deafness due to tinnitus in the deaf ear (Vermeire et al., 2008; Buechner et al., 2010; Firszt et al., 2012). The effects of congenital or early onset of unilateral hearing are less well explored.

Many previous studies have investigated the plasticity of the brain following cochlear implantation and have described, both in humans and in an animal model, sensitive developmental periods for plasticity (review in Kral and Sharma, 2012). When hearing is imbalanced (as caused by early unilateral hearing loss following periods of binaural hearing), the auditory system reorganizes (Bilecen et al., 2000; King et al., 2001; Langers et al., 2005; Popescu and Polley, 2010; Kral et al., 2013). Central reorganizations have been suggested previously in cases including sequential cochlear implantations in children (Peters et al., 2007; Graham et al., 2009; Gordon et al., 2013; Illg et al., 2013). The outcomes for the implantation of the second ear critically depend on the age at implantation of the first ear and the delay between the implantations (Sharma et al., 2007; Graham et al., 2009; Illg et al., 2013). Recently, two studies elucidated the mechanisms behind such phenomena. In the first study, a sensitive period for the reorganization of aural preference at the cortex ipsilateral to the first implanted ear has been demonstrated using electrophysiological methods in cats (Kral et al., 2013). This study uncovered the mechanism behind the critical dependence of the outcome of the second implantation on age at first implantation. The second study confirmed and extended the findings using electroencephalographic recordings in sequentially-implanted children (Gordon et al., 2013).

The present study directly compares the hemispheric effects of unilateral hearing. Congenitally deaf (white) cats were selected from a colony of deaf white cats using an early hearing screening procedure described earlier (Heid et al., 1998). Some animals were implanted with a cochlear implant during early development, so that stimulation onset was possible from 2.5 to 6 months of age, covering the age of synaptic development of deaf cats (**Figure 1**, Kral and Sharma, 2012). Two animals were born unilaterally deaf (Kral et al., 2013) and were used as models of very early asymmetric hearing (single-sided deafness).

The present study demonstrates that reorganizations following unilateral hearing (deafness) show a specificity for the hemisphere. The cortex ipsilateral to the hearing ear demonstrates a functional shift toward the hearing ear (Kral et al., 2013). On the other hand, at the hemisphere contralateral to the hearing ear a reduction of the responses to the deaf ear was observed. Despite some ear-specific effects in onset latency, the morphology of the local field potentials (LFPs) showed more pronounced differences between hemispheres than differences observed on the same hemisphere when comparing the responses to stimulation of the deaf and the hearing ear. This demonstrates hemispheric specificity of the reorganizations. Finally, reorganizations observed in onset latency demonstrated a shorter sensitive period for plasticity in the hemisphere ipsilateral to the hearing ear when compared to the contralateral hemisphere.

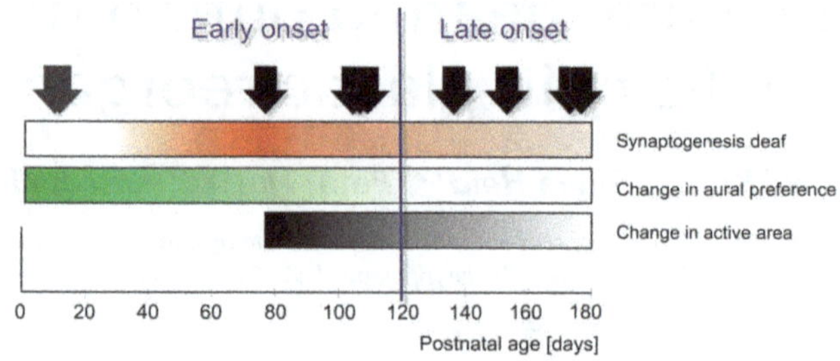

FIGURE 1 | Onset of unilateral hearing in ten animals (arrows) compared with the developmental time-line of deaf cat auditory system as reflected in the auditory cortex. The intensity of the color represents the extent of the given change. "Functional synaptogenesis" (development of synaptic function, measured by current source density analyses of evoked responses in the cortex, thus reflecting synaptic counts combined with synaptic function) in binaurally deaf animals has been shown to be delayed by 1.5 months compared to that in hearing animals, with a maximum of evoked synaptic currents around 3 months (Kral et al., 2005, red). Previous studies in congenitally deaf cats demonstrated two sensitive periods: one for reorganization reflected at cortex ipsilateral to hearing ear (green), terminating between 3.5 and 4.2 months (Kral et al., 2013), the other sensitive period for increase in activated volume of tissue ("active area") in the contralateral field A1 (and the corresponding response latencies; black), terminating between 5 and 6 months (Kral et al., 2002; Kral and Sharma, 2012). In the present study, distinction between early and late onset was based on sensitive period of aural preference (Kral et al., 2013), whereas sensitive period for expansion of the active area extends beyond this timeframe. Gray arrows: unilaterally congenitally deaf animals; black arrows: binaurally deaf animals, implanted with a unilateral cochlear implant at different postnatal times.

Table 1 | Implantations, age at final experiments and investigated cortex for the animals in the study.

Animal	Age at onset of unilateral hearing [months]	Age at experiment [months]	Contralateral cortex	Ipsilateral cortex
1	Congenital	>12		•
2	Congenital	>12	•	•
3	2.5	4.5	•	•
4	3.5	9	•	•
5	3.5	6.5	•	
6	3.5	5.5	•	
7	4.2	9.2		•
8	5.0	10	•	•
9	6.0	11	•	•
10	6.0	8	•	•

MATERIALS AND METHODS

The present experiments complement a previous study and the methods are described in detail there (Kral et al., 2013). Here, we summarize the most important technical aspects of the method.

ANIMALS

Experiments were performed on 10 cats. In all animals, hearing was strongly asymmetric (**Table 1**): two animals had normal hearing in one ear (hearing thresholds being <40 dB SPL) and were unilaterally congenitally deaf in the other ear (hearing thresholds >110 dB SPL). The remaining animals were binaurally congenitally deaf cats (CDCs) monaurally implanted with a custom-made cochlear implant at the age of 2.5–6.0 months and subjected to chronic electrostimulation. The implantation ages of unilateral animals are given in **Table 1**. Not all stimulus/recording combinations could be investigated in each animal.

All animals obtained from our colony of deaf white cats underwent hearing screening within the fourth week of life. The screening procedure was based on a longitudinal study of hearing in deaf white cats recorded every two days after birth and is described in detail elsewhere (Heid et al., 1998).

All experiments were approved by the local state authorities and were performed in compliance with the guidelines of the European Community for the care and use of laboratory animals (EU VD 86/609/EEC) and the German Animal Welfare Act (TierSchG).

To investigate developmental plasticity in animals with unilateral hearing, chronic stimulation by a cochlear implant was initiated at two different ages, reflecting the results of previous studies (**Figure 1**):

- *early* (2.5 and 3.5 months, early implanted animals), when the naive cortex shows a developmental peak in evoked synaptic activity (Kral et al., 2005) and the animals showed plasticity of aural preference (Kral et al., 2013),
- *late* (after 4.0 months), when synaptic activity in deaf animals fell below the level of hearing controls and the known sensitive period for aural preference has already expired (Kral et al., 2013).

IMPLANTATION AND CHRONIC STIMULATION

Implantations were performed under sterile conditions in anesthetized animals as described previously (Kral et al., 2002). Animals were premedicated with 0.25 mg atropine i.p. and anaesthetized with ketamin hydrochloride (24.5 mg/kg Ketavet, Parker-Davis, Germany) and xylazine hydrochloride (1 mg/kg, Bayer, Germany) with supplementary doses when necessary. The animal's status was monitored by capnometry, electroencephalography, electrocardiogram and pulse oximetry. The bulla was exposed via a retrocochlear cutaneous incision and a subsequent soft separation of the muscles overlying it. The bulla was opened using a drill. The membrane of the round window was carefully removed with a sharp hook and the electrode carrier was implanted through the round window. The implant was fixed using a suture (non-absorbable thread) at the dorsal thickened part of the bulla. The bulla was tightly closed using dental acrylic. The contacting leads for the implant were led subcutaneously and additionally secured at the lambdoideal crista. The contact with the processor was transcutaneous in the interscapular line. At the end of the implantation, the electrical thresholds were determined using brainstem-evoked responses. The transcutaneous penetration site was covered with a jacket containing the processor. Animals were treated with ampicilline (100 mg s.c.) for 7 days post-surgery. Three days after the operation the electrical thresholds were behaviorally tested using pinna reflexes (details in Kral et al., 2002). The signal processor was activated subsequent to animal's full recovery (~7 days after implantation). The moment at which the implant was activated determined the age of onset of asymmetric hearing.

Chronic stimulation was performed using single-channel portable processors with a compressed analogue coding strategy in monopolar stimulation. Stimulation was applied continuously without interruption (on a 24/7 basis; for details see supplementary material in Kral et al., 2013). To exclude the effects of stimulation duration, three animals were stimulated for two months (~1440 h of implant stimulation), one animal for three months (~2160 h of implant stimulation) and four animals were stimulated for five months (~3600 h of implant stimulation). The animals were trained to respond to a brief tone of 732 Hz frequency by picking up a reward at a specified location on 5 days a week (20 stimulus presentations per session). The success rate exceeded 50% after 7–21 days of training in all animals and confirmed that the animals used the acoustic input to actively control behavior.

ACUTE EXPERIMENTS: STIMULATION AND RECORDING

For acute experiments, all animals were premedicated with 0.25 mg atropine i.p. and initially anaesthetized with ketamin hydrochloride (24.5 mg/kg Ketavet, Parker-Davis, Germany) and propionylpromazine phosphate (2.1 mg/kg Combelen, Bayer, Germany) or xylazine hydrochloride (1 mg/kg, Bayer, Germany). The animals were then tracheotomized and artificially ventilated with 50% O_2 and 50% N_2O, with a 0.2–1.5% concentration of isoflurane (Lilly, Germany) added to maintain a controlled depth of anesthesia (Kral et al., 1999). It was monitored using heart-rate, end-tidal CO_2, muscle tone and EEG signals. End-tidal CO_2 was maintained below 4%. Core temperature was kept above 37.5°C using a homeothermic blanket. The animals' status was monitored further by blood gas concentration measurements, pH, bicarbonate concentration and base excess, glycaemia and oxygen saturation. A modified Ringer's solution containing bicarbonate (dosage based on the base excess) was infused i.v. The internal state was monitored by testing capillary blood every 12 h.

The animal's head was fixed in a stereotactic holder (Horsley-Clarke). Both bullae and ear canals were exposed. In order to record evoked auditory brainstem responses, a small trephination was drilled at the vertex and a silver-ball electrode (diameter 1 mm) was attached epidurally. Hearing status was tested at the beginning of the experiments. So as to prevent electrophonic responses, the hair cells in normal-hearing ears were destroyed by intracochlear instillation of 300 μl 2.5% neomycine sulphate solution over a 5 min. period and subsequent rinsing using Ringer's solution. The absence of hearing was subsequently confirmed by the absence of brainstem-evoked responses.

Stimulation in the final acute experiments was performed using cochlear implants inserted bilaterally into the cochleae. In chronically electrically stimulated animals, the chronic implant was used for stimulation at the "hearing" ear. The stimulus was a biphasic pulse (200 μs/phase) applied through the apicalmost electrode contact at 10 dB above the lowest cortical threshold (see Kral et al., 2009).

For recording, a trephination above the auditory cortex was performed and the dura was opened. First, within a grid of 3 × 3 positions, LFPs were recorded using low-impedance electrodes to determine the lowest cortical threshold for stimulation with a biphasic pulse (200 μs/phase) applied through the apicalmost electrode of the implant. Mapping of cortical responses was performed using glass microelectrodes ($Z \approx 6\,M\Omega$) that were moved along the auditory cortex with a micromanipulator (1 μm precision) at the cortical surface. Stimulus was 10 dB above the lowest cortical thresholds, the current level at which electrically-evoked LFPs reach the saturation point. By choosing that intensity the whole active volume of the cortex can be determined. The signals were amplified 5000–10,000 times, bandpass filtered (0.01–10 kHz), digitized (at a sampling rate of 25 kHz) and 50 responses were averaged to determine the mean LFP at each recording position. First, contralateral cortex was investigated, followed by the ipsilateral cortex. The tested combinations of recording site and stimulation site are shown in **Table 1**.

DATA PROCESSING

From the more than 100 recordings at the cortical surface within field A1 and adjacent fields, cortical activation maps were constructed (**Figure 2**).

The electrical artifacts from the stimulation occurred between 0.0 and 0.6 ms post-stimulus and did not influence the response (latency > 7 ms). The signal before the response (500 ms duration in each animal) was characterized by computing its mean and standard deviation. The threshold of mean ± 4*standard deviation was then used for detecting neuronal responses. The threshold attained absolute values of 10–20 μV.

Using this measure, onset latencies were detected for the first positive response (P_a component, **Figure 3**) of the LFPs. For each recording position of the surface maps, these data were determined for crossed and uncrossed stimulation. Normality of the data was tested using the Jarque-Bera test (5% significance level) and if confirmed, a two-tailed *t*-test was carried out; if it failed, a Wilcoxon-Mann-Whitney test (both at 5% significance level) was used. Additionally, for each position a paired difference of the onset latency was computed. The medians were used as population measures since the latency values showed a significantly skewed distribution. Comparisons between the experimental groups were performed by applying the Wilcoxon-Mann-Whitney test (two-tailed, 5% significance level).

Peak amplitudes of P_a components were determined using an automated procedure (based on the time derivatives of the signals). Amplitudes below 50 μV were discarded from the processing to minimize the effect of noise on small amplitude signals.

Some analyses were performed exclusively from six positions within the area with the largest responses (the "hot-spot," Kral et al., 2009). These responses were averaged and used in comparisons. For this, a sliding window of 2 ms was used, comparisons were performed using the Wilcoxon-Mann-Whitney two-tailed *t*-test at $\alpha = 0.1\%$, adjusted to multiple comparisons using the false detection rate procedure (Benjamini and Hochberg, 1995).

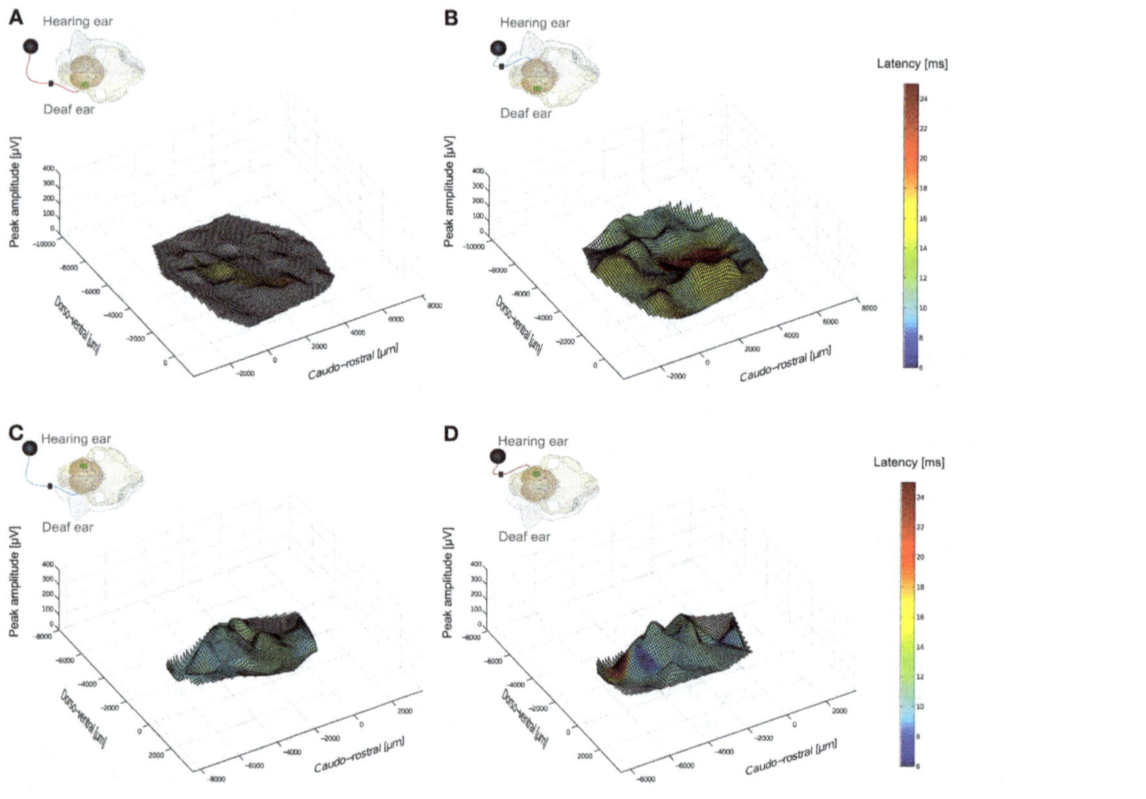

FIGURE 2 | Hemispheric specificity of amplitude effects in cortical responses of a unilaterally congenitally deaf animal investigated at the ipsilateral and contralateral cortex. Insets indicate stimulation-recording configurations. In the inset, small loudspeaker indicates hearing side, and green spot the cortex in which recordings are made. Blue and red wires indicate ear stimulated with a cochlear implant. Largest peak amplitudes and peak latencies (color) are shown as a function of recording position. Responses below 50 μV were not considered and are shown without coloring. **(A)** cochlear implant stimulation at the contralateral (deaf) ear, recording at hemisphere contralateral to hearing ear. Few responses above 50 μV were observed. **(B)** in the same animal, stimulation of hearing ear extensively activated the whole contralateral primary auditory cortex. **(C,D)** at cortex ipsilateral to hearing ear, stimulation of both deaf (left) and hearing (right) ear resulted in strong activation of portions of auditory cortex.

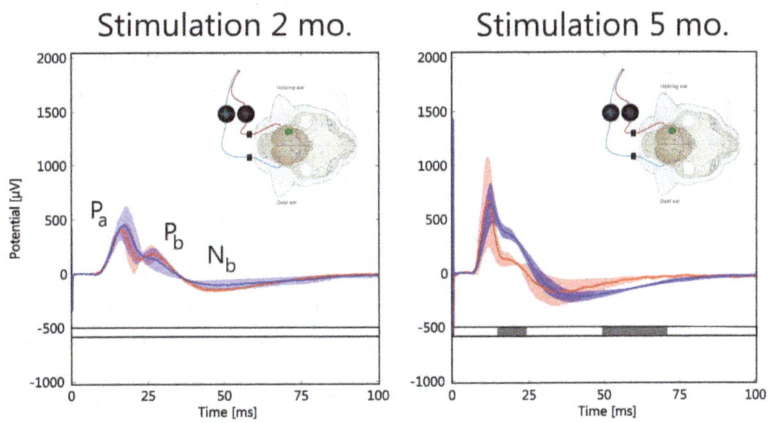

FIGURE 3 | Effect of stimulation duration (2 and 5 months) on morphology of mean local field potentials (LFPs) from hot spots in two early-implanted animals. Inset shows configuration: recording was at the ipsilateral cortex (green spot), stimulation of hearing and deaf ear. Response color denotes stimulation site (red: uncrossed stimulation, blue: crossed stimulation); shaded area is the temporally smoothed region of one standard deviation around mean. Gray bar below curve indicates statistical significance of difference between red and blue curve using a running two-tailed Wilcoxon-Mann-Whitney test (2 ms window, $\alpha = 0.001$, corrected by the false detection rate procedure). Increasing stimulation duration increased overall amplitudes of responses, but more so for hearing ear. Additionally, latencies decreased with stimulation duration. Statistically significant portions are at P_b and N_b regions.

The comparison of the morphology of mean LFP was assessed using the dissimilarity index (DI, Kral et al., 2009):

$$DI = 0.5 \cdot \sum_T \left| \frac{\mathrm{LFP}_1(T)}{\sum_t |\mathrm{LFP}_1(t)|} - \frac{\mathrm{LFP}_2(T)}{\sum_t |\mathrm{LFP}_2(t)|} \right|$$

This index considers the morphology of the LFPs irrespective of the amplitude. A dissimilarity index can reach values between 0 and 1, whereas 0 represents identical LFPs. Identical but time-reversed signals yield a high dissimilarity index due to the sample-by-sample comparison.

RESULTS

The present comparisons concentrated on LFP morphology and onset latency. First, the response maps and morphology of the LFPs are described, followed by onset latency comparisons.

TERMINOLOGY

In the present paper, the terms *contralateral* and *ipsilateral* are always used with reference to the side of the "chronically" hearing ear. The *hearing ear* may be either normal hearing (in unilaterally congenitally deaf animals) or born deaf and implanted at a later age (in the chronically electrically stimulated animals). The ipsilateral cortex is the one on the same side of the brain as the hearing ear.

On the other hand, the term "*crossed*" is used relative to the side of a given recording or stimulation and always refers to the "opposite" side of the brain. The term "*uncrossed*" refers to the same side as the ear stimulated or the cortex in which recordings were made.

Thus, if the left ear was the hearing ear, and a probe stimulus was presented at the right (i.e., the deaf) ear, the crossed response refers to the response recorded at the left cortex and the uncrossed response refers to that at the right cortex. In this case, the ipsilateral cortex is then the left one and the contralateral cortex is the right one.

SPATIAL AND TEMPORAL CORTICAL RESPONSE PATTERN

Crossed and uncrossed responses compared at the same cortex tend to result in different LFPs in normal hearing animals, with crossed responses showing larger amplitudes and shorter latencies (Kral et al., 2009). In binaurally deaf animals, this difference was diminished in amplitudes and absent in latencies (Kral et al., 2009). The congenitally unilaterally deaf animal exhibited a remarkable pattern of activity when the hemispheres were compared directly (**Figure 2**). The cortex ipsilateral to the hearing ear showed responses to both the hearing as well as the deaf ear (Kral et al., 2013). The cortex contralateral to the hearing ear, on the other hand, showed very weak responses to the stimulation of the deaf ear following congenital unilateral deafness despite good responsiveness to the hearing ear.

To minimize the effect of different spatial position when comparing responses at the contralateral and the ipsilateral cortex, further analysis was concentrated on hot spots: the areas of largest responses. These were considered as being the cortical representation of the stimulated region in the cochlea and were therefore considered the functionally corresponding sites in the cortex. From a total area of 1.5 mm^2 within the hot spot, all LFPs were averaged (~6 recording positions; **Figure 3**).

First, the effect of stimulation duration was compared in early-implanted animals (**Figure 3**, animals 3 and 4, **Table 1**): Longer experience with a unilateral cochlear implant increased the amplitudes of the responses in the hot spot, and more so for the hearing ear; however, responses to both the hearing and the deaf ear increased. At longer latencies (component P_b and later), more significant differences for the two stimulation sites were observed than at short latencies (**Figure 3**; see also below).

Crossed responses to stimulation of the deaf ear and to stimulation of the hearing ear were compared next (**Figure 4**). For crossed responses the maximum amplitudes were of a similar order of magnitude for both ears, although significant interindividual variability was noted in the maximum potential. However, in the congenitally unilaterally deaf animal, a marked difference in the morphology of the response was observed at longer latencies (**Figure 4**, top). In particular, component P_b was well separated from the P_a component when the deaf ear was stimulated (**Figure 4** top, red curve), whereas the components appeared fused when the hearing ear was stimulated (**Figure 4** top, blue curve). A morphological difference of this nature was less expressed in late-implanted animals, particularly since P_b could not always be identified (**Figure 4**, lower panel).

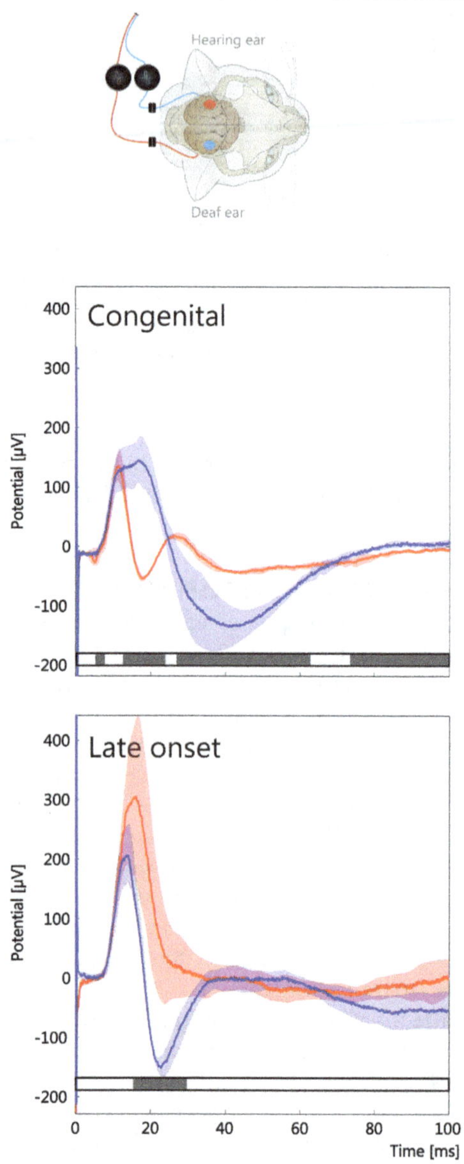

FIGURE 4 | Crossed responses in a congenitally unilaterally deaf animal and a late-implanted animal (stimulation duration 5 months). Stimulation of hearing ear and recording at contralateral cortex shown in blue, for deaf ear and recording at the ipsilateral hemisphere in red, shaded area is the temporally smoothed region of one standard deviation around mean. Gray bars below curve indicate statistical significance of a running two-tailed Wilcoxon-Mann-Whitney test ($\alpha = 0.001$, corrected by false detection rate procedure, 2 ms window). Ear-specific effects were observed in both animals; however, regions of statistical significance were larger in the congenital onset case. Maximum amplitudes in both compared animals were within 200–400 μV, as reported previously (Kral et al., 2009).

At the ipsilateral hemisphere early-implanted animals had uncrossed responses larger than crossed ones (**Figure 5A**). This was not observed in the late-implanted animals (**Figure 5C**, comp. Kral et al., 2013). The crossed and uncrossed mean response had similar morphology when considered at the same hemisphere (comparisons within the panels **A–D** in **Figure 5**). At the cortex contralateral to the hearing ear, a marked difference in amplitude of the crossed and uncrossed response was evident in the congenitally unilaterally deaf animal (**Figure 5B**; see also **Figure 2**). Nonetheless, even in this case it was apparent that the LFP morphology within a hemisphere was more similar than between hemispheres. In total, the responses at the same hemisphere (comparisons within panels **Figures 5A–D**) were more similar than those compared between hemispheres (comparisons between panels in **Figures 5A,B** or **Figures 5C,D**), irrespective of the age of onset.

To quantify this observation, dissimilarity index for P_a/P_b complex was computed for different intrahemispheric and interhemispheric comparisons (**Figure 6**). A Kruskal-Wallis test demonstrated a significant effect of the configuration ($p = 0.01$). For the crossed and uncrossed responses at the ipsilateral hemisphere, the LFP morphology was similar (a small DI of 0.16 ± 0.08, $n = 6$). However, comparing the crossed response of the contralateral hemisphere to the uncrossed response of the ipsilateral hemisphere resulted in larger difference (same animals, $DI = 0.38 \pm 0.12$, two-tailed Wilcoxon-Mann-Whitney test, $p = 0.010$). Further, crossed responses (compared between hemispheres) showed a high dissimilarity index of similar magnitude as the latter comparison ($DI = 0.41 \pm 0.15$, $p = 0.749$). The dissimilarity index at the contralateral hemisphere for the crossed vs. uncrossed comparison was not different from the same at the ipsilateral hemisphere ($DI = 0.16 \pm 0.08$ vs. 0.16 ± 0.05, $p = 1.000$). Thus, interhemispheric comparisons resulted in larger DIs than intrahemispheric comparisons. Taken together, these results demonstrate that the cortical response shows hemispheric specificity in morphology irrespective of the ear that is stimulated. Although the largest DIs were found in the congenitally unilaterally deaf animal (**Figures 5A,B**), the correlation with onset age was not significant in DI measures ($\alpha = 5\%$).

ONSET LATENCIES

A previous study demonstrated high plasticity of LFP onset latency and its sensitivity to developmental modifications (Kral et al., 2013). This measure showed lower variance over cortical positions and animal than peak amplitudes, so that interhemispheric comparisons were statistically testable and recording positions biased less to the comparisons. For these reasons, further comparisons were performed using onset latencies of LFPs. In the previous study (Kral et al., 2013), we performed paired

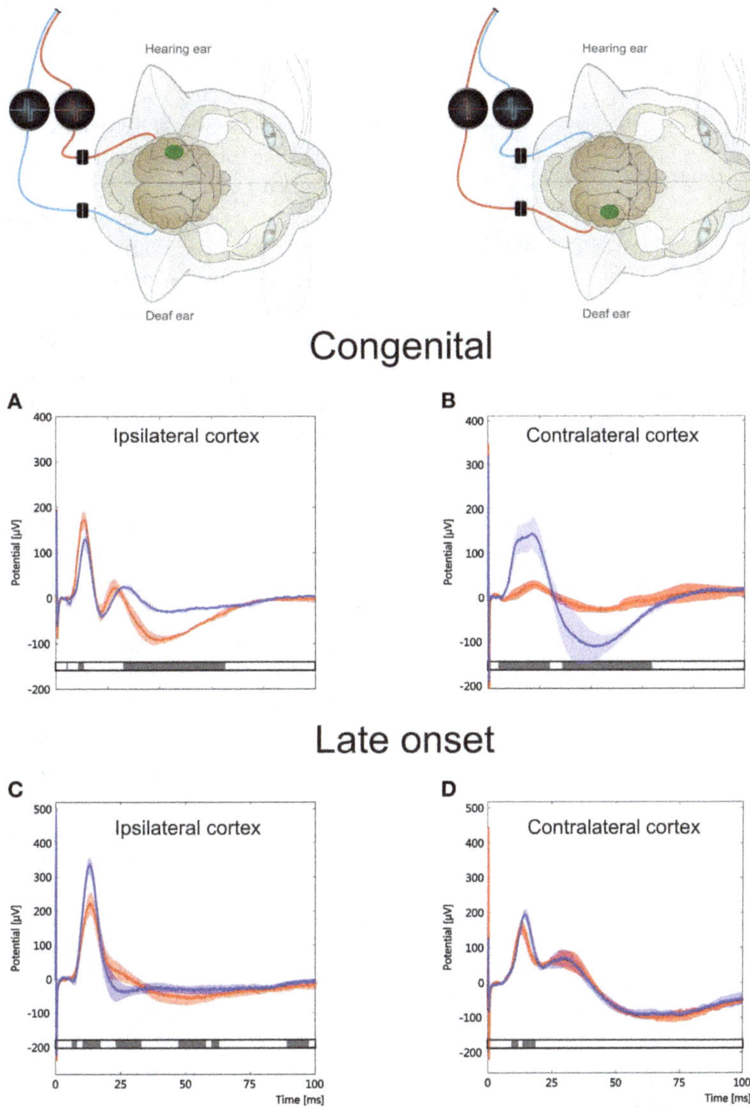

FIGURE 5 | Comparison of crossed and uncrossed responses at both hemispheres in a congenitally unilaterally deaf animal (A,B) and a late implanted animal (C,D). Inset shows stimulus configuration; green spot shows recorded hemisphere. Crossed response is denoted in blue, uncrossed response in red; shaded area is the temporally smoothed region of one standard deviation around mean. Gray bar below curve indicates statistical significance of a running two-tailed Wilcoxon-Mann-Whitney test ($\alpha = 0.001$, corrected by false detection rate procedure, 2 ms window). Morphology of LFPs shows temporal regions of significant difference in all configurations, but more so in the congenitally unilaterally deaf animal. Further, morphology is more different between hemispheres than within one hemisphere. Note differences in ordinate. Early-implanted animals had larger maximal amplitudes than congenital unilateral and late-implanted animals. The absolute LFP amplitude showed a high interindividual variability.

comparisons at the ipsilateral cortex; in the present study, we had to perform unpaired comparisons (between hemispheres and animals).

First, the effect of stimulation duration and implantation age on onset latencies of crossed responses was determined at the contralateral hemisphere for stimulation of the hearing ear (**Figure 7**). In animals implanted early (3.5 months), as expected, stimulation duration was associated with a decrease in median onset latency, demonstrating that onset latency does change as a result of the stimulation. Moreover, increasing implantation age decreased the effect of stimulation on contralateral onset latency after 5 months of chronic electrical stimulation, changing from 9.1 ± 1.89 ms (median ± absolute deviation of the median) at 3.5 months to 9.95 ± 1.00 ms at 5.0 months to finally reach 10.5 ± 2.63 at 6 months onset (significant increases with increasing age of onset, two-tailed Wilcoxon-Mann-Whitney test at $\alpha = 0.05$). Therefore, onset latency reflects the amount of hearing experience and age of onset and thus represents a good measure of plastic adaptation caused by the stimulation.

Next, onset latencies of crossed responses were compared between hemispheres in four animals with a stimulation duration of 5 months (**Figure 8**). Here, stimulation of the hearing ear

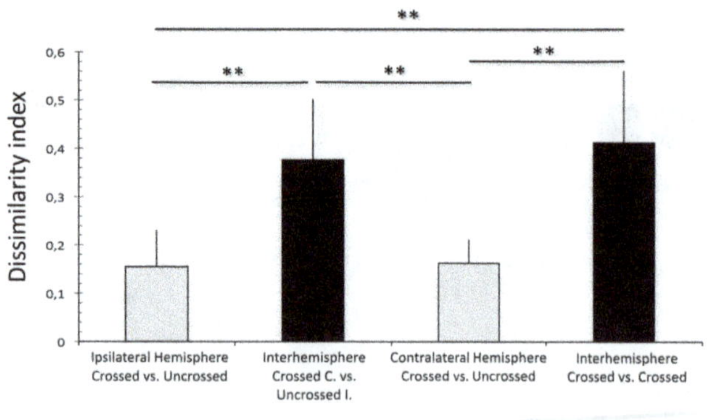

FIGURE 6 | Dissimilarity index computed between mean LFPs within one hemisphere (gray) and between hemispheres (black). Interhemisphere comparisons result in significantly higher dissimilarity index than within-hemisphere comparisons. Two-tailed Wilcoxon-Mann-Whitney test, $^{**}p < 0.01$.

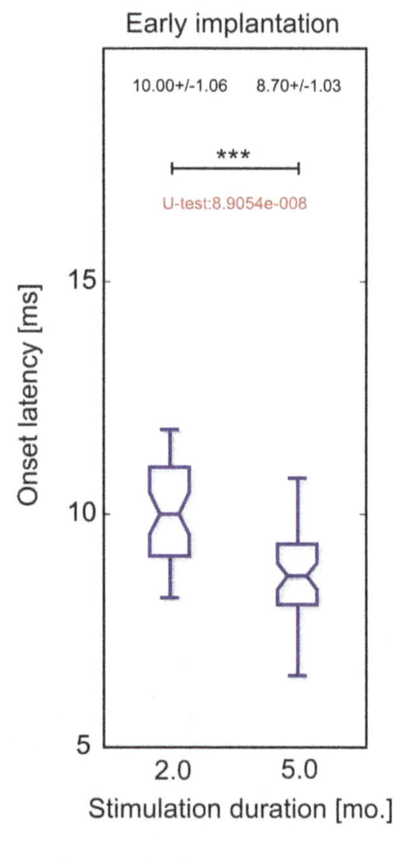

FIGURE 7 | Onset latency at the cortex contralateral to hearing ear in response to stimulation of hearing ear in two animals implanted at 3.5 months. One was stimulated for 2 months and the other for 5 months. Longer stimulation resulted in shorter-onset latency (two-tailed Wilcoxon-Mann-Whitney test, $^{***}\sim p < 0.001$).

resulted in shorter crossed response latencies than that of the deaf ear. The effect was significant in early onset animals and disappeared in late-implanted animals. However, when considering the crossed pathway of the deaf ear, the latency of the congenital and the late implanted animals were similar and we could not detect any consistent age-of-onset effect. Consequently, with regard to onset latency, the effect of stimulation in crossed responses is confined to the hearing ear; the influence on the crossed response of the deaf ear was weak. Remember that the amplitudes were, however, similar for the crossed response of the deaf and the hearing ear (**Figure 4**).

Finally, the onset latencies for the responses to the stimulated (hearing) ear were compared between the cortices (**Figure 9**). This comparison was performed on one congenitally unilaterally deaf and five implanted animals, two with early and three with late implantation. In the animals with early onset of asymmetric hearing, the latencies were short and not different at the contralateral and ipsilateral cortex, with a tendency toward shorter latencies for ipsilateral (uncrossed) response. This is highly unusual, as in all hearing cats the situation was the reverse and significant (Kral et al., 2013). However, in late-implanted animals, the latencies tended to be longer (see **Figure 9**), and in two out of three animals tested, contralateral onset latency was significantly smaller than the ipsilateral onset latency (in the remaining animal it was not significant, but with a tendency toward shorter contralateral response, **Figure 9**). That demonstrates that in the late implantation, there is some profit from the stimulation, but it is more confined to the crossed response. In early implantation, there is benefit to both the uncrossed and crossed response. In this respect, the afferent pathway to the contralateral cortex has a longer sensitive period than the one to the ipsilateral cortex.

To verify this outcome, the difference in medians of uncrossed and crossed responses to the hearing ear was compared between early and late onset of asymmetric hearing (**Figure 10**). In early-onset animals, uncrossed response showed a shorter onset latency, resulting in a negative mean difference in all three animals, but the difference became positive in all three cases of late implantations (Wilcoxon-Mann-Whitney two-tailed test, $p = 0.044$, **Figure 10**). This further demonstrates that the benefit to the uncrossed response is confined to early-onset asymmetric hearing.

DISCUSSION

The present manuscript describes hemispheric specificity of effects of unilateral hearing following congenital deafness. It demonstrates that in early-onset unilateral hearing, both the ipsilateral and the contralateral hemisphere reorganize and strengthen the responses to stimulation of the hearing ear, giving it an advantage over the deaf ear. In the early-onset animals, the ipsilateral hemisphere responded more strongly to stimulation of the hearing ear. The morphology of the LFPs demonstrated that the reorganizations following unilateral deafness were hemisphere-specific (**Figure 6**).

The uncrossed pathway appeared more susceptible to developmental alteration of hearing balance than the crossed pathway, although both the crossed and uncrossed responses to the hearing ear were changed by the stimulation. In late implantations, the uncrossed response did not show similar reorganization, and it was largely the crossed pathway of the hearing ear that still benefited from stimulation, although less than in early implanted animals (**Figures 8**, **9**). The uncrossed pathway was more sensitive to age of onset than was the crossed pathway, demonstrating

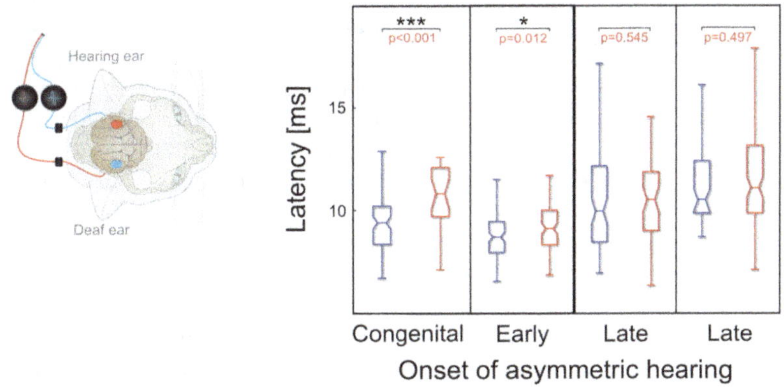

FIGURE 8 | Onset latency for crossed responses; color denotes configuration. Blue denotes the hearing ear. In animals with early onset of unilateral hearing, crossed response for hearing ear was significantly shorter than that for the deaf ear (two-tailed Wilcoxon-Mann-Whitney test). This was not the case for late-onset animals. Onset latency for stimulation of deaf ear did not show any systematic dependence on onset of asymmetric hearing, whereas onset latency for hearing ear became longer in cases of late-onset asymmetric hearing. ***$\sim p < 0.001$; *$\sim p < 0.05$.

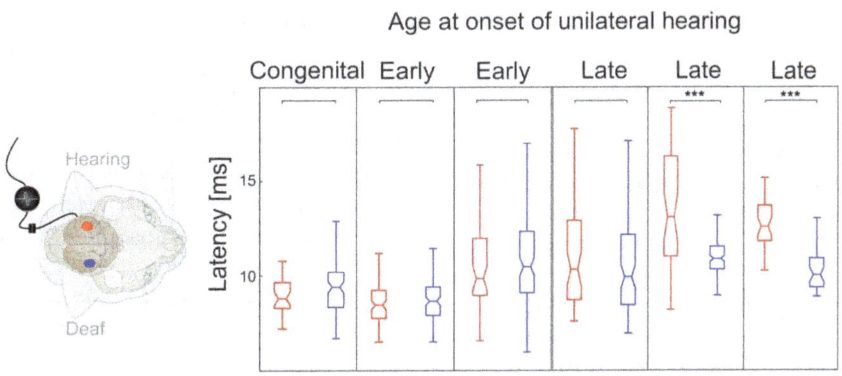

FIGURE 9 | Comparison of crossed and uncrossed responses for hearing ear. Color denotes hemisphere in which recordings are made (red: ipsilateral, blue: contralateral). In all early-onset animals, ipsilateral hemisphere showed a nominally smaller median onset latency, but difference was not statistically significant (two-tailed Wilcoxon-Mann-Whitney test). In all late-onset animals, contralateral hemisphere showed a smaller median latency, but in only two of three animals was the difference statistically significant (two-tailed Wilcoxon-Mann-Whitney test). Note that both ipsilateral and contralateral latencies were greater in late-onset animals. ***$\sim p < 0.001$.

a shorter sensitive period. The mutual relationship between the hearing ear and the hemisphere investigated is critically important when assessing developmental auditory plasticity.

METHODOLOGICAL DISCUSSION

The present study compared the effects of stimulation at both hemispheres. There are several limitations to the present approach that merit discussion. First of all, comparisons between hemispheres preclude pairwise testing. Although the present study used an approach validated by several previous studies performing interindividual comparisons (Klinke et al., 1999; Kral et al., 2002, 2006), the present approach is more limited than the pairwise comparison (Kral et al., 2013). The present experiments took 48 h in most animals, with the possibility of a state change during the procedure. However, even though recordings at the ipsilateral cortex were performed later, the responses to stimulation were not systematically different in hemispheres exposed later than those exposed earlier (e.g., for the hearing ear or the amplitudes of crossed responses; see examples in **Figures 2, 4** and **5**). Furthermore, onset latencies systematically changed depending on experience and on which ear was stimulated, and not on time of recording (later-exposed cortices showed shorter onset latencies in early-implanted animals and longer ones in the late-implanted animals), so that a change of state during the experiments can be ruled out. In total, we have no indication of any systematic shifts in the general state of the animals during recordings.

Degeneration of spiral ganglion cells is unlikely to have contributed to the findings here, as there was no significant spiral ganglion cell loss in the implanted (basal) region of the cochlea within the first 2 years of life in congenitally deaf cats, and even at an older age there was less degeneration in the basal cochlea (Heid et al., 1998). Moreover, stimulation of the deaf ear in unilateral animals resulted in much smaller responses at the hemisphere contralateral to the hearing ear, but at the ipsilateral cortex the responses to the deaf ear were comparable to the

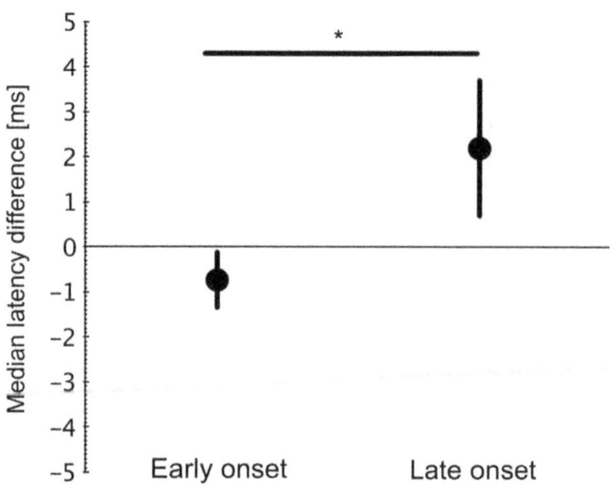

FIGURE 10 | Difference between median latencies (uncrossed–crossed response) for hearing ear. All three early-onset animals had negative differences (uncrossed < crossed), whereas all late-onset animals had positive differences (uncrossed > crossed). Two-tailed Wilcoxon-Mann-Whitney test, $p = 0.04$ ($^{*}\sim p < 0.05$).

responses to the hearing ear (**Figures 2, 6**), showing not only the hemispheric specificity of plastic reorganization, but also ruling out any significant influence of peripheral ear-specific effects.

Finally, age at final experiment did not significantly contribute to the present findings. The cortical developmental sequence in deaf and hearing cats with respect to electrically evoked responses terminates at ~6 months (Kral et al., 2005; for similar data on acoustic stimulation, see Eggermont, 1996; for data on onset latencies, see supplementary material in Kral et al., 2013). Only two of the 10 investigated animals were younger (animals no. 3 and 6 in **Table 1**). Omitting these two animals from the comparisons did not affect any finding of the study. Overall, we can also rule out age at experiment as a confounding factor.

Finally, it has to be considered that the effects measured at the ipsilateral cortex need not necessarily arise in the ipsilateral hemisphere, but may have an origin in the contralateral hemisphere before pathway crossing. For the sake of simplicity, however, we will not complicate the considerations below by including this aspect.

DISCUSSION OF RESULTS

The present study is well in agreement with previous investigations on the subject. The notion of auditory sensitive periods in neuronal plasticity (review in Kral, 2013) has been established for deaf, cochlear-implanted animals (Kral et al., 2001, 2002, 2013) and cochlear-implanted children (Ponton and Eggermont, 2001; Sharma et al., 2002, 2005), as well as for hearing animals (Zhang et al., 2002; Nakahara et al., 2004; de Villers-Sidani et al., 2008). However, sensitive periods are not observed in all plastic reorganizations in the brain (Noreña et al., 2006; Eggermont, 2013; Pienkowski et al., 2013).

Early neonatal unilateral ablation studies suggested a reorganization of the auditory brain toward the hearing ear (Nordeen et al., 1983; Kitzes and Semple, 1985), although it has not been possible to stimulate the ablated ear and compared it with the hearing ear, and no developmental study has been undertaken.

The reorganization reported here and in previous studies is in accord with results from cochlear-implanted children (Peters et al., 2007; Zeitler et al., 2008; Graham et al., 2009; Gordon et al., 2013; Illg et al., 2013). Early second implantations are important in terms of retaining the potential to reverse the aural preference, whereas the effects were observed after more than 1 year of unilateral use (in early implantations at 1.74 years, Gordon et al., 2013; in single-sided deafness, see Scheffler et al., 1998; Bilecen et al., 2000; Langers et al., 2005; Burton et al., 2012; Maslin et al., 2013). As the greatest effects were observed in congenitally unilaterally deaf animals in the present study, before cortical synaptogenesis has set in in cats (Kral et al., 2013), implantation at ages of less than 1 year of life (peak of synaptogenesis between 1 and 4 years, comparison cat-human in Kral and O'Donoghue, 2010) can be expected to generate substantially larger effects in children than those described to date. It has to be stressed here, however, that although age at first implantation is important for the outcome in pediatric cochlear implantation, some benefit from the second ear is found even in cases of longer interimplant delay (Zeitler et al., 2008; Illg et al., 2013). This corresponds to the present observation that in no case was the response to the deaf ear eliminated completely (see also Kral et al., 2013). Nonetheless, lesser responses for the deaf ear at the contralateral cortex supports the suggestion that the deaf ear is placed at a disadvantage in competition for cortical resources particularly in individuals with early onset-unilateral hearing (Kral et al., 2013).

Importantly, the outcome shows specificity for the ear that has received input (**Figures 2, 4, 8**). Both onset latency (**Figure 8**) and amplitudes (Kral et al., 2013) of the responses appeared different for different ears, but a more detailed analysis demonstrated that the morphology (disregarding amplitudes) is more hemispheric-specific than ear-specific (**Figures 5, 6**). Nonetheless, a lesser response was observed for the deaf ear, particularly at the contralateral hemisphere in the congenital animal (**Figure 2**). At the ipsilateral hemisphere, a pairwise comparison demonstrated smaller responses for the deaf ear (Kral et al., 2013). Pairwise testing was unfortunately not possible for the present interhemispheric comparisons, so that small differences may went unnoticed.

Subcortical reorganization with deafness and cochlear implants has been described before (Snyder et al., 1991; Shepherd et al., 1999; Ryugo et al., 2005; O'Neil et al., 2010). Nevertheless, several studies indicate that cortical plasticity is higher than subcortical (Ma and Suga, 2005; Popescu and Polley, 2010), and that the former plays the controlling role via efferent systems (Ma and Suga, 2005). Interestingly, despite pronounced developmental effects observed in other measures, the dissimilarity index did not show a clear developmental pattern. For the present experiments, this means that it is more the balance of aural inputs that is developmentally modulated and less the way in which the inputs are processed after converging on the same neuronal elements. Further it shows that the plasticity mechanism is similar at all ages, only the extent of the effect fades with increasing age, and fades out faster at the ipsilateral hemisphere. The present study indicates a subcortical site for reorganization following unilateral deafness (before or at the point of binaural convergence).

The uncrossed response latency for stimulation of the hearing ear became smaller than the crossed response latency, so that the difference in medians was negative, but only in the early-implanted animals (**Figures 9, 10**). This finding could indicate a loss of inhibition at the ipsilateral cortex in early-implanted animals, allowing uncrossed inputs to be pulled to much shorter latency (Zhou et al., 2012). In normal, binaural hearing animals, the uncrossed response evokes inhibition more frequently, whereas the crossed response is more excitatory (Zhang et al., 2004). The present observations can therefore be explained by a specific down-regulation of inhibition in unilateral hearing at the hemisphere ipsilateral to the hearing ear (Vale et al., 2004), as it may explain the shorter latency, larger uncrossed response for the hearing ear, as compared with the longer-latency, smaller uncrossed response for the deaf ear. Different recruitment of inhibition in the ipsilateral and contralateral hemisphere would then also affect the morphology of the LFPs differentially for the different hemispheres. The relatively large drop in onset latency in early-onset animals (uncrossed response in the ipsilateral hemisphere) can be alternatively explained only by an increase in synaptic conduction in many synapses; this, however, fails to explain the hemispheric specificity of the outcomes on LFP morphology. Finally, a downregulation of inhibition in (preferentially) the ipsilateral hemisphere can explain the rapid onset of the effect that is different from the process behind the slower plastic changes in the contralateral hemisphere (**Figure 7**, see also Kral et al., 2002). Previous experiments with unilateral cochlear ablation also suggest that the mechanism underlying ipsilateral adaptations in the midbrain differs from that underlying contralateral adaptations (Vale et al., 2004). Future studies on unit activity in congenitally unilaterally deaf and unilaterally implanted animals may demonstrate this by showing the reduction or absence of suppressive binaural interaction in the ipsilateral hemisphere and its presence in the contralateral hemisphere.

Inhibitory synaptic transmission matures later than excitation (review in Kral et al., 2013) and is likely one of the mechanisms explaining the shorter sensitive period for the uncrossed response. In this sense the longer onset latency with increasing implantation age at the ipsilateral hemisphere could be related to the fact that in early-implanted animals, the developmental process of inhibitory transmission was not yet finalized when the hearing asymmetry started and could be therefore more modulated by unilateral hearing. In late-implanted animals the unilateral hearing set in after the development of inhibition has terminated. Plasticity observed before this point is likely to involve changes on both inhibitory and excitatory transmission, whereas later plasticity likely depends more on excitatory synapses with smaller contribution of inhibitory synapses. That can explain the different sensitive periods at the ipsilateral and contralateral hemisphere.

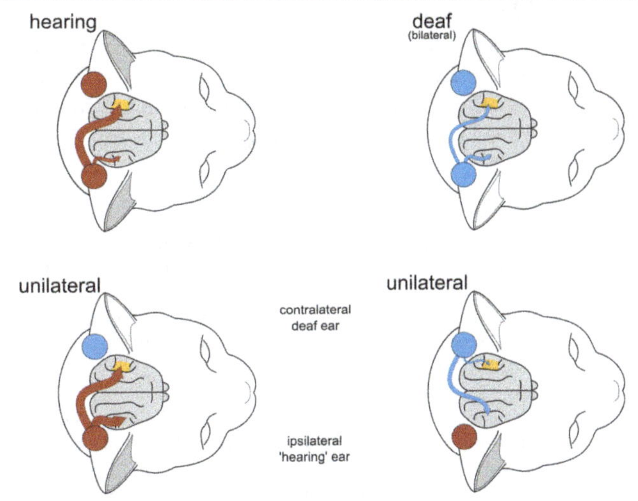

FIGURE 11 | Graphical summary of results from this and two previous studies (Kral et al., 2009, 2013). In binaurally deaf animals, contralaterality was reduced. In early-onset unilaterally deaf animals, hearing ear resulted in reduced contralaterality (when assessed from crossed and uncrossed response for hearing ear), whereas deaf ear showed increased contralaterality (when assessed from crossed and uncrossed response for deaf ear) due to reduced uncrossed response.

Stimulation of the hearing ear generates strong responses both at the ipsilateral and the contralateral hemisphere (for human data, see Bilecen et al., 2000; Hanss et al., 2009; Burton et al., 2012; Gordon et al., 2013). Stimulation of the deaf ear activates the crossed pathway but does so only weakly for the uncrossed pathway. The contralateral preference of the deaf ear is strengthened due to reduction of the uncrossed responses, the contralateral preference of the hearing ear being reduced because of to strengthening of the uncrossed responses (**Figure 11**). The present findings therefore provide an explanation of the mechanism behind the outcomes of human imaging studies (Bilecen et al., 2000; Gordon et al., 2013).

CONCLUSION

The present study supports the concept of several sensitive developmental periods by demonstrating a shorter sensitive period for reorganization at the ipsilateral hemisphere as compared with the contralateral hemisphere. It shows more extensive changes in uncrossed responses than in the crossed responses in early-onset animals. Furthermore, it shows that unilateral deafness results in an asymmetric brain, with different hemispheres showing differential responses for both the deaf and the hearing ear. The hemisphere ipsilateral to the hearing ear most likely downregulates inhibition, by that specifically decreasing onset latency of the response to the hearing ear. This effect is not found in the contralateral hemisphere.

The deaf ear is, however, not completely 'disconnected' from the cortex following single-sided deafness. The hemisphere ipsilateral to the hearing ear preserves responsiveness to the deaf ear, although with a preference for the hearing ear. Finally, the present results support a greater 'separation' of the ears in early onset unilateral hearing.

ACKNOWLEDGMENTS

The study was supported by the German Research Foundation (DFG; Cluster of Excellence Hearing4all and DFG Grant Kr 3370/1-3). The authors want to thank Peter Baumhoff, MSc., for designing **Figure 11** and the insets of **Figures 2–5, 8** and **9**.

REFERENCES

Benjamini, Y., and Hochberg, Y. (1995). Controlling the false discovery rate: a practical and powerful approach to multiple testing. *J. R Stat. Soc. B* 57, 289–300. doi: 10.2307/2346101

Bilecen, D., Seifritz, E., Radü, E. W., Schmid, N., Wetzel, S., Probst, R., et al. (2000). Cortical reorganization after acute unilateral hearing loss traced by fMRI. *Neurology* 54, 765–767. doi: 10.1212/WNL.54.3.765

Buechner, A., Brendel, M., Lesinski-Schiedat, A., Wenzel, G., Frohne-Buechner, C., Jaeger, B., et al. (2010). Cochlear implantation in unilateral deaf subjects associated with ipsilateral tinnitus. *Otol. Neurotol.* 31, 1381–1385. doi: 10.1097/MAO.0b013e3181e3d353

Burton, H., Firszt, J. B., Holden, T., Agato, A., and Uchanski, R. M. (2012). Activation lateralization in human core, belt, and parabelt auditory fields with unilateral deafness compared to normal hearing. *Brain Res.* 1454, 33–47. doi: 10.1016/j.brainres.2012.02.066

de Villers-Sidani, E., Simpson, K. L., Lu, Y. F., Lin, R. C., and Merzenich, M. M. (2008). Manipulating critical period closure across different sectors of the primary auditory cortex. *Nat. Neurosci.* 11, 957–965. doi: 10.1038/nn.2144

Eggermont, J. J. (1996). Differential maturation rates for response parameters in cat primary auditory cortex. *Aud. Neurosci.* 2, 309–327.

Eggermont, J. J. (2013). On the similarities and differences of non-traumatic sound exposure during the critical period and in adulthood. *Front. Syst. Neurosci.* 7:12. doi: 10.3389/fnsys.2013.00012

Eiserman, W. D., Hartel, D. M., Shisler, L., Buhrmann, J., White, K. R., and Foust, T. (2008). Using otoacoustic emissions to screen for hearing loss in early childhood care settings. *Int. J. Pediatr. Otorhinolaryngol.* 72, 475–482. doi: 10.1016/j.ijporl.2007.12.006

Firszt, J. B., Holden, L. K., Reeder, R. M., Waltzman, S. B., and Arndt, S. (2012). Auditory abilities after cochlear implantation in adults with unilateral deafness: a pilot study. *Otol. Neurotol.* 33, 1339–1346. doi: 10.1097/MAO.0b013e318268d52d

Gordon, K. A., Wong, D. D., and Papsin, B. C. (2013). Bilateral input protects the cortex from unilaterally-driven reorganization in children who are deaf. *Brain* 136, 1609–1625. doi: 10.1093/brain/awt052

Graham, J., Vickers, D., Eyles, J., Brinton, J., Al Malky, G., Aleksy, W., et al. (2009). Bilateral sequential cochlear implantation in the congenitally deaf child: evidence to support the concept of a 'critical age' after which the second ear is less likely to provide an adequate level of speech perception on its own. *Cochlear Implants Int.* 10, 119–141. doi: 10.1002/cii.419

Hanss, J., Veuillet, E., Adjout, K., Besle, J., Collet, L., and Thai-Van, H. (2009). The effect of long-term unilateral deafness on the activation pattern in the auditory cortices of French-native speakers: influence of deafness side. *BMC Neurosci.* 10:23. doi: 10.1186/1471-2202-10-23

Heid, S., Hartmann, R., and Klinke, R. (1998). A model for prelingual deafness, the congenitally deaf white cat–population statistics and degenerative changes. *Hear. Res.* 115, 101–112. doi: 10.1016/S0378-5955(97) 00182-2

Illg, A., Giourgas, A., Kral, A., Büchner, A., Lesinski-Schiedat, A., and Lenarz, T. (2013). Speech comprehension in children and adolescents after sequential bilateral cochlear implantation with long interimplant interval. *Otol. Neurotol.* 34, 682–689. doi: 10.1097/MAO.0b013e31828bb75e

Imig, T. J., and Adrián, H. O. (1977). Binaural columns in the primary field (A1) of cat auditory cortex. *Brain Res.* 138, 241–257. doi: 10.1016/0006-8993(77)90743-0

King, A. J., Kacelnik, O., Mrsic-Flogel, T. D., Schnupp, J. W., Parsons, C. H., and Moore, D. R. (2001). How plastic is spatial hearing? *Audiol. Neurootol.* 6, 182–186. doi: 10.1159/000046829

Kitzes, L. M., and Semple, M. N. (1985). Single-unit responses in the inferior colliculus: effects of neonatal unilateral cochlear ablation. *J. Neurophysiol.* 53, 1483–1500.

Klinke, R., Kral, A., Heid, S., Tillein, J., and Hartmann, R. (1999). Recruitment of the auditory cortex in congenitally deaf cats by long- term cochlear electrostimulation. *Science* 285, 1729–1733. doi: 10.1126/science.285.5434.1729

Kral, A. (2013). Auditory critical periods: a review from system's perspective. *Neuroscience* 247, 117–133. doi: 10.1016/j.neuroscience.2013.05.021

Kral, A., Hartmann, R., Tillein, J., Heid, S., and Klinke, R. (2001). Delayed maturation and sensitive periods in the auditory cortex. *Audiol. Neurootol.* 6, 346–362. doi: 10.1159/000046845

Kral, A., Hartmann, R., Tillein, J., Heid, S., and Klinke, R. (2002). Hearing after congenital deafness: central auditory plasticity and sensory deprivation. *Cereb. Cortex* 12, 797–807. doi: 10.1093/cercor/12.8.797

Kral, A., Hubka, P., Heid, S., and Tillein, J. (2013). Single-sided deafness leads to unilateral aural preference within an early sensitive period. *Brain* 136, 180–193. doi: 10.1093/brain/aws305

Kral, A., and O'Donoghue, G. M. (2010). Profound deafness in childhood. *N. Engl. J. Med.* 363, 1438–1450. doi: 10.1056/NEJMra0911225

Kral, A., and Sharma, A. (2012). Developmental neuroplasticity after cochlear implantation. *Trends Neurosci.* 35, 111–122. doi: 10.1016/j.tins.2011.09.004

Kral, A., Tillein, J., Hartmann, R., and Klinke, R. (1999). Monitoring of anaesthesia in neurophysiological experiments. *Neuroreport* 10, 781–787. doi: 10.1097/00001756-199903170-00022

Kral, A., Tillein, J., Heid, S., Hartmann, R., and Klinke, R. (2005). Postnatal cortical development in congenital auditory deprivation. *Cereb. Cortex* 15, 552–562. doi: 10.1093/cercor/bhh156

Kral, A., Tillein, J., Heid, S., Klinke, R., and Hartmann, R. (2006). Cochlear implants: cortical plasticity in congenital deprivation. *Prog. Brain Res.* 157, 283–313. doi: 10.1016/S0079-6123(06)57018-9

Kral, A., Tillein, J., Hubka, P., Schiemann, D., Heid, S., Hartmann, R., et al. (2009). Spatiotemporal patterns of cortical activity with bilateral cochlear implants in congenital deafness. *J. Neurosci.* 29, 811–827. doi: 10.1523/JNEUROSCI.2424-08.2009

Langers, D. R., van Dijk, P., and Backes, W. H. (2005). Lateralization, connectivity and plasticity in the human central auditory system. *Neuroimage* 28, 490–499. doi: 10.1016/j.neuroimage.2005.06.024

Ma, X., and Suga, N. (2005). Long-term cortical plasticity evoked by electric stimulation and acetylcholine applied to the auditory cortex. *Proc. Natl. Acad. Sci. U.S.A.* 102, 9335–9340. doi: 10.1073/pnas.0503851102

Maslin, M. R., Munro, K. J., and El-Deredy, W. (2013). Source analysis reveals plasticity in the auditory cortex: evidence for reduced hemispheric asymmetries following unilateral deafness. *Clin. Neurophysiol.* 124, 391–399. doi: 10.1016/j.clinph.2012.07.016

Middlebrooks, J. C., Clock, A. E., Xu, L., and Green, D. M. (1994). A panoramic code for sound location by cortical neurons. *Science* 264, 842–844. doi: 10.1126/science.8171339

Nakahara, H., Zhang, L. I., and Merzenich, M. M. (2004). Specialization of primary auditory cortex processing by sound exposure in the "critical period." *Proc. Natl. Acad. Sci. U.S.A.* 101, 7170–7174. doi: 10.1073/pnas.0401196101

Nordeen, K. W., Killackey, H. P., and Kitzes, L. M. (1983). Ascending projections to the inferior colliculus following unilateral cochlear ablation in the neonatal gerbil, Meriones unguiculatus. *J. Comp. Neurol.* 214, 144–153. doi: 10.1002/cne.902140204

Noreña, A. J., Gourévitch, B., Gourevich, B., Aizawa, N., and Eggermont, J. J. (2006). Spectrally enhanced acoustic environment disrupts frequency representation in cat auditory cortex. *Nat. Neurosci.* 9, 932–939. doi:10.1038/nn1720

O'Neil, J. N., Limb, C. J., Baker, C. A., and Ryugo, D. K. (2010). Bilateral effects of unilateral cochlear implantation in congenitally deaf cats. *J. Comp. Neurol.* 518, 2382–2404. doi: 10.1002/cne.22339

Peters, B. R., Litovsky, R., Parkinson, A., and Lake, J. (2007). Importance of age and postimplantation experience on speech perception measures in children with sequential bilateral cochlear implants. *Otol. Neurotol.* 28, 649–657. doi: 10.1097/01.mao.0000281807.89938.60

Pienkowski, M., Munguia, R., and Eggermont, J. J. (2013). Effects of passive, moderate-level sound exposure on the mature auditory cortex: spectral edges, spectrotemporal density, and real-world noise. *Hear. Res.* 296, 121–130. doi: 10.1016/j.heares.2012.11.006

Ponton, C. W., and Eggermont, J. J. (2001). Of kittens and kids: altered cortical maturation following profound deafness and cochlear implant use. *Audiol. Neurootol.* 6, 363–380. doi: 10.1159/000046846

Popescu, M. V., and Polley, D. B. (2010). Monaural deprivation disrupts development of binaural selectivity in auditory midbrain and cortex. *Neuron* 65, 718–731. doi: 10.1016/j.neuron.2010.02.019

Reale, R. A., Brugge, J. F., and Chan, J. C. (1987). Maps of auditory cortex in cats reared after unilateral cochlear ablation in the neonatal period. *Brain Res.* 431, 281–290.

Ryugo, D. K., Kretzmer, E. A., and Niparko, J. K. (2005). Restoration of auditory nerve synapses in cats by cochlear implants. *Science* 310, 1490–1492. doi: 10.1126/science.1119419

Scheffler, K., Bilecen, D., Schmid, N., Tschopp, K., and Seelig, J. (1998). Auditory cortical responses in hearing subjects and unilateral deaf patients as detected by functional magnetic resonance imaging. *Cereb. Cortex* 8, 156–163. doi: 10.1093/cercor/8.2.156

Sharma, A., Dorman, M. F., and Kral, A. (2005). The influence of a sensitive period on central auditory development in children with unilateral and bilateral cochlear implants. *Hear. Res.* 203, 134–143. doi: 10.1016/j.heares.2004.12.010

Sharma, A., Dorman, M. F., and Spahr, A. J. (2002). A sensitive period for the development of the central auditory system in children with cochlear implants: implications for age of implantation. *Ear Hear.* 23, 532–539. doi: 10.1097/00003446-200212000-00004

Sharma, A., Gilley, P. M., Martin, K., and Roland, P. (2007). Simultaneous versus sequential bilateral implantation in young children: effects on central auditory system development and plasticity. *Audiol. Med.* 5, 218–223. doi: 10.1080/16513860701659479

Shepherd, R. K., Baxi, J. H., and Hardie, N. A. (1999). Response of inferior colliculus neurons to electrical stimulation of the auditory nerve in neonatally deafened cats. *J Neurophysiol* 82, 1363–1380.

Snyder, R. L., Rebscher, S. J., Leake, P. A., Kelly, K., and Cao, K. (1991). Chronic intracochlear electrical stimulation in the neonatally deafened cat. II. Temporal properties of neurons in the inferior colliculus. *Hear. Res.* 56, 246–264. doi: 10.1016/0378-5955(91)90175-9

Vale, C., Juiz, J. M., Moore, D. R., and Sanes, D. H. (2004). Unilateral cochlear ablation produces greater loss of inhibition in the contralateral inferior colliculus. *Eur. J. Neurosci.* 20, 2133–2140. doi: 10.1111/j.1460-9568.2004.03679.x

Vermeire, K., Nobbe, A., Schleich, P., Nopp, P., Voormolen, M. H., and Van de Heyning, P. H. (2008). Neural tonotopy in cochlear implants: an evaluation in unilateral cochlear implant patients with unilateral deafness and tinnitus. *Hear. Res.* 245, 98–106. doi: 10.1016/j.heares.2008.09.003

Watkin, P., and Baldwin, M. (2012). The longitudinal follow up of a universal neonatal hearing screen: the implications for confirming deafness in childhood. *Int. J. Audiol.* 51, 519–528. doi: 10.3109/14992027.2012.673237

Zeitler, D. M., Kessler, M. A., Terushkin, V., Roland, T. J., Svirsky, M. A., Lalwani, A. K., et al. (2008). Speech perception benefits of sequential bilateral cochlear implantation in children and adults: a retrospective analysis. *Otol. Neurotol.* 29, 314–325. doi: 10.1097/MAO.0b013e3181662cb5

Zhang, J., Nakamoto, K. T., and Kitzes, L. M. (2004). Binaural interaction revisited in the cat primary auditory cortex. *J. Neurophysiol.* 91, 101–117. doi: 10.1152/jn.00166.2003

Zhang, L. I., Bao, S., and Merzenich, M. M. (2002). Disruption of primary auditory cortex by synchronous auditory inputs during a critical period. *Proc. Natl. Acad. Sci. U.S.A.* 99, 2309–2314. doi: 10.1073/pnas.261707398

Zhou, Y., Mesik, L., Sun, Y. J., Liang, F., Xiao, Z., Tao, H. W., and et al. (2012). Generation of spike latency tuning by thalamocortical circuits in auditory cortex. *J. Neurosci.* 32, 9969–9980. doi: 10.1523/JNEUROSCI.1384-12.2012

2

Training changes processing of speech cues in older adults with hearing loss

Samira Anderson[1,2†], Travis White-Schwoch[1,2], Hee Jae Choi[1,2] and Nina Kraus[1,2,3,4,5]*

[1] Auditory Neuroscience Laboratory, Department of Communication Sciences and Disorders, Northwestern University, Evanston, IL, USA
[2] Department of Communication Sciences, Northwestern University, Evanston, IL, USA
[3] Institute for Neuroscience, Northwestern University, Evanston, IL, USA
[4] Department of Neurobiology and Physiology, Northwestern University, Evanston, IL, USA
[5] Department of Otolaryngology, Northwestern University, Evanston, IL, USA

Correspondence:
Nina Kraus, Auditory Neuroscience Laboratory, Northwestern University, 2240 Campus Drive, Evanston, IL 60208, USA
e-mail: nkraus@northwestern.edu
www.brainvolts.northwestern.edu

†Present address:
Samira Anderson, Department of Hearing and Speech Sciences, University of Maryland, College Park, USA

Aging results in a loss of sensory function, and the effects of hearing impairment can be especially devastating due to reduced communication ability. Older adults with hearing loss report that speech, especially in noisy backgrounds, is uncomfortably loud yet unclear. Hearing loss results in an unbalanced neural representation of speech: the slowly-varying envelope is enhanced, dominating representation in the auditory pathway and perceptual salience at the cost of the rapidly-varying fine structure. We hypothesized that older adults with hearing loss can be trained to compensate for these changes in central auditory processing through directed attention to behaviorally-relevant speech sounds. To that end, we evaluated the effects of auditory-cognitive training in older adults (ages 55–79) with normal hearing and hearing loss. After training, the auditory training group with hearing loss experienced a reduction in the neural representation of the speech envelope presented in noise, approaching levels observed in normal hearing older adults. No changes were noted in the control group. Importantly, changes in speech processing were accompanied by improvements in speech perception. Thus, central processing deficits associated with hearing loss may be partially remediated with training, resulting in real-life benefits for everyday communication.

Keywords: auditory plasticity, speech envelope, aging, hearing loss, speech perception, temporal fine structure, temporal coding

INTRODUCTION

Hearing loss is associated with reduced quality of life in older adults, affecting social and emotional well-being (Heine and Browning, 2002). The effects of hearing loss are especially noticeable in noisy backgrounds with multiple talkers (Dubno et al., 1984; Jin and Nelson, 2010). Many factors contribute to age-related deficits in speech-in-noise perception, including cochlear pathology (Dubno et al., 1984), impairments in central auditory processing (Phillips et al., 2000), and decreased cognitive resources (Pichora-Fuller, 2003; Wingfield et al., 2005; Peelle et al., 2010). Perceptual and neurophysiologic studies have demonstrated that central auditory processing is compromised by aging and hearing loss (Gordon-Salant et al., 2006; Clinard et al., 2010; Lister et al., 2011; Anderson et al., 2012). Hearing aid amplification improves audibility but cannot restore central auditory function (Tremblay et al., 2003). Training-driven neuroplasticity, which can partially reverse the effects of age-related deficits in temporal resolution in humans (Anderson et al., 2013c) and animals (de Villers-Sidani et al., 2010), may provide a means for treating abnormal central function processing associated with hearing loss.

One chief barrier to the wider use of amplification has been that hearing aids often make speech louder without improving clarity, especially in background noise (Johnson and Dillon, 2011). This phenomenon may arise from the effects of hearing loss on central processing of speech. Two acoustic aspects of speech, the slowly varying temporal envelope and the rapidly varying temporal fine structure (TFS), have been extensively studied (Ardoint et al., 2010; Hopkins and Moore, 2011). Although the envelope appears to be the dominant cue for understanding speech in quiet and in steady-state noise, both the envelope and TFS may play a role when listening to speech in fluctuating noise (Shannon et al., 1995; Moore, 2008). However, the role of TFS for understanding speech in fluctuating noise remains an area of debate (Oxenham and Simonson, 2009). In an animal model, sensorineural hearing loss is associated with enhanced envelope coding in the auditory nerve (Kale and Heinz, 2010) and midbrain (Anderson et al., 2013a). Perceptual studies also suggest exaggerated encoding of the envelope in humans with unilateral hearing loss (Moore et al., 1996) and potentially reduced ability to use TFS cues (Lorenzi et al., 2006). These effects might explain the hearing impaired listener's complaint that speech is loud yet unclear (Johnson and Dillon, 2011).

Because hearing aid amplification primarily addresses loss of audibility associated with cochlear pathology, there is a need to develop novel methods for counteracting the deleterious effects of hearing loss on central processing. Here, we assessed whether auditory-based cognitive training can be used to partially restore the imbalance of speech cue representation associated with exaggerated envelope encoding. Since both TFS (Sheft et al., 2008) and

envelope (Swaminathan and Heinz, 2012) cues play an important role in consonant perception, we hypothesized that directed attention to the fast-changing consonant-vowel (CV) transition within an adaptive training paradigm results in reweighing of speech cue representation, such that the TFS becomes more salient. To test this hypothesis, we randomly assigned older adults with and without hearing loss to complete 8 weeks of computerized training. We evaluated subcortical representation of envelope and TFS cues before and after training in addition to speech perception in noise, auditory short-term memory, and auditory attention.

MATERIALS AND METHODS

PARTICIPANTS

We recruited 58 (35 female) participants (ages 55–79) for a study examining training for speech-in-noise processing. Pure-tone audiometric thresholds were obtained bilaterally at octave intervals 0.125–8 kHz and at 3 and 6 kHz. No left/right asymmetries or interaural click-evoked auditory brainstem response Wave V differences ($\geq$0.2 ms) were noted. No participants had a history of neurologic conditions and all participants had normal IQs [$\geq$85 on the WASI (Zhu and Garcia, 1999)]. Participants provided informed consent for procedures that were approved by the Northwestern Institutional Review Board and were paid for their time.

Participants were divided into normal-hearing and hearing-impaired subgroups. The normal-hearing participants had hearing thresholds $\leq$25 dB HL through 6 kHz and the participants with hearing loss had hearing thresholds $\leq$80 dB HL through 8 kHz. See **Figure 1** for average thresholds in the normal-hearing and hearing-impaired groups. Participants from both hearing groups were randomly assigned to complete either auditory-based cognitive training or active control training (Smith et al., 2009). Both involved training on an in-home computer, 1 h/day, 5 days/week, for 8 weeks. The *auditory training* group completed Brain Fitness™ cognitive training (Posit Science Corporation, San Francisco, CA) consisting of six modules designed to increase the speed and accuracy of auditory processing: (1) time-order judgments of frequency-modulated sweeps, (2) discriminating between pairs of confusable syllables, (3) recognizing sequences of confusable syllables and words, (4) matching pairs of confusable syllables and words, (5) implementing sequences of commands, and (6) answering questions from stories (see Smith et al., 2009 for details). In the first module, an adaptively decreasing inter-stimulus interval challenges processing speed. In subsequent modules, focused attention is directed to adaptively expanding and contracting CV transitions. The overall goal of the training is to improve sensory function, based on the idea that an increase in the quality of neural information flowing through peripheral and central sensory systems may lead to better cognitive function (Schneider and Pichora-Fuller, 2000). Completion of training was verified through automated online logs. The *active control* group watched educational DVDs and completed multiple-choice questions about the content. See **Figure 2** for a schematic of the experimental design. Training groups (and hearing subgroups) were matched for sex, age, hearing, click-evoked wave V brainstem latency, IQ, and test-retest intervals (**Table 1**).

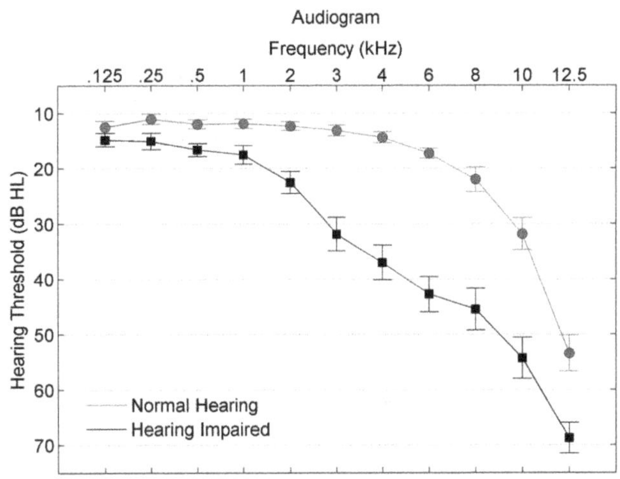

FIGURE 1 | Average hearing thresholds are plotted from 0.125–8 kHz for participants with normal hearing (gray circles) and with hearing loss (black squares), with error bars ± 1 SE.

BEHAVIORAL ASSESSMENTS

Perceptual—speech perception in noise

The QuickSIN is a non-adaptive measure of speech perception in noise. Sentences are presented in a background of four-talker babble and the SNR decreases by 5 dB for each sentence. Participants receive a point for correctly repeating target words. The total number of points is subtracted from 25.5 to arrive at a final SNR loss [or the increase in SNR required to achieve 50% correct performance compared to normal performance of 0 dB SNR; see Killion et al. (2004)].

Cognitive

Two subtests of the Woodcock-Johnson III Cognitive Test Battery (Woodcock et al., 2001) were used to obtain an age-normed cluster score for auditory short-term memory: Numbers Reversed and Memory for Words. The attention score was based on the sustained index of overall attention (visual and auditory) on the IVA+: Integrated Visual and Auditory Continuous Performance Test (BrainTrain, North Chesterfield, VA). Due to equipment malfunction, we are missing attention data from 3 participants in the *auditory training* group and 1 participant in the *active control* group.

ELECTROPHYSIOLOGY

Stimulus

We duplicated the electrophysiologic methods previously used to document enhanced envelope coding in older adults with hearing loss (Anderson et al., 2013a), using the protocol that produced the greatest hearing loss effects. The stimulus was a 40-ms syllable [da] synthesized in a Klatt-based synthesizer (Klatt, 1980). It began with a 5-ms onset burst followed by a CV transition and was perceived as a full CV syllable although it lacked a steady-state vowel. After the initial onset burst, the fundamental frequency (F_0) of the stimulus rose linearly from 103 to 125 Hz while the formants shifted as follows: F_1: 220 $\rightarrow$ 720 Hz; F_2: 1700 $\rightarrow$ 1240 Hz; F_3: 2580 $\rightarrow$ 2500 Hz. The fourth

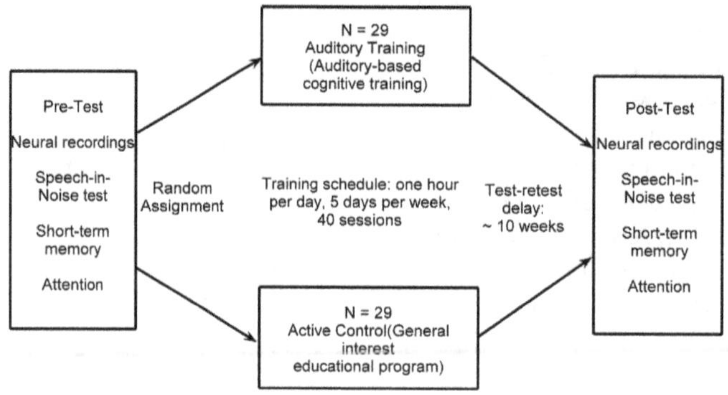

FIGURE 2 | A summary of the experimental design.

Table 1 | Means and *SDs* are provided for age, IQ, and hearing (PTA dB HL; average hearing threshold 0.5–4 kHz) for all participants in the *Auditory Training* and *Active Control* groups and the subgroups of normal hearing and hearing impaired.

Mean (*SD*)	Auditory training			Active control		
	Total ($N = 29$)	Normal hearing ($N = 14$)	Hearing impaired ($N = 15$)	Total ($N = 29$)	Normal hearing ($N = 14$)	Hearing impaired ($N = 15$)
Age	64.11 (5.78)	60.86 (3.74)	67.36 (5.72)	64.07 (5.22)	62.86 (3.34)	65.29 (6.50)
IQ	118.43 (12.15)	117.00 (12.30)	119.36 (12.43)	120.00 (14.23)	118.36 (14.28)	122.56 (14.61)
Hearing (dB HL)	20.64 (11.29)	11.36 (3.18)	28.25 (8.19)	18.3 (7.83)	13.43 (3.20)	22.87 (8.19)
Sex (males)	9	5	4	14	8	6

The groups are matched on all listed variables (all p's > 0.10).

(3600 Hz) and fifth (4500 Hz) formants remained constant for the duration of the stimulus. A spectrogram and Fourier transform of the stimulus waveform are presented in **Figures 3A,B**, respectively.

To partially equate for the effects of hearing loss, the [da] stimulus was individually amplified based on the National Acoustics Laboratory-Revised algorithm (NAL-R; Byrne and Dillon, 1986) using a custom program in MATLAB (The MathWorks, Inc., Natick, MA). The amplified presentation level did not exceed 90 dB SPL or the participants' loudness discomfort thresholds. We have previously found that the amplification procedure improves morphology without distorting spectral components of the response (Anderson et al., 2013b). In addition, although we found enhanced encoding in brainstem responses to both amplified and unamplified stimuli, the differences were clearest for the amplified stimuli (Anderson et al., 2013a); therefore, we expected to see the greatest treatment effects in response to the amplified stimuli. Repeated hearing tests verified that there were no changes in hearing after 8 weeks and therefore all participants received the same amplified stimulus before and after training.

Recording

The [da] was presented binaurally in pink noise at +10 dB SNR. Stimuli were presented at 80 dB SPL for normal hearing listeners and amplified stimuli for participants with hearing loss were presented at an intensity of up to 90 dB SPL, with most stimuli in the range of 80–83 dB SPL. Stimuli were presented via the Bio-Logic Navigator Pro System (Natus Medical, Inc., Mundelein, IL) at a rate of 10.9 Hz (inter-stimulus interval of 52 ms) through electromagnetically shielded insert earphones (ER-3A, Etymotic Research, Elk Grove Village, IL). A vertical montage of four Ag-AgCl electrodes (Cz active, Fpz ground, earlobe references) was used with all contact impedances <5 kΩ. A criterion of $\pm$ 23 μV was used for online artifact rejection. Two blocks of 3000 artifact-free sweeps were collected in each condition for each participant and averaged using an 85.3-ms window, including a 15.8-ms prestimulus period. Responses were sampled at 12 kHz and were online bandpass filtered from 100 to 2000 Hz (Butterworth filter, 12 dB/octave, zero phase-shift) to minimize disruption by the low-frequency cortical response and to sample energy up to the phase-locking limits of the brainstem (Liu et al., 2006).

The [da] was presented in alternating polarities, allowing for the creation of responses comprised of both the sum and the difference of the two polarities (Campbell et al., 2012). When creating the summed frequency following response (FFR), the non-inverting envelope component of the response is enhanced while the inverting TFS component is minimized; conversely, for the subtracted responses the inverting TFS component is enhanced while the non-inverting envelope component is substantially reduced (Aiken and Picton, 2008). While this analysis is a somewhat different operationalization of envelope and TFS representation than is used in some other studies, the selection of measures of envelope and TFS representation is driven by the model organization and site of interest (Shamma and Lorenzi,

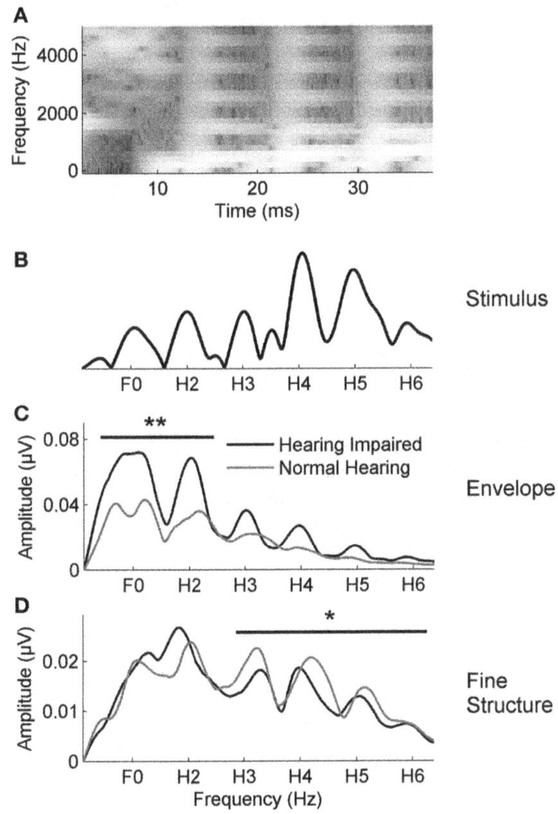

FIGURE 3 | (A) The spectrogram of the 40-ms syllable [da]. Fast Fourier transforms were calculated from 20 to 42 ms for the stimulus **(B)** and in responses to the envelope **(C)** and the TFS **(D)** in noise. The average responses for the participants with normal hearing (gray) and with hearing loss (black) are displayed. The group with hearing loss has higher amplitudes in the envelope-dominated low frequencies (F_0–H_2) in noise relative to the group with normal hearing **(C)**; conversely, the group with normal hearing has higher amplitudes in the fine structure dominated higher frequencies (H_3–H_6) than the group with hearing loss **(D)**. $^*p < 0.05$, $^{**}p < 0.01$.

2013), and adding/subtracted brainstem responses to alternating polarities is a typical method used in analyzing human FFRs (Aiken and Picton, 2008; Gockel et al., 2011; Anderson et al., 2013a). Nevertheless, we note that the relationship between envelope/TFS representation reflected in the FFR, perceptual measures, and auditory nerve coding remains an avenue for future research. Spectral amplitudes were calculated using fast Fourier transforms (FFTs) over 60 Hz bins around the frequencies of interest, which included the fundamental frequency (F_0) and its integer harmonics. The time region chosen for this calculation was 20–42 ms, corresponding to the most periodic time region of the FFR.

STATISTICAL ANALYSIS

A Multivariate Analysis of Variance (MANOVA) was used to assess hearing group differences in the envelope and TFS. The F_0 and H_2 amplitudes from the added polarities (henceforth F_{0ADD}–H_{2ADD}) were entered as dependent variables in the MANOVA to represent the envelope, as these lower frequency spectral peaks dominate the envelope-following FFR. The H_3–H_6 amplitudes from the subtracted polarities (H_{3SUB}–H_{6SUB}) were entered as dependent variables to represent the TFS, which is more prominent in relatively higher frequencies in the FFR. A repeated measures ANOVA was used to compare envelope-dominated (F_{0ADD}–H_{2ADD}) and TFS-dominated (H_{3SUB}–H_{6SUB}) frequency encoding, QuickSIN SNR scores, and memory and attention measures before and after training.

RESULTS

EFFECTS OF HEARING LOSS ON ENCODING SPEECH ENVELOPE/TFS

The combined participants with hearing loss from both groups had greater representation of the envelope (F_{0ADD} and H_{2ADD}) than participants with normal hearing [$F_{(1, 57)} = 7.218$, $p = 0.002$] (**Figure 3C**), replicating a previous study demonstrating greater subcortical representation of the envelope in response to speech in noise in older adults with hearing loss (Anderson et al., 2013a). In contrast to the Anderson et al. study (2013a), however, we also found reduced representation of the TFS (H_{3SUB}–H_{6SUB}) in the older adults with hearing loss [$F_{(1, 57)} = 3.066$, $p = 0.024$] (**Figure 3D**). The current study comprised 58 participants vs. the 30 participants in the previous study; therefore, the new finding of significant differences in TFS representation in the current study may be attributed to increased power and is in fact consistent with Henry and Heinz (2012), who found a reduction in TFS coding in noise in auditory nerve fibers of chinchillas with noise-induced hearing loss.

TRAINING: NEUROPHYSIOLOGICAL CHANGES

In the group with hearing loss, we found a training group × test session interaction [$F_{(1, 30)} = 4.351$, $p = 0.023$], with a significant reduction in envelope encoding (F_{0ADD} to H_{2ADD}) occurring within the *auditory training* group [$F_{(1, 14)} = 3.843$, $p = 0.049$] but not the *active control* group [$F_{(1, 14)} = 0.381$, $p = 0.691$] (see **Figures 4A,B**). We also analyzed the pre and post data of the groups with normal hearing and found no training group × test session interaction [$F_{(1, 27)} = 0.803$, $p = 0.459$] and no changes in either group (all p's > 0.1) (see **Figures 4C,D**). Although there was no training group × hearing group × test session interaction [$F_{(1, 57)} = 2.239$, $p = 0.117$], there was a hearing group × test session interaction in the *auditory training* group [$F_{(1, 29)} = 3.573$, $p = 0.043$] that was not present in the *active control* group [$F_{(1, 29)} = 0.136$, $p = 0.874$] (see **Figures 4E,F**), suggesting that the auditory training effect was specific to the participants with hearing loss. Representation of the TFS (H_{3SUB}–H_{6SUB}) did not change for either hearing impaired or normal hearing participants of either training group (all p's > 0.1) (**Figure 5**). **Figures 6, 7** display mean F_{0ADD} and H_{2ADD} and mean H_{3SUB}–H_{6SUB} amplitudes, respectively, for individual participants. It is evident from these figures that individuals with hearing loss have greater variability than individuals with normal hearing.

TRAINING: BEHAVIORAL CHANGES

Summary: There were significant training-induced changes in speech-in-noise perception, memory, and attention across hearing groups in the *auditory training* group. The training effects

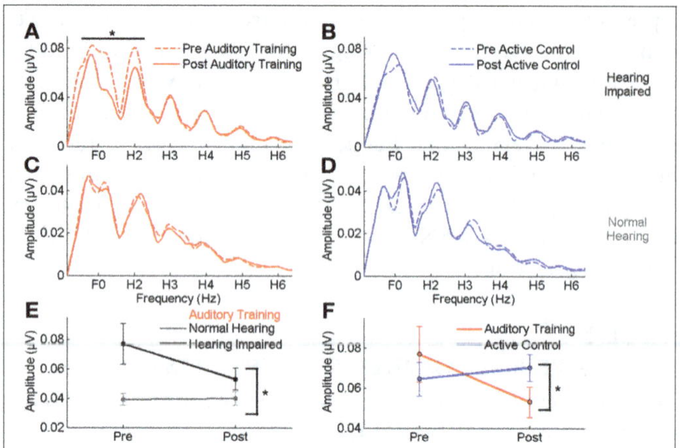

FIGURE 4 | (A,B) A comparison of pre- (dotted lines) and post-training responses (solid lines) to speech in noise to the envelope (F_0–H_2) in the *auditory training* (red) and *active control* (blue) groups with hearing loss, demonstrating a significant reduction in response to the envelope in the *auditory training* group. **(C,D)** No reduction was seen in response to the envelope in either group with normal hearing. **(E)** A significant hearing × session interaction was noted in the *auditory training* group, demonstrating that the change was specific to the participants with hearing loss. **(F)** A significant group × session interaction in the groups with hearing loss indicating a reduction in the representation of the F_0 in the *auditory training* group only. $^*p < 0.05$. Error bars: ± 1 SE.

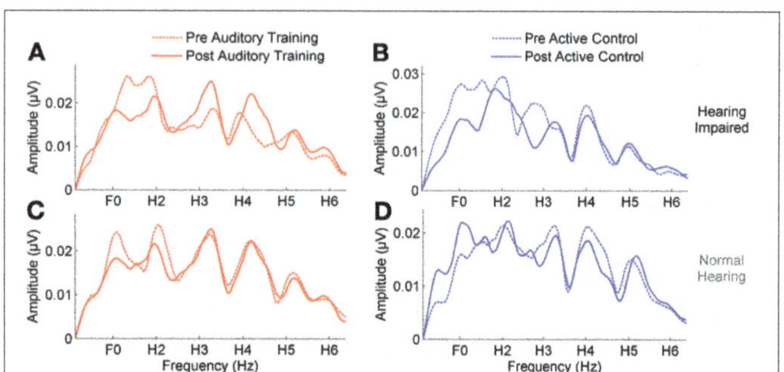

FIGURE 5 | (A,B) A comparison of pre- (dotted lines) and post-training responses (solid lines) to speech in noise to the fine structure (H_3–H_6) in the *auditory training* (red) and *active control* (blue) groups with hearing loss, demonstrating no change in either group. **(C,D)** No change was seen in response to the fine structure in either group with normal hearing.

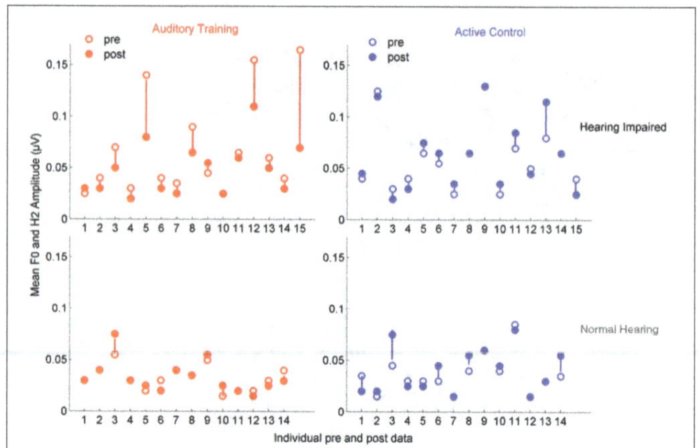

FIGURE 6 | Mean F_{0ADD} and H_{2ADD} amplitudes are displayed for individual pre- (open circles) and post-data (closed circles) for the auditory training (red) and active control (blue) groups. Visual observation of the data reveals that there is greater pre-training variability in both groups with hearing loss and in the degree of change in the auditory training group with hearing loss.

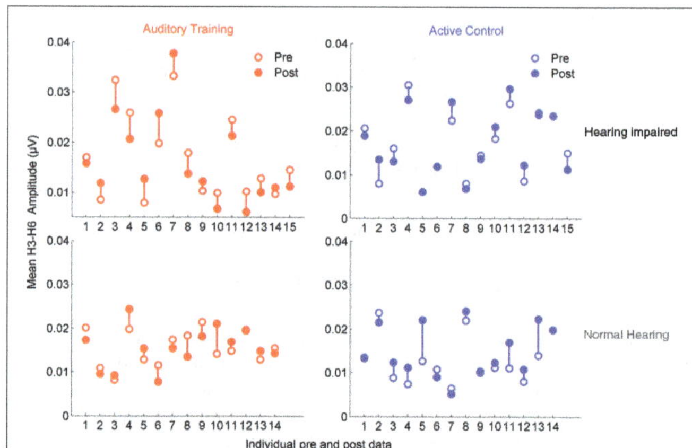

FIGURE 7 | Mean H_{3SUB} and H_{6SUB} amplitudes are displayed for individual pre- (open circles) and post-data (closed circles) for the auditory training (red) and active control (blue) groups. Similar to the data for the envelope, the data demonstrates greater variability in both groups with hearing loss for pre-test data, but there is no systematic change with training as was found for the envelope.

specific to hearing status varied depending on the task. The improvement in speech-in-noise performance was specific to the hearing impaired group, the memory change was found only in the normal hearing group, and attention improved in both groups. There were no corresponding changes in the *active control* group.

For speech-in-noise performance (QuickSIN), there was a significant training group × test session interaction [$F_{(1, 57)} = 5.191$, $p = 0.027$], with improvement noted in the *auditory training* group [$F_{(1, 28)} = 13.394$, $p = 0.001$] but not in the *active control* group [$F_{(1, 28)} = 1.678$, $p = 0.206$]. This change was largely driven by the improvement in performance in the auditory training group with hearing loss [$F_{(1, 14)} = 12.220$, $p = 0.004$]; the improvement in the normal-hearing group was not significant [$F_{(1, 14)} = 3.041$, $p = 0.105$]. Neither hearing group in the *active control* group changed with training (all p's > 0.1). There was a decrease in the QuickSIN of 1.22 dB in the *auditory training* group with hearing loss—given four lists, this number is below the 1.9 dB necessary for a critical difference between conditions with an 95% confidence interval (Killion et al., 2004). However, a 1 dB decrease in SNR corresponds to approximately a 10% increase in word recognition—a difference that is likely to be noticeable to the listener (Middelweerd et al., 1990). It should also be noted that the participants with hearing loss did not have more than a mild SNR loss—less than 7 dB—so greater gains might be expected from individuals with greater deficits.

Similarly, for short-term memory there was a significant training group × test session interaction [$F_{(1, 57)} = 6.042, p = 0.017$], with improvements in the *auditory training* group [$F_{(1, 28)} = 9.800$, $p = 0.004$] but not the *active control* group [$F_{(1, 28)} = 0.158$, $p = 0.694$]. For memory, however, the changes were only significant in the group with normal hearing [$F_{(1, 28)} = 7.648$, $p = 0.016$] but not in the group with hearing loss [$F_{(1, 28)} = 2.630$, $p = 0.127$] and neither hearing group in the *active control* group changed (all p's > 0.1).

Finally, for attention, there was a significant training group × test session interaction [$F_{(1, 50)} = 3.765$, $p = 0.043$], with improvements in the *auditory training* group [$F_{(1, 25)} = 17.941$, $p < 0.001$] but not the *active control* group [$F_{(1, 24)} = 0.623$, $p = 0.438$]. In this case, there were significant improvements for both the subgroups with normal hearing [$F_{(1, 11)} = 8.182$, $p = 0.016$] and with hearing loss of the *auditory training* group [$F_{(1, 12)} = 9.339$, $p = 0.009$]. Again, there were no changes for members of either hearing subgroup of the *active control* group (all p's > 0.1). See **Figure 8** for interaction plots of behavioral changes. Please refer to **Table 2** for means and standard deviations of pre- and post-training changes in behavioral measures for the normal hearing and hearing impaired participants of the *auditory training* and *active control* groups.

DISCUSSION

Here we show that the imbalance in neurophysiological processing of speech cues associated with hearing loss is malleable and reversible with training in older adults. The results are summarized as follows: first, compared to normal hearing individuals, older adults with hearing loss have excessively large envelope encoding of speech in noise. Second, training that targets the CV transition reduces envelope representation in individuals with hearing loss to levels in line with those of normal-hearing individuals. Finally, the training-induced changes in neurophysiology are accompanied by gains in speech-in-noise perception, attention, and short-term memory, although it should be noted that the change in speech-in-noise perception was modest, and would not be considered clinically significant (Killion et al., 2004). Nevertheless, we note that an improvement of 1 dB SNR corresponds to approximately 10% word intelligibility in noise (Middelweerd et al., 1990), so the changes may be perceived as beneficial to the listener.

Our results confirm previous findings of exaggerated representation of envelope cues in animal and human models of sensorineural hearing loss (Kale and Heinz, 2010; Henry and Heinz, 2012; Anderson et al., 2013a), providing a possible explanation for the observation that the hearing impaired listener perceives speech as loud but unclear (Jin and Nelson, 2010). At present, the

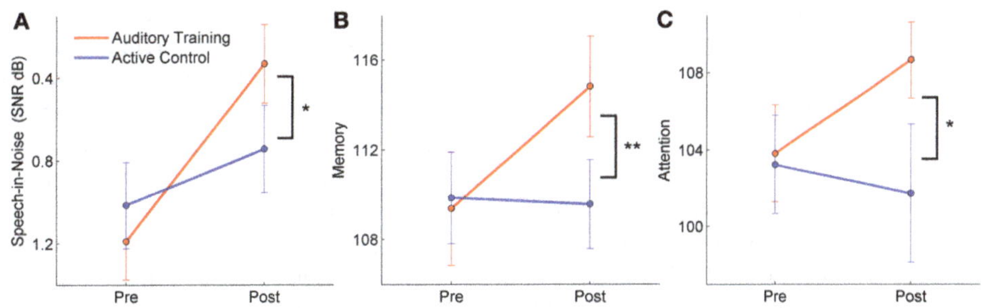

FIGURE 8 | Pre and post-training perceptual and cognitive scores for participants with both normal hearing and hearing loss (group × session interactions). The *auditory training* group improved in speech-in-noise perception **(A)**, memory **(B)**, and attention **(C)**, whereas there were no changes in the *active control* group. *$p < 0.05$, **$p < 0.01$. Error bars: ± 1 SE.

Table 2 | Means and *SDs* are provided for pre- and post-test scores for speech-in-noise perception, auditory short-term memory and attention for the *Auditory Training* and *Active Control* groups, including the subgroups of participants with normal hearing and with hearing loss.

Mean (*SD*)	Session	Auditory training			Active control		
		Total (*N* = 29)	Normal hearing (*N* = 14)	Hearing impaired (*N* = 15)	Total (*N* = 29)	Normal hearing (*N* = 14)	Hearing impaired (*N* = 15)
Speech-in-noise perception	Pre	1.51 (1.44)	0.72 (0.82)	2.04 (1.38)	1.13 (1.16)	0.93 (1.26)	1.31 (1.07)
	Post	0.65 (1.27)	0.25 (1.08)	0.84 (1.32)	0.91 (1.22)	0.63 (1.14)	1.18 (1.27)
Memory	Pre	09.28 (14.24)	104.71 (12.77)	113.53 (14.62)	110.38 (11.65)	113.53 (14.62)	109.80 (7.72)
	Post	114.24 (13.08)	111.43 (14.32)	116.57 (11.67)	109.72 (11.34)	116.57 (11.67)	108.07 (10.87)
Attention	Pre	103.48 (14.47)	99.08 (17.44)	107.00 (10.96)	103.62 (15.48)	100.00 (16.51)	107.11 (12.27)
	Post	108.25 (11.81)	104.50 (12.38)	112.00 (10.30)	99.35 (23.61)	100.46 (24.90)	105.37 (24.24)

mechanisms underlying this exaggerated representation in auditory brainstem are unknown; however, evidence from auditory nerve suggests a peripheral etiology arising from reduced outer hair cell compression in cases of mild to moderate hearing loss and from inner hair cell damage (steeper input-output functions) in cases of moderate to severe hearing loss (Kale and Heinz, 2010). The fact that envelope coding changed with training suggests that there may also be a top-down central gain effect resulting from auditory deprivation (Munro and Blount, 2009). However, there was no change in TFS coding in the training group. The effects of hearing loss on envelope and TFS representation are a function of complex interactions among cochlear function, stimulus presentation level, and SNR (Henry and Heinz, 2012). One possibility is that a change in TFS coding was too subtle to be observed at the single SNR we used. Another important consideration is the nature of the training: all of the training stimuli were presented in quiet, not in noise. It is possible that this presentation technique favored envelope coding, which is maladaptively enhanced even in quiet in listeners with cochlear hearing loss (Anderson et al., 2013a). Further investigation to establish the effects of hearing loss at different presentation levels and SNRs is warranted, as a better understanding of the mechanisms underlying abnormal stimulus encoding will help guide future treatment efforts.

The results of our study contrast with those of two previous studies that found training-induced increases in envelope coding in normal-hearing young adults using different types of training: pitch discrimination training (Carcagno and Plack, 2011) and recognition of speech presented in babble and other challenging conditions (Song et al., 2012). The key difference between these studies and ours is that our study population included individuals with hearing impairment. Given the differences between normal-hearing and hearing-impaired listeners in performance on perceptual tasks, neurophysiological encoding of sound, and reliance on cognitive mechanisms for speech intelligibility (Lorenzi et al., 2006; Anderson et al., 2013a; Humes et al., 2013), it is not necessarily surprising that there are different effects of auditory training. Another important difference is the training itself. The training in our study directed attention to fast-changing sounds in high memory load situations and occurred in quiet. It may be that training on recognition of speech in noise, such as in the Song et al. study, produces more robust gains in speech-in-noise perception and different outcomes when comparing pre and post envelope and TFS coding. As another example, FFR neural representation of the F_0 is correlated with behavioral pitch discrimination, (Krishnan et al., 2010; Marmel et al., 2013); therefore, enhanced neural representation of cues contributing to the perception of pitch may underlie the training-induced gains in pitch discrimination found by Carcagno and Plack (2011). Thus, outcomes may vary depending on the type of training and the targeted population.

We propose, therefore, that the training effects in this study were influenced by neural mechanisms specific to older adults with hearing loss. Both aging (Turner et al., 2005; Schatteman et al., 2008) and hearing loss (Vale and Sanes, 2002; Dong et al., 2009) appear to cause an imbalance in excitatory and inhibitory function, likely affecting stimulus encoding. However, this imbalance is at least partially reversed in animal models of auditory training (de Villers-Sidani et al., 2010) and acoustic experience (Turner et al., 2013). Although we are unable to verify these effects in humans, we speculate that the training-induced changes were facilitated by alterations in the balance of neurotransmitter levels to allow for precise encoding of subtle CV differences. That said, just as it is difficult to disambiguate between peripheral (i.e., outer hair cell loss and peripheral neuropathy) vs. central mechanisms of hearing loss, it is difficult to say with certainty which mechanisms were targeted by training.

Our training was designed to strengthen sensory function through attention to meaningful sound; specifically, focusing attention on CV transitions in speech may drive top-down modulation, which occurred in five of the six training modules. Animal models have demonstrated that directed attention to behaviorally-relevant stimuli is necessary for neural and behavioral plasticity (Fritz et al., 2005, 2007). In our study, we found that neural response changes were accompanied by improvements in attention. A functional connection between prefrontal and auditory cortices provides a basis for efferent activation during difficult tasks that require focused attention (Raizada and Poldrack, 2007). A tentative connection has also been suggested between prefrontal cortex and auditory brainstem based on fMRI studies (Roelfsema et al., 2010). Although our methodology does not allow us to draw similar conclusions, we propose that rapid TFS cues may become more salient when sensory and cognitive demands drive a prefrontal-brainstem connection to adjust subcortical encoding of these cues.

A number of questions remain unanswered. We did not include anyone in our study who wore hearing aids, because hearing aids themselves may induce plasticity in auditory processing (Munro et al., 2007; Munro and Merrett, 2013). Therefore, the use of amplification itself can be considered a form of training. Hornickel et al. (2012) demonstrated that assistive listening devices engender improved trial-to-trial consistency in brainstem firing, presumably by directing attention to a more robust and noise-free representation of the stimulus. Future work should compare the neural effects of amplification alone vs. amplification plus training. In addition, more work should be done to determine the persistence of training effects and the time course of learning. A number of approaches were employed in our training protocol, involving strictly bottom-up discrimination training and combined memory and perceptual training exercises. It would be important to identify the aspects of training that were primarily responsible for engendering plasticity. We note that there is a great deal of individual variability in the participants with hearing loss, both in terms of pre-training spectral amplitudes and in the degree of change. In future work, it will be important to identify sources of variability, and the factors that contribute to success in individuals.

Finally, although neither envelope nor TFS representation changed in the normal hearing group, this group did experience changes in attention and short-term memory. Therefore, we assume the normal-hearing participants experienced training-induced biological changes that were not observed using the current envelope/TFS technique. The lack of observed improvement in memory in the group with hearing loss may be due to the auditory nature of our assessment measure. Although the presentation level was adjusted to a comfortable volume for each participant, it may be that peripheral hearing loss limited performance, even in the post-training session, given the known effects of hearing loss on verbal short-term memory (McCoy et al., 2005; Verhaegen et al., 2013). The speech-in-noise perception scores (QuickSIN) of normal hearing groups would be considered clinically normal—less than 3 dB SNR loss (Killion et al., 2004), and so the lack of improvement in this group probably stems from a ceiling effect. Further investigation is needed to determine the mechanisms of training-induced improvements in individuals with normal hearing.

These results have implications for management of hearing loss problems in older adults. Although provision of audibility is a necessary foundation for the treatment of hearing difficulties, we assert that auditory training is just as important. The combination of amplification and auditory training may lead to improved speech clarity in noise without distortion from overamplification.

ACKNOWLEDGMENTS

We thank Trent Nicol, Karen Chan, and Alexandra Parbery-Clark for their critical reviews of the manuscript. Supported by the NIH (R01 DC010016) and the Knowles Hearing Center.

REFERENCES

Aiken, S. J., and Picton, T. W. (2008). Envelope and spectral frequency-following responses to vowel sounds. *Hear. Res.* 245, 35–47. doi: 10.1016/j.heares.2008.08.004

Anderson, S., Parbery-Clark, A., White-Schwoch, T., Drehobl, S., and Kraus, N. (2013a). Effects of hearing loss on the subcortical representation of speech cues. *J. Acoust. Soc. Am.* 133, 3030–3038. doi: 10.1121/1.4799804

Anderson, S., Parbery-Clark, A., White-Schwoch, T., and Kraus, N. (2013b). Auditory brainstem response to complex sounds predicts self-reported speech-in-noise performance. *J. Speech Lang. Hear. Res.* 56, 31–43. doi: 10.1044/1092-4388(2012/12-0043)

Anderson, S., White-Schwoch, T., Parbery-Clark, A., and Kraus, N. (2013c). Reversal of age-related neural timing delays with training. *Proc. Natl. Acad. Sci. U.S.A.* 110, 4357–4362. doi: 10.1073/pnas.1213555110

Anderson, S., Parbery-Clark, A., White-Schwoch, T., and Kraus, N. (2012). Aging affects neural precision of speech encoding. *J. Neurosci.* 32, 14156–14164. doi: 10.1523/JNEUROSCI.2176-12.2012

Ardoint, M., Sheft, S., Fleuriot, P., Garnier, S., and Lorenzi, C. (2010). Perception of temporal fine-structure cues in speech with minimal envelope cues for listeners with mild-to-moderate hearing loss. *Int. J. Audiol.* 49, 823–831. doi: 10.3109/14992027.2010.492402

Byrne, D., and Dillon, H. (1986). The National Acoustic Laboratories' (NAL) new procedure for selecting the gain and frequency response of a hearing aid. *Ear Hear.* 7, 257–265. doi: 10.1097/00003446-198608000-00007

Campbell, T., Kerlin, J., Bishop, C., and Miller, L. (2012). Methods to eliminate stimulus transduction artifact from insert earphones during electroencephalography. *Ear Hear.* 33, 144–150. doi: 10.1097/AUD.0b013e3182280353

Carcagno, S., and Plack, C. (2011). Subcortical plasticity following perceptual learning in a pitch discrimination task. *J. Assoc. Res. Otolaryngol.* 12, 89–100. doi: 10.1007/s10162-010-0236-1

Clinard, C. G., Tremblay, K. L., and Krishnan, A. R. (2010). Aging alters the perception and physiological representation of frequency: evidence from human frequency-following response recordings. *Hear. Res.* 264, 48–55. doi: 10.1016/j.heares.2009.11.010

de Villers-Sidani, E., Alzghoul, L., Zhou, X., Simpson, K. L., Lin, R. C. S., and Merzenich, M. M. (2010). Recovery of functional and structural age-related changes in the rat primary auditory cortex with operant training. *Proc. Natl. Acad. Sci. U.S.A.* 107, 13900–13905. doi: 10.1073/pnas.1007885107

Dong, S., Mulders, W., Rodger, J., and Robertson, D. (2009). Changes in neuronal activity and gene expression in guinea-pig auditory brainstem after unilateral partial hearing loss. *Neuroscience* 159, 1164–1174. doi: 10.1016/j.neuroscience.2009.01.043

Dubno, J. R., Dirks, D. D., and Morgan, D. E. (1984). Effects of age and mild hearing loss on speech recognition in noise. *J. Acoust. Soc. Am.* 76, 87–96. doi: 10.1121/1.391011

Fritz, J., Elhilali, M., and Shamma, S. (2005). Active listening: task-dependent plasticity of spectrotemporal receptive fields in primary auditory cortex. *Hear. Res.* 206, 159–176. doi: 10.1016/j.heares.2005.01.015

Fritz, J. B., Elhilali, M., David, S. V., and Shamma, S. A. (2007). Does attention play a role in dynamic receptive field adaptation to changing acoustic salience in A1? *Hear. Res.* 229, 186–203. doi: 10.1016/j.heares.2007.01.009

Gockel, H., Carlyon, R., Mehta, A., and Plack, C. (2011). The frequency following response (FFR) may reflect pitch-bearing information but is not a direct representation of pitch. *J. Assoc. Res. Otolaryngol.* 12, 767–782. doi: 10.1007/s10162-011-0284-1

Gordon-Salant, S., Yeni-Komshian, G. H., Fitzgibbons, P. J., and Barrett, J. (2006). Age-related differences in identification and discrimination of temporal cues in speech segments. *J. Acoust. Soc. Am.* 119, 2455–2466. doi: 10.1121/1.2171527

Heine, C., and Browning, C. J. (2002). Communication and psychosocial consequences of sensory loss in older adults: overview and rehabilitation directions. *Disabil. Rehabil.* 24, 763–773. doi: 10.1080/09638280210129162

Henry, K. S., and Heinz, M. G. (2012). Diminished temporal coding with sensorineural hearing loss emerges in background noise. *Nat. Neurosci.* 15, 1362–1364. doi: 10.1038/nn.3216

Hopkins, K., and Moore, B. C. J. (2011). The effects of age and cochlear hearing loss on temporal fine structure sensitivity, frequency selectivity, and speech reception in noise. *J. Acoust. Soc. Am.* 130, 334–349. doi: 10.1121/1.3585848

Hornickel, J., Zecker, S. G., Bradlow, A. R., and Kraus, N. (2012). Assistive listening devices drive neuroplasticity in children with dyslexia. *Proc. Natl. Acad. Sci. U.S.A.* 109, 16731–16736. doi: 10.1073/pnas.1206628109

Humes, L. E., Kidd, G. R., and Lentz, J. J. (2013). Auditory and cognitive factors underlying individual differences in aided speech-understanding among older adults. *Front. Syst. Neurosci.* 7:55. doi: 10.3389/fnsys.2013.00055

Jin, S. H., and Nelson, P. B. (2010). Interrupted speech perception: the effects of hearing sensitivity and frequency resolution. *J. Acoust. Soc. Am.* 128, 881. doi: 10.1121/1.3458851

Johnson, E. E., and Dillon, H. (2011). A comparison of gain for adults from generic hearing aid prescriptive methods: impacts on predicted loudness, frequency bandwidth, and speech intelligibility. *J. Am. Acad. Audiol.* 22, 441–459. doi: 10.3766/jaaa.22.7.5

Kale, S., and Heinz, M. (2010). Envelope coding in auditory nerve fibers following noise-induced hearing loss. *J. Assoc. Res. Otolaryngol.* 11, 657–673. doi: 10.1007/s10162-010-0223-6

Killion, M., Niquette, P., Gudmundsen, G., Revit, L., and Banerjee, S. (2004). Development of a quick speech-in-noise test for measuring signal-to-noise ratio loss in normal-hearing and hearing-impaired listeners. *J. Acoust. Soc. Am.* 116, 2395–2405. doi: 10.1121/1.1784440

Klatt, D. (1980). Software for a cascade/parallel formant synthesizer. *J. Acoust. Soc. Am.* 67, 971–995. doi: 10.1121/1.383940

Krishnan, A., Bidelman, G., and Gandour, J. T. (2010). Neural representation of pitch salience in the human brainstem revealed by psychophysical and electrophysiological indices. *Hear. Res.* 268, 60–66. doi: 10.1016/j.heares.2010.04.016

Lister, J. J., Roberts, R. A., and Lister, F. L. (2011). An adaptive clinical test of temporal resolution: age effects. *Int. J. Audiol.* 50, 367–374. doi: 10.3109/14992027.2010.551218

Liu, L.-F., Palmer, A. R., and Wallace, M. N. (2006). Phase-locked responses to pure tones in the inferior colliculus. *J. Neurophysiol.* 95, 1926–1935. doi: 10.1152/jn.00497.2005

Lorenzi, C., Gilbert, G., Carn, H., Garnier, S., and Moore, B. C. J. (2006). Speech perception problems of the hearing impaired reflect inability to use temporal fine structure. *Proc. Natl. Acad. Sci. U.S.A.* 103, 18866–18869. doi: 10.1073/pnas.0607364103

Marmel, F., Linley, D., Carlyon, R. P., Gockel, H. E., Hopkins, K., and Plack, C. J. (2013). Subcortical neural synchrony and absolute thresholds predict frequency discrimination independently. *J. Assoc. Res. Otolaryngol.* 14, 757–766. doi: 10.1007/s10162-013-0402-3

McCoy, S. L., Tun, P. A., Cox, L. C., Colangelo, M., Stewart, R. A., and Wingfield, A. (2005). Hearing loss and perceptual effort: downstream effects on older adults' memory for speech. *Q. J. Exp. Psychol. A* 58, 22–33. doi: 10.1080/02724980443000151

Middelweerd, M., Festen, J., and Plomp, R. (1990). Difficulties with speech intelligibility in noise in spite of a normal pure-tone audiogram. *Int. J. Audiol.* 29, 1–7. doi: 10.3109/00206099009081640

Moore, B. C. J. (2008). The role of temporal fine structure processing in pitch perception, masking, and speech perception for normal-hearing and hearing-impaired people. *J. Assoc. Res. Otolaryngol.* 9, 399–406. doi: 10.1007/s10162-008-0143-x

Moore, B. C. J., Wojtczak, M., and Vickers, D. A. (1996). Effect of loudness recruitment on the perception of amplitude modulation. *J. Acoust. Soc. Am.* 100, 481–489. doi: 10.1121/1.415861

Munro, K. J., and Blount, J. (2009). Adaptive plasticity in brainstem of adult listeners following earplug-induced deprivation. *J. Acoust. Soc. Am.* 126, 568–571. doi: 10.1121/1.3161829

Munro, K. J., and Merrett, J. F. (2013). Brainstem plasticity and modified loudness following short-term use of hearing aids. *J. Acoust. Soc. Am.* 133, 343–349. doi: 10.1121/1.4770234

Munro, K. J., Pisareva, N. Y., Parker, D. J., and Purdy, S. C. (2007). Asymmetry in the auditory brainstem response following experience of monaural amplification. *Neuroreport* 18, 1871–1874. doi: 10.1097/WNR.0b013e3282f1b003

Oxenham, A. J., and Simonson, A. M. (2009). Masking release for low- and high-pass-filtered speech in the presence of noise and single-talker interference. *J. Acoust. Soc. Am.* 125, 457–468. doi: 10.1121/1.3021299

Peelle, J. E., Troiani, V., Wingfield, A., and Grossman, M. (2010). Neural processing during older adults' comprehension of spoken sentences: age differences in resource allocation and connectivity. *Cereb. Cortex* 20, 773–782. doi: 10.1093/cercor/bhp142

Phillips, S. L., Gordon-Salant, S., Fitzgibbons, P. J., and Yeni-Komshian, G. (2000). Frequency and temporal resolution in elderly listeners with good and poor word recognition. *J. Speech Lang. Hear. Res.* 43, 217–228.

Pichora-Fuller, M. K. (2003). Cognitive aging and auditory information processing. *Int. J. Audiol.* 42, 26–32. doi: 10.3109/14992020309074641

Raizada, R. D. S., and Poldrack, R. A. (2007). Challenge-driven attention: interacting frontal and brainstem systems. *Front. Hum. Neurosci.* 1:3. doi: 10.3389/neuro.09.003.2007

Roelfsema, P. R., van Ooyen, A., and Watanabe, T. (2010). Perceptual learning rules based on reinforcers and attention. *Trends Cogn. Sci.* 14, 64. doi: 10.1016/j.tics.2009.11.005

Schatteman, T. A., Hughes, L. F., and Caspary, D. M. (2008). Aged-related loss of temporal processing: altered responses to amplitude modulated tones in rat dorsal cochlear nucleus. *Neuroscience* 154, 329–337. doi: 10.1016/j.neuroscience.2008.02.025

Schneider, B., and Pichora-Fuller, K. (2000). "Implications of perceptual deterioration for cognitive aging research," in *The Handbook of Aging and Cognition*, eds F. M. I. Craik and T. A. Salthouse (Mahwah, NJ: Lawrence Erlbaum Associates), 155–219.

Shamma, S., and Lorenzi, C. (2013). On the balance of envelope and temporal fine structure in the encoding of speech in the early auditory system. *J. Acoust. Soc. Am.* 133, 2818. doi: 10.1121/1.4795783

Shannon, R. V., Zeng, F.-G., Kamath, V., Wygonski, J., and Ekelid, M. (1995). Speech recognition with primarily temporal clues. *Science* 270, 303. doi: 10.1126/science.270.5234.303

Sheft, S., Ardoint, M., and Lorenzi, C. (2008). Speech identification based on temporal fine structure cues. *J. Acoust. Soc. Am.* 124, 562–575. doi: 10.1121/1.2918540

Smith, G. E., Housen, P., Yaffe, K., Ruff, R., Kennison, R. F., Mahncke, H. W., et al. (2009). A cognitive training program based on principles of brain plasticity: results from the improvement in memory with plasticity-based adaptive cognitive training (IMPACT) study. *J. Am. Geriatr. Soc.* 57, 594–603. doi: 10.1111/j.1532-5415.2008.02167.x

Song, J. H., Skoe, E., Banai, K., and Kraus, N. (2012). Training to improve hearing speech in noise: biological mechanisms. *Cereb. Cortex* 22, 1180–1190. doi: 10.1093/cercor/bhr196

Swaminathan, J., and Heinz, M. G. (2012). Psychophysiological analyses demonstrate the importance of neural envelope coding for speech perception in noise. *J. Neurosci.* 32, 1747–1756. doi: 10.1523/JNEUROSCI.4493-11.2012

Tremblay, K., Piskosz, M., and Souza., P. (2003). Effects of age and age-related hearing loss on the neural representation of speech cues. *Clin. Neurophysiol.* 114, 1332–1343. doi: 10.1016/S1388-2457(03)00114-7

Turner, J. G., Hughes, L. F., and Caspary, D. M. (2005). Affects of aging on receptive fields in rat primary auditory cortex layer V neurons. *J. Neurophysiol.* 94, 2738–2747. doi: 10.1152/jn.00362.2005

Turner, J. G., Parrish, J. L., Zuiderveld, L., Darr, S., Hughes, L. F., Caspary, D. M., et al. (2013). Acoustic experience alters the aged auditory system. *Ear Hear.* 34, 151–159. doi: 10.1097/AUD.0b013e318269ca5b

Vale, C., and Sanes, D. H. (2002). The effect of bilateral deafness on excitatory and inhibitory synaptic strength in the inferior colliculus. *Eur. J. Neurosci.* 16, 2394–2404. doi: 10.1046/j.1460-9568.2002.02302.x

Verhaegen, C., Collette, F., and Majerus, S. (2013). The impact of aging and hearing status on verbal short-term memory. *Neuropsychol. Dev. Cogn. B Aging Neuropsychol. Cogn.* doi: 10.1080/13825585.2013.832725. [Epub ahead of print].

Wingfield, A., Tun, P. A., and McCoy, S. L. (2005). Hearing loss in older adulthood. *Curr. Dir. Psychol. Sci.* 14, 144–148. doi: 10.1111/j.0963-7214.2005.00356.x

Woodcock, R. W., McGrew, K. S., and Mather, N. (2001). *Woodcock-Johnson III Tests of Cognitive Abilities* Itasca, IL: Riverside Publishing.

Zhu, J., and Garcia, E. (1999). *The Wechsler Abbreviated Scale of Intelligence (WASI)*. New York, NY: Psychological Corporation.

3

Across-frequency combination of interaural time difference in bilateral cochlear implant listeners

Antje Ihlefeld[1,2]*, Alan Kan[1] and Ruth Y. Litovsky[1]

[1] *Waisman Center, University of Wisconsin, Madison, WI, USA*
[2] *Center for Neural Science, New York University, New York, NY, USA*

Correspondence:
Antje Ihlefeld, Center for Neural Science, New York University, 4 Washington Place, New York, NY 10003, USA
e-mail: ai33@nyu.edu

The current study examined how cochlear implant (CI) listeners combine temporally interleaved envelope-ITD information across two sites of stimulation. When two cochlear sites jointly transmit ITD information, one possibility is that CI listeners can extract the most reliable ITD cues available. As a result, ITD sensitivity would be sustained or enhanced compared to single-site stimulation. Alternatively, mutual interference across multiple sites of ITD stimulation could worsen dual-site performance compared to listening to the better of two electrode pairs. Two experiments used direct stimulation to examine how CI users can integrate ITDs across two pairs of electrodes. Experiment 1 tested ITD discrimination for two stimulation sites using 100-Hz sinusoidally modulated 1000-pps-carrier pulse trains. Experiment 2 used the same stimuli ramped with 100 ms windows, as a control condition with minimized onset cues. For all stimuli, performance improved monotonically with increasing modulation depth. Results show that when CI listeners are stimulated with electrode pairs at two cochlear sites, sensitivity to ITDs was similar to that seen when only the electrode pair with better sensitivity was activated. None of the listeners showed a decrement in performance from the worse electrode pair. This could be achieved either by listening to the better electrode pair or by truly integrating the information across cochlear sites.

Keywords: cochlear implant, interaural time difference, envelope ITD, across-frequency integration, spatial sound

INTRODUCTION

Interaural time differences (ITDs), which occur due to different arrival times of sound energy in the left and right ear, are paramount for localizing the direction of a sound source and for attending to speech in a mixture of surrounding sound (Darwin and Hukin, 1999; Kidd et al., 2005). However, bilateral cochlear implant (CI) listeners do not rely much on ITDs when localizing sound (e.g., Seeber and Fastl, 2008). Moreover, studies on speech intelligibility in situations with background sound demonstrate that binaural processing effects in bilateral CI users are either absent, or much smaller compared to normal-hearing (NH) listeners (Litovsky et al., 2006, 2009; Loizou et al., 2009). This suggests that when compared to NH listeners, CI listeners struggle to effectively utilize ITDs (Ihlefeld and Litovsky, 2012). One of the key challenges for CI listeners is to understand speech in situations with background sound, where ITDs can greatly aid speech understanding in NH listeners. Because speech is a broadband signal, binaural preservation of cues through multi-channel stimulation is ultimately required for restoring speech intelligibility in CI listeners in natural, multi-source environments. A first step toward the goal of restoring multi-channel binaural cues is to examine ITD sensitivity in CI listeners when multiple cochlear sites are simultaneously stimulated, and this is the focus of the current study.

Most CI listeners can resolve ITDs in the signal envelopes, at least for 100% modulated pulse trains in quiet, but are insensitive to fine structure ITDs transmitted by high carrier rates (Lawson et al., 1998; van Hoesel and Tyler, 2003; Laback et al., 2004). Previous work shows that CI listeners can discriminate envelope-ITDs with thresholds as small as 50 μs (van Hoesel et al., 2009), with an overall sensitivity that shows U-shaped tuning as a function of envelope modulation frequency and peak sensitivity around 100 Hz (Noel and Eddington, 2013). However, when stimulation rate is low, there is generally reduced potency of fine structure ITD cues in bilateral CI listeners, and it is common to observe idiosyncratic differences in ITD sensitivity across cochlear sites (Litovsky et al., 2012). One reason is that within each ear, electric fields from stimulating electrodes can spread to nearby sites, resulting in reduced sensitivity to stimulation at desired electrodes (e.g., Bierer, 2010). Moreover, within and across listeners, there are interaural differences in neural survival and electrode placement which leads to reduced ITD sensitivity (Kan et al., 2013). Differences in envelope ITD sensitivity across stimulation sites could affect how CI listeners interpret broadband envelope ITD information.

In addition to these idiosyncratic factors, the acoustic environment could also influence across-electrode integration of envelope ITD. From an acoustic perspective, usefulness of envelope-ITDs is known to have limits. ITD robustness can be much reduced in everyday environments, where sound energy reflected from walls and ceiling, and energy from competing acoustic sources superpose with target sound. Reverberation often reduces the modulation depth of a target source relative to quiet anechoic conditions, decreasing both speech identification and sound localization performance (Houtgast and Steeneken, 1984; Watkins, 2005; Ihlefeld and Shinn-Cunningham, 2011; Ruggles and Shinn-Cunningham, 2011). Under anechoic conditions, potency of envelope-ITDs depends on the rise time of the slope of the envelope and on the duration of gaps in the envelope, both of which generally vary with modulation depth (Klein-Hennig et al., 2011; Laback et al., 2011; Dietz et al., 2013). This raises the question of how the auditory system can accommodate interference from reduced modulation depth in CI listeners. The effects of demodulation may be even more detrimental on performance for CI than for NH listeners. Indeed, when bilateral CI listeners localize sounds in a noisy background, the signal to noise ratio at which they can effectively utilize envelope-ITDs is much higher than for NH listeners (for a recent review, see van Hoesel, 2012).

Few previous studies have systematically investigated the role of modulation depth for ITD sensitivity in CI listeners. Early work on bilateral CI listening reported results for single-site stimulation in one CI listener, whose ITD sensitivity improved with increasing modulation depth (van Hoesel and Tyler, 2003). More recent work on CI listeners shows that, for trapezoidally amplitude modulated 1515 pps carriers, envelope-ITD sensitivity improves with decreasing duty cycle of the envelope (Laback et al., 2011). CI simulations with NH listeners confirm this effect of duty cycle and further suggest that envelope-ITD sensitivity improves monotonically at low modulation depths, then saturates beyond a critical modulation depth (Bernstein and Trahiotis, 2011; Klein-Hennig et al., 2011; Laback et al., 2011; Dietz et al., 2013).

It is notable that previous work on CI envelope-ITDs has focused on single-site stimulation (van Hoesel and Tyler, 2003; Laback et al., 2011; Noel and Eddington, 2013). However, most natural sounds have broadband energy. For CI stimulation it is therefore desirable to provide envelope-ITDs concurrently at multiple sites along the cochlear array. The current study examines broadband ITD sensitivity in bilateral CI listening, when stimulation occurs at two cochlear sites, and when ITDs are consistent across sites. The aim was to examine the integration of envelope-ITD cues that are spectrally remote due to their positioning at two anatomically different places along the cochlear arrays. Two experiments compared envelope-ITD sensitivity in CI listeners for stimulation that was at a single site vs. dual-site stimulation.

Previous work showed that some CI listeners depend heavily on onset ITD cues (Laback et al., 2007; van Hoesel, 2008). Unlike ongoing cues, due to their transient nature, onset cues do not offer multiple independent "looks" and thus do not provide the opportunity to combine sensory information across time. For an optimal listener, the availability of ongoing cues should improve performance relative to having only onset cues (Hafter and Dye, 1983). To gauge the relative importance of onset cues on integrating binaural cues across electrodes, Experiment 1 measured performance with onset cues; Experiment 2 tested four listeners with "good" binaural sensitivity as determined by data from Experiment 1, with attenuated onset cues.

Of interest was how bilateral CI users who are stimulated at two sites along the cochlear array extract binaural cues, in particular if, due to neural-electrode interface or neural survival issue, these listeners have different sensitivity to binaural cues at the two sites. In one potential scenario, these listeners might only process the binaural cue that is most salient. Thus, CI listeners may interpret binaural cues from the two cochlear sites as one aggregate spatial percept, and their performance with two binaural pairs of electrodes is not expected to increase relative to the single-site stimulation. We also consider the possibility that dual-site stimulation may increase a listener's uncertainty as to what cues to listen to, causing mutual interference and reducing ITD saliency. In this second scenario, ITD sensitivity would decrease in the aggregate sound compared to listening to the better single-site alone. Another possible outcome would be that of enhanced performance with dual-site vs. single-site electrodes; this might occur if CI listeners can combine ITD cues from multiple pairs of electrodes that are treated as independent channels of information.

Here we provide behavioral evidence buttressing the early finding that envelope-ITD sensitivity improves with increasing modulation depth (van Hoesel and Tyler, 2003). Furthermore, we show that when two cochlear sites jointly convey ITD information, CI listeners perform no worse than when they listen to the better single site. Six out of eight tested bilateral CI listeners either showed an improvement in ITD d'-sensitivity when two cochlear regions were stimulated jointly, or their performance was similar to that with the better of the two electrode pairs. None of these six listeners showed consistent interference from the worse electrode pair. Two additional performers, with very poor ITD sensitivity, showed neither consistent improvement nor decrement in performance for dual- vs. single-site stimulation.

MATERIALS AND METHODS

LISTENERS

Eight bilateral CI users with Nucleus devices participated in the study and were paid for their time. All testing was administered according to the guidelines of the Institutional Review Board of the University of Wisconsin-Madison. **Table 1** lists details of their clinical etiology.

STIMULI

Custom-written software (implemented in Matlab, The Mathworks, Natick, MA) was used to present the stimuli and record listeners' responses. Stimuli were delivered with two synchronized Nucleus Implant Communicators (Cochlear Ltd., Sydney, NSW, Australia). Prior to testing human listeners, we confirmed the proper function of the custom-written stimulation software, by projecting the output from two test implants to an oscilloscope across a range of ITDs. Moreover, as a precaution at the beginning of each testing day, we checked proper function of our equipment with an oscilloscope.

Each stimulus consisted of a 300-ms long, 1000 pps pulse train that was 100-Hz sinusoidally amplitude-modulated (**Figure 1**). Electrodes were activated in monopolar configuration. Pulses

Table 1 | Clinical etiology, device: nucleus 24-electrodes.

CI listener	IAZ	IBB	IBF	IBK	IBP	IBU	IAJ	IBR
Etiology	Unknown	Progressive sensori-neural	Hereditory	Hereditory	Hereditory	Bacterial meningitis	Unknown	Progressive sensori-neural
Age (years)	77	45	62	57	70	64	65	56
Use duration (months)	R(49) L(72)	R(57) L(36)	R(63) L(45)	R(48) L(48)	R(25) L(96)	R(86) L(79)	R(84) L(168)	R(7) L(4)
Stimulation rate per channel (Hz)	1200	1800	900	1800	1800	900	1200	900

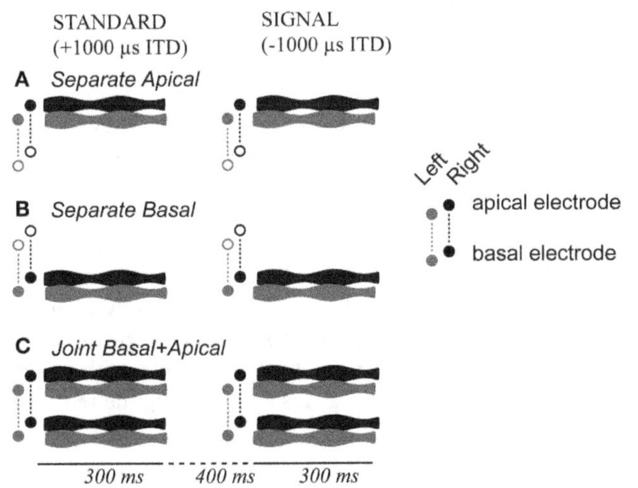

FIGURE 1 | Task and stimulus design. Stimuli could be presented via either **(A)** basal-only, **(B)** apical only, or **(C)** dual-site electrode configuration. The two cochlear sites are shown in the vertical dimension of each panel, left and right ear are shown in gray and black, time is shown along the horizontal dimension.

were biphasic, with phase duration of 25 or 50 μs, depending on the comfortable loudness range of each CI listener (cf. **Table 2**). Envelopes (E) of each amplitude modulated pulse train were as follows:

$$E(t) = I_{\max} - m/200 * (I_{\max} - I_{\min}) * [1 + \cos(2 * pi * f * t)], (1)$$

where $I_{\max}$ and $I_{\min}$ are the maximal and minimal amplitudes in clinical units, respectively, m denotes the modulation depth in percent, f equals 100 Hz, and t denotes time. $I_{\min}$ equaled detection threshold (T-level) for a 1000 pps pulse train with 0% modulation depth. $I_{\max}$ was set such that, for single-site stimulation, the overall stimulus loudness was the same across modulation depths (see Loudness Calibration Procedures below). Throughout testing, $I_{\max}$ was held fixed for each electrode and modulation depth. As a result, component stimulation levels in the dual-site stimulus were identical to the single-site cases. The starting phase of the envelope equaled zero.

1000 pps pulse trains were multiplied with the envelope and waveforms were time-delayed across ears, generating 1000 or 2000 μs ITDs. We initially presented 1000 μs ITD, expecting that it would lead to perfect performance at 100% modulation depth (van Hoesel et al., 2009). However, some listeners were unable to do the task with 1000 μs ITD during initial training. Those listeners were tested with 2000 μs ITD instead.

CALIBRATION PROCEDURES

Three types of calibration procedure were performed. First, a bilateral pitch-matching task was conducted to select electrodes whose combined stimulation produced binaurally fused percepts (see Methods in Litovsky et al., 2010). Second, a loudness-balancing task was performed to ensure that all single-site stimuli were presented at a similar overall loudness. Third, an interaural level difference (ILD) centering was conducted so that the sounds were perceived roughly in the center of the head for an ITD of zero.

Pitch matching

For bilateral pitch matching, we initially selected two basal and two apical electrodes in the left ear. For each of these left-ear electrodes, we selected five right-ear electrodes whose clinical frequency stimulation ranges were close to that of the left ear. With a 1000 pps unmodulated pulse train stimulus, we sequentially stimulated the left ear electrode followed by one of its potential pitch matched electrodes in the right ear and asked the listener to categorize the perceived pitch of the second stimulus by determining whether, relative to the first stimulus, it was heard as: much lower, slightly lower, similar, slightly higher, or much higher. Twenty trials were collected per electrode pair for each listener. To reduce the possibility of range effects, all potential apical and basal pairs were presented in random order. This pitch comparison task resulted in one basal and one apical bilateral pair of electrodes that listeners most consistently rated similar in perceived pitch across ears. **Table 2** lists the electrode numbers for each listener comprising left-right pairs.

Loudness balancing

Each listener performed a series of loudness balancing calibrations (Landsberger and McKay, 2005). For each loudness-balancing track, two sounds, a fixed loudness reference and a level-adjustable target, were presented sequentially in two stimulus intervals. The level-adjustable target was initially set to a quiet level. The listener controlled the stimulus and increased the target level $I_{\max,\text{Target}}$ until the target sounded louder than the reference, then decreased the target level until the target

Table 2 | The left and right (L/R) electrodes in each pair, the threshold level I_{min} in clinical units (cu), and the most comfortable level I_{max}, for 0% modulation depth at 1000 pps.

CI listener	IAZ	IBB	IBF	IBK	IBP	IBU	IAJ	IBR
Basal	8/8	8/8	6/7	6/8	4/6	9/6	6/9	4/5
I_{min} [cu]	117/127	111/133	123/113	148/115	140/145	118/113	147/172	125/112
I_{max} [cu]	174/150	178/178	176/169	215/185	173/169	147/157	176/195	149/154
Apical	18/18	20/19	18/18	16/18	20/21	20/18	19/20	18/20
I_{min} [cu]	120/128	110/138	132/129	165/132	142/106	130/111	123/171	110/130
I_{max} [cu]	156/158	169/185	179/180	225/183	168/153	150/155	139/201	168/172

sounded softer than the reference, followed by another increase in level until both reference and target sounded equally loud. Two tracks were recorded, and subsequently the roles of the two sounds were reversed and testing was repeated for two additional tracks. The signed difference between the target and reference, averaged across all four tracks was then added to the initial reference level, resulting in the loudness-balanced target level.

This loudness balancing was initially performed with 1000 pps unmodulated pulse trains, once across the two left-ear electrodes, and once across the two right-ear electrodes. The resulting sounds were near most comfortable level (C-level) on all four electrodes. In each ear, the basal and apical electrodes were then presented jointly at current levels that were a few dB below these loudness balanced current levels, and their levels were gradually increased together until they sounded comfortably loud when presented jointly. Specifically, for the dB scaling, the output level in current level units (CLU) was converted into units of Ampere, scaled in dB and then converted back in to CLU.

ILD centering

Loudness balancing tracks were followed by ILD centering where all four electrodes were stimulated simultaneously, and the listener was asked to adjust the perceived intracranial location of the sound until it was perceived to be in the center of the head. The adjustment was made by lowering the stimulus level on the side that dominated perceived laterality of the sound image.

After ILD centering, another round of loudness balancing measurements followed. For each of the four electrodes, the modulated sound was adjusted with the loudness balancing routine described above, balancing unmodulated 1000 pps with each of 100, 20, and 60% modulation depth (in that order). Specifically, the reference sound was the unmodulated 1000 pps train presented at the C-level that would have produced an ILD-centered percept for dual-site stimulation. I_{min} was set to the T-level for 1000 pps at that electrode. Modulation depth was held constant. Listeners balanced I_{max} of the modulated sound. I_{max}-values for 10, 40, and 80% modulation depth were then linearly interpolated. As a final verification, we presented all four electrodes jointly at 100% modulation depth, and asked listeners to report the intracranial perceived location. All listeners reported that they perceived a dominant intracranial image approximately near midline. Note that due to monaural loudness summation, the dual-site, ILD-centered C-levels were smaller or equal to the C-levels for electrodes stimulated in isolation. Moreover, some listeners showed bilateral asymmetries, whereby they reduced the level of their better ear well below that ear's isolated C-level in order to obtain a centered intracranial image.

TESTING PROCEDURES

Pitch-matched, loudness-balanced, ILD-centered stimuli were used for ITD discrimination testing. Using a 2I-2AFC task, on each trial, left-leading and right-leading ITDs were presented in random order, separated by a 400 ms inter-stimulus interval (ISI). The listener's task was to identify whether the overall sound image moved from left to right or from right to left across the two stimulus intervals. The order of the intervals with left-leading and right-leading stimulus varied randomly from trial to trial. For training purposes, each listener performed the first two blocks of testing at each electrode condition with correct-response feedback. No feedback was given during the remainder of the experiment.

Psychometric functions

For each channel, we measured percent correct as a function of *m*, the envelope's modulation depth. On each trial, *m* was chosen randomly from one of the possible modulation depths. To prevent learning effects, all values of *m* were tested once before being presented again. We initially tested seven modulation depths: 0, 10, 20, 40, 60, 80, and 100%. Occasionally, listeners clearly performed at floor or ceiling levels for some of these modulation depths. For these listeners we focused data collection on the most informative modulation depths. We presented 15 trials per block, and held the electrode configuration and modulation depth constant within each block. Blocks were grouped in triplets. Each triplet consisted of one modulation depth, presented at one apical-only, one basal-only, and one dual-site apical-basal configuration; these configurations were interleaved in a Latin Square Balanced design across blocks. Modulation depth varied randomly across triplet groups and was balanced in Latin Square design. All modulation depths and electrode configurations were tested once before everything was repeated with new randomization. There were four overall repeats of all testing conditions, resulting in 60 trials per electrode configuration and modulation depth and CI listener. All listeners completed the testing within 1 day. During training, even in the easiest, 100% modulated condition, two listeners (IAJ, and IBR) struggled to discriminate between movement from $+1000\,\mu s$ ITD to $-1000\,\mu s$ ITD vs. the opposite direction. Those listeners were tested with $\pm 2000\,\mu s$ ITD instead.

Time permitting, listeners who could perform the ITD discrimination task with $\pm 1000\,\mu s$ ITD participated in a second

ITD discrimination experiment with ramped onsets and offsets. Compared to Experiment 1, the only difference in Experiment 2 was that the stimulus onsets and offsets were ramped with raised-cosine ramps of 100 ms rise and 100 ms fall time. Four listeners completed Experiment 2.

DATA ANALYSIS

For each listener and experimental condition, percent correct scores were calculated and converted into d'-values. Probabilities of hits for each stimulus interval, P_1 and P_2, were estimated and, to prevent numeric instabilities, bracketed within the range of $1/N$ and $1 - 1/N$, where N equals 60, the number of trials. Response biases were removed and unbiased d'-values were calculated by averaging the normal deviates of these probabilities (Klein, 2001):

$$d' = \sqrt{2} * \left[z\left(P_1\right) + z\left(P_2\right)\right]/2. \qquad (2)$$

For an optimal listener, with independent internal peripheral noises and no central decision making noise, predicted performance in the dual-site conditions equals

$$d'_{\text{pred}} = \sqrt{d_b'^2 + d_a'^2} \qquad (3)$$

where d'_b and d'_a are the d' sensitivities in the basal and apical single-site conditions (e.g., Gockel et al., 2010).

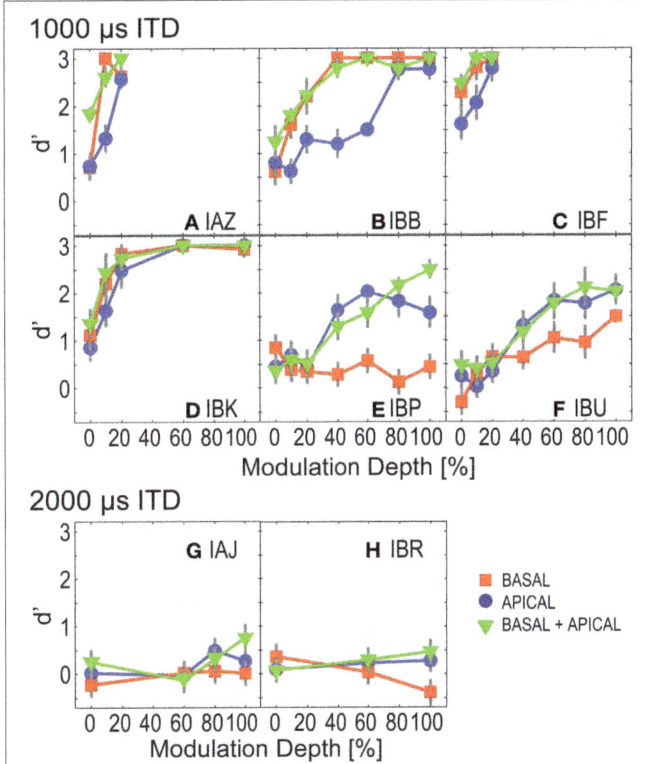

FIGURE 2 | ITD sensitivity as a function of modulation depth for Experiment 1. Each panel shows results for one listener. Basal-only, apical-only, and dual-site electrode configurations are shown by the different symbols. Panels show performance of "good" listeners **(A–F)** and poorer performers **(G–H)**.

RESULTS

PSYCHOMETRIC FUNCTIONS

Figure 2 shows ITD discrimination performance as a function of modulation depth for each of the eight listeners. Panels **A–F** show d' performance for those listeners who could discriminate ±1000 μs ITD, whereas panels **G,H** show data from the two listeners who could not discriminate ±1000 μs and were therefore tested with ITDs of ±2000 μs. Basal-only, apical-only, and dual-site electrode conditions are denoted by square, circle, and triangle symbols. Error bars, where large enough to be visible, show one standard error of the individual d', assuming binomially distributed response rates.

For the six listeners with "good" sensitivity to ITDs (**Figures 2A–F**), performance generally improved with increasing modulation depth. An exception is IBP whose performance was near chance for the basal electrodes. Four of these listeners performed better for basal than for apical electrodes (squares fall above circles for IAZ, IBB, IBF, and IBK), while the other two listeners performed better at the apical electrodes (IBP and IBU).

None of the listeners performed consistently worse in the dual-site than in the single-site conditions (in **Figure 2**, triangles generally fall above or coincide with squares and circles). Occasionally, performance in the dual-site conditions fell slightly below that of the better single site. Specifically, for IBB at 40 and 80% modulation depth, and for IBP at 0, 40, and 60% modulation depth, d' sensitivity at the better single-site marginally outperformed dual-site stimulation. However, this was not a consistent trend. Performance was then examined across listeners, to assess whether dual-site stimulation is better than single-site alone. We considered only those modulation depths where all "good" listeners performed the task for all electrode configurations, i.e., modulation depths smaller than or equal to 20%. Repeated measures ANOVA resulted in significant effects of electrode configuration and modulation depth [$F_{(2, 10)} = 11.487$ and 9.128, $p = 0.003$ and 0.025 with Greenhouse–Geisser correction, for electrode configuration and modulation depth].

Post-hoc least significant difference (LSD) testing revealed significant differences between all pairwise comparisons of electrode configurations ($p = 0.026$, 0.025, 0.016 for basal vs. apical, basal vs. dual-site, and apical vs. dual-site). Specifically, performance in the basal condition was slightly better than in the apical condition (by an estimated marginal mean difference of 0.4 d'-units), indicating that the nominal high-frequency places of stimulation were more sensitive to ITD than the low-frequency places. Moreover, performance in the dual-site condition was slightly and consistently better than in the basal- and apical-only conditions (by estimated marginal mean differences of 0.2 and 0.5 d'-units). This suggests that as a group in the dual-site configuration listeners were not simply basing their decision on the apical pair or the basal pair.

The minimal required modulation depth to reach ceiling performance varied strongly across listeners, with IAZ and IBF performing at $d' = 3$ with as shallow as 20% modulation depth, and IBP and IBU not approaching ceiling performance until 100% modulation depth.

A noteworthy caveat, overall dynamic ranges varied across listeners, perhaps contributing some of the observed variance in the ITD discrimination performance. To address this potential confound, all dual-site-configuration curves were fitted with probit functions. To that end, the d'-values in Equation (1) were inverse transformed, and the resulting unbiased percent correct scores were then fit with probit functions. For each listener and electrode, dynamic ranges were calculated as the dB difference between I_{min} and I_{max} current amplitudes at 100% modulation depth. The slopes in the dual-site electrode conditions vs. each listener's smallest dynamic range in dB were not significantly correlated ($R^2 = 0.01$, $p = 0.99$). Probit mean and dynamic range were also not significantly correlated ($R^2 = 0.56, p = 0.24$). This suggests that overall dynamic range did not dramatically affect ITD performance.

CONSIDERING THE OPTIMAL LISTENER MODEL

When apical and basal electrodes were presented jointly, all listeners tended to perform similarly to what would be expected based on optimal integration of the ITD information across the two electrode pairs [Equation (2)]; however, subsequent statistical analysis failed to differentiate between true integration and listening to stimuli presented only to the site with better ITD sensitivity.

Pooled across all listeners and the three lowest modulation depths (0, 10, and 20%), theoretically optimal d' and observed dual-site d' were highly correlated ($R^2 = 0.931$, $p < 0.0001$). Moreover, when contrasting predicted and observed performance in the dual-site conditions, repeated measures ANOVA found no significant differences between predicted values and observed values [$F_{(1, 5)} = 6.380$, $p = 0.53$]; and a significant effect of modulation depth [$F_{(2, 10)} = 7.758$, $p = 0.009$]. However, when comparing better electrode with dual-site performance, those d'-values were also highly correlated ($R^2 = 0.91$, $p < 0.0001$), and repeated measures ANOVA also did not reveal a statistically significant difference between the two conditions [$F_{(1, 5)} = 0.14$; $p = 0.14$, and $p = 0.01$, for better electrode vs. joint performance, and $F_{(2, 10)} = 7.32$, $p = 0.01$ for modulation depth]. Thus, two different interpretations are consistent with these findings. One interpretation suggests that the six "good" listeners were indeed able to optimally combine information across pairs of electrodes. Alternatively, these listeners simply extracted information from the electrode pair with better ITD sensitivity.

POORER PERFORMERS

For the two more poorly performing listeners (subjects IAJ and IBR), d' was overall close to chance (zero), even with $\pm 2000\,\mu$s ITD (**Figures 2G,H**). At 80 and 100% modulation depth, for the dual-site electrode conditions, subject IAJ's performance was qualitatively better than chance. A paired t-test comparing apical, basal, and dual-site performance showed a significant difference between 0 and 100% modulation depth [$t_{(df=2)} = -4.5$, $p = 0.05$]. However, paired t-tests did not reveal significant differences between the three electrode configurations [$t_{(df=3)} = -0.2$, $p = 0.9$ for basal vs. dual-site; $t_{(df=3)} = -1.6$, $p = 0.2$ for apical vs. dual-site]. Subject IBR's d'-data show that at 80 and 100% modulation depth this listener was somewhat able to discriminate left- and right-leading stimuli. However, d' was negative for the basal conditions, indicating that this listener consistently reported the opposite directions for these sounds. IBR's results did not differ significantly across stimulus conditions [$t_{(df=2)} = 0.2$, $p = 0.9$, paired t-test for 0 vs. 100% modulation depth; $t_{(df=2)} = 0.2$, $p = 0.9$ for apical vs. dual-site; $t_{(df=2)} = 0.4$, $p = 0.8$ for basal vs. dual-site]. In summary, the results suggest that of the two more poorly-performing listeners, one was more sensitive to ITDs in the modulated condition than in the unmodulated condition.

ONSET CUES

For the four best-performing listeners (IAZ, IBB, IBF, and IBK, **Figures 2A–D**), even at 0% modulation depth, performance was better than chance; for each of the electrode configurations, t-tests for measured d'-values vs. $d' = 0$ revealed statistically significantly results [$t_{(df=5)} = 2.6$, $p = 0.05$ for basal; $t_{(df=5)} = 4.1$, $p = 0.009$ for apical; $t_{(df=5)} = 4.0, p = 0.01$ for dual-site]. These results suggest that the four best-performing listeners were able to exploit onset ITD information, consistent with previous findings (Laback et al., 2007; van Hoesel, 2008).

To estimate how well listeners could discriminate ITDs with attenuated onsets, Experiment 2 tested four of the "good" listeners with conditions that were identical to those tested in Experiment 1, except that the stimuli were ramped on and off with 100 ms windows. **Figure 3** shows d'-performance for the ramped conditions. The overall pattern in performance is similar to that in **Figure 2**. Performance increases monotonically as a function of modulation depth. Moreover, at each modulation depth, performance in the dual-site electrode configurations is

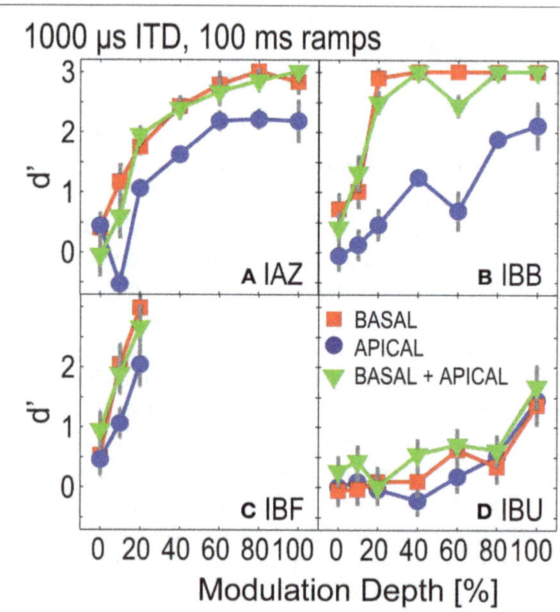

FIGURE 3 | ITD sensitivity as a function of modulation depth for ramped stimuli in Experiment 2. Each panel **(A–D)** shows results for one listener. Basal-only, apical-only, and dual-site electrode configurations are shown by the different symbols.

similar to or better than that of the better electrode. Repeated measures ANOVA considering only those modulation depths that had been tested in all listeners and electrode configurations (0, 10, and 20%) found significant effects of modulation depth [$F_{(2, 6)} = 6.648$, $p = 0.030$] and of electrode configuration [$F_{(2, 6)} = 6.740$, $p = 0.029$]. However, *post-hoc* LSD indicated no significant differences between any of the pairwise comparisons across electrode configurations ($p = 0.091$ for basal vs. apical, $p = 0.692$ for basal vs. dual-site, and, $p = 0.055$ for apical vs. dual-site). Pairwise comparisons across modulation depths also found no significant differences with *post-hoc* LSD ($p = 0.137$ for 0–10%; $p = 0.070$ for 0–20%; and $p = 0.088$ for 10–20%).

Figure 4 shows performance in the ramped conditions as a function of performance in the un-ramped conditions (one data point plotted per modulation depth). Overall, performance in the ramped conditions was worse than that in the un-ramped conditions (points fall below the diagonal). Repeated measures ANOVA, considering only those three modulation depths that were tested for all four listeners in both the ramped and un-ramped conditions, found no significant effect of ramping [$F_{(1, 3)} = 7.619$, $p = 0.07$]. Main factors of electrode configuration and modulation depth remained significant [$F_{(2, 6)} = 10.783$, $p = 0.01$; $F_{(2, 6)} = 11.596$; $p = 0.009$ for electrode configuration and modulation depth]. Note that unlike the data points in **Figure 4**, this analysis only considers performance above 20% modulation depth, where all listeners were tested. The effect of ramping is non-significant, however, it appears that at least for some listeners ramping can affect performance (e.g., IAZ, where all points fall below the diagonal in **Figure 4A**).

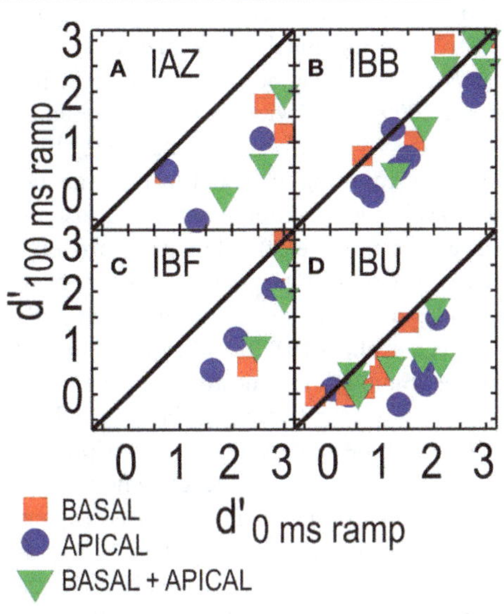

FIGURE 4 | ITD sensitivity for stimuli with and without ramp, from Experiment 1 and 2, respectively. Each panel **(A–D)** shows results for one listener. Basal-only, apical-only, and dual-site electrode configurations are shown by the different symbols. Repeated symbols reflect the fact that performance is shown across a range of modulation depths.

DISCUSSION

Natural sounds have broadband energy, giving rise to ITDs along the full spectral range. In order to present binaural cues with fidelity for broadband sounds, it is necessary for CIs to present ITDs concurrently at multiple electrodes that are placed along the cochlear array. Current bilateral CIs present sounds, and therefore ITDs, through envelope information. However, in everyday acoustic settings, sound envelopes are often de-modulated by competing sources and by reverberant energy. In these adverse listening conditions, both CI sound localization and speech intelligibility suffer compared to NH performance (e.g., van Hoesel, 2012). The current study examined how CI listeners were able to combine envelope-ITD information across two concurrent stimulation sites, when modulation depth was parametrically varied. We compared ITD sensitivity across apical and basal cochlear regions when these two regions were stimulated either alone or jointly.

Consistent with early findings for one CI listener (van Hoesel and Tyler, 2003), our results show that ITD sensitivity increased with larger modulation depth for six out of eight CI listeners. Previously, when presented with transposed stimuli, ITD sensitivity in NH listeners decreased and perceived intracranial laterality moved frontally with smaller modulation depth (Bernstein and Trahiotis, 2011). The current results are consistent with the interpretation that, for CI listeners, similar to NH listeners, the intracranial localization strength was more distinctly available with steeper modulations.

There is some disagreement in the literature on CI listeners about whether binaural performance varies with stimulation site (apical or basal). One previous study found no difference across stimulation sites, for high-rate pulse trains (6000 pps) that were sinusoidally modulated at 100 Hz (van Hoesel et al., 2009). The absence of a stimulation site effect is consistent with findings in NH listeners who show similar ITD sensitivity to transposed tones with high frequency carriers and low-frequency pure tones, which stimulate the basal and apical regions of the cochlea, respectively (van de Par and Kohlrausch, 1997). The current study supports those findings. In particular, while each listener had a better electrode pair, there was no consistent across-listener trend that would differentiate apical and basal results: four out of six "good" listeners performed worse at the apical than at the basal pair, for two listeners the reverse was true. Similar findings have been reported for un-modulated low-rate pulsatile stimulation (Litovsky et al., 2010). That study had examined basal, middle, and apical for 100 pps and found no effect of place. However, other data shows that listeners performed better with basal than with apical stimulation, as tested with low-rate pulse trains (100 pps; Best et al., 2011).

Here, basal-alone and apical-alone levels at each electrode pair were usually below C-level for that pair when played in isolation. ITD sensitivity can decrease with decreasing stimulation level (van Hoesel, 2007). Here, we loudness-balanced the stimuli across cochlear stimulation sites. Therefore, it is unlikely that observed differences in ITD sensitivity across basal and apical stimulation sites are an artifact of the stimulus level choices. Instead, differential ITD sensitivity could be due to across-site differences in neural survival and biological or surgical factors, including proximity of electrodes and nerve (Litovsky et al., 2010, 2012). Our results show that in the dual-site electrode configurations, performance was always better than that of the electrode pair producing poorer performance. By loudness-balancing we ensured that performance was not simply dominated by the louder and therefore more salient pair of electrodes.

While previous work demonstrates that interactions across cochlear sites can influence performance for conflicting ITD cues for both acoustic and electric hearing (McFadden and Pasanen, 1975; Best et al., 2011), here, both pairs of electrodes were situated in a more basal position relative to where neurons with best frequencies in the 600–700 Hz range are typically located, and both provided non-conflicting envelope-ITDs, making it unlikely that binaural interference would affect listeners' performance. Indeed, to the extent that binaural interference may have influenced ITD sensitivity, performance in the dual-site conditions should have been worse than that of the single-site basal conditions. No such binaural interference was observed. In fact, the electrode pair with worse performance did not drive performance below that of the electrode pair with good performance in any of the dual-site stimulation conditions, showing that listeners do not suffer from interference even when one electrode pair provides poorly represented spatial information.

An important issue regarding many previous studies with bilaterally implanted CI users is the consideration of subject selection criteria. In a number of prior studies, listeners had been pre-selected based on their abilities to perform a binaural task with low-rate stimuli (e.g., Laback and Majdak, 2008; van Hoesel, 2008; van Hoesel et al., 2009). Here, listeners were not pre-selected according to performance criteria, which may help explain the fact that some listeners could not perform the task with 1000 μs at 100% modulation depth, even though this has not been reported in the literature before.

A potential confound to note is that modulation depth was measured in percentage of the dynamic range between I_{min} and I_{max}, and this range differed across listeners (**Table 2**). A listener with a large difference between I_{min} and I_{max} may have performed better because the sounds were modulated over a wider dynamic range than for a listener with a small dynamic range. However, because the dynamic range was not significantly correlated with task performance, we deem this possibility unlikely.

Some listeners were able to perform the ITD discrimination task even at 0% modulation depth. This is consistent with previous work demonstrating that some listeners can utilize onset cues of high-rate pulse trains to discriminate ITDs, even in the absence of post-onset ITD information (Laback et al., 2007; van Hoesel, 2008; Noel and Eddington, 2013). Similarly, in another previous study using an ITD discrimination task, when tested with 800 and 1200 pps stimuli and 600 μs ITD, CI listeners could perform the task above chance (Laback and Majdak, 2008). Note that in these prior studies, CI listeners were discriminating between 0 ITD and left or right-leading ITD in a 2AFC paradigm (Laback et al., 2007; Laback and Majdak, 2008; Noel and Eddington, 2013), or they were asked to indicate perceived intracranial position (van Hoesel, 2008). Here, CI listeners judged the direction of a change in ITD of 2000 or 4000 μs, so the task was considerably easier than in those previous studies.

Experiment 2 tested the usefulness of onset cues by ramping the sounds on and off. Ramping altered the stimuli in two ways. It should have resulted in a more staggered stimulation of the neural population than with the non-ramped stimuli, reducing the potential usefulness of onset cues. In addition, the ramp shortened the perceived duration of the sound. Here, when stimuli were ramped, one listener (IAZ) performed clearly worse than when stimuli were not ramped, whereas other listeners showed less appreciable change in performance. Here, because the ±1000 μs ITD was an integer multiple of the period of the 1000 pps carrier signal, ongoing temporal fine structure ITDs did not provide unambiguous information about source direction. The relatively robust performance with attenuated onsets is consistent with the previous finding that some listeners can utilize ongoing envelope-ITDs (Noel and Eddington, 2013). Moreover, it suggests that strategies for weighting the onset and running portions of each stimulus differ across listeners. These results are relevant when considering previous work on onset weighting. Using stimuli with a dichotic onset pulse followed by three diotic pulses, Laback et al. (2007) demonstrated that with increasing pulse rate CI listeners tend to rely more strongly on onset cues. Similarly, post-onset pulses exerted stronger effects on CI listeners' ITD sensitivity at 100 pps than they did at 300 and 600 pps (van Hoesel, 2008). These studies share that onset and post-onset pulses carried conflicting ITD information. In contrast, here, all pulses had the same ITD. Therefore, here, post-onset pulses are likely to have helped listeners perform the ITD discrimination task, even when onsets were attenuated.

Recent findings suggest that binaural sensitivity can be poorer when nearby electrodes cause energetic masking (Lu et al., 2010). Moreover, in an ITD discrimination task, the binaural bandwidth eliciting a robust ITD on a target electrode was estimated to be about five times greater in CI than in NH (Poon et al., 2009). Specifically, to decrease ITD sensitivity by a factor of 2 (binaural half-width), the mismatch in cochleotopic position across ears in CI users is 3.7 mm as opposed to 0.7 mm in NH listeners (Poon et al., 2009). This widened binaural bandwidth in CI users as compared to NH listeners could imply higher susceptibility to energetic masking also within one ear. Furthermore, in a binaural masking level difference task, CI listeners' abilities to detect a tone on a target electrode pair improved when fewer electrodes carried the masking signal, even when those additional masking electrodes were outside the nominal critical band for the target electrode (Lu et al., 2010). In addition, the extent of channel interaction, as estimated from auditory nerve evoked potentials in several listeners, was negatively correlated with binaural benefit (Lu et al., 2010). These studies show that peripheral interaction can impact binaural sensitivity, especially when spacing between neighboring electrodes is small. To limit the impact of performance asymmetries across the cochlea due to energetic masking, here, we chose electrodes that were spaced relatively widely. Still, in Experiment 1, each listener had a better electrode pair, similar to previous reports (Laback et al., 2011). Specifically, for three listeners who were tested in both experiments, that better pair was the same across both experiments. Often the differences between apical and basal stimulation within that listener were pronounced with a sizeable difference in midpoints of the underlying psychometric functions. An additional analysis using dB modulation depth along the abscissa (not shown) did not produce qualitatively different trends, nor could we identify a parameter in the level map of the CI listeners that could explain these within-listener differences.

SUMMARY AND CONCLUSIONS

The current study reinforces and extends findings from previous studies on sensitivity to envelope ITD in bilateral CI listeners. Specifically, when discriminating envelope-ITDs of 100 Hz modulated high-rate pulse trains, a CI listener's performance improves with increasing modulation depth. Moreover, consistent with previous work, most CI listeners performed clearly better at one of the two stimulation sites (Laback et al., 2007; van Hoesel, 2008). However, whether the apical or the basal stimulation site produced higher percent correct scores did not vary consistently across listeners. Finally, some listeners could discriminate 1000 μs ITDs for an unmodulated 1000 pps train, whereas others struggled with this task. Moreover, when comparing the ramped to the non-ramped conditions, listeners varied in their ability to utilize onset cues. Together, these findings provide further evidence to previous work that listeners differ in how strongly they weigh onset and ongoing cues of the stimulus (Laback et al., 2007; van Hoesel, 2008).

Results show that CI listeners did not perform worse when two electrode pairs jointly transmitted ITD information, compared to listening to the better of the two pairs. This finding is consistent with the interpretation that CI listeners either truly integrated ITD information across the two stimulation sites or that they performed based on the electrode pair carrying more salient ITD information. Performance asymmetries between the two stimulation sites make it difficult to conclusively differentiate between these two explanations. Together these findings provide evidence that CI listeners can sustain ITD sensitivity for two-site stimulation compared to single-site stimulation. The current results are encouraging in that no interference from the worse electrode pair was observed.

REFERENCES

Bernstein, L. R., and Trahiotis, C. (2011). Lateralization produced by envelope-based interaural temporal disparities of high-frequency, raised-sine stimuli: empirical data and modeling. *J. Acoust. Soc. Am.* 129, 1501–1508. doi: 10.1121/1.3552875

Best, V., Laback, B., and Majdak, P. (2011). Binaural interference in bilateral cochlear-implant listeners. *J. Acoust. Soc. Am.* 130, 2939–2950. doi: 10.1121/1.3641400

Bierer, J. A. (2010). Probing the electrode-neuron interface with focused cochlear implant stimulation. *Trends Amplif.* 14, 84–95. doi: 10.1177/1084713810375249

Darwin, C. J., and Hukin, R. W. (1999). Auditory objects of attention: the role of interaural time differences. *J. Exp. Psychol. Hum. Percept. Perform.* 25, 617–629. doi: 10.1037/0096-1523.25.3.617

Dietz, M., Wendt, T., Ewert, S. D., Laback, B., and Hohmann, V. (2013). Comparing the effect of pause duration on threshold interaural time differences between exponential and squared-sine envelopes (L). *J. Acoust. Soc. Am.* 133, 1. doi: 10.1121/1.4768876

Gockel, H., Carlyon, R. P., and Plack, C. J. (2010). Combining information across frequency regions in fundamental frequency discrimination. *J. Acoust. Soc. Am.* 4, 2466–2478. doi: 10.1121/1.3327811

Hafter, E. R., and Dye, R. H. Jr. (1983). Detection of interaural differences of time in trains of high–frequency clicks as a function of interclick interval and number. *J. Acoust. Soc. Am.* 73, 644–651. doi: 10.1121/1.388956

Houtgast, T., and Steeneken, H. J. M. (1984). A review of the MTF concept in room acoustics and its use for estimating speech intelligibility in auditoria. *J. Acoust. Soc. Am.* 77, 1069–1077. doi: 10.1121/1.392224

Ihlefeld, A., and Litovsky, R. Y. (2012). Interaural level differences do not suffice for restoring spatial release from masking in simulated cochlear implant listening. *PLoS ONE* 7:e45296. doi: 10.1371/journal.pone.0045296

Ihlefeld, A., and Shinn-Cunningham, B. G. (2011). Effect of source spectrum on sound localization in an everyday reverberant room. *J. Acoust. Soc. Am.* 130, 1530–1541. doi: 10.1121/1.3596476

Kan, A., Stoelb, C., Litovsky, R. Y., and Goupell, M. J. (2013). Effect of mismatched place-of-stimulation on binaural fusion and lateralization in bilateral cochlear-implant users. *J. Acoust. Soc. Am.* 134, 2923–2936. doi: 10.1121/1.4820889

Kidd, G. Jr., Arbogast, T. L., Mason, C. R., and Gallun, F. J. (2005). The advantage of knowing where to listen. *J. Acoust. Soc. Am.* 118, 3804–3815. doi: 10.1121/1.2109187

Klein, S. (2001). Measuring, estimating, and understanding the psychometric function: a commentary. *Percept. Psychophys.* 63, 1421–1455. doi: 10.3758/BF03194552

Klein-Hennig, M., Dietz, M., Hohmann, V., and Ewert, S. D. (2011). The influence of different segments of the ongoing envelope on sensitivity to interaural time delays. *J. Acoust. Soc. Am.* 129, 3856–3872. doi: 10.1121/1.3585847

Laback, B., and Majdak, P. (2008). Binaural jitter improves interaural time-difference sensitivity of cochlear implantees at high pulse rates. *Proc. Natl. Acad. Sci. U.S.A.* 105, 814–817. doi: 10.1073/pnas.0709199105

Laback, B., Majdak, P., and Baumgartner, W. D. (2007). Lateralization discrimination of interaural time delays in four-pulse sequences in electric and acoustic hearing. *J. Acoust. Soc. Am.* 121, 2182–2192. doi: 10.1121/1.2642280

Laback, B., Pok, S. M., Baumgartner, W. D., Deutsch, W. A., and Schmid, K. (2004). Sensitivity to interaural level and envelope time differences of two bilateral cochlear implant listeners using clinical sound processors. *Ear Hear.* 25, 488–500. doi: 10.1097/01.aud.0000145124.85517.e8

Laback, B., Zimmermann, I., Majdak, P., Baumgartner, W. D., and Pok, S. M. (2011). Effects of envelope shape on interaural envelope delay sensitivity in acoustic and electric hearing. *J. Acoust. Soc. Am.* 130, 1515. doi: 10.1121/1.3613704

Landsberger, D. M., and McKay, C. M. (2005). Perceptual differences between low and high rates of stimulation on single electrodes for cochlear implantees. *J. Acoust. Soc. Am.* 117, 319–327. doi: 10.1121/1.1830672

Lawson, D. T., Wilson, B. S., Zerbi, M., van den Honert, C., Finley, C. C., Farmer, J. C., et al. (1998). Bilateral cochlear implants controlled by a single speech processor. *Am. J. Otol.* 19, 758–761.

Litovsky, R., Parkinson, A., Arcaroli, J., and Sammeth, C. (2006). Simultaneous bilateral cochlear implantation in adults: a multicenter clinical study. *Ear Hear.* 27, 714. doi: 10.1097/01.aud.0000246816.50820.42

Litovsky, R. Y., Goupell, M. J., Godar, S., Grieco-Calub, T., Jones, G. L., Garadat, S. N., et al. (2012). Studies on bilateral cochlear implants at the University of Wisconsin's Binaural Hearing and Speech Laboratory. *J. Am. Acad. Audiol.* 23, 476–494. doi: 10.3766/jaaa.23.6.9

Litovsky, R. Y., Jones, G. L., Agrawal, S., and van Hoesel, R. (2010). Effect of age at onset of deafness on binaural sensitivity in electric hearing in humans. *J. Acoust. Soc. Am.* 127, 400–414. doi: 10.1121/1.3257546

Litovsky, R. Y., Parkinson, A., and Arcaroli, J. (2009). Spatial hearing and speech intelligibility in bilateral cochlear implant users. *Ear Hear.* 27, 714–31. doi: 10.1097/01.aud.0000246816.50820.42

Loizou, P. C., Hu, Y., Litovsky, R. Y., Yu, G., Peters, R., Lake, J., et al. (2009). Speech recognition by bilateral cochlear implant users in a cocktail-party setting. *J. Acoust. Soc. Am.* 125, 372–383. doi: 10.1121/1.3036175

Lu, T., Litovsky, R. Y., and Zeng, F. G. (2010). Binaural masking level differences in actual and simulated bilateral cochlear implant listeners. *J. Acoust. Soc. Am.* 127, 1479–1490. doi: 10.1121/1.3290994

McFadden, D., and Pasanen, E. G. (1975). Lateralization at high frequencies based on interaural time differences. *J. Acoust. Soc. Am.* 59, 634–639. doi: 10.1121/1.380913

Noel, V. A., and Eddington, D. K. (2013). Sensitivity of bilateral cochlear implant users to fine-structure and envelope interaural time differences. *J. Acoust. Soc. Am.* 133, 2314–2328. doi: 10.1121/1.4794372

Poon, B. B., Eddington, D. K., Noel, V., and Colburn, H. S. (2009), Sensitivity to interaural time difference with bilateral cochlear implants: development over time and effect of interaural electrode spacing. *J. Acoust. Soc.* 126, 806–815. doi: 10.1121/1.3158821

Ruggles, D., and Shinn-Cunningham, B. G. (2011). Spatial selective auditory attention in the presence of reverberant energy: individual differences in normal-hearing listeners. *J. Assoc. Res. Otolaryngol.* 12, 395–405. doi: 10.1007/s10162-010-0254-z

Seeber, B. U., and Fastl, H. (2008). Localization cues with bilateral cochlear implants. *J. Acoust. Soc. Am.* 123, 1030–1042. doi: 10.1121/1.2821965

van de Par, S., and Kohlrausch, A. (1997). A new approach to comparing binaural masking level differences at low and high frequencies. *J. Acoust. Soc. Am.* 101, 1671–1680. doi: 10.1121/1.418151

van Hoesel, R. J. M. (2007). Sensitivity to bilateral timing in bilateral cochlear implant users. *J. Acoust. Soc. Am.* 121, 2192–2206. doi: 10.1121/1.2537300

van Hoesel, R. J. M. (2008). Observer weighting of level and timing cues in bilateral cochlear implant users. *J. Acoust. Soc. Am.* 124, 3861–3872. doi: 10.1121/1.2998974

van Hoesel, R. J. M. (2012). Contrasting benefits from contralateral implants and hearing aids in cochlear implant users. *Hear. Res.* 288, 100–113. doi: 10.1016/j.heares.2011.11.014

van Hoesel, R. J. M., Jones, G. M., and Litovsky, R. Y. (2009). Interaural time-delay sensitivity in bilateral cochlear implant users: effect of pulse rate, modulation rate, and place of stimulation. *J. Assoc. Res. Otolaryngol.* 10, 557–567. doi: 10.1007/s10162-009-0175-x

van Hoesel, R. J. M., and Tyler, R. S. (2003). Speech perception, localization, and lateralization with bilateral cochlear implants. *J. Acoust. Soc. Am.* 113, 1617–1630. doi: 10.1121/1.1539520

Watkins, A. J. (2005). Perceptual compensation for effects of reverberation in speech identification. *J. Acoust. Soc. Am.* 118, 249–262. doi: 10.1121/1.1923369

4

Lexico-semantic and acoustic-phonetic processes in the perception of noise-vocoded speech: implications for cochlear implantation

Carolyn McGettigan[1,2]*, Stuart Rosen[3] and Sophie K. Scott[2]*

[1] *Department of Psychology, Royal Holloway, University of London, Egham, UK*
[2] *Institute of Cognitive Neuroscience, University College London, London, UK*
[3] *Department of Speech, Hearing and Phonetic Sciences, University College London, London, UK*

Correspondence:
Carolyn McGettigan, Department of Psychology, Royal Holloway, University of London, Egham Hill, Egham TW20 0EX, UK
e-mail: Carolyn.McGettigan@rhul.ac.uk;
Sophie K. Scott, Institute of Cognitive Neuroscience, University College London, London WC1N 3AR, UK
e-mail: sophie.scott@ucl.ac.uk

Noise-vocoding is a transformation which, when applied to speech, severely reduces spectral resolution and eliminates periodicity, yielding a stimulus that sounds "like a harsh whisper" (Scott et al., 2000, p. 2401). This process simulates a cochlear implant, where the activity of many thousand hair cells in the inner ear is replaced by direct stimulation of the auditory nerve by a small number of tonotopically-arranged electrodes. Although a cochlear implant offers a powerful means of restoring some degree of hearing to profoundly deaf individuals, the outcomes for spoken communication are highly variable (Moore and Shannon, 2009). Some variability may arise from differences in peripheral representation (e.g., the degree of residual nerve survival) but some may reflect differences in higher-order linguistic processing. In order to explore this possibility, we used noise-vocoding to explore speech recognition and perceptual learning in normal-hearing listeners tested across several levels of the linguistic hierarchy: segments (consonants and vowels), single words, and sentences. Listeners improved significantly on all tasks across two test sessions. In the first session, individual differences analyses revealed two independently varying sources of variability: one lexico-semantic in nature and implicating the recognition of words and sentences, and the other an acoustic-phonetic factor associated with words and segments. However, consequent to learning, by the second session there was a more uniform covariance pattern concerning all stimulus types. A further analysis of phonetic feature recognition allowed greater insight into learning-related changes in perception and showed that, surprisingly, participants did not make full use of cues that were preserved in the stimuli (e.g., vowel duration). We discuss these findings in relation cochlear implantation, and suggest auditory training strategies to maximize speech recognition performance in the absence of typical cues.

Keywords: speech perception, individual differences, cochlear implants

INTRODUCTION

A cochlear implant (CI) is a hearing aid that converts acoustic sound energy into electrical stimuli to be transmitted to the auditory nerve, via an array of electrodes arranged tonotopically along the basilar membrane of the inner ear (Rubinstein, 2004). Although the implant restores some degree of hearing to profoundly deaf individuals, the substitution of thousands of inner hair cells with, at most, tens of electrodes means that the transmitted signal is greatly impoverished in spectral detail. CI devices give a weak sense of voice pitch and transmit fewer discriminable steps in amplitude, and there is often a mis-match between frequencies being transmitted by the individual electrodes and those best received at the position of contact on the basilar membrane. Thus, particularly for post-lingual recipients of an implant (i.e., those who lost their hearing after the acquizition of language), the listener must learn to make sense of an altered and unfamiliar sound world. This process of adaptation and perceptual learning after cochlear implantation can take a long time, with widely varying levels of success (Pisoni, 2000; Sarant et al., 2001; Munson et al., 2003; Skinner, 2003). Much research relating to implantation has therefore been concerned with identifying predictive markers of success, and appropriate training regimes to optimize post-implantation outcomes.

A growing body of studies has employed acoustic simulations of CIs to model post-implantation adaptation in normal-hearing participants. Vocoding is an acoustic transformation that produces speech with degraded spectral detail by replacing the original wideband speech signal with a variable number of amplitude-modulated carriers, such as noise bands (noise-vocoding) or sine waves (tone vocoding). Here, the carriers simulate the electrodes of the CI to create a re-synthesized speech signal that is spectrally impoverished, yet maintains relatively intact amplitude envelope cues (Shannon et al., 1995). Here, increasing the number of bands (or channels) increases the spectral resolution, with a concomitant increase in intelligibility of transformed sounds. As with the studies in CI recipients, it has been shown that normal-hearing participants also exhibit considerable individual variability in performance with CI simulations (Nogaki et al., 2007; Stacey and Summerfield, 2007; Eisner et al., 2010).

An important issue for clinicians testing and training CI recipients is the selection of appropriate materials (Loebach and Pisoni, 2008; Loebach et al., 2008, 2009). The main day-to-day context for spoken communication is spontaneous face-to-face conversation, so it is natural to consider training paradigms similar to that situation. For example, connected discourse tracking (CDT), using face-to-face repetition of a story told by an experimenter, has been shown to yield significant improvements in the recognition of severely degraded speech in hearing participants (Rosen et al., 1999). However, delivery of this kind of training is very labor-intensive (though a recent study comparing live CDT with a computer-based approach showed equivalent training benefits from the two training routines; Faulkner et al., 2012). Thus, training and assessment routines typically involve the recognition of laboratory recordings of materials such as sentences, words and simple syllables. There is some evidence that improvements with one kind of test material can generalize to another. For example, Loebach and Pisoni (2008) found that training participants with exposure and feedback on either words, sentences or environmental sounds gave improvements in performance that generalized to the other tasks. In a very small group of three CI recipients, Fu et al. (2005) found that training with CV and CVC syllables (where "C" stands for Consonant, and "V" for Vowel) led to improved test performance on sentence recognition. However, the picture is not straightforward: Loebach and Pisoni (2008) found that generalization was most effective between materials of the same class (e.g., words to words, sentences to sentences), and that training on speech materials did not afford any improvements in recognition of environmental sounds. This may depend on the nature of the vocoding transformation, as this severely degrades spectral detail important for recognizing some environmental sounds—similarly, training on vocoded sentence materials gave poor generalization to the recognition of talkers (Loebach et al., 2009).

Imbalances in learning transfer may also be affected by the behavior of the listener. Loebach et al. (2008) found that training on talker identification afforded greater generalization to vocoded sentence transcription than training on talker gender identification. The authors suggest this is because the more difficult task of talker identification led to greater attentional engagement of the listeners with the acoustic properties of vocoded speech. Similarly, Loebach et al. (2010) and Davis et al. (2005) found that training participants with semantically anomalous sentences was just as effective as training with meaningful sentences, while Hervais-Adelman et al. (2008) found equivalent improvements in performance after training with vocoded nonwords as observed with real-word training. Loebach et al. (2010) suggest this is because the absence of semantic cues engages a more analytic listening mode in the listener, where attention is directed to the acoustic-phonetic aspects of the signal rather than "synthetic," higher-order processes focused on linguistic comprehension. Although they acknowledge that sentence and word materials afford greater ecological validity (Loebach et al., 2010), Loebach and colleagues suggest that encouraging analytic, acoustic-phonetic, listening can afford better generalization of learning across a range of materials.

Another way to view the data from these training studies is that there are potentially both "analytic" and "synthetic" factors at play when listeners adapt to degraded speech input. However, the extent to which these operate independently is not known, and it may be that some listeners would stand to benefit more from training on higher-order processes for employment in the recognition of ecologically valid, linguistic materials encountered in day-to-day life. A study by Grant and Seitz (2000) showed that use of "top–down" contextual information—what Loebach and colleagues would consider a "synthetic" process—varies across individuals. They presented 34 hearing-impaired listeners with filtered sentences from the IEEE corpus (e.g., "Glue the sheet to the dark blue background"; IEEE, 1969), and their constituent keywords in isolation, at three different intelligibility levels. Using Boothroyd and Nittrouer's (1988) equation explaining the relationship between word recognition in sentences and in isolation, Grant and Seitz (2000) calculated individual k-factor scores—representing the listener's ability to use semantic and morpho-syntactic information in the sentence to identify the words within it—and observed considerable variability in this parameter across their listening population. In further support of multiple factors underlying speech recognition, Surprenant and Watson's (2001) large-scale study of individual variability in speech-in-noise recognition indicated that performance is far from identical across different linguistic levels—Pearson's correlation coefficients between speech-in-noise recognition of CV-units, words and sentences and a clear-speech syllable identification task ranged from only 0.25 to 0.47 in their experiment. Therefore, extracting patterns of covariance, and measuring how these change with learning, could offer additional insight into the underlying perceptual processes supporting adaptation to a CI or simulation. For example, close correlation of speech recognition at segment, word and sentence level may indicate a unified "analytic" strategy, whereas statistical independence of sentence stimuli from words and segments could reflect considerable importance for top–down syntactic and semantic processing strategies in recognizing vocoded sentences.

In the current experiment, we tested a group of normal-hearing adults in the transcription of noise-vocoded sentences, words and segments at a range of difficulty levels (operationalized in terms of the number of vocoding bands), with the following objectives:

- *To explore patterns of covariation across the linguistic hierarchy*—segment, word, sentence—in order to characterize the number and nature of factors underlying the recognition of vocoded speech. We predicted that individual scores across the five tasks would be significantly correlated, but that individuals' differing abilities to use "top–down"/"synthetic" and "bottom–up"/"analytic" processes would limit the strength of these correlations.
- *To measure long-term perceptual learning of vocoded speech*—by re-testing participants after 1–2 weeks. There were several aims here:

i. To assess whether adaptation to noise-vocoded speech can be maintained over several days without exposure.
ii. To compare the size of any adaptation effects across stimulus type.
iii. To explore whether adaptation / additional exposure alters listening strategies (as measured using analyses of covariation).

Davis et al. (2005) found that transcription of vocoded sentences improved significantly within 30 items of exposure, in the absence of feedback. Therefore, to minimize design complexity and optimize the exploitation of individual differences analyses, learning in the current experiment was operationalized as the improvement in performance from Session 1 to Session 2, without involvement of explicit training procedures.

- *To quantify the efficiency of "analytic" listening*—Loebach et al. (2010) suggested that failure to attend to critical acoustic properties of vocoded stimuli may limit the transfer of learning. Our final objective was to use information transfer (IT) analyses of consonant and vowel perception to quantify the reception of acoustic-phonetic features, and to directly assess the degree to which the acoustic cues present in the stimulus are being used by untrained listeners.

Previous work on the learning of vocoded speech has tended to train and test participants at a fixed level of degradation (i.e., number of bands; Davis et al., 2005; Hervais-Adelman et al., 2008; Loebach and Pisoni, 2008; Eisner et al., 2010). Given the considerable variation in individual performance with vocoded stimuli, this runs the risk of floor or ceiling effects in the data. For the current experiment, we adopted an approach used by Shannon et al. (2004), who tested across a range of difficulty levels (numbers of channels) and fitted logistic functions to describe performance on a range of noise-vocoded speech recognition tasks. In the current experiment, curves were fitted to the recognition data for each participant, by task and by session—estimates of 50% thresholds, representing performance across a range of difficulty, could then be extracted for use in further analysis of learning effects and covariation across tasks and time.

METHOD

PARTICIPANTS

Participants were 28 monolingual speakers of British English (12 male), with no language or hearing problems. The participants were recruited from the UCL Department of Psychology Subject Pool using an age inclusion criterion of 18–40 years old (individual date of birth information was not collected). All participants were naïve to noise-vocoded speech.

MATERIALS

Listeners were tested on perception of 5 different stimulus types, all vocoded with 1, 2, 4, 8, 16, and 32 bands (where 1 is most degraded, and 32 the most intelligible). The items were also available in undistorted form. All materials were recorded by a female speaker of Standard Southern British English in a soundproof, anechoic chamber. Recordings were made on a Digital Audio Tape recorder (Sony 60ES) and fed to the S/PDIF digital input of an M-Audio Delta 66 PC soundcard. The files were then downsampled at a rate of 44100 Hz to mono.wav files with 16-bit resolution using Cool Edit 96 software (Syntrillium Software Corporation, USA). The vocoding algorithm followed the general scheme described by Shannon et al. (1995), with analysis and output filters between 100–5000 Hz and envelope extraction via half-wave rectification and low-pass filtering at 400 Hz.

The stimulus sets were as follows:

- **Simple Sentences.** One-hundred-and-forty items from the BKB sentence corpus (Bench et al., 1979), each with three keywords (e.g., The *clown* had a *funny face*).
- **Low Predictability Sentences.** One-hundred-and—forty items from the IEEE sentence corpus (IEEE, 1969), each with five keywords (e.g., The *birch canoe slid* on the *smooth planks*).
- **Single Words.** One-hundred-and-forty items from the phonemically-balanced Boothroyd AB lists (e.g., gas, mice, whip; Boothroyd, 1968).
- **Consonants.** Seventeen consonants: b, d, f, g, dʒ, k, l, m, n, p, s, ʃ, t, v, w, j, z. One token of each consonant was recorded in the context /ɑː/-C-/ɑː/, where C is a consonant e.g., *apa, aga, ala*.
- **Vowels.** Seventeen vowels: æ, eɪ, ɑː, ɛː, iː, iə, e, ɪ, aɪ, ɜ, ɒ, əʊ, uː, ɔː, aʊ, ɔɪ, ʌ. One token of each vowel was recorded in the context */b/-V-/d/*, where V is the vowel e.g., *bad, beard, boyed.*

DESIGN AND PROCEDURE

Twenty-seven listeners made two visits to the lab, separated by 7–15 days ($M = 10.44$ days, $SD = 2.69$), while the twenty-eighth participant could only return after 78 days. All stimulus presentation routines were programmed and run in MATLAB v7.1 (The Mathworks, Inc., Natick, MA).

- **Sentences and Words.** For each task (Simple Sentences, Low Predictability Sentences and Words, respectively), each session featured a set of 70 different items with 10 at each difficulty level. Within each task, one set of 70 items was labeled as Set A and another 70 distinct items as Set B. Fourteen participants received Set A items in Session 1, while the remainder received Set B items in Session 1. Within-session, a pseudorandomization routine ensured that the 70 items (i.e., their linguistic content) were completely randomized across the task, but that within each chronological block of 7 sentences there was an example from each difficulty level.
- **Consonants and Vowels.** The consonants and vowels were tested separately. Each of the tokens was repeated at all of the seven difficulty levels, and the whole list of items was fully randomized. Exposure to the difficulty levels was not chronologically constrained.

In each session, the tasks were administered in the order: BKB sentences, IEEE sentences, words, consonants, vowels. All test materials were presented over Sennheiser HD25-SP headphones in a quiet room, at a fixed volume setting using QuickMix (Version 1.06; Product Technology Partners, Cambridge, UK). The sentences and words tasks were open-set recognition tasks. Each stimulus was played once and the participant gave a typed report of the item content. Responses were self-timed.

The listener was encouraged to type as much as possible from what they heard (and that partial answers were acceptable), but were also told that it was fine to leave a blank response bar if the item was completely unintelligible. The consonants and vowels tasks each adopted a 17-alternative forced-choice paradigm. The response choices were presented on a printed sheet which remained in view for the duration of the task. In these two tasks, listeners were encouraged not to leave any gaps, even when they were completely unsure of the answer.

ANALYSIS

For each participant, performance on the tasks was scored as the proportion of keywords/items correct at each distortion level. For the sentences, a scoring system was adopted in which deviations in tense and number agreement on nouns (i.e., if the participant reported "men" when the actual keyword was "man") and verbs (i.e., if the participant reported "carries" or "carried" when the correct word was "carry") were allowed. The reasoning behind this approach was to allow for errors that may have resulted from the participant's attempts to report a grammatically correct sentence for each item. For example, if the participant hears the first keyword in "the cup hangs on a hook" as "cups," then he/she may choose to report "hang" as the second keyword, in order to maintain number agreement. For both the Sentences and Words, typographic errors that produced homophones of the target word e.g., "bare" and "bear" were permitted.

Psychometric performance curves

Logistic curve-fitting was performed on group data (by task and session), and on each individual data set (by participant, task, and session) using the psignifit software package (Wichmann and Hill, 2001a,b). For superior fits, the distortion levels (number of bands) were converted into their $\log_{10}$ equivalents (as used by Shannon et al., 2004). Data from undistorted stimuli were not included. The equation used for fitting is shown in **Figure 1**.

In the output of the fitting procedure, the alpha parameter corresponds to the number of bands giving 50% of maximum performance, and was extracted from each fitted curve for use in subsequent analyses. Lower alpha values indicate better performance. Beta is inversely proportional to the curve steepness. The parameter gamma corresponds to the base rate of performance (or "guessing rate"), while lambda reflects the "lapse rate" i.e., a lowering of the upper asymptote to allow for errors unrelated to the stimulus level. The software takes a constrained maximum-likelihood approach to fitting, where all four variables are free to vary, but where, in this case, gamma and lambda are constrained between 0.00 and 0.05. For the forced-choice tasks (Consonants and Vowels), the gamma parameter was set to 1/17.

$$(f(x:\alpha,\beta,\gamma,\lambda)) = \gamma + \frac{1-\gamma-\lambda}{1+e^{-(x/\alpha)^{\beta}}}$$

FIGURE 1 | Equation used to estimate psychometric functions describing the relationship between number of bands and speech intelligibility. α, alpha; β, beta; γ, gamma; λ, lambda. "x" in this study was the log of the number of channels in the noise vocoder.

Information transfer analyses

The forced-choice nature of the consonant and vowel tasks means that the data could be arranged into confusion matrices for use in an Information Transfer (IT) analysis (e.g., Miller and Nicely, 1955). IT analysis makes use of confusions (e.g., /b/ is mistaken for /d/) in speech identification tasks to measure the extent to which phonetic features (e.g., place of articulation, presence/absence of voicing) in the stimuli are transmitted accurately to the listener. The data are typically quantified in terms of the proportion or percentage of available bits of information in the stimuli that are accurately received by the listener. If no confusions are made in the participant's identification of a certain feature (e.g., vowel length), the IT score would be 1 or 100%, and correspondingly, if the participant's responses do not vary lawfully with the actual feature value, the score would be 0.

Unfortunately, as the participants' responses were made by typing the answers, rather than by selecting onscreen response options, some participants in the current experiment deviated from the forced-choice response constraints. This could take the form of omitted responses (which often occurred at particularly difficult distortion levels) or responses from outside the closed list. As a consequence, all data sets that included any omissions or deviations from the forced-choice options were not included in the IT analysis.

Consonants. A total of 14 data sets were entered into the IT analysis for consonant recognition. The feature matrix used included voicing, place and manner, and is shown in **Table 1**.

Unconditional IT feature analyses were run within the FIX analysis package (Feature Information XFer, University College London, UK; http://www.phon.ucl.ac.uk/resource/software.html). The amount of Information transferred for Voicing, Place, and Manner (as a proportion of the amount input for each of the features) was recorded for (i) group confusion

Table 1 | Feature matrix for IT analysis of the Consonants task.

	B	d	f	g	dʒ	k	l	m	n	p	s	ʃ	t	v	w	j	z
Voicing	+	+	−	+	+	−	+	+	+	−	−	−	−	+	+	+	+
Manner	plos	plos	fric	plos	aff	plos	app	nas	nas	plos	fric	fric	plos	fric	app	app	fric
Place	bil	alv	lad	vel	paa	vel	alv	bil	alv	bil	alv	paa	alv	Lad	lav	pal	alv

For Voicing, the '+' and '−' signs correspond to present and absent voicing, respectively. For Manner, plos, plosive; fric, fricative; aff, affricate; app, approximant; nas, nasal. For Place, bil, bilabial; alv, alveolar; lad, labiodental; paa, postalveolar; vel, velar; lav, labialized velar; pal, palatal.

matrices constructed at 1, 2, 4, 8, 16, and 32 bands, for Session 1 and Session 2 separately and (ii) for individual confusion matrices collapsed across 1–32 bands, for Session 1 and Session 2 separately. For the particular set of consonants used, there were 0.937 bits of information available for Voicing, 2.542 bits for Place of articulation and 2.095 bits for Manner of articulation.

Vowels. A total of 14 data sets were entered into the IT analysis for vowel recognition. The feature matrix used included vowel height, backness, roundedness, length, and whether the vowel was a monophthong or diphthong (**Table 2**).

IT feature analyses were run, using the FIX analysis package, for (i) group confusion matrices constructed at 1, 2, 4, 8, 16, and 32 bands, for Session 1 and Session 2 separately and (ii) for individual confusion matrices collapsed across 1–32 bands, for Session 1 and Session 2 separately. In all analyses, there were 3.264 bits of information available for vowel Height, 2.816 bits for Backness, 1.452 bits for Roundedness, 0.874 bits for Length and 0.937 bits for Mono—vs. Diphthong status.

All other reported statistical analyses were carried out in SPSS (version 19; IBM, Armonk, NY).

RESULTS

This section falls into two parts. In the first, psychometric performance functions are fitted to each individual's performance, and individual differences analyses of curve position used to characterize group performance across and within the two sessions. The second part uses IT analyses to explore the perception of consonants and vowels and relate this to recognition of sentences and words.

MEASURING PROFILES OF LEARNING AND COVARIANCE

Figure 2 shows a plot of the group performance functions for the open-set [2(a)] and closed-set [forced-choice; 2(b)] tasks in each session.

For analysis, the alpha scores generated in the curve fitting procedure were operationalized as the Threshold Number of Bands (TNB) for each participant, in each task, in each session. **Figure 3** shows that there was an overall decrease in TNBs on the five tasks between Session 1 and 2. A repeated-measures ANOVA analysis was run on the TNBs, with Session and Task as within-subjects factors. A between-subjects factor, Version (which coded the order of presentation of the item sets) was also included. There was a significant effect of Session [$F_{(1, 26)} = 35.094$, $p < 0.001$], a significant effect of Task [$F_{(4, 104)} = 117.18$, $p < 0.001$), and a non-significant interaction of these two factors ($F < 1$), indicating that the degree of improvement was not significantly different across tasks.

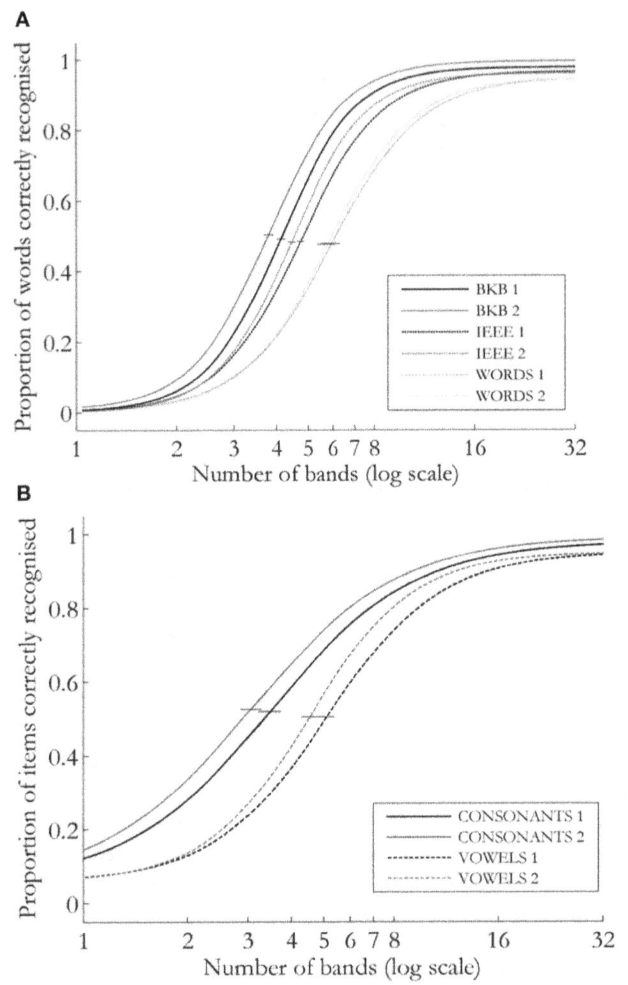

FIGURE 2 | Logistic curves describing group performance on the speech recognition tasks for (A) open-set tasks (sentences and words) and (B) consonants and vowels. Error bars show 95% confidence limits around α.

Table 2 | Feature matrix for IT analysis of the Vowels task.

	æ	eɪ	ɑː	ɛː	iː	ɪə	e	ɪ	aɪ	ɜ	ɒ	əʊ	uː	ɔː	aʊ	ɔɪ	ʌ
Height	no	cm-fc	o	om	c	nc-m	cm	nc	o-nc	om	o	m-nc	c	om	o-nc	om-nc	om
Backness	f	f-nf	b	f	f	nf-c	f	nf	f-nf	c	b	c-nb	b	b	f-nb	b-nf	b
Roundedness	n	n	n	n	n	n	n	n	n	n	y	ny	y	y	ny	yn	n
Length	s	l	l	l	l	l	s	s	l	l	s	l	l	l	l	l	s
Diphthong?	n	y	n	n	n	y	n	n	y	n	n	y	n	n	y	y	n

For Height, o, open; no, near-open; om, open-mid; m, mid; cm, close-mid; nc, near-close; c, close. For Backness, b, back; nb, near-back; c, central; nf, near-front; f, front. For Roundedness, y, rounded and n, unrounded. For Length, s, short and l, long. For Diphthong, y, diphthong and n, monophthong. Dashes indicate the separation of the diphthong descriptions into monophthongal elements, in temporal order.

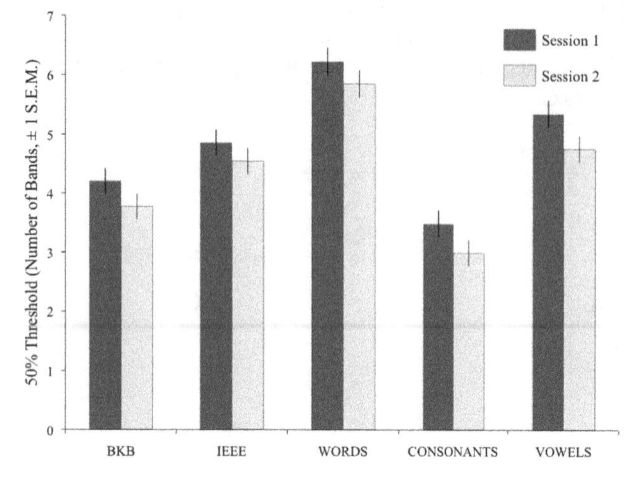

FIGURE 3 | Mean TNBs (Threshold Number of Bands) for speech recognition across the five tasks, and across the two test sessions. Error bars show ±1 standard error of the mean.

Table 3 | Pearson's correlation coefficients between the five tasks in the experiment, across the two testing session.

	BKB	IEEE	Words	Cons	Vowels
(A) SESSION 1					
BKB	–	0.356*	0.259^	0.003	−0.100
IEEE		-	0.323*	0.069	−0.056
Words			–	0.417*	0.331*
Cons				–	0.302^
Vowels					–
(B) SESSION 2					
BKB	–	0.277^	0.333*	0.299^	0.236
IEEE		–	-0.025	0.393*	0.296^
Words			–	0.015	0.057
Cons				–	0.317^
Vowels					–

Cons, Consonants; $^{\wedge}p < 0.10$, $^{*}p < 0.05$.

Table 4 | Results of factor analyses on individual TNBs (Threshold Number of Bands).

	Factor 1	Factor 2
(A) SESSION 1		
BKB		0.605
IEEE		0.593
Words	0.705	0.469
Consonants	0.558	
Vowels	0.562	
(B) SESSION 2		
BKB	0.520	0.344
IEEE	0.545	
Words		0.946
Consonants	0.642	
Vowels	0.491	

Only factor loadings over 0.3 are shown.

The between-subjects effect of Version was non-significant ($F < 1$), as were the two-way interactions of Version with Session [$F_{(1, 26)} = 1.33$, $p = 0.260$] and Version with Task [$F_{(1, 104)} = 1.16$, $p = 0.333$]. There was, however, a significant three-way interaction of Version, Session and Task [$F_{(4, 104)} = 5.57$, $p < 0.001$]; while most conditions across both versions showed a mean improvement from Session 1 to Session 2, Version A participants showed a trend in the opposite direction on the IEEE task, while the Version B participants showed a very small decrease in mean performance on the Words task from Session 1 to Session 2.

There was evidence of several significant relationships across tasks for the TNB scores. **Table 3A** shows the one-tailed Pearson's correlation matrix for TNB scores in Session 1. These show significant (and marginally significant) correlations between the two sentence tasks, and between the consonants and vowels tasks, while the words correlated reasonably well with all other tasks.

A common factor analysis was run on the threshold data, with maximum likelihood extraction and varimax rotation. The rotated factor matrix is shown in **Table 4A**, for those factors producing eigenvalues above 1. Two components were extracted. In the rotated matrix, the first component accounted for 22.6% of the variance, while the second component accounted for 19.2%. The pattern of correlations for TNB scores in Session 2 no longer fitted the processing framework suggested by the Session 1 data (see **Table 3B**), with the Words task now somewhat separate from the others. A common factor analysis was run on the data as for the Session 1 scores. This converged on two components—see **Table 4B**. In this analysis, Factor 1 accounted for 24.4% of the variance, where Factor 2 accounted for a further 20.4%.

EXPLORING ANALYTIC LISTENING USING IT ANALYSIS

Consonants

The results of the pooled group analysis are plotted in **Figure 4**, showing the proportion of Information transferred for each feature, across each difficulty level. The plots give a readily interpretable visual representation of the "cue-trading" behavior of the listeners as spectral information is manipulated, and as a result of perceptual learning.

Figure 5 shows the results of the individual analyses for each feature and session collapsed across difficulty level. A repeated-measures ANOVA gave significant effects of Session [$F_{(1, 13)} = 13.52$, $p = 0.003$] and Feature [$F_{(2, 26)} = 64.13$, $p < 0.001$]. A significant interaction of these two factors [$F_{(1.38, 26)} = 4.16$, $p = 0.046$; Greenhouse-Geisser corrected] was explored using 3 *post-hoc t*-tests with Bonferroni correction (significance level $p < 0.017$). These indicated a significant increase in IT for Manner [$t_{(13)} = 2.97$, $p = 0.002$] and Voicing [$t_{(13)} = 2.97$, $p = 0.011$] from Session 1 to Session 2, but not for Place [$t_{(13)} = 2.17$, $p = 0.049$].

The individual-subject IT scores for voicing, place and manner in each session were entered as predictors in linear regression analyses on the TNB scores for the five tasks. In Session 1, a significant model with Place and Voicing as predictors offered the best account of consonant recognition [R^2adj. = 0.750; $F_{(2, 11)}$ = 21.71, $p = 0.001$]. Performance on the vowels task was best predicted by Voicing [R^2adj. = 0.295; $F_{(1, 12)}$ = 6.44, $p = 0.026$]. In Session 2, Manner and Place predicted TNB scores on the Consonants task [R^2adj. = 0.580; $F_{(1, 12)}$ = 9.98, $p = 0.003$], while Manner scores predicted TNB scores on the IEEE sentences [R^2adj. = 0.270; $F_{(1, 12)}$ = 5.80, $p = 0.033$]. There were no other significant models.

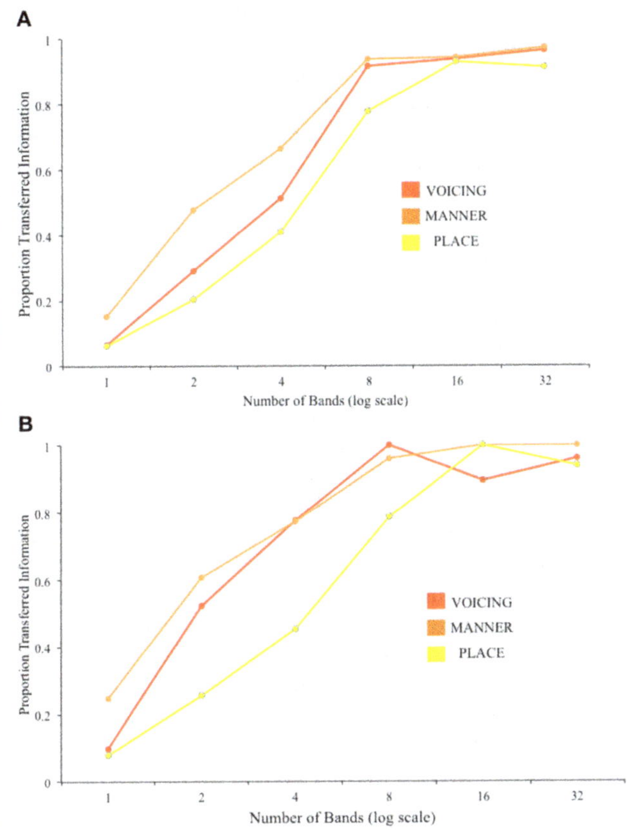

FIGURE 4 | Results of the group IT analysis on consonant perception for (A) Session 1 and (B) Session 2.

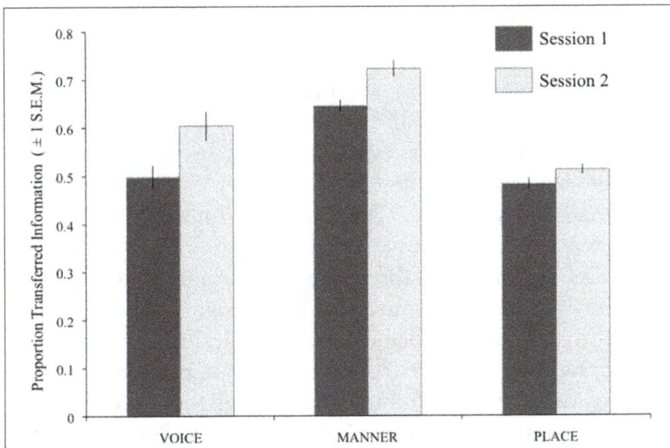

FIGURE 5 | Results of the IT analysis on consonant perception, using individual participant data. For each feature, the darker bars show the results for Session 1, and the paler bars show the results for Session 2. Error bars show ±1 standard error of the mean.

Vowels

The results of the pooled group IT (**Figure 6**) show that vowel Length information is the best transferred (as a proportion of the information input about this feature) of the five features at low spectral resolutions (1, 2, and 4 bands), with the other features more closely bunched. At greater spectral resolutions (16 and 32 bands), this discrepancy is reduced.

Figure 7 shows the results of the individual analyses for each Feature and Session collapsed across difficulty level). A repeated-measures ANOVA gave significant effects of Session [$F_{(1, 13)}$ = 23.17, $p < 0.001$] and Feature [$F_{(1.12, 52)}$ = 34.34, $p < 0.001$; Greenhouse-Geisser corrected) with no interaction of the two factors.

The individual-subject IT scores for each feature in each session were entered as predictors in linear regression analyses on the TNB scores for the five tasks. In Session 1, a significant model featured Height as the sole predictor of TNB scores on the Vowels task [R^2adj. = 0.743; $F_{(1, 12)}$ = 38.68, $p < 0.001$]. In

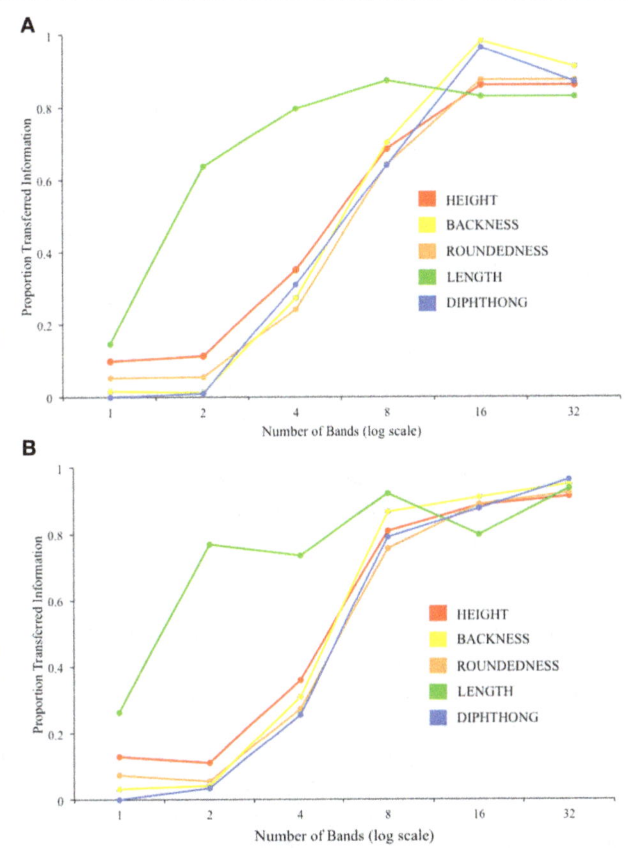

FIGURE 6 | Results of the group IT analysis on vowel perception for (A) Session 1 and (B) Session 2.

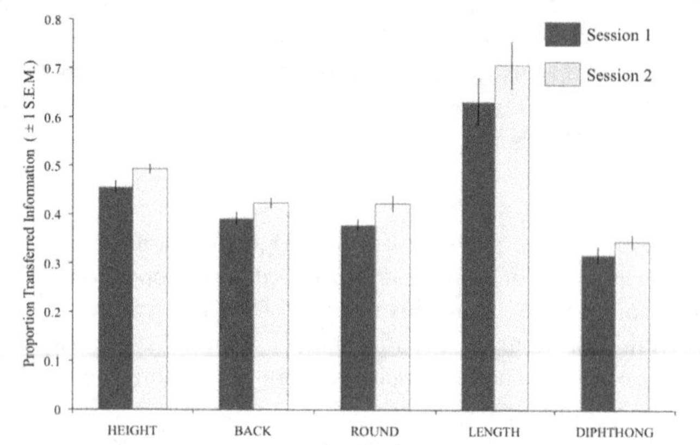

FIGURE 7 | Results of the IT analysis on vowel perception, using individual participant data. For each feature, the darker bars show the results for Session 1, and the paler bars show the results for Session 2. Error bars show ±1 standard error of the mean. BACK, backness; ROUND, roundedness.

Session 2, a significant model with Height and Length [R^2adj. = 0.772; $F_{(1, 12)} = 28.51$, $p < 0.001$] gave the best prediction of TNB scores on the Vowels task, and a model with Length emerged as significant for scores on the BKB sentences [R^2adj. = 0.308; $F_{(1, 12)} = 6.80, p = 0.023$]. There were no other significant models.

DISCUSSION

The current data showed evidence for improved recognition of noise-vocoded sentences, words and segments, when re-tested after a 1–2 week period of no exposure, and without any explicit training. Using individual differences as the starting point for analyses, we identified a pattern of covariance across levels of the linguistic hierarchy, which changed with learning. Analyses of confusion data revealed that participants in the experiment improved on the reception of acoustic-phonetic features by Session 2, but exhibited inefficient use of cues available in the vocoded signal. Further, these suggested predictive roles for specific phonetic features in the perception of noise-vocoded stimuli.

UNDERSTANDING NOISE-VOCODED SEGMENTS, WORDS AND SENTENCES: EFFECTS OF LEARNING AND TASK

We found that performance improved significantly between Session 1 and Session 2 of the experiment, and by an equivalent amount across tasks. As the experiment was primarily designed to explore individual differences and patterns of covariance across tasks and time, we chose to run the five speech tests in a fixed order for both sessions. Given that the task order was not counterbalanced across the group, we therefore cannot conclude whether the observed improvements are due to within-session exposure or between-session consolidation—for example, the BKB test occurred at the start of each session, and so the improvement observed by Session 2 may reflect adaptation during the remaining four tasks in Session 1 and before the delay period. However, taken across all tasks, the significant improvement in performance is, at least, a demonstration of medium-term retention of adaptation to noise-vocoded speech in the absence of exposure or training. We also note that, for the sentences and words tasks, the improved performance reflects perceptual learning at an acoustic-phonetic level, as recognition in Session 2 was tested using novel tokens (Davis et al., 2005).

UNDERSTANDING NOISE-VOCODED SEGMENTS, WORDS AND SENTENCES: EXPLORING COVARIANCE

Simple correlations between the tasks in each session showed, like Surprenant and Watson (2001), rather modest evidence for covariation of individual thresholds across the tasks (**Table 3**). This once again demonstrates that there is no straightforward, unitary approach to recognizing degraded speech across levels of the linguistic hierarchy. However, a factor analysis of Session 1 TNB scores suggested some systematicity—this revealed two similarly-weighted, orthogonal factors in the Session 1 threshold data, with sentences and words loading on one factor, and words and segments loading on the other. This suggests two independent modes of listening: a "top–down" mode making use of lexical, syntactic and semantic information to generate hypotheses about stimulus identity, and a "bottom–up" mode concerned with acoustic-phonetic discriminations. Notably, the words task occupies an intermediate status, by loading on both "top–down" and "bottom–up" factors. By Session 2, when performance had improved, all tasks but one—Words—patterned together. It appears that once the initial learning of sound-to-representation mappings has taken place, the listener can begin to approach most stimulus types in a similar way. In this sense, we suggest that the *nature* of the underlying factors was different in Session 2, such that these could no longer be well described by a greater involvement of "top–down" or "bottom–up" processes. However, we note that, in both session, the factors only accounted for a proportion of the variance, and therefore we cannot rule out the influence of additional factors underlying performance.

The plot in **Figure 2** shows that the Words task was the most difficult of the open-set tasks in both sessions, with listeners requiring a greater amount of spectral detail (i.e., larger numbers of bands) in order to reach the 50% performance threshold. Within the open-set tasks, the overall amount of exposure to vocoded material across seventy sentences is much greater than for seventy monosyllabic words. However, Hervais-Adelman et al. (2008) showed that, even when matched for number of words of exposure, learning is still slower for noise-vocoded words than for sentences. These authors interpret such findings in terms of the relative richness of the "teaching signal" that assists learning. In the current experiment, the listener could draw upon many sources of knowledge against which to test hypotheses for sentence recognition—lexical, syntactic and semantic (Miller, 1947). Furthermore, the segment recognition tasks provided a learning frame-work through their forced-choice design. In contrast, the recognition of monosyllabic, degraded words could be constrained by the expectation of real lexical items, but with many monosyllables having several real-word neighbors (bat, cat, sat, fat etc.), any error in phonemic identification could lead to the participant making the wrong "guess" in their response to difficult items. In line with Hervais-Adelman et al., we argue that the nature of the Words task will have made it most difficult within each testing session, but also limited the potential for improved performance with learning. By the second testing session, listeners have established a sufficient level of acoustic-to-phonemic mapping that, in combination with expectancy constraints, allowed for improved performance on the sentences and segments tasks. However, the recognition of single words could not be performed using the same listening strategies(s).

EXPLORING ACOUSTIC-PHONETIC PROCESSING: INFORMATION TRANSFER FOR CONSONANTS AND VOWELS

The forced-choice design of the consonants and vowels tasks allowed us to explore performance in terms of the perception of phonetic features, using an IT analysis. The outcomes of IT analyses on the consonants and vowels recognition data are generally in agreement with the findings of several previous studies using noise-vocoded speech (Dorman et al., 1990, 1997; Shannon et al., 1995; Dorman and Loizou, 1998; Iverson et al., 2007). However, the current study enabled the assessment of two extra dimensions: the effect of perceptual learning on the extraction of feature information, and the relationship of feature processing to performance on the five speech recognition tasks.

The group IT analysis of the consonants data suggested that, numerically, place was the most poorly transferred feature, with no improvement across sessions. Dorman et al. (1990) tested identification of consonants by CI patients. They reasoned that, given the good temporal resolution by implants, envelope-borne information would be well transferred while the poor resolution offered by a small number of electrodes (6 in the device tested in their study) would limit the transfer of spectral information. Envelope information potentially cues listeners to voicing and manner, while transmission of place information is dependent on high-rate temporal structure (fluctuation rates from around 600 to 10 kHz) cueing spectro-temporal dynamics including the ability to resolve formants in the frequency domain; (Rosen, 1992). In CIs and their simulations, frequency resolution can be very poor in the region of formant frequencies, such that both F1 and F2 may be represented by the output of only one channel/electrode. Even if the first two formants can be resolved, the ability to differentiate one speech sound from the other can depend on within—formant transitions in frequency, for example in the discrimination of /b/ and /d/. The ability to make discriminations based on formant-carried frequency information in noise-vocoded speech will depend on the ability of listeners to compare the relative amplitude outputs of the different bands. A study by Shannon et al. (1995) with normal-hearing listeners exposed to noise-vocoded speech demonstrated that, after several hours of exposure, voicing and manner were almost completely transferred from spectral resolutions of 2 bands and upwards, while place IT was around 30% with 2 bands and did not exceed 70% by 4 bands. It should be noted that the three phonetic features of voicing, place and manner are not completely independent of each other, and there is likely to be some degree of overlap in the corresponding acoustic features. Dorman et al. (1990) point out that the amount of transferred place information should vary with the amount transferred about manner, as some manner cues facilitate place recognition e.g., frication manner (i.e., a wideband noise in the signal) potentially allows relatively easy discrimination between /s/ or /ʃ/ and /f/ or /θ/, as the former pair can be 15dB more intense than the latter.

The slightly more marked improvement in reception of voicing information than for the other two features in the current task can perhaps be explained by considering the acoustic nature of the noise-vocoded stimulus. Voicing can be weakly signaled by relatively slow envelope fluctations—for example, through detection of the longer silent periods in voiceless than voiced plosives, or in the greater amplitude of voiced compared to voiceless obstruents. However, voicing is also signaled by periodicity, that is, temporal regularity in the speech waveform carried by fluctuations primarily between 50 and 500 Hz (Rosen, 1992). This information is reasonably well preserved after the vocoding scheme used in the present experiment, where the amplitude envelope was low-pass filtered at 400 Hz. The between-session improvement shown for voicing at low band numbers could reflect the participants' increased ability to use the available temporal information in the stimulus to assist performance in the absence of cues to place of articulation that are more dependent on spectral resolution. However, voicing information is also carried by cues to overall spectral balance, as voicing is weighted toward low frequencies. These cues become apparent as soon as at least a second band of information is added to the noise-vocoded stimulus. We note that the duration of the preceding vowel in naturally-produced VCV stimuli can be a cue to voicing in the upcoming consonant. However, the mean preceding vowel duration was not significantly different between tokens with voiced and voiceless consonants in our task [$t_{(15)} = 1.09$, $p = 0.292$].

It is clear that the transmission of spectral shape information, as is required for identification of height, backness, roundedness, and diphthongs, is a limiting factor in recognition of noise-vocoded vowels, and that these four features are closely related in terms of recognition. However, as neither the amplitude envelope nor the duration of the signal is distorted by the noise-vocoding procedure, the information on vowel length should have been readily transmitted at all channels. Indeed, at lower numbers of bands, length was the most well recognized feature in the vowels task. However, overall recognition of this feature was well below 100%, and variable across the participant group. Regression models identified length as a significant predictor of scores on the other speech tasks, suggesting that timing and rhythmic information are of importance in perception of noise-vocoded speech. Our findings are similar to those by Iverson et al. (2007), who measured IT for vowel length in CI users and normal-hearing listeners listening to a CI simulation. Both listening groups in the Iverson et al. study showed sub-optimal IT. The authors propose that, given the excellent preservation of durational information in noise-vocoding, participants should be able to show 100% IT for length, even at low spectral resolutions. Therefore, while the evidence suggests that timing and rhythm may be important for successful perception of some forms of noise-vocoded speech, listeners may require more guidance and training in order to make better use of durational cues.

RECOGNITION OF NOISE-VOCODED SPEECH OVER PARTICIPANT, TASK, AND TIME—IMPLICATIONS FOR TRAINING AND COCHLEAR IMPLANTATION

The current study presents a number of findings relevant to more applied settings such as training regimes for CI recipients. We identified that, on initial exposure to noise-vocoded speech, the pattern of covariance across tasks was suggestive of two different "levels" of processing—one lexico-semantic (or "top–down"), and the other more acoustic-phonetic (or "bottom–up"). The words task was implicated in both of these factors. Isolated monosyllabic items such as "mice" and "gas" have lexical and semantic content, and the expectation of meaningful tokens can constrain the listener's candidate pool of targets in the recognition task. However, with all the items bearing the same CVC structure, and without any higher-order syntactic and semantic cues, the listener must also engage an analytical, acoustic-phonetic approach in order to successfully identify the words. It may be this demand on both approaches that makes the words task the most difficult in the set. Loebach and colleagues (Loebach and Pisoni, 2008; Loebach et al., 2008, 2009, 2010) argue that training in analytical, acoustic-phonetic listening offers the most promising route for adaptation to distorted speech. In a test of vocoded sentence perception they observed equivalent transfer of learning after training with semantically anomalous sentences as from training with real sentences. They suggest that this reflects an increased demand for attention to acoustic-phonetic aspects of the signal (rather than higher-order syntactic or semantic cues) when listening to the anomalous stimuli—their implication is that learning at this level can then be readily transferred to other stimulus types (Loebach et al., 2010). However, they also find that transfer is greatest between stimuli of the same linguistic class (Loebach and Pisoni, 2008). We have identified two sources of variability, of similar explanatory power, underlying the recognition of noise-vocoded speech. We suggest that both listening "strategies" should potentially yield benefits for adaptation, and that the effects observed by Loebach and colleagues may be associated with more generalized attentional engagement rather than the superior effects of analytic listening. Nogaki et al. (2007) partly ascribe the variability within normal-hearing participants listening to CI simulations to variable levels of enthusiasm and involvement in difficult listening tasks, and contrast this with the keener sense of urgency shown by CI patients, for whom successful training has important consequences for their quality of life. An experimental modulation of attentional engagement with noise-vocoded speech might offer greater insight into how this might differentially affect top–down and bottom–up aspects of listening. In the context of cochlear implantation, it is important to recognize that most of what we hear in everyday speech takes the form of connected phrases and sentences. Therefore, identifying methods of engaging attention in higher-order aspects of linguistic processing, such as the use of semantic and syntactic cues to "fill in the gaps" in difficult listening situations, may yield benefits of a similar magnitude to more bottom–up strategies.

We also identified targets for improved bottom–up processing of noise-vocoded speech from the current dataset. The use of IT analyses to explore acoustic-phonetic processing produced findings unattainable from basic recognition scores. We identified significant predictive roles for voicing and vowel length information in recognizing noise-vocoded stimuli across the linguistic hierarchy. Both of these properties were well represented at low spectral resolutions in the current stimuli—in particular, vowel length information was fully present even with one band. However, although perception of these features showed marked improvement over time, **Figures 4–7** show that listeners' accuracy in recognizing these features was much less than 100% in both sessions. This suggests that, in the absence of specific guidance or instruction, listeners continue to rely on typically dominant cues to phoneme identification (e.g., formant frequencies in vowels) at the expense of other information that is more reliably preserved in the degraded signal. Based on this result, and similar findings from Iverson et al. (2007), we suggest that if CIs are to be trained in analytic listening to aid perceptual learning, this should be targeted at the acoustic cues that are most likely to be preserved when transmitted through the device. We suggest that focused training on perception of duration, amplitude modulation, and spectral balance cues could be used to improve acoustic-phonetic processing from the bottom–up by maximizing the usefulness of the information in the acoustic signal.

CONCLUSION

The current study offers some insight into the existence of overlapping lexico-semantic and acoustic-phonetic processes underlying the adaptation to a CI simulation in normal-hearing participants. We suggest that both "top–down" and "bottom–up" listening strategies have potential validity in settings such as training for recipients of CIs. To improve "analytic" processing, we suggest that training should involve targeted attentional engagement with acoustic cues that are well preserved in the degraded stimulus. Further work is necessary to evaluate the benefits of such an approach. When considering all of the findings, however, we must acknowledge that the speech transformation used in the current study forms only a basic approximation to the signal perceived by most users of CIs. The process of implantation can result in incomplete insertion of the electrode array and damage to parts of the basilar membrane (yielding "dead regions"), both of which have consequences for the mapping of sound to the auditory nerve. Such effects can be simulated through additional transformations in the noise-vocoding technique (e.g., Rosen et al., 1999; Smith and Faulkner, 2006), and future work will need to determine whether the current findings are borne out for these more degraded signals.

ACKNOWLEDGMENTS

This work was supported by an Economic and Social Research Council +3 Postgraduate Studentship (PTA-030-2004-01065) awarded to Carolyn McGettigan.

REFERENCES

Bench, J., Kowal, A., and Bamford, J. (1979). The BKB (Bamford-Kowal-Bench) sentence lists for partially-hearing children. *Br. J. Audiol.* 13, 108–112. doi: 10.3109/03005367909078884

Boothroyd, A. (1968). Developments in speech audiometry. *Sound* 2, 3–10.

Boothroyd, A., and Nittrouer, S. (1988). Mathematical treatment of context effects in phoneme and word recognition. *J. Acoust. Soc. Am.* 84, 101–114. doi: 10.1121/1.396976

Davis, M. H., Johnsrude, I. S., Hervais-Adelman, A., Taylor, K., and McGettigan, C. (2005). Lexical information drives perceptual learning of distorted speech: evidence from the comprehension of noise-vocoded sentences. *J. Exp. Psychol. Gen.* 134, 222–441. doi: 10.1037/0096-3445.134.2.222

Dorman, M. F., and Loizou, P. C. (1998). The identification of consonants and vowels by cochlear implant patients using a 6-channel continuous interleaved sampling processor and by normal-hearing subjects using simulations of processors with two to nine channels. *Ear Hear.* 19, 162–166. doi: 10.1097/00003446-199804000-00008

Dorman, M. F., Loizou, P. C., and Rainey, D. (1997). Speech intelligibility as a function of the number of channels of stimulation for signal processors using sine-wave and noise-band outputs. *J. Acoust. Soc. Am.* 102, 2403–2411. doi: 10.1121/1.419603

Dorman, M. F., Soli, S., Dankowski, K., Smith, L. M., McCandless, G., and Parkin, J. (1990). Acoustic cues for consonant identification by patients who use the Ineraid cochlear implant. *J. Acoust. Soc. Am.* 88, 2074–2079. doi: 10.1121/1.400104

Eisner, F., McGettigan, C., Faulkner, A., Rosen, S., and Scott, S. K. (2010). Inferior frontal gyrus activation predicts individual differences in perceptual learning of cochlear-implant simulations. *J. Neurosci.* 30, 7179–7186. doi: 10.1523/JNEUROSCI.4040-09.2010

Faulkner, A., Rosen, S., and Green, T. (2012). Comparing live to recorded speech in training the perception of spectrally shifted noise-vocoded speech. *J. Acoust. Soc. Am.* 132, EL336–EL342. doi: 10.1121/1.4754432

Fu, Q. J., Galvin, J., Wang, X., and Nogaki, G. (2005). Moderate auditory training can improve speech performance of adult cochlear implant patients. *Acoust. Res. Lett. Online* 6, 106–111. doi: 10.1121/1.1898345

Grant, K.W., and Seitz, P. F. (2000). The recognition of isolated words and words in sentences: individual variability in the use of sentence context. *J. Acoust. Soc. Am.* 107, 1000–1011. doi: 10.1121/1.428280

Hervais-Adelman, A., Davis, M. H., Johnsrude, I. S., and Carlyon, R. P. (2008). Perceptual learning of noise vocoded words: effects of feedback and lexicality. *J. Exp. Psychol. Hum. Percept. Perform.* 34, 460–474. doi: 10.1037/0096-1523.34.2.460

IEEE. (1969). IEEE recommended practice for speech quality measurements. *IEEE Trans. Audio Electroacoust.* 17, 225–246. doi: 10.1109/TAU.1969.1162058

Iverson, P., Smith, C., and Evans, B. (2007). Vowel recognition via cochlear implants and noise vocoders: effects of formant movement and duration. *J. Acoust. Soc. Am.* 120, 3998–4006. doi: 10.1121/1.2372453

Loebach, J. L., and Pisoni, D. B. (2008). Perceptual learning of spectrally degraded speech and environmental sounds. *J. Acoust. Soc. Am.* 123, 1126–1139. doi: 10.1121/1.2823453

Loebach, J. L., Bent, T., and Pisoni, D. B. (2008). Multiple routes to the perceptual learning of speech. *J. Acoust. Soc. Am.* 124, 552–561. doi: 10.1121/1.2931948

Loebach, J. L., Pisoni, D. B., and Svirsky, M. A. (2009). Transfer of auditory perceptual learning with spectrally reduced speech to speech and nonspeech tasks: implications for cochlear implants. *Ear Hear.* 30, 662–674. doi: 10.1097/AUD.0b013e3181b9c92d

Loebach, J. L., Pisoni, D. B., and Svirsky, M. A. (2010). Effects of semantic context and feedback on perceptual learning of speech processed through an acoustic simulation of a cochlear implant. *J. Exp. Psychol. Hum. Percept. Perform.* 36, 224–234. doi: 10.1037/a0017609

Miller, G., and Nicely, P. (1955). An analysis of perceptual confusions among some English consonants. *J. Acoust. Soc. Am.* 27, 338–352. doi: 10.1121/1.1907526

Miller, G. A. (1947). The masking of speech. *Psychol. Bull.* 44, 105–129. doi: 10.1037/h0055960

Moore, D. R., and Shannon, R. V. (2009). Beyond cochlear implants: awakening the deafened brain. *Nat. Neurosci.* 12, 686–691. doi: 10.1038/nn.2326

Munson, B., Donaldson, G. S., Allen, S. L., Collison, E. A., and Nelson, D. A. (2003). Patterns of phoneme perception errors by listeners with cochlear implants as a function of overall speech perception ability. *J. Acoust. Soc. Am.* 113, 925–935. doi: 10.1121/1.1536630

Nogaki, G., Fu, Q. J., and Galvin, J. J. 3rd. (2007). Effect of training rate on recognition of spectrally shifted speech. *Ear Hear.* 28, 132–140. doi: 10.1097/AUD.0b013e3180312669

Pisoni, D. B. (2000). Cognitive factors and cochlear implants: some thoughts on perception, learning, and memory in speech perception. *Ear Hear.* 21, 70–78. doi: 10.1097/00003446-200002000-00010

Rosen, S. (1992). Temporal information in speech - acoustic, auditory and linguistic aspects. *Philos. Trans. R. Soc. Lond. B Biol. Sci.* 336, 367–373. doi: 10.1121/1.428215

Rosen, S., Faulkner, A., and Wilkinson, L. (1999). Adaptation by normal listeners to upward spectral shifts of speech: implications for cochlear implants. *J. Acoust. Soc. Am.* 106, 3629–3636. doi: 10.1098/rstb.1992.0070

Rubinstein, J. T. (2004). How cochlear implants encode speech. *Curr. Opin. Otolaryngol. Head Neck Surg.* 12, 444–448. doi: 10.1097/01.moo.0000134452.24819.c0

Sarant, J. Z., Blamey, P. J., Dowell, R. C., Clark, G. M., and Gibson, W. P. (2001). Variation in speech perception scores among children with cochlear implants. *Ear Hear.* 22, 18–28. doi: 10.1097/00003446-200102000-00003

Scott, S. K., Blank, C. C., Rosen, S., and Wise, R. J. (2000). Identification of a pathway for intelligible speech in the left temporal lobe. *Brain* 123, 2400–2406. doi: 10.1093/brain/123.12.2400

Shannon, R. V., Fu, Q. J., and Galvin, J. 3rd. (2004). The number of spectral channels required for speech recognition depends on the difficulty of the listening situation. *Acta Otolaryngol. Suppl.* 552, 50–54. doi: 10.1080/03655230410017562

Shannon, R. V., Zeng, F. G., Kamath, V., Wygonski, J., and Ekelid, M. (1995). Speech recognition with primarily temporal cues. *Science* 270, 303–304. doi: 10.1126/science.270.5234.303

Skinner, M. W. (2003). Optimizing cochlear implant speech performance. *Ann. Otol. Rhinol. Laryngol. Suppl.* 191, 4–13.

Smith, M. W., and Faulkner, A. (2006). Perceptual adaptation by normally hearing listeners to a simulated "hole" in hearing. *J. Acoust. Soc. Am.* 120, 4019–4030. doi: 10.1121/1.2359235

Stacey, P. C., and Summerfield, A. Q. (2007). Effectiveness of computer-based auditory training in improving the perception of noise-vocoded speech. *J. Acoust. Soc. Am.* 121, 2923–2935. doi: 10.1121/1.2713668

Surprenant, A. M., and Watson, C. S. (2001). Individual differences in the processing of speech and nonspeech sounds by normal-hearing listeners. *J. Acoust. Soc. Am.* 110, 2085–2095. doi: 10.1121/1.1404973

Wichmann, F. A., and Hill, N. J. (2001a). The psychometric function: I. Fitting, sampling, and goodness of fit. *Percept. Psychophys.* 63, 1293–1313. doi: 10.3758/BF03194544

Wichmann, F. A., and Hill, N. J. (2001b). The psychometric function: II. Bootstrap-based confidence intervals and sampling. *Percept. Psychophys.* 63, 1314–1329. doi: 10.3758/BF03194545

5

How age and linguistic competence alter the interplay of perceptual and cognitive factors when listening to conversations in a noisy environment

Meital Avivi-Reich, Meredyth Daneman and Bruce A. Schneider*

Human Communication Laboratory, Department of Psychology, University of Toronto Mississauga, Mississauga, ON, Canada

Correspondence:
Bruce A. Schneider, Human Communication Laboratory, Department of Psychology, University of Toronto Mississauga, Room: CCT 4073, 3359 Mississauga Road N., Mississauga, ON L5L 1C6, Canada
e-mail: bruce.schneider@utoronto.ca

Multi-talker conversations challenge the perceptual and cognitive capabilities of older adults and those listening in their second language (L2). In older adults these difficulties could reflect declines in the auditory, cognitive, or linguistic processes supporting speech comprehension. The tendency of L2 listeners to invoke some of the semantic and syntactic processes from their first language (L1) may interfere with speech comprehension in L2. These challenges might also force them to reorganize the ways in which they perceive and process speech, thereby altering the balance between the contributions of bottom-up vs. top-down processes to speech comprehension. Younger and older L1s as well as young L2s listened to conversations played against a babble background, with or without spatial separation between the talkers and masker, when the spatial positions of the stimuli were specified either by loudspeaker placements (real location), or through use of the precedence effect (virtual location). After listening to a conversation, the participants were asked to answer questions regarding its content. Individual hearing differences were compensated for by creating the same degree of difficulty in identifying individual words in babble. Once compensation was applied, the number of questions correctly answered increased when a real or virtual spatial separation was introduced between babble and talkers. There was no evidence that performance differed between real and virtual locations. The contribution of vocabulary knowledge to dialog comprehension was found to be larger in the virtual conditions than in the real whereas the contribution of reading comprehension skill did not depend on the listening environment but rather differed as a function of age and language proficiency. The results indicate that the acoustic scene and the cognitive and linguistic competencies of listeners modulate how and when top-down resources are engaged in aid of speech comprehension.

Keywords: age, nonnative listeners, speech comprehension, spatial separation, hearing, multitalker discourse, auditory-cognitive interaction, hearing loss

INTRODUCTION

Conversations with friends, co-workers, healthcare providers, and others often occur in noisy environments (e.g., malls, restaurants, stores, offices) in which there are a number of different sound sources that could interfere with one's ability to communicate effectively. In particular, the presence of other talkers, who are not part of the conversation, can be particularly distracting when one is trying to follow a conversation between two or more people. Such multi-talker auditory scenes increase the complexity of both the perceptual and cognitive processes required for comprehension. To effectively follow a multi-talker conversation, the listener needs to perceptually segregate the talkers from one another, efficiently switch attention from one talker to another, keep track of what was said by whom, extract the meaning of each utterance, store this information in memory for future use, integrate incoming information with what each conversational participant has said or done in the past, and draw on the listener's own knowledge of the conversation's topic to extract general themes and ideas (Murphy et al., 2006; Schneider et al., 2010). In other words, fully comprehending what is going on in a conversation requires the smooth and rapid coordination of a number of auditory and cognitive processes. Hence, it is not surprising that people in general find such situations stressful, and that older individuals, whose auditory and cognitive systems may be in decline, and even young, healthy listeners who are operating in their second or third language, find such situations particularly devastating.

To experimentally determine the reasons why people may find it difficult to follow conversations in noisy situations, we need laboratory simulations of ecologically-relevant listening environments and tasks, where we can control and manipulate relevant variables such as the nature and number of competing sound sources, their spatial locations, and the signal-to-noise ratios (SNRs) under which they are presented. By far, most of the studies designed to evaluate the relative contribution of perceptual and cognitive factors in hearing involve simple word or sentence recognition (see review by Humes et al., 2012). In such studies the target stimuli are either words or sentences and the listeners are simply asked to repeat them (e.g., George et al., 2007; Francis, 2010). The ability to repeat target words is taken as indicating speech is understood (Humes and Dubno, 2010). Comprehending what is happening in a conversation, as we have argued above, requires much more than simply being able to repeat the words being spoken. Hence, there is a substantial difference between speech recognition and speech comprehension (Schneider, 2011). A review of studies taking a correlational approach to the relationships among perception, cognition and speech recognition suggests that individual differences in speech recognition cannot be explained fully by the auditory or the cognitive factors that have been considered (age, pure tone thresholds, spectral and temporal processing, intensity coding, and cognitive processing; see Houtgast and Festen, 2008 for a review). Such studies, while they provide important information that may shed light on some of the processes needed for speech recognition (e.g., stream segregation, morpheme identification, lexical access), are limited with respect to their ability to address the role played by the higher-order cognitive processes required to successfully comprehend a conversation (e.g., attention switching, information integration, memory).

Although following a conversation in complex auditory scenes is a challenging task for all listeners, this task seems to be disproportionally harder for older adults (Murphy et al., 2006), and most likely for people listening in their second language (L2). Difficulties experienced by older adults could reflect age-related declines in the auditory, cognitive, and/or linguistic processes supporting spoken language comprehension. Age related changes occurring at different levels of the auditory system (e.g., elevated hearing thresholds, loss of neural synchrony, see Schneider, 1997; Schneider and Pichora-Fuller, 2000 for reviews), may also be accompanied by age-related changes in the cognitive processes related to speech comprehension. The cognitive aging literature notes that there are age-related reductions in the ability to focus attention and inhibit irrelevant sources (Hasher and Zacks, 1988; for a review, see Schneider et al., 2007), as well as evidence suggesting a general slowing of cognitive processing (e.g., Salthouse, 1996). Recent studies show that stream segregation may take a longer time to emerge in older adults than in younger adults in the presence of speech and speech-like maskers (Ben-David et al., 2012). In addition, although linguistic knowledge has been found to be relatively preserved in older age (Burke and Shafto, 2008), it is possible that under stressful and difficult listening situations, older adults may experience reduced capability to utilize their linguistic knowledge and skills in order to enhance speech comprehension because of age-related declines in executive functions (Clarys et al., 2009). Such age-related changes in auditory and cognitive processes may require a reorganization of the way information is processed in the brain. A number of studies have shown that older adults often engage different neural circuitry than that employed by younger adults when performing a task (Harris et al., 2009; Wong et al., 2009). Hence it is likely the relative contribution of different auditory and cognitive processes will be affected by aging (Schneider et al., 2010; Wingfield and Tun, 2007). One of the objectives of the current research is to determine how age, linguistic status, and the nature of the auditory scene differentially engage the perceptual and cognitive processes that contribute to speech comprehension.

A couple of relatively recent studies examined age-related changes in speech comprehension using longer and more complex tasks such as monologs and dialogs in order to gain a fuller understanding of the contribution of both the cognitive and perceptual processes involved in speech comprehension, and possible interactions among them. Schneider et al. (2000) asked both younger and older adults to listen to monologs and answer multiple-choice questions regarding their content at the end of each one. The results showed that age-related declines in the ability to process and remember a monolog could be eliminated when individual adjustments are made to compensate for speech recognition thresholds in younger and older listeners. Murphy et al. (2006) adapted Schneider et al.'s methodology to study the ability of younger and older adults to follow two-talker conversations instead of single-talker monologs. They selected a series of engaging one-act plays, each involving dialog between two characters of the same gender. Participants listened to the dialogs either in quiet or in a background of multi-talker babble noise. After listening to a 10–15 min dialog, participants answered a set of 10 multiple-choice questions that tested their comprehension and/or memory of details about the conversation. In Experiments 1–3, the talkers were separated by 9° or 45° azimuth in order to simulate a typical conversation between two talkers who necessarily have different spatial locations. However, in a control experiment, no such spatial separation was present (equivalent to a radio play). Their results indicated that older adults were able to answer fewer questions than younger adults in this listening-to-conversation task when both age groups were tested under identical stimulus conditions (Experiment 1) and that this age difference could be reduced but not eliminated when the listening situation is adjusted to make it equally difficult for younger and older adults to hear individual words when the two talkers are spatially separated (Experiments 2 and 3). The results of their last experiment (Experiment 4) showed that the age effect could be eliminated when listening situations were individually adjusted and there was no spatial separation present between talkers.

These results provided some evidence that older adults are indeed less skilled than younger adults at extracting and remembering information from a two-person conversation if adjustments have not been made for their poorer speech recognition thresholds. In addition, the consistent age difference, which was found as long as spatial separation between the two talkers was present, even after compensations had been made for the older listeners' deficits in hearing individual words, suggests that older adults might not be able to benefit as much from the full range of acoustic cues available with real spatial separation. A number of studies have shown that the improvement in speech reception thresholds that occurs when targets and maskers are spatially-separated rather than co-located, is significantly larger for young normal-hearing adults than for older, hearing-impaired adults (Neher et al., 2011). This inability of older and/or hearing-impaired adults to benefit from spatial separation could make it more difficult for them to establish and maintain stream segregation. In turn, increased stream segregation difficulties are likely to reduce the fidelity of the bottom-up, acoustic information, thereby requiring a greater degree of attentional investment at the perceptual level (Neher et al., 2009). As a result a change in the balance between the contributions of bottom-up vs. top-down processes may occur to compensate for the loss of fidelity in the neural representation of the acoustic signal. It is reasonable to assume that as a result of the changes mentioned, more weight will be given to top-down processes as the use of bottom-up information becomes limited. In particular, when there is interference with the bottom-up, stimulus-driven processes leading to lexical access, the listener may come to depend more on those top-down processes, such as vocabulary knowledge, that could be used to aid lexical access. Hence we might expect to find the correlation between vocabulary knowledge and speech comprehension to increase as the auditory scene becomes more complex. In addition, the deployment of attentional resources to aid lexical access could make it more difficult for listeners to engage higher-order modality-independent processes (such as those involved in reading comprehension) to help them to understand and retain what they have heard. However, to our knowledge, there have been no attempts to investigate the degree to which listening difficulties alter the relative balance between bottom-up and top-down processing in ecologically-valid listening situations, nor have there been attempts to determine the degree to which the contribution of different levels of processing to speech comprehension in such situations are modulated by the characteristics of the auditory scene, and the age and linguistic competence of the listener.

In order to further explore the sources of the age difference in the ability to comprehend and recall a dialog when two talkers are spatially separated, we used the precedence effect to change the virtual location of each talker. A number of studies have shown that if the same sound is played over two loudspeakers located to the left and right of the listener, with the sound on the left loudspeaker lagging behind that on the right, the listener perceives the sound as emanating from the right and vice versa (e.g., Rakerd et al., 2006). Because the sound is played over both loudspeakers, a virtual spatial separation is achieved without altering the SNR at each ear. Hence a perceived spatial separation can be achieved even though there is a substantial reduction in the auditory cues supporting spatial separation (e.g., no head shadow effect). Moreover, Cranford et al. (1990) have shown that when the precedence effect is used to specify the virtual locations of sounds, both younger and older adults experienced the sound as emanating from the side where the leading loudspeaker was positioned The precedence effect has been used in a number of studies related to informational masking as a way of achieving a perceived (virtual) separation between sound sources without substantially affecting the SNR at each ear of the listener (e.g., Freyman et al., 1999; Li et al., 2004) and it has been shown that both younger and older adults reap the same degree of benefit from perceived separation (Li et al., 2004). However, using the precedence effect to achieve and maintain a virtual spatial separation among sound sources may require that a larger proportion of attentional resources be allocated to stream segregation since the sound sources under the precedence effect are perceived as more diffuse and cannot be precisely located in space. This, in turn, may alter the balance between the top-down and bottom-up processes involved in speech recognition.

Nonnative listeners also constitute a group that experiences considerable difficulty when attempting to follow a conversation in their second language (L2) in the presence of background noise. Nonnative young listeners are not likely to differ from native young listeners using their first language (L1) with respect to basic auditory and cognitive abilities. However, nonnative listeners of a language tend to have lower scores than native listeners on a number of speech-perception measures (Mayo et al., 1997; Bradlow and Pisoni, 1999; Meador et al., 2000; Bradlow and Bent, 2002; Cooke et al., 2008; Rogers and Lopez, 2008; Ezzatian et al., 2010). This difference in performance is influenced by several factors, such as duration of exposure to L2, degree of similarity between L1 and L2, knowledge of the L2 vocabulary and grammatical structure, frequency and extent of L2 use, etc. The acoustic–phonetic characteristics of a second language, which was acquired or learned at a later age than their L1, may not be fully acquired (e.g., Florentine, 1985; Mayo et al., 1997), resulting in a reduced ability to discriminate fine phonemic information, such as phonetic contrasts and phonemic categories which are crucial for successful speech perception (Bradlow and Pisoni, 1999; Meador et al., 2000). In regard to listening in noise, previous literature on young nonnative listeners suggests that nonnative listeners are less able to make use of a language mismatch between masking and target stimuli to facilitate masking release (Brouwer et al., 2012). In the case of nonnative listeners, it is reasonable to assume that the difficulties they experience in L2 environments may be due to the fact their L2 semantic and linguistic processes may not be completely differentiated from the semantic and syntactic processes that are usually invoked when listening in their L1 (Kroll and Steward, 1994).

In the current study we choose to further explore the effect of age and linguistic status on the ability to successfully follow a two-talker conversation (dialog) conducted in a babble background noise with the locations of the sound sources being either virtual or real, and with the two talkers being spatially separated or co-located. Native-English younger and older listeners and young nonnative-English listeners were asked to listen to conversations played against a babble background noise and to answer questions regarding their content. Individual hearing differences were compensated for by creating the same degree of difficulty in identifying individual words in a babble background when there was little or no contextual support for word recognition. Two measures of individual differences in linguistic competence were included; a measure of vocabulary knowledge (the Mill Hill; Raven, 1965) and a measure of reading comprehension skill (the Nelson-Denny; Brown et al., 1981)[1]. If listening difficulty, linguistic status, or age alters the relative contribution of bottom-up and top-down processes, and differentially affects the various stages in the speech processing network, we might expect that the degree to which these two factors are correlated with the ability

[1]These two measures were chosen to tap two different levels of linguistic and cognitive competence. We might expect a vocabulary measure to be related to processes involved with lexical access, whereas reading comprehension would likely tap additional higher-order modality independent processes involved in language comprehension. Other, more specific cognitive and linguistic skills could also be investigated in future studies.

to comprehend and remember dialogs to vary across groups and listening conditions.

MATERIALS AND METHODS

PARTICIPANTS

The participants were 24 normal hearing younger adults who are native-English listeners (mean age: 21.26 years; *SD*: 3.02), 24 normal hearing older adults who are native–English listeners (mean age: 69.7 years; *SD*: 4.6), and 24 normal hearing young adults who are nonnative-English listeners (mean age: 21.04 years; *SD*: 1.71). Native-English listeners were all born and raised in a country in which the primary language was English and were not fluent in any other language at the time of participation. Nonnative-English listeners were those who first became immersed in an English speaking environment after the age of 14. One older listener, who found the noisy background in the study to be uncomfortable, withdrew from the experiment and had to be replaced. The young participants were volunteers recruited from the students and staff at the University of Toronto Mississauga. The older participants were volunteers from the local community. All participants were asked to complete a questionnaire regarding their general health, hearing, vision, and cognitive status. Only participants who reported that they were in good health and had no history of serious pathology (e.g., stroke, head injury, neurological disease, seizures, and the like) were included. All participants reported having a normal or corrected vision and were asked to use their correcting lenses when necessary. None of the participants had any history of hearing disorders, and none used hearing aids. The studies reported here were approved by the Ethics Review Board of the University of Toronto.

During each participant's first session at the lab we administrated audiometric thresholds, the Nelson-Denny reading comprehension test (Brown et al., 1981) and the Mill Hill test of vocabulary knowledge (Raven, 1965). The dialogs, along with the babble thresholds and the low-context R-SPIN thresholds were administered over the next two experimental sessions (three dialogs per session). Tests were administered in a double-walled sound-attenuating chamber. All participants were paid $10/h for their participation.

HEARING MEASURES

Audiometric testing

Pure-tone air-conduction thresholds were measured at nine frequencies (0.25–8 kHz) for both ears using an Interacoustics Model AC5 audiometer (Interacoustic, Assens, Denmark). All younger participants were required to have pure tone air-conduction thresholds 15 dB HL or lower, between 0.25 and 8 kHz in both ears. Young participants with a threshold of 20 dB HL at a single frequency were not excluded from the study. Older participants were required to have a pure tone thresholds 25 dB HL or lower from 0.25 to 3 kHz and 35 dB HL or lower for frequencies <6 kHz. Participants who demonstrated unbalanced hearing (more than a 15 dB difference between ears under one or more frequencies) were excluded from participation. Older adults with hearing in the range described are usually considered to have normal hearing for their age. However, it is acknowledged that older adults' hearing changes and deteriorates with age and is not equivalent to that of younger adults (Wingfield et al., 1985; Fitzgibbons and Gordon-Salant, 1996; Wingfield, 1996; Schneider and Pichora-Fuller, 2001; Glyde et al., 2011). The average audiograms for the three groups of participants are shown for the right and the left ears in **Figure 1**. The two groups of young adults had equivalent hearing levels at all frequencies. Hearing levels for older adults were about 7 dB poorer than those of the younger adults at frequencies ≤3 kHz, with the younger-older difference increasing as a function of frequency for frequencies >3 kHz.

Babble threshold test

The adaptive two-interval forced choice procedure employed by Schneider et al. (2000) was used to measure individual detection thresholds for the 12-talker babble masker used in this experiment. In this procedure, a 1.5 s babble segment was randomly presented in one of two intervals which were separated by a 1.5-s silent period. Two lights on the button box indicated the occurrence of each interval, and the listener's task was to identify the interval containing the babble segment by pressing the corresponding button. Immediate feedback was provided after each press. We used an adaptive two down one up procedure (Levitt, 1971) to determine the babble threshold corresponding to the 79% point on the psychometric function. Two different babble thresholds were determined for each individual. First, a babble threshold was determined when the babble was presented over a single central loudspeaker. The sound levels of the speech signals for the condition in which the voices of both talkers were presented only over the central loudspeaker (no separation, single loudspeaker condition) were individually set to be 45 dB above this babble threshold (sensation level, SL, of 45 dB). A second babble threshold was determined when the babble was played simultaneously over two loudspeakers located 45° to the right and left of the listeners. This babble threshold was used to adjust the intensity of speech signal to 45 dBSL for the conditions in which voices were presented over both lateral loudspeakers. For a graphic illustration of the two babble conditions see **Figure 2**, first column on the left.

R-SPIN test

In this test participants are asked to immediately repeat the last word of individual sentences presented to them in a multi-talker

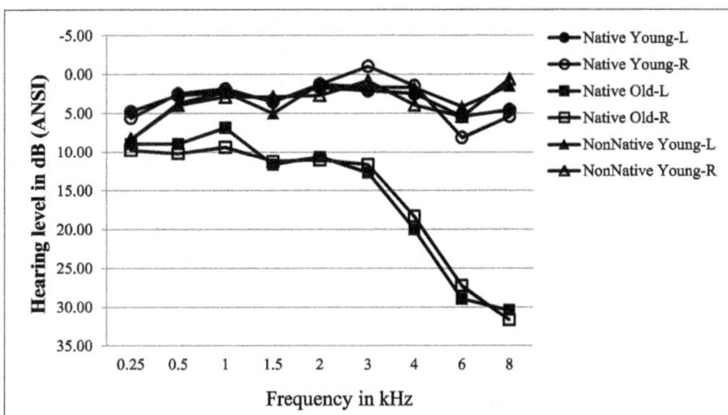

FIGURE 1 | Average audiograms for the three groups of participants are shown for the right and the left ears. ANSI, American National Standards Institute.

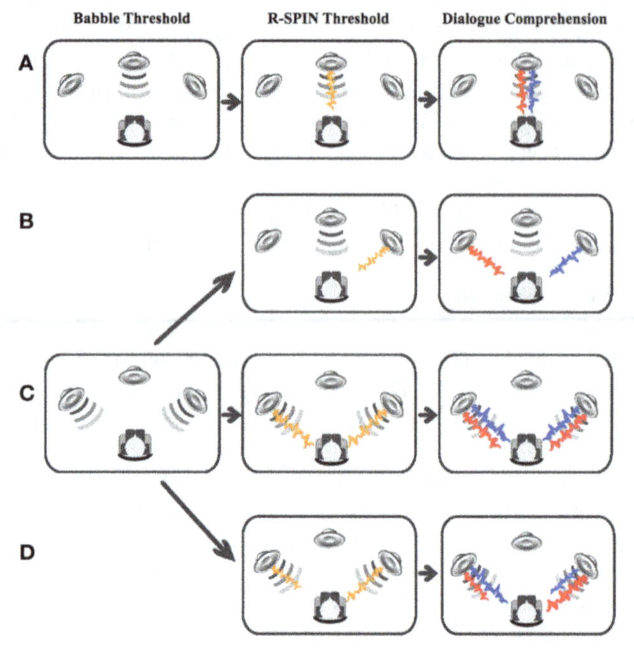

FIGURE 2 | The left column specifies the two babble thresholds collected, and under what conditions they were used to adjust the signal level; the middle column specifies the conditions under which R-SPIN thresholds were obtained; and the right column illustrates the four dialog comprehension test conditions in the experiment. The top row **(A)** specifies the babble, R-SPIN and dialog comprehension scenarios for the real no-separation condition. The three other conditions share the same babble threshold but differ from each other in respect to the R-SPIN and the dialog comprehension tasks. The second row from the top **(B)** illustrates the R-SPIN and dialog comprehension for the real spatial separation condition, the third row **(C)** illustrates the settings for the virtual no-separation and the fourth **(D)** specifies the settings for the virtual spatial separation. Orange stands for R-SPIN, red stands for talker 1, blue for talker 2, and gray for babble.

babble background. As in Schneider et al. (2000) and Murphy et al. (2006), we used the Revised Speech Perception in Noise (R-SPIN) test (Bilger et al., 1984) to individually determine the SNR producing 50% correct identification of final words of low-context sentences (e.g., Jane was thinking about the van.) presented in multitalker babble under both real and virtual location conditions. In the real no-separation condition, both the babble and R-SPIN sentences were played over the central loudspeaker. In the real separation conditions, the babble was presented over the central loudspeaker and the R-SPIN sentences were presented over the right loudspeaker. In the virtual no separation condition, both the babble and R-SPIN sentences were presented simultaneously over both loudspeakers. In the virtual separation conditions the babble was presented over both lateral loudspeakers simultaneously with the R-SPIN sentences also presented over both loudspeakers but with the sentences presented over the right loudspeaker leading the sentences presented over the left loudspeaker by 3 ms. Hence R-SPIN thresholds were determined for each of the conditions under which participants were tested. The R-SPIN thresholds estimated were rounded to units of 1 dB before being integrated into the calculation of the individually adjusted SNR which was used for presentation of the dialogs. If the estimated R-SPIN threshold was calculated to be exactly half way between two integer values rounding was conducted toward alleviating the SNR difficulty (e.g., 3.5 dB SNR was rounded to 4 dB SNR and −3.5 dB SNR to −3 dB SNR). For a graphic illustration of the four R-SPIN conditions see **Figure 2**, second column from the left.

Dialog comprehension task

Each participant was asked to listen to six dialogs presented in babble noise in a sound-attenuating chamber. These dialogs were created and previously used by Murphy et al. (2006). Each dialog was based on a published one-act play and had only two characters; in three of the six dialogs, the two characters were female, and in the other three, the two characters were male. At the end of each dialog, which was 10–15 min long, the participant was presented with a series of 10 multiple-choice questions regarding the contents of that dialog (for more information regarding the dialogs and the questions see Murphy et al., 2006). There were four conditions in the experiment: (a) Real spatial separation with the babble presented over the central loudspeaker, with the voice of one of the talkers presented over the left loudspeaker, and the voice of the other talker presented over the right loudspeaker; (b) Real, no spatial separation, with the babble, and the voices of the two talkers presented over the central loudspeaker only; (c) Virtual no spatial separation with the babble and two voices being played simultaneously over both lateral loudspeakers; (d) Virtual spatial separation with the babble presented simultaneously over both lateral loudspeakers, and the two voices also presented over both lateral loudspeakers with the perceived location of the two talkers manipulated using the precedence effect (the voice of talker one over the left loudspeaker playing 3 ms in advance over the same voice playing over the right loudspeaker, with the opposite timing arrangement for the second voice). For a graphic illustration of the four dialog comprehension conditions, see **Figure 2** rightmost column. Half of the participants were tested in conditions a and c (separation conditions), the other half in conditions b and d (no separation conditions). Hence in this design, virtual vs. real location was a within-subject factor and spatial location was a between-subjects factor. The participants in each group were randomly assigned to one of the two spatial location conditions. The dialogs were presented in babble at an SNR which was individually adjusted per participant and condition based on his or her babble threshold and R-SPIN results according to the following calculations:

Dialogs were presented at babble threshold + 45 dB; Babble was presented at babble threshold + 45 dB − R-SPIN threshold + 21 dB.

At the end of each dialog, participants were asked to answer a set of 10 multiple-choice questions with four alternatives that were also constructed and previously used by Murphy et al. (2006). Each question referred to a specific item of information that was mentioned explicitly only once during the dialog.

LANGUAGE PROFICIENCY MEASURES

Vocabulary knowledge

Participants were asked to complete the Mill Hill vocabulary test (Raven, 1965), which is a 20-item synonym test. In this test participants were required to match each test item with its closest synonym from six listed alternatives. No time restrains were applied. The extent of a person's vocabulary represents knowledge that can be used to facilitate word recognition. When listening becomes difficult, and the fidelity of the bottom-up information contributing to word identification becomes questionable, we might expect the role played by top-down knowledge (e.g., the extent of an individual's vocabulary) to increase. Hence we might expect the correlation between vocabulary knowledge and the number of dialog questions correctly answered to increase with listening difficulty.

Reading comprehension skill

The Nelson-Denny test (Brown et al., 1981) was used to assess the reading comprehension skills of each participant. In this test the participants had to read through a series of eight independent passages and answer multiple-choice questions regarding the content of the passages. This test includes a total of 36 questions and was limited to 20 min. Participants were instructed to complete as many questions as possible within the time given.

The six dialogs were administered over two sessions, three dialogs per session. Sessions were typically 1.5–2 h in duration and were completed within 2 weeks.

RESULTS

Table 1 presents the gender breakdown, mean age, educational level, Mill Hill test of vocabulary knowledge and Nelson-Denny test of reading comprehension results for each age group. One of the nonnative-English listeners had an R-SPIN threshold of 22 dB SNR in the virtual no separation condition. Since this value was more than three standard deviations above the mean for that group, this value was identified as an outlier and was replaced by the average R-SPIN threshold of the nonnative-English listeners group after excluding the outlier (6 dB SNR)[2].

R-SPIN THRESHOLDS

Figure 3 plots the average 50% correct R-SPIN thresholds (dB) as a function of separation condition and group for the native-English younger listeners (dotted rectangles), the native-English older listeners (lined rectangles), and the nonnative-English young listeners (solid rectangles). The SNR levels required for 50% correct repetition of the last word in low-context sentences was highest when there was no spatial separation vs. when there was a separation between the target sentences and the babble background, and were on average lower for real than for virtual locations. The R-SPIN thresholds also appear to be higher for young nonnative-English listeners than for older native-English listeners, who, in turn, had higher thresholds than the younger native listeners. In addition, the advantage due to spatial separation is larger when spatial location is real than when it is virtual. The benefit of separation over no separation on average was larger

Table 1 | Demographic information (Mean Age and Years of Education, Gender Distribution, Mean Vocabulary, and Reading Comprehension Scores) and Mean Babble and R-SPIN thresholds for the participants in the two separation conditions divided into the three groups tested.

	Separation con.							No-separation con.						
	Younger natives		Older natives		Young nonnatives		$p < 0.05$	Younger natives		Older natives		Young nonnatives		$p < 0.05$
	M	*SD*	*M*	*SD*	*M*	*SD*		*M*	*SD*	*M*	*SD*	*M*	*SD*	
Age	21.09	2.17	68.83	3.33	21.33	1.50	A, C	21.42	2.19	70.58	5.20	20.75	1.91	A, C
Education	15.58	2.27	15.85	2.44	14.67	1.50		16.17	2.29	14.58	2.39	14.25	1.48	B
Gender	10 F + 2 M		11 F + 1 M		9 F + 3 M			10 F + 2 M		7 F + 5 M		9 F + 3 M		
Vocabulary (max = 20)	13.25	2.34	15.00	1.35	8.58	2.11	A, B,C	14.33	1.23	15.25	2.22	9.17	3.64	B, C
Reading comprehension (max = 36)	26.33	7.13	19.92	3.90	18.08	5.73	A, B	24.42	4.87	22.92	7.59	15.83	7.27	B, C
Babble threshold from central loudspeaker (dB SPL)								9.82	3.24	15.72	6.70	10.41	2.60	A, C
Babble threshold from lateral loudspeakers (dB SPL)	5.23	1.47	11.68	4.02	6.40	3.08	A, C	6.19	3.13	11.91	7.48	6.27	2.92	A, C
R-SPIN threshold for real condition (dB)	−3.76	2.65	−1.52	2.29	−0.66	2.51	A, B	1.86	1.56	2.32	1.56	6.54	2.87	B, C
R-SPIN threshold for virtual condition (dB)	−1.40	1.62	1.30	1.40	4.13	1.72	A, B, C	1.36	0.92	1.92	1.47	7.29	4.72	B, C

Statistically significant differences between groups are noted.

Max, maximum; dB, decibel; SPL, sound pressure level; R-SPIN, Revised Speech Perception in Noise.

A, A statistically significant difference between Younger Native-English and Older Native-English listeners.

B, A statistically significant difference between Younger Native-English and Young Nonnative-English listeners.

C, A statistically significant difference between Older Native-English and Young Nonnative-English listeners.

[2] Analyses were done for both the R-SPIN thresholds and the number of correct answers, in which the participant was excluded completely. All the results which were statistically significant in the analyses reported in this paper remained significant and all the results which were statistically insignificant remained as such. We have chosen to replace this one data point with the group average in order to minimize the loss of data.

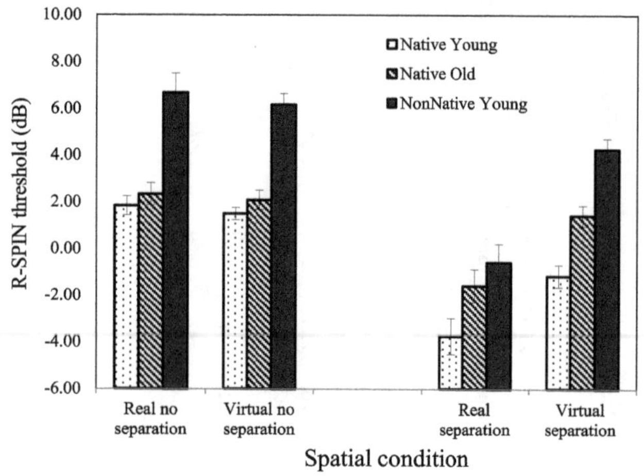

FIGURE 3 | Average R-SPIN thresholds (dB) calculated under each of the four spatial conditions. Standard error bars are shown.

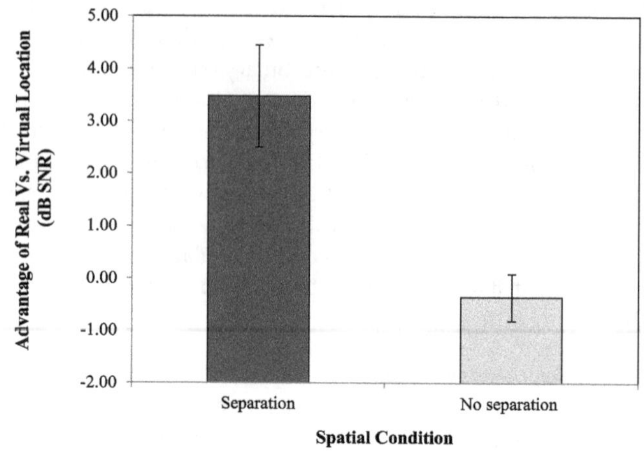

FIGURE 4 | Average advantage of real vs. virtual location cues (R-Spin threshold virtual—R-SPIN threshold real) for the two types of separation (target sentences and babble separated vs. co-located). Standard error bars are shown.

for the young nonnative-English listeners (5.18 dB) than both the younger (4.2 dB) and older natives-English listeners (2.18 dB).

A repeated measures ANOVA with two separation conditions (yes/no) and three groups (younger and older native-English listeners and young nonnative-English listeners) as between-subjects factors, and with the two types of spatial location (real/virtual) as a within-subject factor confirmed this description, showing a significant main effect of Separation Condition [$F_{(1, 66)} = 97.613$, $p < 0.000$], Group [$F_{(2, 66)} = 51.539$, $p < 0.000$] and Type of Location [real vs. virtual; $F_{(1, 66)} = 30.451$, $p < 0.000$] as well as a two-way Group by Separation interaction [$F_{(2, 66)} = 3.559$, $p = 0.034$] and a Type of Location by Separation interaction [$F_{(1, 66)} = 46.367$, $p < 0.000$]. No other effects were significant. *Post-hoc* tests with Sidak adjustment found that all three groups differed significantly from one another ($p < 0.005$ for all three pairwise comparisons).

To better illustrate the nature of the Separation by Type of Location interaction, **Figure 4** shows the advantage of real vs. virtual location cues (R-Spin threshold virtual—R-SPIN threshold real) for the two types of separation (target sentence and babble separated vs. co-located). This figure clearly indicates the advantage of real over virtual location is larger when the target sentence and babble were perceived to be spatially separated than when they were perceived to be co-located.

Figure 5 suggests that the Group by Separation interaction is due to the fact that the benefit due to spatial separation is smaller for older native listeners than either of the younger groups. An examination of the group by spatial separation interaction for older vs. younger native listeners found the benefit due to spatial separation to be significantly smaller for older natives than for younger natives [Group × Separation interaction: $F_{(1, 44)} = 6.127$, $p = 0.017$]. The Group × Separation interaction was also significant when the two groups were older natives and young nonnatives [$F_{(1, 44)} = 4.927$, $p = 0.032$], but not when young native listeners were compared to young nonnative listeners [$F_{(1, 44)} < 1$]. **Figure 5** also suggests that when there is no separation, the R-SPIN thresholds are equivalent for both younger and

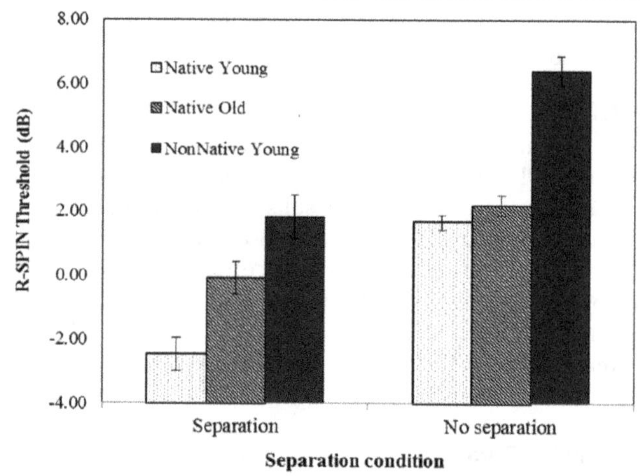

FIGURE 5 | Average R-SPIN thresholds (dB) calculated under each of the two spatial location conditions for each of the three groups. Error bars are shown.

older native listeners. A separate ANOVA on the no-separation condition revealed a significant effect of group [$F_{(2, 32)} = 38.154$, $p < 0.001$] with *post-hoc* tests with Sidak adjustment indicating that the nonnative English listeners differed significantly from both native groups ($p < 0.001$ in both cases) but that that the younger and older native English listeners did not differ significantly from one another. A comparable analysis of the data from the Separation Condition revealed a significant Group effect [$F_{(2, 33)} = 20.842$, $p < 0.001$] with the *post-hoc* tests with Sidak adjustment revealing that all three groups differed significantly from one another ($p < 0.03$ for all pairwise comparisons).

DIALOG COMPREHENSION RESULTS

The main finding of interest was that once the SNR levels were adjusted based on the R-SPIN results, only small differences were found between the three groups tested in the amount of questions correctly answered (see **Figure 6**). In general the native-English young listeners seemed to perform slightly better than either the native-English older listeners or the nonnative-English young listeners. However, a 2-within-subject (real vs. virtual) × 2-between-subject (separation vs. no-separation) by 3-between-subject (younger and older native-English listeners, nonnative-English young listeners) ANOVA revealed only a significant main effect of Separation [$F_{(1, 66)} = 4.671$, $p = 0.034$] with performance being better when the voices were separated rather than co-located.

THE CONTRIBUTION OF VOCABULARY KNOWLEDGE AND READING COMPREHENSION TO DIALOG COMPREHENSION

We explored the degree to which the different levels of the factors (Separation, Group and Type of Location) were differentially associated with individual differences in vocabulary knowledge and in reading comprehension skill. First we examined whether individual differences in vocabulary knowledge were more predictive of the number of dialog comprehension questions answered correctly when the cues to spatial location were real, as opposed to virtual. **Figure 7** relates the percentage of questions correctly answered as a function of vocabulary score separately for the virtual location conditions (upper panel), and the real location conditions (lower panel). In this figure, the vocabulary scores were first centered within each group of participants to normalize the vocabulary scores across the six groups of participants. Percent correct answers were also normalized within each of the 12 conditions in the experiment to eliminate the contribution of any residual effects of conditions on performance. Before conducting these regression analyses, we first removed any effect that individual differences in reading comprehension had on performance (see Appendix A). This allowed us to evaluate the effects of individual differences in vocabulary once the effects of reading comprehension on performance had been removed. **Figure 7** shows that slope of the line relating percent correct to vocabulary knowledge is considerably higher for virtual location than real location. A regression analysis (see Appendix A) found vocabulary knowledge to be significantly related to dialog comprehension for the virtual conditions but not for the real location conditions, with the difference in correlation between the two (the interaction between vocabulary and Type of Location) also being significant [$F_{(1, 142)} = 4.70$, $p = 0.03$]. However, similar regression analyses failed to find any evidence that the relationship of vocabulary knowledge to percent correct differed between the no-separation conditions and the separation conditions, or among the three groups of participants (native-English younger listeners, native-English older listeners, and nonnative-English young listeners).

A similar analysis was conducted to examine the contribution of reading comprehension skill to dialog comprehension. In particular, before evaluating the contribution of reading comprehension to performance, we first moved any effect that individual differences in vocabulary had on performance. The results of this analysis indicated that the contribution of reading comprehension skill to dialog comprehension did not differ between the virtual and real location conditions, nor did the contribution

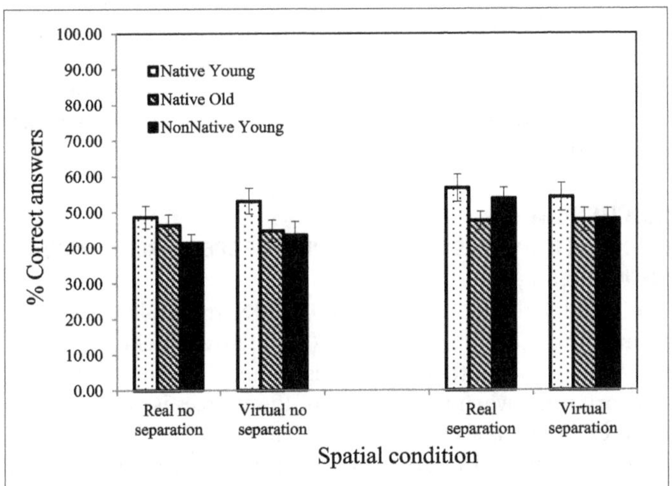

FIGURE 6 | Average percentage of correctly answered questions calculated under each of the four spatial conditions for each of the three groups. Error bars are shown.

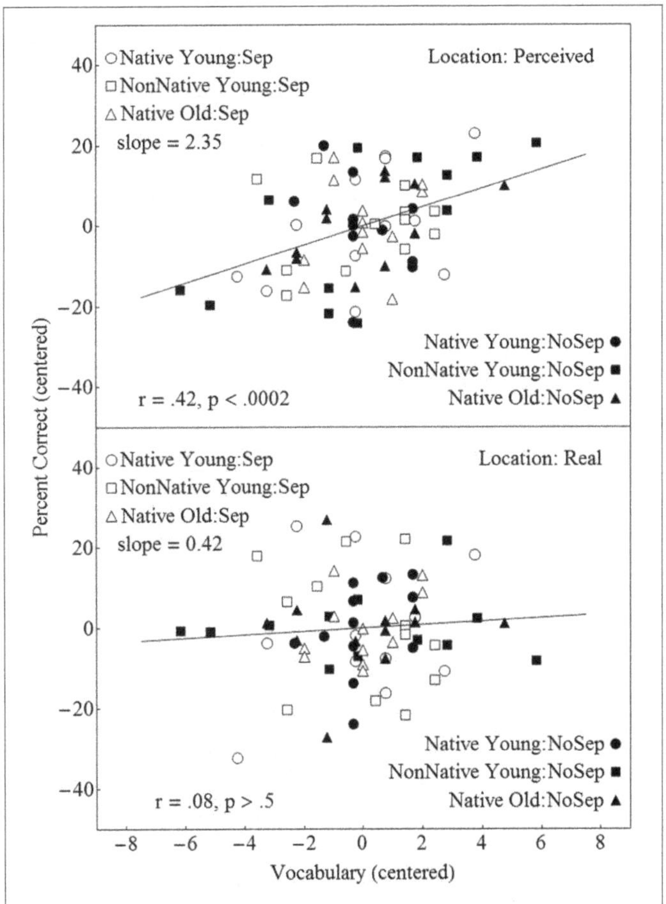

FIGURE 7 | Percentage of correctly answered dialog questions plotted against the individual performance on the Mill Hill vocabulary test after the contribution of reading comprehension to performance had been removed. Both the adjusted number of questions answered and the Mill Hill scores are centered within each group. A least squares regressions line is presented for each of the two types of location.

differ between the no-separation and separation conditions. However, the contribution of reading comprehension skill to performance on the dialog comprehension task did differ across the three groups. **Figure 8** shows that reading comprehension was positively correlated with performance for the native-English younger listeners only. A regression analysis (see Appendix A) indicated that the strength of the relationship differed among the three groups, with Bonferroni—corrected pairwise comparisons confirming that the slopes differed significantly between young native-English and nonnative-English listeners.

We also examined whether either the vocabulary scores or the reading comprehension scores were related to R-SPIN in each of the 12 conditions (3 Groups × 2 Spatial Locations × 2 Types of Location). Similar analyses to those conducted for the percentage of correctly answered dialog questions failed to find any evidence that either vocabulary knowledge or reading comprehension skill could account for individual differences in the R-SPIN threshold values.

COMPARISON OF CURRENT DATA TO PREVIOUS DATA

Two of the conditions in the current study replicate two similar conditions which were found in the Murphy et al. (2006) study. In both the Murphy et al. and the current study, younger and older native-English listeners were volunteers recruited from the University Community and local neighborhood community, respectively. No nonnative-English listeners were tested in Murphy et al. The real separation condition in the present study is comparable to the high babble noise condition where the dialogs were presented from loudspeakers at 45° azimuth in Experiment 3 of Murphy et al. and the real no spatial separation condition replicates the condition in which the dialogs were presented once the spatial separation was removed in the last experiment reported (experiment 4) by Murphy et al. The R-SPIN thresholds and the dialog comprehension results of these two comparable conditions from both studies were analyzed separately using a Univariate Analysis of Variance with Age, Experiment and Separation as between-subjects variables. The results of this analysis revealed a significant main effect of Age [$F_{(7,\,88)} = 4.296$, $p = 0.041$] but not of Experiment [$F_{(1,\,88)} = 0.963$, $p = 0.329$] nor Separation [$F_{(1,\,88)} = 0.210$, $p = 0.648$] on dialog comprehension performance. In addition there were no significant two- or three-way interactions among these three factors. Hence there is no evidence that the participants in this experiment differed in performance from those in Murphy et al.

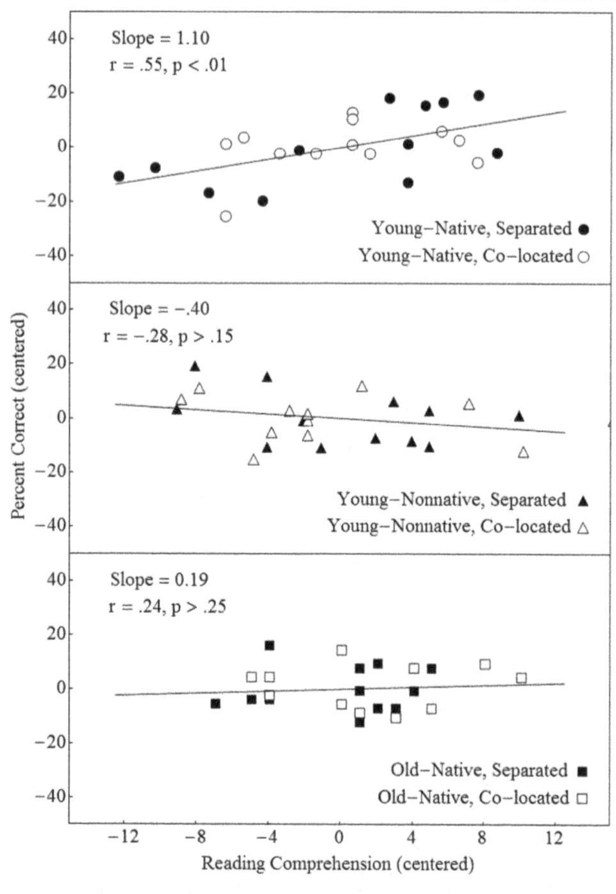

FIGURE 8 | Percentage of correctly answered dialog questions plotted against the individual performance on the Nelson-Denny reading comprehension test after the contribution of vocabulary to performance had been removed. Both the adjusted number of questions answered and the Nelson Denny scores are centered within each group. A least squares regressions line is presented for each of the three groups.

A similar analysis which compared the R-SPIN thresholds calculated under the two comparable conditions in the two studies showed a significant effect of Age [$F_{(1,\,88)} = 125.94, p < 0.001$] and Separation [$F_{(1,\,88)} = 504.45$, $p < 0.001$]. As for the dialog comprehension performance, no significant effect of Experiment was found [$F_{(1,\,88)} = 0.089$, $p = 0.89$], however a significant interaction was found between Age and Experiment [$F_{(1,\,88)} = 21.4$, $p = 0.039$]. The latter interaction is probably a result of the younger adults in the current study performing slightly worse than the younger adults who participated in Murphy et al. and the older adults in the current study performing slightly better than the older adults who participated in Murphy et al. when there was no spatial separation. Overall, the evidence suggests that the current study successfully replicated the study conducted by Murphy et al. (2006) in regard to the two comparable conditions, and that participants in this study did not differ significantly from the participants in Murphy et al. with respect to their performance in both the dialog comprehension task and the R-SPIN word recognition task in those conditions which were comparable across the two experiments.

DISCUSSION

USING THE R-SPIN RESULTS AS AN INDEX OF SPEECH RECOGNITION DIFFICULTIES

The R-SPIN results indicate that R-SPIN thresholds are lower for real than for virtual location (see **Figure 3**). This is consistent with the hypothesis that it is more difficult to parse the auditory scene when the location of the sources is virtual rather than real. There is also evidence (see **Figure 4**) that the advantage of real over virtual location of stimuli is considerably larger in the presence of spatial separation. The R-SPIN results also indicate that nonnative-English young listeners and native-English older listeners find it more difficult to recognize words in babble than young native-English listeners (see **Figure 3**). Moreover the results show that older adults benefit less from spatial separation than native-English and nonnative-English younger listeners (see **Figure 5**).

The results also show that when the target sentence and babble appear to be co-located, younger and older native-English listeners have similar R-SPIN thresholds that are significantly lower than those of the nonnative-English listeners. However, when the target sentences and the babble are perceived to be separated younger native-English listeners have significantly lower thresholds than the older natives-English listeners, who, in turn, have lower thresholds than the nonnative-English listeners. This suggests that when target and masker are co-located, normal-hearing older, and younger native-English listeners do not differ with respect to speech recognition in a background of babble, but that both groups have lower speech-recognition thresholds than do young nonnative-English listeners. However, speech recognition in the presence of spatial separation is better for younger than for older native-English listeners.

Overall, the results of the R-SPIN word recognition task show that when there are cues to spatially separate the target from the masker, word recognition in older native-English listeners and young nonnnative-English listeners is inferior to that of younger native-English listeners. When listeners of those two groups attempt to communicate in real-life situations where sound sources are often spatially separated, they will experience greater difficulty with respect to word recognition. In older native-English listeners, this increased difficulty most likely is due to the reduction in the quality of the bottom-up information leading to word recognition. In young nonnative-English listeners, difficulties in word recognition are likely due to the increased difficulty they experience in segregating language streams in their L2 (Cooke et al., 2008; Ezzatian et al., 2010).

DIALOG COMPREHENSION RESULTS

The dialog comprehension results demonstrated that when R-SPIN thresholds were used to adjust for individual differences in the ability to recognize words without supportive context, no effects due to Type of Location (real vs. virtual), or Group (young native-English listeners, older native-English listeners, young nonnative-English listeners) were found. However, the main effect of Separation was significant even though the SNRs were adjusted based on the R-SPIN thresholds. Listeners on average performed significantly better under spatial separation conditions than when sources were co-located. This suggests that spatial separation (real or perceived) facilitates the comprehension and retention of information obtained from the dialogs even when lexical access is presumably equated across the co-located and spatially separated conditions using the R-SPIN adjustment procedure. For example, spatial separation between the talkers may facilitate the association of the incoming information with a specific talker as well as facilitate its retention. However, it is not possible to determine from the present data the precise mechanisms responsible for this spatial separation effect. One possible reason why the R-SPIN adjustment in the spatial separation condition did not eliminate the Separation effect in the dialogs might be that R-SPIN thresholds were determined for a single voice emanating from the right of the listener with the babble occupying a central location. In the separation condition for the dialogs, however, a voice could be on the left or right depending on who was speaking, with the babble emanating from the center. Hence, spatial separation in the dialog condition could have facilitated switching attention back and forth from the right to left depending on who was speaking. The fact that the R-SPIN test did not require the listener to switch attention from one side to other may explain why it was not successful in eliminating the Separation effect in the dialog portion of this study.

The results from the younger and older adults in the real location conditions of the present study were found to be consistent with the results from the equivalent conditions in the Murphy et al. (2006) study. The age difference found when we combined the real location conditions of these two studies supports the hypothesis that older adults might not be as good as younger adult at using the full range of interaural cues to either obtain or maintain stream segregation when sources are separated in space. Older adults frequently need to communicate in multi-talker daily situations taking place in a noisy environment, and naturally they have to do so without any SNR adjustments to accommodate for any individual age-related changes in hearing. The results described here emphasize the notion that in addition to age related difficulties in word recognition, older adults might have a limited toolbox of acoustic cues to assist them when attempting to meet a speech comprehension challenge in real-life situations (e.g., listening to a movie in a surround sound environment). This reduction in the ability to benefit from the acoustic cues provided by physical separation among sound sources is likely to have even greater implications in the presence of a hearing impairment (Neher et al., 2009).

THE RELATIONSHIP BETWEEN AGE, LINGUISTIC COMPETENCE, AND SPEECH COMPREHENSION PERFORMANCE

Given the differences in word recognition across groups and acoustic situations found in the current study, we might expect that different processes are differentially engaged in order to compensate for the specific individual deficits in word recognition when listening to dialog. To examine this we took the two measures of linguistic competence and looked to see the extent to which those measures were correlated with performance under each of the acoustic settings used in the current study. This examination, which was done for both the R-SPIN results as well as for the dialog comprehension results separately, can be used to help identify the relative importance of bottom-up and top-down influences on speech comprehension, and how the pattern of interactions among these factors are modulated by the nature of the acoustic scene.

Specifically, we looked at each of the six groups (12 younger natives in the separation condition; 12 younger native-English listeners in the no-separation condition; 12 young nonnative-English listeners in the separation condition; 12 young nonnative-English listeners in the no-separation condition; 12 older native-English listeners in the separation condition; and 12 older native-English listeners in the no-separation condition) to determine the contribution of the two linguistic measures to performance (number of questions correctly answered) within each group and condition (see Appendix A for further details). This analysis showed that both the vocabulary and the reading comprehension tests results were related to the average number of questions correctly answered ($r = 0.32$, $p = 0.007$, and $r = 0.38$, $p < 0.001$, for reading comprehension skill and vocabulary knowledge, respectively), but that these slopes did not differ across groups. More interestingly, the results of the analysis indicated that there was a significant correlation between vocabulary knowledge and the number of dialog questions correctly answered under the virtual location conditions but not under the real spatial location conditions (see **Figure 7**), and that this interaction between the Type of Location and Vocabulary was significant (the slopes of the lines differed significantly from each other). We would like to suggest a hypothesis which could explain this finding. An early stage in speech comprehension involves obtaining lexical access to the meaning of words. It has been shown that both bottom-up and top-down processes are involved in word recognition. We can hypothesize that the degree to which top-down processes are engaged in lexical access is modulated by acoustic factors. When listening is relatively easy, we might expect successful lexical access with minimal assistance from top-down processes. However, when listening becomes difficult, we might expect that the top-down processes involved with lexical access to be more fully engaged. When sources are located virtually in space using the precedence effect, they give the impression that their location is diffuse, and there are fewer acoustic cues that can be used to segregate the different acoustic streams than when source location is real (Freyman et al., 1999; Li et al., 2004). Therefore, it is reasonable to expect that under such conditions, obtaining and maintaining stream segregation will be more demanding, and it is possible that the bottom-up processes involved in lexical access will be less reliable because of occasional intrusions from the competing streams. The R-SPIN results indicate that word-recognition is indeed more effortful under virtual as opposed to real location conditions (on average, 50% thresholds are 1.56 dB higher for virtual than for real location conditions), and might require a greater engagement of top-down lexical processes in order to maintain word-recognition accuracy. Hence we would expect that the relative contribution of top-down processes to lexical access to be greater for virtual than for real spatial location conditions. When there is relatively little need to draw on top-down, knowledge-driven processes to obtain lexical access, we would expect a small or negligible contribution of individual differences in the efficacy of these processes to performance. However, when the draw on top-down processes is heavy, then we would expect that some of the variance in performance to be accounted for by individual differences in the efficacy of these processes. Hence we might expect that the contribution of vocabulary knowledge to dialog comprehension performance to increase with level of listening difficulty, as it appears to do in this experiment.

It is also interesting to speculate on the reasons why the relationship between reading comprehension skill and dialog comprehension performance did not differ between real and virtual location conditions (see Appendix A). One possibility is that the linguistic and cognitive skills tapped by the reading comprehension measure are separate from those involved in lexical access. Bottom-up lexical access in these experiments is obtained exclusively through the auditory channel. We can hypothesize that reading comprehension taps higher-order processes that are modality independent and are related to the integration of information, extraction of themes, etc., and therefore are unlikely to be as affected by parameters of the acoustic scene such as whether the location type is real or virtual. On the other hand, we did find group differences with respect to the relationship between reading comprehension and the number of dialog questions answered correctly (**Figure 8**). Specifically reading comprehension was found to be positively and significantly correlated with performance only in younger native-English listeners

The fact that, in young native-English listeners, individual differences in reading comprehension skills account for a significant portion of the variance in the number of dialog questions correctly answered, indicates that there are higher-order, modality-independent skills that contribute to both reading and listening comprehension in this population. The lack of correlation in older native-English listeners suggests that listening comprehension in difficult listening situations depends on a different set of modality-specific processes that are engaged to compensate for the loss of fidelity in the auditory processing system. In other words in younger native-English listeners, listening comprehension is akin to reading comprehension once lexical access has been achieved. In older native-English listeners and in young nonnative-English listeners, the same degree of listening comprehension (the number of dialog questions correctly answered did not differ across groups) appears to be achieved in a different way. This is consistent with the notion that different neural circuitry supports speech comprehension in different populations (e.g., Harris et al., 2009; Wong et al., 2009).

There may be different reasons why reading comprehension appears to contribute little to individual differences in performance in the older native-English listeners and young nonnative-English listeners. The Nelson-Denny reading comprehension test was developed and standardized for younger native-English listeners and might not be as valid when testing other populations such as older adults or nonnative-English speakers. Because the Nelson-Denny is a time-limited task, it might not adequately reflect individual differences in reading comprehension in older adults whose reading speed is substantially slower than that of younger adults (Rodríguez-Aranda, 2003). It is also unlikely to be a good measure of individual differences in reading competence in young nonnative-English adults either because they too are likely slower readers, or because this test does not adequately gauge the linguistic and cognitive skills used by nonnative-English speakers in comprehending written language. In addition, the draw on attentional resources in young nonnative-English speakers may be higher than in younger and older native-English speakers because lexical access in nonnative speakers most likely requires the activation and integration of information from both their L1 and L2 lexicons (Kroll and Steward, 1994). Moreover, the execution of the higher-order tasks involved in listening comprehension by L2 listeners, such as extracting themes, integrating information with past knowledge, and storing this information for future use may partially be executed in their L1. With respect to older adults, a number of cognitive aging theorists hypothesize that they have a more limited pool of attentional resources than do younger adults (Craik and Byrd, 1982). Alternatively, age-related changes in hearing may place a greater demand on attentional resources in older than in younger adults. Either or both of these factors would result in a greater degree of attentional focus within the auditory domain in older native listeners compared to younger native listeners. As a result, speech comprehension in older adults may depend more on processes that are specific to the auditory modality when listening becomes difficult.

To determine whether the failure to find a relationship between reading comprehension and performance in older native-English listeners when listening becomes difficult reflects an increased dependence on modality-specific processes in listening comprehension tasks, we examined the contribution of the reading comprehension performance to the number of correctly answered questions when older native-English listeners were asked to perform a similar task under less demanding perceptual conditions. As previously mentioned, in a study conducted by Murphy et al. (2006), both younger and older listeners were asked to listen to the same two-talker conversations under different acoustic setting, one of which was in quiet. We tested the contribution of vocabulary and reading comprehension to the dialog comprehension performance in quiet (see Appendix B for a detailed description of the analysis conducted) and found that the least squares regressions of the adjusted percentage correct scores against reading comprehension for both the younger and older participants were highly significant (see **Figure 9**). Hence, under perceptually easy listening conditions, reading comprehension is as strongly related to performance in older native-English listeners as it is in younger native-English listeners. The results of this analysis is consistent with the hypothesis that the lack of a significant contribution of reading comprehension to performance in older adults in noise reflects an increased dependence on modality specific processes when listening becomes difficult.

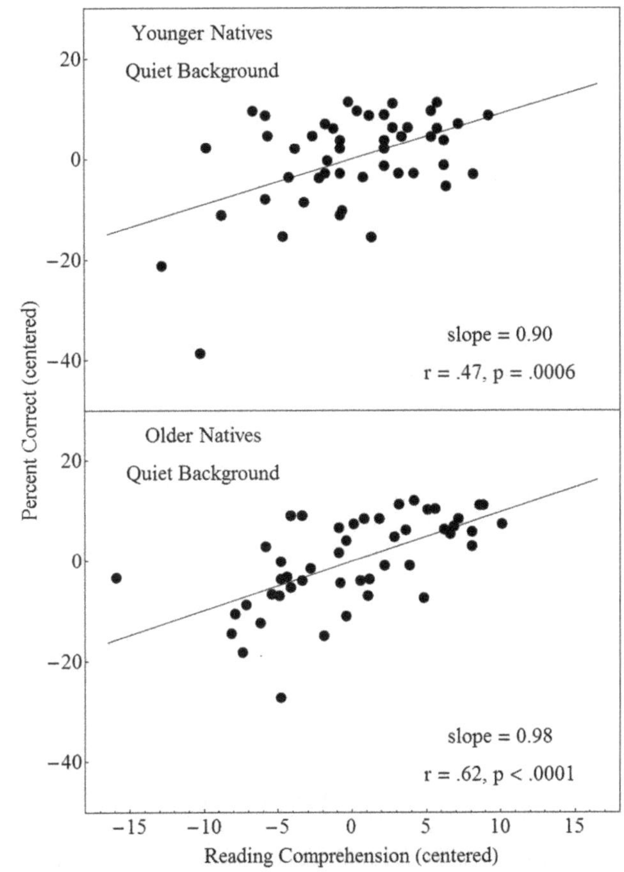

FIGURE 9 | Percentage of correctly answered dialog questions plotted against the individual performance on the Nelson-Denny reading comprehension test after the contribution of vocabulary to performance had been removed when testing was conducted in quiet in the Murphy et al. (2006) study. Both the adjusted number of questions answered and the Nelson Denny scores are centered within each group. A least squares regressions line is presented for each of two groups.

TOWARD A GENERAL MODEL OF RESOURCE ALLOCATION IN SPEECH COMPREHENSION

The differential contribution of vocabulary to dialog performance under virtual vs. real location conditions suggests that difficult listening conditions require that attentional resources be deployed in aid of scene analysis and word recognition. In addition, the relative weight given to bottom-up and top-down processes contributing to lexical access may be shifted in favor of top-down influences when listening becomes difficult. Previous theories such as the Ease of Language Understanding Model (ELU) have proposed that lexical access is impeded or slowed when listening becomes difficult (Rönnberg et al., 2013). Hence, more attentional and working memory resources are required to support lexical access. The current results suggest that the demand on such resources is modulated by the nature of the acoustic scene, which, in turn, affects the engagement of the more central, modality independent cognitive resources involved in language comprehension. Let us assume that the virtual location conditions require additional attentional resources be deployed to locate the diffused sources in space, depleting the pool of the resources available for phoneme identification and bottom-up lexical access. The notion here is that with real spatial location, the task of locating the stimuli is easy whereas virtual localization requires a larger amount of attentional processing. Now consider the problem facing the executive. When full auditory attentional resources can be devoted to lexical access and the bottom-up acoustic information is reliable and sufficient, the executive will trust the output from bottom-up lexical processing, and give less weight to top-down, knowledge-driven factors such as vocabulary knowledge. However, when lower-level attentional resources are required to locate the sound sources, this additional burden reduces the reliability of the information produced through bottom-up lexical processes. In that case, the executive may places more weight on the top-down processes involved in lexical access to compensate for the missing or corrupted bottom-up information.

The hypothesis presented here suggests that depending on the acoustic scene the listening strategy may change the relative engagement of the different processes involved in speech comprehension. The idea that listeners may systematically downplay the contribution of acoustic detail and increase their reliance on lexical-semantic knowledge has been previously suggested by Mattys et al. (2009, 2010) and Mattys and Wiget (2011). Mattys et al. (2009, 2010), Mattys and Wiget (2011) demonstrated a shift which they refer to as a cognitive-load-induced "lexical drift" in cases of high cognitive load (CL) due to an additional secondary task even when no actual energetic masking or additional auditory information is involved (e.g., a secondary visual task). For example, Mattys and Wiget (2011) measured the magnitude of lexical bias on phoneme identification under CL and no CL by adding a secondary visual search task to increase CL. Their results suggested that the CL interferes with detailed phonetic analysis which leaves the listener with impoverished encoding of the auditory input and a greater need to rely on lexical knowledge in order to compensate for the missing information. The collaborative evidence provided by Mattys et al. (2009, 2010) as well as by Mattys and Wiget (2011) and the current study support the existence of a dynamic rather than stationary processing strategy which changes depending on the listening situation, and the age and linguistic status of the listener.

Individual differences in top-down lexical knowledge, as indexed by the Mill-Hill vocabulary test, may be expected to account for a greater proportion of the variance in speech comprehension when the accuracy of the bottom-up processes involved in lexical access is compromised by listening difficulty or by age. Hence we would not expect to find Mill-Hill scores to be related to comprehension in good listening conditions with only a single talker. However, as the listening situation becomes more complex and harder to analyze (competing sound sources, diffused virtual locations rather than compact coherent ones, etc.), the more likely it is that top-down lexical processes will be engaged, and individual differences in speech comprehension to be related to measures of top-down lexical processing. Note also that the complexity of the listening situation need not affect processes subsequent to word recognition. Hence measures indexing the contribution of higher-order processes involved in language comprehension (e.g., integration of information across talkers and with stored knowledge) might not be affected by the acoustic parameters of the auditory scene.

The behavioral evidence that the nature of the acoustic scene, and the age and linguistic competence of the listener, modify the engagement of different auditory and cognitive processes involved in speech comprehension is consistent with recent findings from brain-imaging studies. These studies demonstrate that the degree to which the different neural networks involved in speech comprehension are activated, is modulated by the degree of stimulus complexity, type of task, and age. Previous neuroimaging studies which attempted to map the brain areas involved in speech perception and comprehension demonstrated a frontal-temporal network in which temporal regions subserve bottom-up processes, whereas frontal regions subserve top-down processes (Zekveld et al., 2006). This network seems to be differentially activated depending on the nature of the auditory stimuli and the complexity of the task (Benson et al., 2001; Zekveld et al., 2006). In addition, neural activation seems to not only be affected by the characteristics of the stimuli and task, but also by the characteristics of the listeners as well. Harris et al. (2009) examined the performance of both younger and older adults on word recognition task in which the intelligibility of the stimuli was manipulated using low-pass filtering. Their results showed no age differences in the auditory cortex but differences were found in the anterior cingulate cortex which is presumed to be associated with attention. Age related differences were also found in the Wong et al. (2009) study in which younger and older adults were asked to identified single words in quiet and in two multi-talker babble noise conditions (SNR = 20, −5). The fMRI results for older adults showed reduced activation in the auditory cortex but increased activation in the prefrontal and precuneus regions which are associated with working memory and attention. The increased cortical activities in the general cognitive regions were positively correlated with the behavioral results in the older adults. Wong et al. interpreted this correlation, as well as a more diffused activation involving frontal and ventral brain found in the older adults, as an indication of a possible compensatory strategy used in older age. These studies provide evidence for possible age related changes in the involvement of the different brain regions engaged in speech recognition in noise. As Scott and McGettigan (2013) note in their recent review of the neural processing of masked speech, "Further outstanding challenges will be to identify cortical signatures that are masker specific and that might be recruited for both energetic/modulation masking and informational masking,. . .and address the ways that aging affects the perception of masked speech while controlling for intelligibility (page 65, last paragraph)".

In general then, we would expect that the auditory and cognitive processes that are engaged in speech comprehension to be modulated by a number of factors including but not limited to: (1) the complexity of the auditory scene, (2) the nature of the speech material, (3) the task demands placed on the individual, and (4) individual differences in the auditory, linguistic, and cognitive skills and knowledge available to the listener. Future studies which will further examine how one or more of these factors modulate the contribution of auditory and cognitive processes are required. It could be interesting, for example, to conduct a similar study using other background noises such as speech spectrum noise or competing conversations, which differ in the levels of energetic and informational masking created, to further explore the effect masking type may have on the involvement of the different processes which support speech comprehension.

ACKNOWLEDGMENTS

This work was supported by Canadian Institutes of Health Research grants (MOP-15359, TEA-1249) and by a European Research Area in Ageing 2 grant. We would like to thank Jane Carey, Michelle Bae, and James Qi for their assistance in conducting these experiments.

REFERENCES

Ben-David, B. M., Tse, V. Y. Y., and Schneider, B. A. (2012). Does it take older adults longer than younger adults to perceptually segregate a speech target from a background masker? *Hear. Res.* 290, 55–63. doi: 10.1016/j.heares.2012.04.022

Benson, R. R., Whalen, D. H., Richardson, M., Swainson, B., Clark, V. P., Lai, S., et al. (2001). Parametrically dissociating speech and nonspeech perception in the brain using fMRI. *Brain Lang.* 78, 364–396. doi: 10.1006/brln.2001.2484

Bilger, R. C., Nuetzel, J. M., Rabinowitz, W. M., and Rzeczkowski, C. (1984). Standardization of a test of speech perception in noise. *J. Speech Hear. Res.* 27, 32–38.

Bradlow, A. R., and Bent, T. (2002). The clear speech effect for non-native listeners. *J. Acoust. Soc. Am.* 112, 272–284. doi: 10.1121/1.1487837

Bradlow, A. R., and Pisoni, D. B. (1999). Recognition of spoken words by native and non-native listeners: talker-, listener-, and item-related factors. *J. Acoust. Soc. Am.* 106, 2074–2085. doi: 10.1121/1.427952.

Brouwer, S., Van Engen, K. J., Calandruccio, L., and Bradlow, A. R. (2012). Linguistic contributions to speech-on-speech masking for native and non-native listeners: language familiarity and semantic content. *J. Acoust. Soc. Am.* 131, 1449–1464. doi: 10.1121/1.3675943

Brown, J. I., Bennett, J. M., and Hanna, G. (1981). *The Nelson-Denny Reading Test.* Chicago, IL: Riverside.

Burke, D. M., and Shafto, M. A. (2008). *Language and Aging. The Handbook of Aging and Cognition.* 3rd Edn. New York, NY: Psychology Press.

Clarys, D., Bugaiska, A., Tapia, G., and Baudouin, A. (2009). Ageing, remembering, and executive function. *Memory* 17, 158–168. doi: 10.1080/09658210802188301

Cooke, M., Garcia Lecumberri, M. L., and Barker, J. (2008). The foreign language cocktail part problem: energetic and informational masking effects in non-native speech perception. *J. Acoust. Soc. Am.* 123, 414–427. doi: 10.1121/1.2804952

Craik, F. I. M., and Byrd, M. (1982). "Aging and cognitive deficits: the role of attentional resources," in *Aging and Cognitive Processes*, eds F. I. M Craik and S. E. Trehub (New York, NY: Plenum), 191–211.

Cranford, J. L., Boose, M., and Moore, C. A. (1990). Effects of aging on the precedence effect in sound localization. *J. Speech Hear. Res.* 33, 654–659.

Ezzatian, P., Avivi, M., and Schneider, B. A. (2010). Do nonnative listeners benefit as much as native listeners from spatial cues that release from speech masking? *Speech Commun.* 5, 919–929. doi: 10.1016/j.specom.2010.04.001

Fitzgibbons, P., and Gordon-Salant, S. (1996). Auditory temporal processing in elderly listeners: speech and non-speech signals. *J. Am. Acad. Audiol.* 7, 183–189.

Florentine, M. (1985). Speech perception in noise by fluent, non-native listeners. *Proc. Acoust. Soc. Jpn.* H-85–H-116.

Francis, A. L. (2010). Improved segregation of simultaneous talkers differentially affects perceptual and cognitive capacity demands for recognizing speech in competing speech. *Atten. Percept. Psychophys.* 72, 501–516. doi: 10.3758/APP.72.2.501

Freyman, R. L., Helfer, K. S., McCall, D. D., and Clifton, R. K. (1999). The role of perceived spatial separation in the unmasking of speech. *J. Acoust. Soc. Am.* 106, 3578–3588. doi: 10.1121/1.428211

George, E. L., Zekveld, A. A., Kramer, S. E., Goverts, S. T., Festen, J. M., and Houtgast, T. (2007). Auditory and nonauditory factors affecting speech reception in noise by older listeners. *J. Acoust. Soc. Am.* 121, 2362–2375. doi: 10.1121/1.2642072

Glyde, H., Hickson, L., Cameron, S., and Dillon, H. (2011). Problems hearing in noise in older adults: a review of spatial processing disorder. *Trends Amplif.* 15, 116–126. doi: 10.1177/1084713811424885

Harris, K. C., Dubno, J. R., Keren, N. I., Ahlstrom, J. B., and Eckert, M. A. (2009). Speech recognition in younger and older adults: a dependency on low-level auditory cortex. *J. Neurosci.* 29, 6078–6087. doi: 10.1016/j.heares.2007.01.021

Hasher, L., and Zacks, R. T. (1988). "Working memory, comprehension and aging: a review and a new view," in *The Psychology of Learning and Motivation*, Vol. 22, ed G. H. Bower (San Diego, CA: Academic Press), 193–225.

Houtgast, T., and Festen, J. M. (2008). On the auditory and cognitive functions that may explain an individual's elevation of the speech reception threshold in noise. *Int. J. Audiol.* 47, 287–295. doi: 10.1080/14992020802127109

Humes, L. E., and Dubno, J. R. (2010). "Factors affecting speech understanding in older adults," in *Springer Handbook of Auditory Research: the Aging Auditory System: Perceptual Characterization and Neural Bases of Presbycusis*, eds S. Gordon-Salant, R. D. Frisina, A. N. Popper, and R. R. Fay (New York, NY: Springer), 211–258.

Humes, L. E., Dubno, J. R., Gordon-Salant, S., Lister, J. J., Cacace, A. T., Cruickshanks, K. J., et al. (2012). Central presbycusis: a review and evaluation of the evidence. *J. Am. Acad. Audiol.* 23, 635–666. doi: 10.3766/jaaa.23.8.5

Kroll, J. F., and Steward, E. (1994). Category interference in translation and picture naming: evidence for asymmetric connections between bilingual memory representations. *J. Mem. Lang.* 33, 149–174. doi: 10.1006/jmla.1994.1008

Levitt, H. (1971). Transformed up-down methods in psychoacoustics. *J. Acoust. Soc. Am.* 49, 467–477. doi: 10.1121/1.1912375

Li, L., Daneman, M., Qi, J. G., and Schneider, B. A. (2004). Does the information content of an irrelevant source differentially affect speech recognition in younger and older adults? *J. Exp. Psychol. Hum. Percept. Perform.* 30, 1077–1091. doi: 10.1037/0096-1523.30.6.1077

Mattys, S. L., Brooks, J., and Cooke, M. (2009). Recognizing speech under processing load: Dissociating energetic from informational factors. *Cogn. Psychol.* 59, 203–243. doi: 10.1016/j.cogpsych.2009.04.001

Mattys, S. L., Carroll, L. M., Li, C. K. W., and Chan, S. L. Y. (2010). Effects of energetic and informational load on speech segmentation by native and non-native speakers. *Speech Commun.* 52, 887–899. doi: 10.1016/j.specom.2010.01.005

Mattys, S. L., and Wiget, L. (2011). Effects of cognitive load on speech recognition. *J. Mem. Lang.* 65, 145–160. doi: 10.1016/j.jml.2011.04.00

Mayo, L. H., Florentine, M., and Buus, S. (1997). Age of second language acquisition and perception of speech in noise. *J. Speech Lang. Hear. Res.* 40, 686–693.

Meador, D., Flege, J. E., and Mackay, I. R. A. (2000). Factors affecting the recognition of words in a second language. *Biling. Lang. Cogn.* 3, 55–67. doi: 10.1017/S1366728900000134

Murphy, D. R., Daneman, M., and Schneider, B. A. (2006).Why do older adults have difficulty following conversations? *Psychol. Aging* 21, 49–61. doi: 10.1037/0882-7974.21.1.49

Neher, T., Behrens, T., Carlile, S., Jin, C., Kragelund, L., Petersen, A. S., et al. (2009). Benefit from spatial separation of multiple talkers in bilateral hearing-aid users: Effects of hearing loss, age, and cognition. *Int. J. Audiol.* 48, 758–774. doi: 10.3109/14992020903079332

Neher, T., Laugesen, S., Jensen, N. S., and Kragelund, L. (2011). Can basic auditory and cognitive measures predict hearing-impaired listeners' localization and spatial speech recognition abilities? *J. Acoust. Soc. Am.* 130, 1542–1558. doi: 10.1121/1.3608122

Rakerd, B., Aaronson, N. L., and Hartmann, W. M. (2006). Release from speech-on-speech masking by adding a delayed masker at a different location. *J. Acoust. Soc. Am.* 119, 1597–605. doi: 10.1121/1.2161438

Raven, J. C. (1965). *The Mill Hill Vocabulary Scale.* London: H. K. Lewis.

Rodríguez-Aranda, C. (2003). Reduced writing and reading speed and age-related changes in verbal fluency tasks. *Clin. Neuropsychol.* 17, 203–215. doi: 10.1076/clin.17.2.203.16508

Rogers, C. L., and Lopez, A. S. (2008). Perception of silent-center syllables by native and non-native English speakers. *J. Acoust. Soc. Am.* 124, 1278–1293. doi: 10.1121/1.2939127

Rönnberg, J., Lunner, T., Zekveld, A., Sörqvist, P., Danielsson, H., Lyxell, B., et al. (2013). The Ease of Language Understanding (ELU) model: theoretical, empirical, and clinical advances. *Front. Syst. Neurosci.* 7:31. doi: 10.3389/fnsys.2013.00031

Salthouse, T. (1996). The processing-speed theory of adult age differences in cognition. *Psychol. Rev.* 103, 403–428. doi: 10.1037/0033-295X.103.3.403

Schneider, B. A. (1997). Psychoacoustics and aging: implications for everyday listening. *J. Speech Lang. Pathol. Audiol.* 21, 111–124.

Schneider, B. A. (2011). How age affects auditory-cognitive interactions in speech comprehension. *Audiol. Res.* 1, 34–39. doi: 10.4081/audiores.2011.e10

Schneider, B. A., Daneman, M., and Murphy, D. R. (2000). Listening to discourse in distracting settings: the effects of aging. *Psychol. Aging* 15, 110–125. doi: 10.1037//0882-7974.15.1.110

Schneider, B. A., Li, L., and Daneman, M. (2007). How competing speech interferes with speech comprehension in everyday listening situations. *J. Am. Acad. Audiol.* 18, 578–591. doi: 10.3766/jaaa.18.7.4

Schneider, B. A., and Pichora-Fuller, M. A. (2000). "Implications of perceptual deterioration for cognitive aging research," in *The Handbook of Aging and Cognition, 2nd Edn.*, eds F. I. M. Craik and T. A. Salthouse (New York, NY: Erlbaum), 155–219.

Schneider, B. A., and Pichora-Fuller, M. K. (2001). Age-related changes in temporal processing: implications for listening comprehension. *Semin. Hear.* 22, 227–239. doi: 10.1055/s-2001-15628

Schneider, B. A., Pichora-Fuller, M. K., and Daneman, M. (2010). "The effects of senescent changes in audition and cognition on spoken language comprehension,' in *Springer Handbook of Auditory Research: The Aging Auditory System: Perceptual Characterization and Neural Bases of Presbycusis*, eds S. Gordon-Salant, R. D. Frisina, A. N. Popper, and R. R. Fay (New York, NY: Springer), 167–210.

Scott, S. K., and McGettigan, C. (2013). The neural processing of masked speech. *Hear. Res.* 303, 58–66. doi: 10.1016/j.heares.2013.05.001

Wingfield, A. (1996). Cognitive factors in auditory performance: context, speed of processing, and constraints of memory. *J. Am. Acad. Audiol.* 7, 175–182.

Wingfield, A., Poon, L. W., Lombardi, L., and Lowe, D. (1985). Speed of processing on normal aging: effects of speech rate, linguistic structure, and processing time. *J. Gerontol.* 40, 579–585.

Wingfield, A., and Tun, P. A. (2007). Cognitive supports and cognitive constraints on comprehension of spoken language. *J. Am. Acad. Audiol.* 18, 548–558. doi: 10.3766/jaaa.18.7.3

Wong, P. C. M., Jin, J. X., Gunasekara, G. M., Abel, R., Lee, E. R., and Dhar, S. (2009). Aging and cortical mechanisms of speech perception in noise. *Neuropsychologia* 47, 693–703. doi: 10.1016/j.neuropsychologia.2008.11.032

Zekveld, A. A., Heslenfeld, D. J., Festen, J. M., and Schoonhoven, R. (2006). Top-down and bottom-up processes in speech comprehension. *Neuroimage* 32, 1826–1836. doi: 10.1016/j.neuroimage.2006.04.199

APPENDIX A

EVALUATING THE CONTRIBUTION OF VOCABULARY AND READING COMPREHENSION TO R-SPIN THRESHOLD AND THE AVERAGE PERCENTAGE OF QUESTIONS CORRECTLY ANSWERED IN THE CURRENT STUDY

We first checked to see whether vocabulary and/or reading comprehension was related to the average percentage of questions correctly answered by the 72 participants in the experiment. In this and the other tests conducted here we centered the vocabulary and reading comprehension scores within each of the six groups by subtracting the mean score of a group from each of the measures in the group. The six groups were: the 12 younger native-English listeners in the separation condition; 12 younger native-English listeners in the no-separation condition; 12 young nonnative-English listeners in the separation condition; 12 young nonnative-English listeners in the no-separation condition; 12 older native-English listeners in the separation condition; and 12 older native-English listeners in the separation condition. We also centered the average percentage of questions answered correctly in each of these six groups. Centering in this fashion allowed us to evaluate the relative contribution of vocabulary to performance within each group of participants. A regression analysis found a significant correlation between both vocabulary and performance ($r = 0.38$, $p < 0.001$) and reading comprehension and performance ($r = 0.32$, $p = 0.007$).

After finding that both vocabulary and reading comprehension were related to average percentage of questions correctly answered, we then investigated whether the relationship between the two language measures and the dependent variable interacted with one or more of the three factors. Specifically, we tested three hypotheses concerning the slopes of the lines relating these two measures to percent correct. Before conducting this analysis, we centered the percent correct scores within each of the 12 conditions (2-Separations × 3 Groups × 2 Types of Spatial Location) in order to be able to compare the relative contribution of vocabulary and reading comprehension across these 12 conditions. Because both of the measures of language ability and the dependent variable were centered in all conditions and groups, the linear relationship between the individual measures and the dependent variable in a condition was specified by a single parameter, namely the slope of the line relating the measure to performance. Hence, the full model is specified by

$$Y_{i,j,k,m} = A_{i,\ j,k}V_{i,j,m} + B_{i,j,k}R_{i,j,m} + e_{i,j,k,m} \quad \text{(A1)}$$

where $Y_{i,j,k,m}$ is the centered percent correct score in the ith level of Separation (voices separate vs. co-located), jth Group (younger native-English listeners, older native-English listeners, young nonnative-English listeners), kth Type of Location (real vs. virtual), of the mth individual in Group j and Separation Condition i. $V_{i,j,m}$ and $R_{i,j,m}$ are the centered vocabulary and reading scores for the mth individual from Group j and Separation Condition i, respectively, and the $e_{i,j,k,m}$ are assumed to be random normal deviates with mean = 0, and standard deviation = σ.

To test whether the relationships between the vocabulary and reading comprehension measures and the dependent variable were independent of the Type of Location (real vs. virtual), we defined and fit a model in which

$$Y_{i,j,k,m} = A_k V_{i,j,m} + B_k R_{i,j,m} + e_{i,j,k,m}. \quad \text{(A2)}$$

This model allows for the slopes relating the two language measures to the dependent variable to differ only between the real and virtual spatial location conditions. The best-fitting least-squares parameters of this model are the a_k and the b_k. We then tested the null hypothesis that $A_{k=1} = A_{k=2}$ after adjusting the dependent measure for the estimated contribution of reading comprehension, R, to performance. In this adjusted model the dependent variable is $Y'_{R,i,j,k,m} = Y_{i,j,k,m} - b_k R_{i,j,m}$ This null hypothesis was rejected [$F_{(1,\ 142)} = 4.70, p = 0.03$], indicating that the relationship between the centered vocabulary scores and the dependent variable differed between the real and virtual spatial location conditions. However, when the dependent variable was adjusted for the contribution of vocabulary to performance ($Y'_{V,i,j,k,m} = Y_{i,j,k,m} - a_k V_{i,j,m}$), the null hypothesis that $B_{k=1} = B_{k=2}$, could not be rejected [$F_{(1,\ 142)} < 1$].

To test whether the relationship of both vocabulary and reading comprehension to performance differed between the no-separation and separation conditions, we first averaged over the Within-Subject factor to arrive at a full Between-Subjects model

$$\overline{Y}_{i,j,m} = A_{i,j}V_{i,j,m} + B_{i,j}R_{i,j,m} + \overline{e}_{i,j,m}. \quad \text{(A3)}$$

We then defined a model in which

$$\overline{Y}_{i,j,m} = A_i V_{i,j,m} + B_i R_{i,j,m} + \overline{e}_{i,j,m}. \quad \text{(A4)}$$

This model allows for the slope relating the language measures to the dependent variable to differ only between the situations in which the two voices were separated vs. when they were co-located. We then tested the null hypotheses that $A_{i=1} = A_{i=2}$ after correcting for the contribution of reading comprehension to performance in the same fashion as described above. We also tested the null hypothesis that $B_{i=1} = B_{i=2}$ after correcting for contribution of vocabulary to performance. Neither null hypothesis could be rejected [$F_{(1,\ 70)} < 1$ for $A_{i=1} = A_{i=2}$, and $F_{(1,\ 70)} = 1.42, p = 0.24$ for $B_{i=1} = B_{i=2}$].

To test whether the contribution of vocabulary and reading comprehension to the dependent variable differed among the three groups, we first averaged over the Within-Subject factor and defined a model in which

$$\overline{Y}_{i,j,m} = A_j V_{i,j,m} + B_j R_{i,j,m} + \overline{e}_{i,j,m}. \quad \text{(A5)}$$

This model allows for the slopes relating the two language measures to the dependent variable to differ among the three groups (younger native-English listeners, older native-English listeners, young nonnative-English listeners). We then tested the null hypotheses that $A_{j=1} = A_{j=2} = A_{j=3}$ after correcting for reading comprehension, and $B_{j=1} = B_{j=2} = B_{j=3}$ after correcting for vocabulary. The null hypothesis that $A_{j=1} = A_{j=2} = A_{j=3}$ could not be rejected [$F_{(2,\ 69)} < 1$], but the null hypothesis that $B_{j=1} = B_{j=2} = B_{j=3}$ was rejected [$F_{(2,\ 69)} = 6.23, p <$

0.01] Because the relationship between the reading comprehension score and percent correct (adjusted for the contribution of vocabulary) differed across the three groups, we tested three subhypotheses: (1) younger native-English listeners' slope = young nonnative-English listeners' slope; (2) younger native-English listeners' slope = older native-English listeners' slope; and (3) young nonnative-English listeners' slope = older native-English listeners' slope. Only the difference between younger native-English listeners' and young nonnative-English listeners' slopes was significant [$F_{(1,\,69)} = 12.37$. $p < 0.01$] at the 0.05 level after applying a Bonferroni correction.

It should be pointed out that we obtained exactly the same pattern of results when we independently examined the contributions of reading comprehension and vocabulary to performance, that is, without correcting for the effect of the other language variable on performance.

Recall that R-SPIN thresholds were determined in two conditions: (1) when the precedence effect was used to determine the locations of the voices and babble (virtual location), and (2) when the voices and babble were played over individual loudspeakers (real location). We examined whether either the centered vocabulary measures or the centered reading comprehension scores were related to both sets of centered R-SPIN thresholds. In conducting these tests, we eliminated the young nonnative-English individual in the no-separation group whose R-SPIN threshold for the virtual location condition was more than 3 standard deviations above the mean of that individual's group. None of these four correlations approached significance ($p > 0.2$ in all four cases).

APPENDIX B

EVALUATING THE CONTRIBUTION OF VOCABULARY AND READING COMPREHENSION TO PERFORMANCE IN THE QUIET CONDITIONS OF THE Murphy et al., 2006 STUDY

The same vocabulary and reading comprehension measures taken on the participants in this study were also taken on the 96 participants (48 young, 48 old) in the Murphy et al. (2006) study, which used the same two-person plays. Four experiments (12 younger and 12 older participants in each experiment) were conducted in both quiet and babble. In this analysis, the dependent variable was the percentage of questions answered in the quiet part of all four experiments. The vocabulary, reading comprehension, and number of questions answered correctly were first centered in each of the four experiments for the two age groups. The full model in the analysis of these data was

$$Y_{i,j,m} = A_{i,j}V_{i,j,m} + B_{i,j}R_{i,j,m} + e_{i,j,m} \qquad \text{(A6)}$$

where $Y_{i,j,m}$ is the centered average percentage of questions correctly answered by the m participants in the quiet conditions for Age Group j of Experiment i, and V, R, A, B and e are defined as above. We then defined and fit a model in which the A and B coefficients were the same for all four experiments and differed only with respect to the Age Group to which the participants belonged. Specifically, we defined and fit the model

$$Y_{i,j,m} = A_jV_{i,j,m} + B_jR_{i,j,m} + e_{i,j,m} \qquad \text{(A7)}$$

We then tested and failed to reject the null hypothesis that $B_{j=1} = B_{j=2}$ after adjusting for the contribution of vocabulary to performance as described above [$F_{(1,\,94)} < 1$]. Least Squares regressions of the adjusted percentage correct scores against reading comprehension for both the younger and older participants were highly significant ($\text{slope}_{\text{young}} = 0.90$, $r_{\text{young}} = 0.47$, $p = 0.0006$; $slope_{old} = 0.98$, $r_{\text{old}} = 0.62$, $p < 0.0001$).

After adjusting the centered average percentage of questions correctly answered for the contribution of reading comprehension, there was no evidence of any relationship of the dependent variable to vocabulary ($\text{slope}_{\text{young}} = 0.04$, $r_{\text{young}} = 0.01$, $p > 0.5$; $\text{slope}_{\text{old}} = 0.72$, $r_{\text{old}} = 0.21$, $p > 0.15$).

6

Upregulation of cognitive control networks in older adults' speech comprehension

Julia Erb* and Jonas Obleser*

Max Planck Research Group "Auditory Cognition," Max Planck Institute for Human Cognitive and Brain Sciences, Leipzig, Germany

***Correspondence:**
Julia Erb and Jonas Obleser, Max Planck Research Group "Auditory Cognition," Max Planck Institute for Human Cognitive and Brain Sciences, Stephanstrasse 1A, 04103 Leipzig, Germany
e-mail: jerb@cbs.mpg.de; obleser@cbs.mpg.de

Speech comprehension abilities decline with age and with age-related hearing loss, but it is unclear how this decline expresses in terms of central neural mechanisms. The current study examined neural speech processing in a group of older adults (aged 56–77, $n = 16$, with varying degrees of sensorineural hearing loss), and compared them to a cohort of young adults (aged 22–31, $n = 30$, self-reported normal hearing). In a functional MRI experiment, listeners heard and repeated back degraded sentences (4-band vocoded, where the temporal envelope of the acoustic signal is preserved, while the spectral information is substantially degraded). Behaviorally, older adults adapted to degraded speech at the same rate as young listeners, although their overall comprehension of degraded speech was lower. Neurally, both older and young adults relied on the left anterior insula for degraded more than clear speech perception. However, anterior insula engagement in older adults was dependent on hearing acuity. Young adults additionally employed the anterior cingulate cortex (ACC). Interestingly, this age group × degradation interaction was driven by a reduced dynamic range in older adults who displayed elevated levels of ACC activity for both degraded and clear speech, consistent with a persistent upregulation in cognitive control irrespective of task difficulty. For correct speech comprehension, older adults relied on the middle frontal gyrus in addition to a core speech comprehension network recruited by younger adults suggestive of a compensatory mechanism. Taken together, the results indicate that older adults increasingly recruit cognitive control networks, even under optimal listening conditions, at the expense of these systems' dynamic range.

Keywords: functional MRI, aging, degraded speech, neural adaptation, executive functions, noise-vocoding, cochlear implant simulation, temporal envelope

INTRODUCTION

Speech comprehension can become difficult with age and age-related hearing loss, especially when listening conditions are challenging. Normal-hearing young adults have the capacity to rapidly adapt to degraded speech (Davis et al., 2005; Samuel and Kraljic, 2009; Eisner et al., 2010; Erb et al., 2013). Such short-term perceptual adaptation is not well established in older adults, although it bears particular relevance as older adults are frequently affected by hearing loss. For example, patients with hearing-aids or, more drastically, cochlear implants (CI) need to adapt to an altered and often distorted auditory signal delivered by their device.

In a previous short-term adaptation study in a cohort of young adults (Erb et al., 2013), we have shown that degraded speech processing elicits an increased blood oxygenation level-dependent (BOLD) response in an "executive" network (Eckert et al., 2009) comprising the anterior insula and anterior cingulate cortex (ACC). Also, adaptation to degraded speech was shown to be accompanied by hemodynamic down-regulation in a cortico-thalamic-striatal loop (Erb et al., 2013). In the current functional MRI experiment, we compare these results to a group of older adults with varying degrees of hearing loss to test: (1) whether older listeners are able to (behaviorally) adapt to spectrally severely degraded ("noise-vocoded") speech at a rate comparable to young listeners and (2) how neural processing of degraded speech differs between young and older adults.

There is evidence that rapid perceptual learning is preserved in older adults (Peelle and Wingfield, 2005; Golomb et al., 2007; Gordon-Salant et al., 2010). For example, older adults are able to quickly adapt to an unfamiliar accent (Adank and Janse, 2010) or a foreign accent (Gordon-Salant et al., 2010). Peelle and Wingfield (2005) showed that older adults adapted to temporally degraded ("time-compressed") and noise-vocoded speech at a similar rate as young adults, when starting accuracy was equated.

However, considerable inter-individual variability has been frequently observed in adaptation to vocoded speech (Shannon et al., 2002; Eisner et al., 2010). Especially in older adults, the degree of hearing loss and cognitive aspects might substantially impact adaptation to degraded speech. Working memory is one cognitive factor that has been implicated in degraded speech comprehension by a number of studies (Pichora-Fuller et al., 1995; Burkholder et al., 2005; Jacquemot and Scott, 2006; Eisner et al.,

2010; Piquado et al., 2010; Obleser et al., 2012). For example, Pisoni and Cleary (2003) observed that working memory scores as measured by digit span significantly predicted speech comprehension in pediatric CI users. In older adults, cognitive factors might be even more closely related to degraded speech recognition (Janse and Adank, 2012), because cognitive decline has been shown to co-occur with sensory decline (Lindenberger and Ghisletta, 2009), which in turn leads to degraded auditory conditions. Thus, we expected working memory capacity in older adults to be related to vocoded speech comprehension.

A second factor which heavily affects comprehension is hearing loss. As age-related hearing loss is accompanied by auditory cortex atrophies (Harris et al., 2009; Peelle et al., 2011; Eckert et al., 2012), older adults likely draw on different neural resources for speech comprehension. It is a common observation that older adults recruit additional regions for speech comprehension compared to young adults, although it is unclear whether this reflects an age-related loss of specialization of cortical brain regions (Park et al., 2004) or a compensatory mechanism (Cabeza et al., 2002). Peelle et al. (2010b) noted that during processing of syntactically complex sentences, older adults engaged middle frontal regions in addition to a "core sentence-processing network" (comprising middle temporal gyrus (MTG) and inferior frontal gyrus (IFG); Peelle et al., 2004; Fiebach et al., 2005) recruited by young adults. The authors interpreted this engagement of additional areas as a compensatory process, whereby the older adults managed to maintain performance despite degeneration of the sensory cortices.

In line with this argumentation, older adults have been hypothesized to engage in more effortful processing during speech comprehension (Pichora-Fuller, 2003). Consistently, Eckert et al. (2008) observed an age-related upregulation of cognitive-control-related frontal areas during an easy word recognition task, while younger adults recruited these areas merely in difficult listening conditions. Harris et al. (2009) further showed that incorrect vs. correct word recognition elicited increased activity in the ACC, but more so in older than younger adults, possibly reflecting an age-related upregulation of error monitoring systems (Sharp et al., 2006). Hence, for solving auditory tasks the reliance on cognitive control appears to increase with age.

It is still largely unknown, however, how older adults adapt to degraded speech. In the current functional MRI study, we were primarily interested in how short-term adaptation to degraded speech and the involvement of cognitive control networks in speech processing changes with age. Young and older listeners heard and repeated back 100 degraded (4-band-vocoded) sentences as well as a control set of interspersed clear-speech sentences. Thus, we could identify age differences in the neural processes related to both, physical degradation of speech (degraded vs. clear sentences) and trial-by-trial fluctuations in comprehension (covariation of BOLD responses with degraded speech comprehension success).

MATERIALS AND METHODS

PARTICIPANTS

Sixteen older adults (aged 56–77, mean 67.1 years, 8 female) participated in the study. Their data were analyzed jointly with a cohort of 30 young adults (aged 22–31, mean 25.9 years, 15 female) who had participated in the study reported in Erb et al. (2013). Participants were recruited from the participant database of the Max Planck Institute for Human Cognitive and Brain Sciences according to the following criteria: they were native speakers of German; had no language or neurological disorders; showed dominant right-handedness according to the Edinburgh inventory (Oldfield, 1971) and were naïve to noise-vocoded speech. Younger adults self-reported normal hearing, whereas older adults had normal hearing to moderate hearing loss based on their pure-tone averages which were audiometrically assessed (see below). Participants received financial compensation of € 16, and gave informed consent. Procedures were approved by the local ethics committee (University of Leipzig).

Audiometric evaluation

Older adults' pure-tone thresholds were measured at conventional frequencies from 0.25–8 kHz using an Equinox 2.0 AC-440 audiometer (Interacoustics) in a sound-proof chamber. Older participants' pure-tone average (PTA; defined as the average thresholds in the listener's better ear at 1, 2 and 4 kHz) indicated normal hearing (< 25 dB HL) to moderate hearing loss (40–70 dB HL), whereas high-frequency hearing ranged from normal to severe hearing loss (70–95 dB HL; audiograms are shown in **Figure 1A**). Young participants' hearing acuity was not tested but all of them self-reported normal hearing.

Auditory forward and backward digit span

To measure working memory capacity, all participants were tested with a digit span test, which is part of the revised Wechsler memory scale (WMS-R; Wechsler, 1987). The experimenter read out to the participant lists of single digits between 1 and 9 at a rate of approximately one digit per second. Participants had to immediately repeat the list of digits in the same order (forward digit span) or in the reverse order (backward digit span). The test had seven levels featuring list lengths starting from three digits increasing by one digit up to nine digits for forward digit span, and list lengths from two to eight digits for backward digit span. Each level comprised two items. The participants' response was marked as correct only if all digits were correctly repeated in the required order. The testing stopped when the participant reported none of the items of a level correctly or when all 14 items had been presented. The level at which the test was terminated was taken as the individual forward or backward digit span measure (Wechsler, 1987).

STIMULI AND EXPERIMENTAL DESIGN

Stimuli were German SPIN sentences, which control for the predictability of the final word (Kalikow et al., 1977; Erb et al., 2012). Only low-predictability sentences were used in the present study, such that semantic cues were limited and the listener had to rely primarily on acoustic properties of the sentence to understand it. A complete list of these sentences is available in Erb et al. (2012). The sentences were recorded by a female speaker of standard German in a sound-proof chamber. The length of the recorded sentences varied between 1620 and 2760 ms.

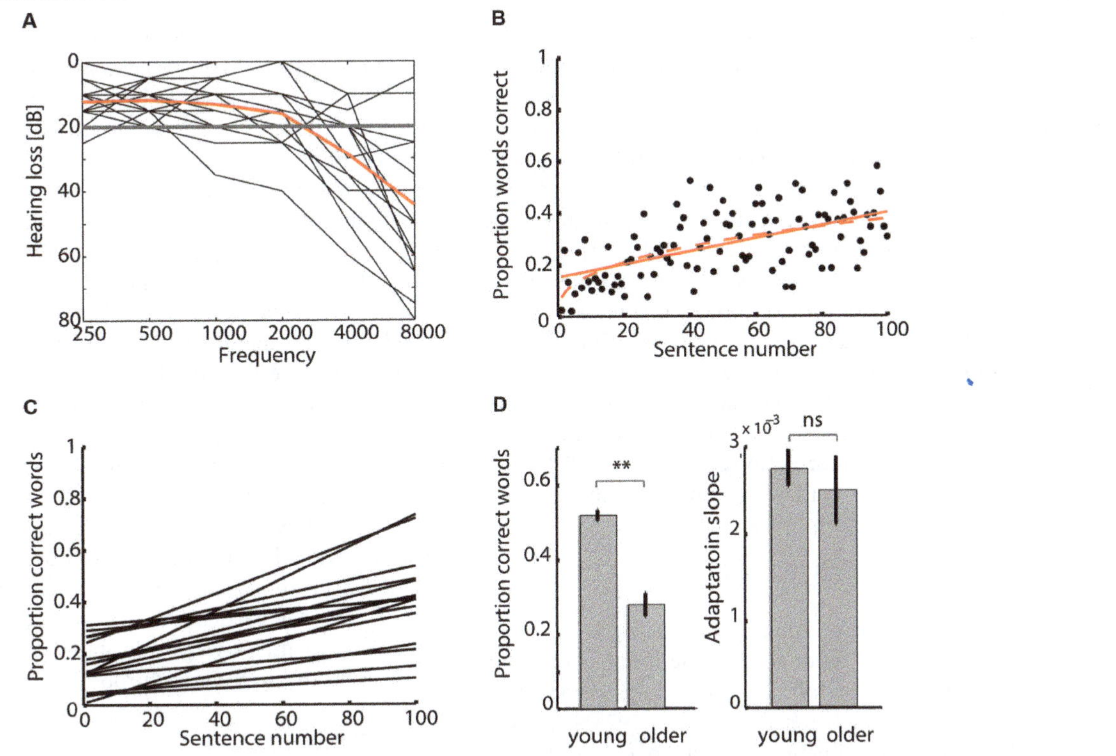

FIGURE 1 | (A) Audiograms of older adults. Older participants are affected by varying degrees of sensorineural hearing loss. Hearing loss for each participant's better ear (black line) and mean over all participants (red line) are shown. **(B)** Mean report scores (averaged over all older participants) with a linear (red solid line) and power law fit (red dashed line). **(C)** Older adults' adaptation curves. Linear fits to report scores show individual differences in adaptation to degraded speech. The slope of the linear fit was taken as measure for perceptual adaptation to degraded speech (adaptation slope). **(D)** Group comparison of mean speech comprehension and adaptation. Young and older adults differ in mean degraded speech comprehension but not adaptation slopes ($^{**}p < 0.001$, *ns* = non-significant).

Sentences were degraded using 4-band noise vocoding. This procedure divides the speech signal into frequency bands, extracts the amplitude envelope from each band and reapplies it to bandpass-filtered noise carriers. Thus, the spectro-temporal fine structure is smeared while the temporal envelope remains preserved. For envelope extraction, we used a second-order, zero-phase Butterworth lowpass-filter with a cutoff frequency of 400 Hz. Noise-vocoding was applied to all sentences in MATLAB 7.11 as described in Rosen et al. (1999) using four frequency bands spanning 70–9000 Hz that were spaced according to Greenwood's cochlear frequency-position function (Greenwood, 1990); for the exact cut-off frequencies of the frequency bands see Erb et al. (2012).

Each trial was approximately 9 s long, but actual trial length varied due to cardiac gating (see below). Trials started with a 1 s silent gap, after which participants heard a sentence lasting for approximately 2.5 s. Following stimulus presentation (3.5 s into the trial), a green light ("go"-signal for response) was visually presented and lasted for 3 s. During this time, participants were to respond by repeating the sentence, but were instructed to stop talking when the green light disappeared in order to avoid movement during scan acquisition. After approximately 1 s of silence, scan acquisition with a TR of 2 s was triggered using cardiac gating. Thus, the onset of auditory stimulation preceded the anticipated scan acquisition by approximately 6.5 s. Verbal responses were recorded for later off-line scoring (Eckert et al., 2009; Harris et al., 2009). Responses were scored as proportions of correctly repeated words per sentence ("report scores", Peelle et al., 2013). Scoring took into account all words of a sentence including function words. The marking scheme was liberal such that errors in declension or conjugation were accepted as correct.

Clear-speech trials were used as a high-level baseline. Clear speech can be assumed to be fully adapted, and therefore to be processed in a stable way over time. This ensured that neural adaptation would not occur in the baseline condition, whereas another type of artificial speech degradation (e.g., rotated speech) might have led to neural adaptation (even in the absence of behavioral adaptation).

Overall, the experiment comprised three conditions, (1) 4-band vocoded sentences ("degraded speech"; 100 trials), (2) clear (non-degraded) sentences ("clear speech"; 24 trials) and (3) trials lacking any auditory stimulation ("silent trials"; 20 trials), summing up to 144 trials in total. Clear speech trials were presented every 5th trial, whereas silent trials were randomly interspersed. Sentences were presented to each participant in one of four different orders; presentation order was counterbalanced across participants.

Individual adaptation curves

To measure individual learning rate, we modeled learning curves in two different ways: as power law or as linear performance increase. It has been claimed that learning curves for short-term adaptation to degraded speech are asymptotic such that perceptual learning follows a power law (Peelle et al., 2010a). However, we had previously shown in young adults, that behavioral adaptation to noise-vocoded speech is better described by linear curves than more complex, power-law fits (Erb et al., 2012, 2013).

Here, to test whether in older adults, a linear or a power law function would better describe the data, both functions were fitted to the individual performance scores over time using a least-squares estimation procedure in MATLAB 7.11 (cf. Erb et al., 2012; for an example linear and power law fit to the older group's average performance see **Figure 1B**). We compared goodness of fit by determining the Bayesian information criterion (BIC; Schwarz, 1978) of the linear and the power law fit within each subject. BIC values were defined as

$$BIC = n \times \ln(\sigma_e^2) + k \times \ln(n) \quad (1)$$

where n is the number of observations (n = 100), σ_e^2 is the error variance or sum of squared residuals, k is the number of fitted parameters (k = 2 for the linear fit, k = 3 for the power law fit). Smaller BIC values indicate a better fit (Schwarz, 1978; Priestley, 1981). The BIC increases as a function of σ_e^2 and of k. Models with higher error variance and more fitted parameters are therefore penalized.

EXPERIMENTAL PROCEDURE

Before participants went into the scanner, they were familiarized with the task by listening to three 8-band vocoded sentences.

To prevent hearing damage due to scanner noise, participants wore Alpine Musicsafe Pro earplugs while in the bore, yielding approximately linear 14-dB reduction in sound pressure up to 8 kHz. Auditory stimuli were delivered through MR-Confon headphones using Presentation software. Presentation level was adjusted for each participant such that loudness was subjectively comfortable and equal across both ears. This ensured that stimuli were presented at a level well above participants' thresholds in the speech range frequencies such that all participants were able to perceive the sentences. Visual prompts were projected on a screen which participants viewed via a mirror.

MRI DATA ACQUISITION

MRI data were collected on a 3-T Siemens Verio scanner. Functional MR images were acquired with a 12-channel head coil using an echo-planar imaging (EPI) sequence [repetition time (TR) ≈ 9000 ms, acquisition time (TA) = 2000 ms, echo time (TE) = 30 ms, flip angle = 90°, 3 mm slice thickness, 30 axial slices (ascending), interslice distance = 1 mm, acquisition matrix of 64 × 64, voxel size = 3 × 3 × 3 mm]. The acquisition matrix was placed such that the x-axis was in line with the anterior–posterior commissure (AC–PC). We used a sparse-sampling procedure, where TR was longer than TA, allowing for silent periods to play stimuli and record responses (Hall et al., 1999).

Cardiac gating was applied to avoid movement artifacts caused by the heartbeat in subcortical structures (Von Kriegstein et al., 2008), in which we were especially interested (Erb et al., 2012, 2013). Participants' heartbeat was monitored using an MR-compatible pulse oximeter (Siemens) attached to their left ring finger. On each trial, after 9 s had elapsed, the scanner waited for the first heartbeat to trigger volume acquisition. Thus, the actual TR was variable.

Following functional imaging, young participants received a T1-weighted structural brain scan with a 32-channel head coil using an MPRAGE sequence [TR = 1300 ms, TE = 3.5 ms, flip angle = 10°, 1 mm slice thickness, 176 sagittal slices, acquisition matrix of 256 × 240, voxel size = 1 mm^3].

Older adults' anatomical scans for registration with the functional images were available through the Institute's brain database. Scanning had been carried out on a 3T Siemens Trio TIM scanner using T1-weighted MPRAGE sequence to acquire 176 sagittal slices, with an acquisition matrix of 256 × 240, yielding a resolution of 1 mm^3.

For one older participant the scanner had become desynchronized with the presentation script, such that he had to be excluded from the functional MRI data analyses, resulting in a total of 15 older participants included in the analyses. In one young participant, we were only able to acquire 136 (as opposed to 144) scans due to technical problems with cardiac gating.

DATA ANALYSIS

Note that all behavioral and MRI analyses of single participants were closely matched to the procedures established previously in the young cohort and published in Erb et al. (2013).

Preprocessing

MRI data were analyzed in SPM8 (Wellcome Trust Centre for Neuroimaging, London, UK). Functional images were realigned and unwarped using a fieldmap, coregistered with the structural scan, segmented and normalized to standard space (Montreal Neurological Institute [MNI] space) using the segmentation parameters, and smoothed with an isotropic Gaussian kernel of 8 mm full-width at half-maximum.

Statistical analyses

MR images were statistically analyzed in the context of the general linear model (GLM). We set up one model to assess effects speech degradation and effects of trial-by-trial-fluctuations in comprehension. In this model, we included two conditions: degraded and clear speech. To avoid overspecification, silent trials were not modeled in the analyses, but solely used for an initial quality check of the data confirming that sound compared to silent trials yielded large clusters of activity in the auditory cortex. Additionally, a parametric modulator of the degraded speech trials was defined, representing the behavioral report scores. A regressor of no interest, containing report latencies, was added in order to account for differences in speech production (analysis explained in detail below). To assess effects of stimulus clarity, we contrasted degraded against clear speech trials. To reveal effects of trial-by-trial fluctuations in speech comprehension, we assessed correlations with the regressor representing report scores. To look for effects of hearing loss, we correlated PTA on the second level with the contrast degraded > clear speech.

Although the present study was designed to image degraded speech perception, parts of the observed activity may be related to speech production or preparation, because participants overtly repeated back what they had understood starting approximately 3.5 s prior to scan acquisition. In particular, participants' verbal responses might have been faster for clear relative to degraded speech trials, perhaps leading to partly imaging the BOLD response to speech production, but more so for clear speech trials. Therefore, differences in report latencies might confound the comparison between degraded and clear speech trials. To control for this potential confound, we calculated report latency relative to the onset of the visual response cue. This measure was included at the first level as one single regressor of no interest in the model. For trials where participants did not produce an overt response, the subject-specific mean report latency was entered instead.

All described analyses were whole-brain analyses. Regressors were modeled using a finite impulse response (FIR) comprising one bin. A high-pass filter with a cutoff of 1024 s was applied to eliminate low-frequency noise. No correction for serial auto-correlation was necessary because of the long TR in the sparse-sampling acquisition.

Second level statistics were calculated using a one-sample *t*-test and group differences were assessed using a two-samples *t*-test. We recognize that comparisons between groups of different sample sizes (here: 15 older adults vs. 30 younger adults) are problematic; especially when variance differs between groups, the group with the larger variance should comprise more samples (Samanez-Larkin and D'Esposito, 2008). There is evidence, however, that BOLD signal variability actually decreases in older adults (Garrett et al., 2010). Further, we wanted to avoid discarding data which were already available for the 30 young adults, resulting in a larger sample size of the young compared to the older adults.

We are aware of the problem that hemodynamics likely change with age (e.g., due to vascular changes), such that simple group differences in the BOLD signal could possibly reflect differences in neurovascular coupling rather than actual differences in neural processing. To overcome this issue, we only tested for age group × condition interactions when assessing age effects on neural processing (Samanez-Larkin and D'Esposito, 2008).

Group inferences are reported at a threshold of $p < 0.001$ and a cluster-extent of $k > 20$ to correct for inflated type I error at the whole-brain level, as based on a Monte Carlo Simulation (Slotnick et al., 2003). *T*-statistic maps were transformed to *Z*-statistic maps using spm_t2z.m, and overlaid and displayed on the ch2 template in MNI space included with MRIcron (Rorden and Brett, 2000).

Regions of interest analyses

In order to extract measures of percent signal change in the regions identified by the whole-brain analyses described above, we defined regions of interest (ROIs) using the SPM toolbox MarsBar (Brett et al., 2002). ROIs were defined as spheres with a radius of 3 mm centered on the identified peak coordinates. Voxels within an ROI were aggregated into a single contrast estimate using the first eigenvariate.

RESULTS

BEHAVIORAL RESULTS

Vocoded speech comprehension

Older adults reported on average 28.0 ± 2.8 (mean ± SEM) % words correctly per degraded sentence. Performance in clear trials was at 98.0 ± 1.4 % correct. In comparison, young adults' degraded speech recognition was substantially better ($t(44) = 8.23$, $p < 0.001$), with on average 51.9 ± 1.4 % words correct per degraded sentence and 99.7 ± 0.2 % correct per clear sentence (**Figure 1D**, left).

Perceptual adaptation

We compared whether a linear or power-law fit would better describe the report scores' increase over time by calculating BIC for each fit and each older participant (**Figures 1B, C**). The BIC scores for the linear fits (median 222.09, range 95.21–268.48) were smaller than those for power law fits (median 226.69, range 99.81–273.09), as shown by a Wilcoxon signed-rank test ($p < 0.001$), indicating that the linear curve better fit the behavioral data. In the young participants, we had also shown that linear fits were more adequate than the power law fits to describe participants' learning curves (see Erb et al., 2013). Thus, the slope of the linear fit (adaptation slope) was taken as a measure of individual perceptual adaptation to degraded speech.

The BIC compares goodness of fit between different models but does not give an estimate of absolute goodness of fit. Absolute goodness of fit as measured by R^2 in the older adults amounted to $R^2 = 0.061 \pm 0.01$ (mean ± SEM) for the power law fit and $R^2 = 0.072 \pm 0.016$ for the linear fit. R^2 did not differ between the linear and the power law fit, as shown by a Mann-Whitney *U*-test ($p = 0.95$). Note however, that a direct comparison of R^2 between different models does not allow for a fair comparison, as R^2 does not take into account the number of fitted parameters.

In order to test whether goodness of fit differed between age groups, we compared R^2 of the linear fits in the two groups. R^2 in the older adults did not differ from R^2 in the younger adults (0.065 ± 0.009), as shown by a Mann-Whitney *U*-test ($p = 0.92$), indicating that the goodness of fit was comparable in older and younger adults. Although these single-subject R^2 values are relatively small (only approximately 7% of the variance is explained by the fitted model), when averaging over the 16 older adults, mean report scores correlated highly with sentence number ($R^2 = 0.32$, $p < 0.001$). Davis et al. (2005) have reported similar correlation coefficients for mean report scores with sentence number in their vocoded speech learning study (but did not report single-subject R^2-values).

To confirm that the slopes of the linear fits were a sensible measure of learning, we used another more traditional measure of learning. For each participant, we subtracted the mean performance over the last 20 trials from the mean performance over the first 20 trials (Bent et al., 2009; Eisner et al., 2010). This performance difference (Δ performance) between the beginning and end of the experiment amounted to 0.22 ± 0.03 proportion correct (mean ± SEM) in the older adults and 0.27 ± 0.02 proportion correct in the younger adults. Across age groups,

Δ performance was highly correlated with the adaptation slopes ($r = 0.91$; $p < 0.001$).

To test whether older and younger adults differed in their rate of learning, we compared both the Δ performance and adaptation slopes between groups. According to a two-samples t-test, there was neither a difference in Δ performance between older and young adults ($t(44) = -1.25$, $p = 0.22$), nor in the adaptation slopes of older ($2.5 \pm 0.39 \times 10^{-3}$, mean ± SEM) and young adults ($2.7 \pm 0.21 \times 10^{-3}$; $t(44) = -0.65$, $p = 0.52$), indicating that both groups were comparable in the rate with which they adapted to degraded speech (**Figure 1D**, right).

Finally, to exclude the possibility that variability in the adaptation curves (shown in **Figure 1C**) was a consequence of the counterbalancing of material across participants (in four different presentation orders), we tested whether presentation order had an effect on adaptation slope. A Kruskal-Wallis test was not significant ($\chi^2(15) = 4.34$, $p = 0.23$), indicating that the fact that different listeners received different materials at different time points did not influence adaptation.

Spearman's correlations

In order to examine whether in older adults, adaptation slope was related to other factors (i.e., age, forward and backward digit span, PTA, mean performance), a two-tailed Spearman's correlation was calculated for all pairs of variables. We adjusted for multiple comparisons by controlling the false discovery rate (Benjamini and Hochberg, 1995), which resulted in a critical $p = 0.019$ at a false discovery rate of $q = 0.05$ ("significant") and $p = 0.039$ at $q = 0.1$ ("non-significant trend").

Within the older adults, adaptation slope correlated positively with backward digit span (**Figure 2A** and **Table 1**), indicating that listeners with a larger working memory capacity adapted faster to degraded speech. Note that this correlation remained significant, when the outlier participant with a slope of 0.006 was removed ($\rho = 0.62$, $p = 0.18$). PTA and age showed a non-significant trend for a negative correlation with adaptation slope, meaning that older age and hearing loss were associated with slower adaptation rates. Similarly, older age and PTA were negatively related to average speech comprehension performance. Finally, age also correlated significantly with PTA, indicating that older adults had greater hearing loss (**Table 1**).

Table 1 | Spearman's correlations between behavioral measures.

	Slope	Age	DSF	DSB	PTA	Perform
Slope		−0.54+	0.37	**0.60***	−0.55+	0.45
Age			0.01	−0.18	**0.65***	**−0.67***
DSF				0.25	−0.26	0.10
DSB					−0.44	0.09
PTA						**−0.61***
Perform						

*Significant correlations are shown in bold: * significant at $q < 0.05$; + significant at $q < 0.1$; Slope: adaptation slope, DSF: digit span forward, DSB: digit span backward, PTA: pure-tone average, Perform: Mean vocoded speech comprehension.*

To analyze more closely the relationship between adaptation slope, age, digit span and hearing loss, we calculated Spearman's partial correlation coefficients between these four variables of interest, with two variables partialled out at a time (**Figure 2B**). Adaptation slope still correlated significantly with backward digit span, even after partialling out age and hearing loss, indicating that the latter could not explain the relationship between working memory and adaptation. The correlation between PTA and age also remained significant in the partial correlation. On the other hand, the non-significant trend for a negative correlation of adaptation slope with hearing loss and age broke down in the partial correlation (**Figure 2B**).

FUNCTIONAL MRI RESULTS IN OLDER ADULTS

The results reported below refer to the group of older adults exclusively. For the cohort of young adults, activation clusters and coordinates of peak activity are described in detail in Erb et al. (2013).

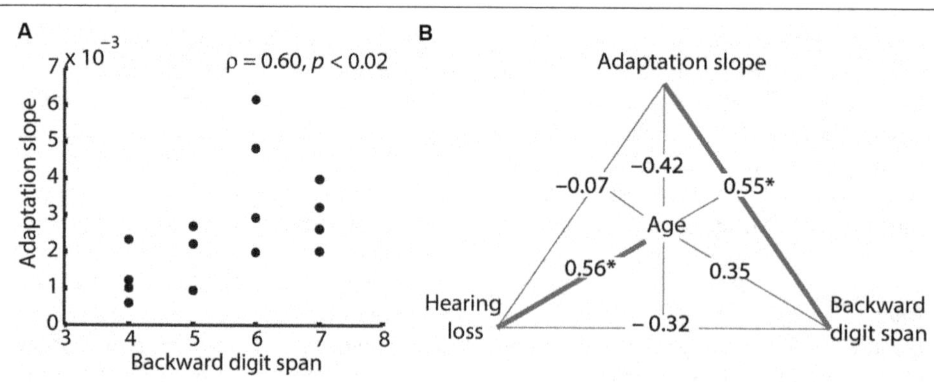

FIGURE 2 | Spearman's correlations between behavioral measures. **(A)** Adaptation slope correlated positively with backward digit span. This correlation remained significant, when the outlier participant with a slope of 0.006 was removed ($\rho = 0.62$, $p = 0.18$). **(B)** Partial correlations between adaptation slope, age, backward digit span and hearing loss (pure-tone average; PTA). Spearman's correlation coefficients are shown. Note that two measures are partialled out at a time; for example, the correlation between adaptation slope and digit span of $\rho = 0.55$ is controlled for age and hearing loss. Only the adaptation–digit span correlation and the age–hearing loss correlation remain significant in the partial correlation. Significant correlations are shown as bold lines (* $p < 0.05$).

Degraded speech processing

To reveal regions that are engaged in degraded speech processing, we compared degraded with clear speech trials. At a cluster-extent corrected threshold of $p < 0.001$, degraded compared to clear speech elicited an increased BOLD signal in the left anterior insula. On the other hand, clear compared to degraded speech yielded higher activations bilaterally in the precentral gyrus spanning the temporal cortices, supramarginal gyrus (SMG), right putamen, posterior cingulate cortex and angular gyrus bilaterally (**Figure 3A**).

Trial-by-trial fluctuations in degraded speech comprehension

To identify areas where the BOLD signal varied with trial-by-trial fluctuations in speech comprehension, we tested for correlations with the behavioral report scores. The hemodynamic response linearly increased with comprehension of degraded speech in bilateral temporal cortices comprising Heschl's gyrus, the middle temporal gyrus, the precentral gyrus bilaterally, the putamen bilaterally, left angular gyrus, and middle frontal gyrus (**Figure 3B**). Although scans might have been sensitive to both speech perception and production, we controlled for report latency (see Section Materials and Methods) to model the hemodynamic response to auditory input rather than speech production. Note, however, that including a regressor for report latency might not completely control for production-related activity, such that motor cortical activity (apparent in **Figures 3A, B**), could be due to more speech production during more intelligible compared to less intelligible trials.

Correlation with hearing loss

We further tested, whether hearing acuity had an influence on neural processing. For the contrast degraded > clear speech, we found a negative correlation with PTA in the right and left anterior insula (**Table 2** and **Figure 3C**). The correlation showed the following pattern: Older adults with better hearing acuity had elevated activity for degraded compared to clear speech. Conversely, listeners with greater hearing loss had an increased BOLD signal for clear relative to degraded speech in the anterior insula (**Figure 3C**, right panel). This Pearson's correlation between insula dynamics and hearing loss was significant even after partialling out age ($r = -0.79$, $p = 0.001$), confirming that the correlation was not driven by age.

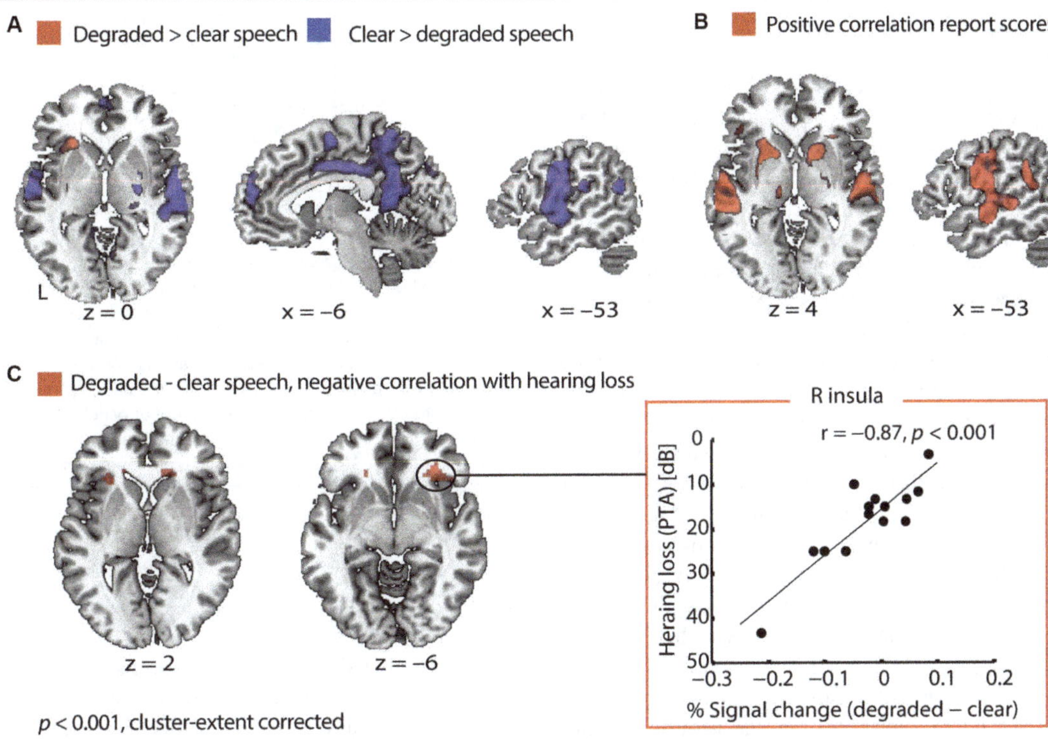

FIGURE 3 | Functional MRI results in older adults. (A) Areas sensitive to speech degradation. In older adults, degraded relative to clear speech perception activated the anterior insula, whereas clear more than degraded speech activated a network comprising the precentral gyrus, the temporal cortices, supramarginal gyrus, right putamen, posterior cingulate cortex and angular gyrus bilaterally. **(B)** Areas varying with speech comprehension. With better speech comprehension on a given trial, activity increased in a network comprising the auditory cortices, precentral gyrus, left angular gyrus, putamen and middle frontal gyrus. There were no negative correlations with trial-by-trial report scores. **(C)** Negative correlation of hearing loss with activity related to degraded speech processing. Pure-tone average (PTA) correlated negatively with the degraded > clear speech contrast in the right and left anterior insula. The plot of this correlation (right panel) shows that older adults with better hearing acuity had an increased BOLD signal for degraded compared to clear speech in the right anterior insula. Conversely, listeners affected by more severe hearing loss had elevated activity for clear relative to degraded speech. The correlation remains significant when removing the outlier participant with a PTA of 43 dB ($r = -0.76$, $p = 0.002$) and when partialling out age ($r = -0.79$, $p = 0.001$). Note that the y-axis is flipped such that better hearing acuity is plotted higher up.

Table 2 | Overview of MRI activation clusters showing a correlation with hearing loss or significant group × condition interactions, thresholded at $p < 0.001$ (cluster-extent corrected).

Location	MNI-Coordinates			*Z*-Score	Extent (mm^3)
Degraded > clear speech, negative correlation with PTA (older adults)					
R anterior insula	33	35	−5	4.38	432
L anterior insula	−30	26	1	4.08	207
Degraded > clear speech, young > older					
L SMA/ACC	−3	26	40	3.58	207
Positive correlation with trial-by-trial comprehension fluctuations, older > young					
R MFG	33	35	34	4.27	754
Positive correlation with trial-by-trial comprehension fluctuations, young > older					
L fusiform gyrus	−30	−43	−11	4.65	855
R cerebellum	12	−49	−35	3.94	477
Posterior cingulate gyrus	0	−58	28	4.49	648

L: left, R: right, ACC: anterior cingulate cortex, MFG: middle frontal gyrus, SMA: supplementary motor area.

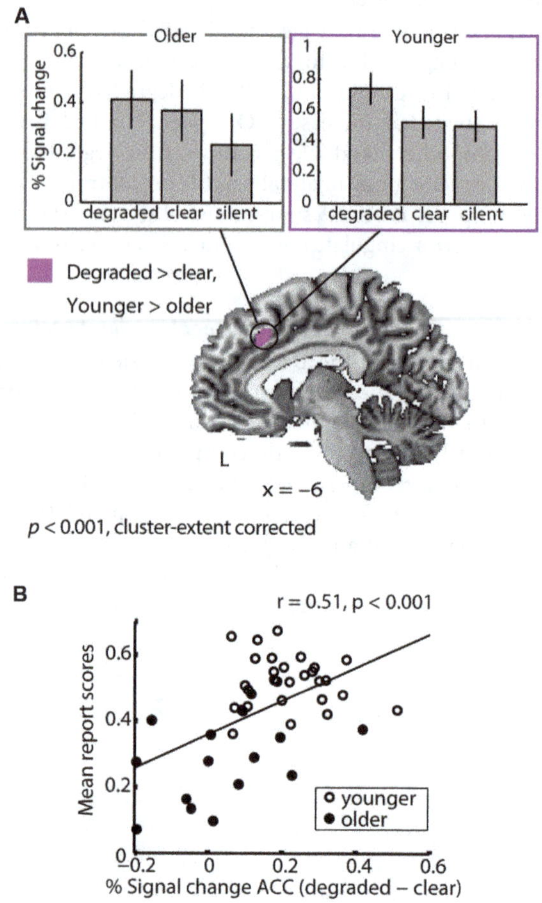

FIGURE 4 | (A) Age group × degradation interaction. Young adults showed a greater difference in anterior cingulate cortex (ACC) activity between degraded and clear speech than older adults. This age group × degradation interaction was driven by a reduced dynamic range in older adults, who displayed increased levels of ACC activation during perception of both clear and degraded speech. This is apparent in the bar graphs showing % signal change for both groups and conditions (upper panel). For comparison, signal change for silent trials is shown, illustrating that older but not younger adults upregulate ACC activity for clear compared to silent trials. **(B)** Correlation of ACC dynamics with performance. A post-hoc ROI analysis showed that across groups, individuals with a better overall degraded speech comprehension (mean report scores) showed a higher differentiation (degraded minus clear speech) in ACC activity.

FUNCTIONAL MRI DIFFERENCES BETWEEN YOUNG AND OLDER ADULTS

Degraded speech processing

Generally, older and younger adults showed largely overlapping activations during degraded speech processing (see Erb et al., 2013 for the activation clusters in young adults). However, the ACC exhibited a group difference: young adults showed a higher increase in ACC activity when comparing degraded to clear speech than older adults did. This age group × degradation interaction was driven by a reduced dynamic range in older adults, who displayed persistently elevated levels of ACC activity in both conditions (**Figure 4A** and **Table 2**).

Extracting individual percentage signal change values from the ACC region of interest (as identified by the age group × degradation interaction) showed that, across groups, activity dynamics in the ACC were related to performance: Individuals with an overall better degraded speech comprehension showed a higher ACC differentiation for degraded vs. clear speech (**Figure 4B**). However, this correlation was driven by age, because the correlation was not significant in both groups separately (Pearson's correlation in young adults: $r = -0.07$, $p = 0.73$; older adults: $r = 0.39$, $p = 0.16$) and the correlation broke down when controlling for age ($r = 0.15$, $p = 0.34$). Within older adults, however, the correlation reached a non-significant trend, when partialling out age ($r = 0.46$, $p = 0.09$). However, the age group × mean performance interaction in the ACC BOLD signal failed to reach significance ($t(41) = 1.5$, $p = 0.14$).

Trial-by-trial fluctuations in degraded speech comprehension

Following up on the comprehension-dependent fluctuations observed in the cohort of young listeners (Erb et al., 2013), we also tested for such fluctuations in the older adults. While observing again substantial overlap between groups, an age group × comprehension interaction, also in prefrontal cortex, was manifest: Older adults' BOLD signal positively correlated with comprehension (i.e., report scores) in the middle frontal gyrus (MFG). Young adults did not show such a correlation in MFG. Young adults, on the other hand, exhibited additional correlations with comprehension in the left fusiform gyrus, right cerebellum and posterior cingulate cortex, where older adults did not show a correlation (**Figure 5** and **Table 2**).

DISCUSSION

The current study intended to compare degraded speech processing between young and older adults to characterize how underlying neural mechanisms change with age. The main results can be summarized as follows: Although degraded speech comprehension overall appeared deteriorated in older adults, both

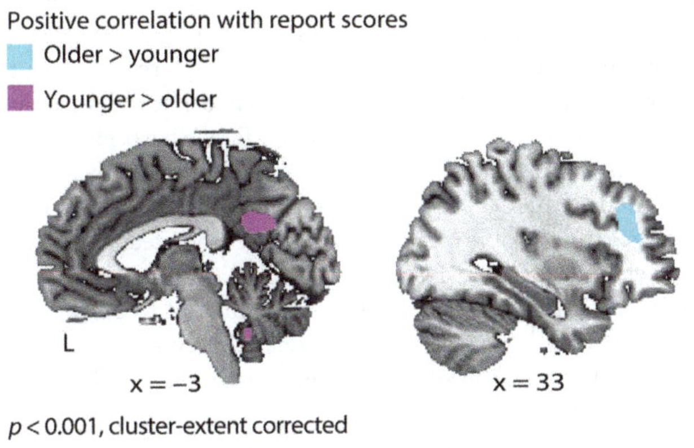

FIGURE 5 | Age group × comprehension interaction. In older adults the hemodynamic response in middle frontal gyrus covaried with comprehension of degraded speech on a trial-by-trial basis (i.e., report scores); young adults did not exhibit such a correlation. Incontrast, young adults showed additional correlations with report scores in the posterior cingulate cortex, left fusiform gyrus and right cerebellum (see **Table 2**).

older and younger adults adapted to degraded speech at the same rate. Within older listeners, better working memory predicted faster adaptation rates and hearing loss predicted worse speech comprehension. Hearing loss was related to a distinct activation pattern in the anterior insula during degraded speech processing. Young listeners showed an expected modulation of ACC activity depending on task difficulty (i.e., degraded greater than clear speech), whereas older adults displayed elevated levels of ACC activity throughout, consistent with a persistent upregulation in this cognitive-control related area. Within the ACC, a greater dynamic range predicted better speech comprehension. Finally, for correctly comprehended degraded speech trials, older listeners recruited middle frontal regions in addition to a core speech comprehension network which younger listeners relied on, most likely reflecting a compensatory mechanism. We will now discuss these results in more detail.

PERCEPTUAL ADAPTATION IS COMPARABLE IN YOUNG AND OLDER ADULTS

Even though degraded speech comprehension was substantially reduced in older listeners, their ability to gradually adapt to degraded speech over the course of the experiment was preserved, as the slopes of their linear fits (adaptation curves) did not differ from young adults (**Figure 1C**). Yet, as the R^2-values were relatively low (but cf. Davis et al., 2005, for comparable R^2-values), it remains questionable what no difference between age groups in a parameter of a badly fitting model actually means. Importantly however, we have shown that a second, model-free measure of learning (Δ performance) is strongly correlated with adaptation slope, and does not differ between age groups either. We take this as evidence that adaptation is comparable in young and older adults.

This result is consistent with a finding by Peelle and Wingfield (2005) who had shown that older adults' (aged 65–78) perceptual learning of both time-compressed and spectrally shifted noise-vocoded speech was comparable to those of young adults: when older adults' starting accuracy was equated with young adults, both groups' speech comprehension improved at the same rate when listening to 20 degraded sentences. Thus, older and younger adults appear to show equivalent behavioral adaptation to degraded speech. However, this does not warrant that the underlying neural mechanisms are identical.

Older listeners with a better short-term memory adapted faster to degraded speech. The correlation of adaptation with backward but not forward digit span reached significance. The latter demands simple maintenance and repetition. In contrast, backward digit span requires the listener to perform an operation on the items held in the memory buffer (i.e., inverse the order of the digits) and has specific demands on central executive mechanisms (Baddeley, 2012), which are supposedly involved in effortful speech perception. Rabbitt (1968) suggested an effortful hypothesis, according to which working memory becomes a limiting factor when perceptual effort is required in degraded speech comprehension: Masked words disrupt the short-term memory buffer, because resources that would otherwise be available for encoding in short-term memory are diverted for perceptual effort (Piquado et al., 2010). Our result lends further support to the hypothesis that such cognitive and perceptual abilities become coupled more tightly at an older age (Baltes and Lindenberger, 1997).

HEARING LOSS DETERIORATES DEGRADED SPEECH COMPREHENSION AND ALTERS INSULA DYNAMICS

One aim here was to identify how individuals with hearing loss recognize and process degraded speech. Unsurprisingly, a decline in hearing acuity was associated with worse average degraded speech comprehension in older adults. This is best explained by the fact that on top of the exogenous signal degradation (i.e., 4-band vocoding), hearing loss endogenously distorts the signal and reduces audibility (Pichora-Fuller and Souza, 2003).

In addition, hearing loss was accompanied by changes in central neural mechanisms. While older adults with worse hearing activated the anterior insula more for clear than degraded speech, better-hearing older listeners had increased anterior insula activity during degraded relative to clear speech perception. Importantly, this activation pattern in the insula could not be explained by age. In Erb et al. (2013), we had shown that younger adults rely on the anterior insula in difficult listening (see Erb et al., 2013). Here, it appears that only better-hearing older adults succeed to recruit the anterior insula in adverse listening conditions, whereas older adults affected by substantial hearing loss show the inverse dynamics. These hearing loss effects were found even though speech was presented at an audible level for each participant, supporting the notion that these are centrally-driven changes.

The insula together with the ACC have commonly been termed the "cingulo-opercular" system (e.g., Harris et al., 2009). Here, an interesting dissociation between insula and ACC dynamics emerges: Anterior insula activation was affected by hearing loss (independent of age), while ACC activity was altered by age (see below).

There is accumulating evidence that the insula plays a crucial role in top-down, executive processes (Eckert et al., 2009; Menon and Uddin, 2010; Sterzer and Kleinschmidt, 2010; Adank, 2012). For example, Wild et al. (2012) showed that in young listeners, the insula exhibited an enhanced BOLD signal when listeners attended to speech (rather than a distracter), and the speech signal was degraded (vocoded rather than clear). Activation in the anterior insula further scaled with task-difficulty of a temporal non-speech auditory task, dependent on attention (Henry et al., 2013).

The current results are somewhat more complicated, as insula engagement depended on the extent of hearing loss; only those listeners with very mild, age-typical hearing loss (< 20 dB HL) exhibit such a pattern, while more hearing-impaired listeners did recruit insular cortex into clear-speech (i.e., already at milder task demands), but less so into degraded-speech processing (higher task demands). Intriguingly, this pattern of insula activation is reminiscent of the Crunch-hypothesis, according to which older adults show a load-dependent inverse *u*-shaped pattern of activity in cognitive-control-related areas (Reuter-Lorenz and Cappell, 2008). While this finding deserves thorough follow-up experimentation, the insula seems to be crucial for cognitive control (Eckert et al., 2009) and the observed alteration of its hemodynamics might add up to declines of the peripheral auditory system and manifest in the observed deterioration in speech recognition.

PERSISTENT UPREGULATION OF ANTERIOR CINGULATE ACTIVITY REFLECTS INCREASED COGNITIVE CONTROL IN OLDER ADULTS

The main objective of the current study was to identify age differences in the neural systems supporting degraded speech processing. We found an age group × degradation interaction in the ACC, where young listeners showed a higher activation difference between degraded and clear speech than older adults. The latter displayed elevated levels of ACC activation during both conditions, indicating a reduced dynamic range in older adults. Thus, the older adults' BOLD signal in the ACC appears to be less informative and flexible, as it is differentiating less between a degraded and clear speech input. This is consistent with an age-related decrease in the variability of the hemodynamic signal (Garrett et al., 2010).

As we intended to compare the results in the older group to the ones obtained in young adults (Erb et al., 2013), we normalized older adults to a young adult (MNI) template. This can be problematic due to group differences in brain morphology. For example, partial volume effects, that is, sampling both grey and white matter in one voxel, may increase in older adults, who commonly exhibit gray matter atrophy in frontal regions. One solution to overcome this problem is to only test for the interaction (Samanez-Larkin and D'Esposito, 2008). As we found an age group × condition interaction in the ACC, it is unlikely that older adults' smaller dynamic range in ACC activity could be driven by the non-diffeomorphic normalization of older adults to a young adult (MNI) template.

Age-related functional and structural changes in frontal lobe systems supporting cognitive control have been previously noted (Cabeza et al., 2004; Colcombe et al., 2005; Sharp et al., 2006; Eckert et al., 2008; Harris et al., 2009). For example, Harris et al. (2009) showed that ACC activity increases for incorrect compared to correct word recognition, but more so in older adults. The authors linked this to auditory cortex architecture, showing that ACC recruitment correlates with age-related neurodegeneration of the auditory cortex. Along the same line, Sharp et al. (2006) showed that aging is accompanied by greater cognitive control, as indexed by higher ACC and prefrontal cortex activity during semantic and syllabic decisions on noise-vocoded words. Both Sharp et al. (2006) and Harris et al. (2009) observed that activity in ACC increased with age and was detrimental to performance. Therefore, they interpreted the age-related increase of ACC activation as upregulation of error monitoring systems (Dosenbach et al., 2006, 2007).

In contrast, the present findings show that a higher dynamic range of ACC activity (i.e., the degree to which the ACC became relatively engaged and disengaged in degraded and clear speech, respectively) was associated with better speech comprehension. However, this correlation was best explained by age, as the correlation broke down when correlating groups separately. The following picture emerges: Dynamic range of ACC activity decreases with age which in turn is detrimental to speech comprehension. Rather than playing a compensatory role for deficits due to aging (Cabeza et al., 2002), the observed ACC dynamics might reflect a generalized upregulation of cognitive control with age irrespective of task difficulty (see also the discussion of dedifferentiation vs. compensation hypothesis below).

COMPENSATORY PREFRONTAL ACTIVITY DURING SPEECH COMPREHENSION IN OLDER ADULTS

For successful speech comprehension, younger adults' activated a perisylvian network (Erb et al., 2013), where the BOLD signal was tightly coupled to actual speech comprehension (i.e., behavioral report scores), rather than acoustic properties of the sentences. Older adults additionally showed a correlation with report scores in middle frontal gyrus. Eckert et al. (2008) similarly demonstrated that older adults engage the MFG when words are most intelligible. However, their design varied speech intelligibility by low-pass filtering words such that effects due to acoustic differences could not be disentangled from actual comprehension. In contrast, the current study held physical stimulus properties constant (i.e., 4-band vocoding) and thus identified regions where activation varied with actual speech comprehension (i.e., behavioral report scores). Therefore, the present data provide evidence that additional MFG activation observed in older adults is related to comprehension rather than physical speech clarity.

Age-related additional recruitment of middle frontal or lateral prefrontal cortex has been repeatedly observed, for example, during working memory tasks (Cabeza et al., 2002), visual attention (Cabeza et al., 2004), word recognition (Eckert et al., 2008), and for processing of syntactically complex sentences (Peelle et al., 2010b). Two hypotheses have been put forward to explain the frequently observed recruitment of additional brain regions by older adults not observed in young adults: The dedifferentiation hypothesis (Baltes and Lindenberger, 1997) interprets the extra activation as difficulties in recruiting specialized neural mechanisms for the relevant task, hence as a loss of neural specialization (Park et al., 2004). Such a generalized non-functional spread of activation has been attributed to a deficit in neurotransmission with a decrease in signal-to-noise ratio in neural firing (Li and Lindenberger, 1999). If this hypothesis is true, engagement of additional regions should not correlate with task performance. On the other hand, the compensation hypothesis suggests that recruitment of additional brain regions plays a compensatory role, for example in counteracting performance decline due to neurodegeneration in specialized brain areas (e.g., the auditory cortex; Harris et al., 2009; Peelle et al., 2011; Eckert et al., 2012), and should therefore improve performance (Cabeza et al., 2002; Heuninckx et al., 2008).

In the current study, engagement of the MFG in older adults covaried with report scores, that is, MFG activity did in fact increase with better performance. We take this as evidence for a compensatory mechanism in older adults, whereby the MFG is recruited in addition to the core speech comprehension network (Erb et al., 2013) when speech comprehension succeeds. In sum, our data contribute to, but cannot solve, the ongoing debate of dedifferentiation vs. compensation, in that the age-group-differences observed in two prefrontal areas, ACC and MFG, are to be interpreted with opposing conclusions regarding the compensation hypothesis by Cabeza et al. (2002, 2004).

CONCLUSIONS

Our results show distinct age-related changes of responses in prefrontal cortex. Higher anterior cingulate and middle frontal gyrus activities are found associated with better performance in adverse listening conditions. However, unlike younger adults, older adults do not succeed in selectively modulating ACC activity depending on listening difficulty, but exhibit generalized upregulated levels of ACC activity also in easy listening conditions. In contrast, MFG activity appears to be truly compensatory, as older adults recruit frontal areas in addition to a speech comprehension network when comprehension succeeds. Moreover, more hearing-impaired older adults involve the anterior insula more even in clear speech comprehension. As all three structures have been linked to cognitive control, the results provide further evidence that older adults increasingly rely on cognitive control networks when adapting to challenging listening conditions, at the potential expense of these systems' dynamic range.

AUTHOR CONTRIBUTIONS

Julia Erb designed and conducted research, analyzed the data and wrote the paper and Jonas Obleser designed research, analyzed the data and wrote the paper.

ACKNOWLEDGMENTS

Research is supported by the Max Planck Society (Max Planck Research group grant to Jonas Obleser). The authors thank their colleagues in the Max Planck Research Group "Auditory Cognition" for initial discussions and two reviewers for their thoughtful comments. Sylvie Neubert and Nicole Pampus helped acquire the behavioral and MR data.

REFERENCES

Adank, P. (2012). The neural bases of difficult speech comprehension and speech production: two activation likelihood estimation (ALE) meta-analyses. *Brain Lang.* 122, 42–54. doi: 10.1016/j.bandl.2012.04.014

Adank, P., and Janse, E. (2010). Comprehension of a novel accent by young and older listeners. *Psychol. Aging* 25, 736–740. doi: 10.1037/a0020054

Baddeley, A. (2012). Working memory: theories, models and controversies. *Annu. Rev. Psychol.* 63, 1–29. doi: 10.1146/annurev-psych-120710-100422

Baltes, P. B., and Lindenberger, U. (1997). Emergence of a powerful connection between sensory and cognitive functions across the adult life span: a new window to the study of cognitive aging? *Psychol. Aging* 12, 12–21. doi: 10.1037/0882-7974.12.1.12

Benjamini, Y., and Hochberg, Y. (1995). Controlling the false discovery rate: a practical and powerful approach to multiple testing. *J. R. Stat. Soc.* 57, 289–300.

Bent, T., Buchwald, A., and Pisoni, D. B. (2009). Perceptual adaptation and intelligibility of multiple talkers for two types of degraded speech. *J. Acoust. Soc. Am.* 126, 2660–2669. doi: 10.1121/1.3212930

Brett, M., Anton, J., Valabregue, R., and Poline, J. (2002). Region of interest analysis using an SPM toolbox. *Presentation at the 8th International Conference on Functional Mapping of the Human Brain, Sendai, Japan,* June 2–6, 2002.

Burkholder, R. A., Pisoni, D. B., and Svirsky, M. A. (2005). Effects of a cochlear implant simulation on immediate memory in normal-hearing adults. *Int. J. Audiol.* 44, 551–558. doi: 10.1080/14992020500243893

Cabeza, R., Anderson, N. D., Locantore, J. K., and Mcintosh, A. R. (2002). Aging gracefully: compensatory brain activity in high-performing older adults. *Neuroimage* 17, 1394–1402. doi: 10.1006/nimg.2002.1280

Cabeza, R., Daselaar, S. M., Dolcos, F., Prince, S. E., Budde, M., and Nyberg, L. (2004). Task-independent and task-specific age effects on brain activity during working memory, visual attention and episodic retrieval. *Cereb. Cortex* 14, 364–375. doi: 10.1093/cercor/bhg133

Colcombe, S. J., Kramer, A. F., Erickson, K. I., and Scalf, P. (2005). The implications of cortical recruitment and brain morphology for individual differences in inhibitory function in aging humans. *Psychol. Aging* 20, 363–375. doi: 10.1037/0882-7974.20.3.363

Davis, M. H., Johnsrude, I. S., Hervais-Adelman, A., Taylor, K., and Mcgettigan, C. (2005). Lexical information drives perceptual learning of distorted speech: evidence from the comprehension of noise-vocoded sentences. *J. Exp. Psychol. Gen.* 134, 222–241. doi: 10.1037/0096-3445.134.2.222

Dosenbach, N. U., Fair, D. A., Miezin, F. M., Cohen, A. L., Wenger, K. K., Dosenbach, R. A., et al. (2007). Distinct brain networks for adaptive and stable task control in humans. *Proc. Natl. Acad. Sci. U S A* 104, 11073–11078. doi: 10.1073/pnas.0704320104

Dosenbach, N. U., Visscher, K. M., Palmer, E. D., Miezin, F. M., Wenger, K. K., Kang, H. C., et al. (2006). A core system for the implementation of task sets. *Neuron* 50, 799–812. doi: 10.1016/j.neuron.2006.04.031

Eckert, M. A., Cute, S. L., Vaden, Jr. I. K., Kuchinsky, S. E., and Dubno, J. R. (2012). Auditory cortex signs of age-related hearing loss. *J. Assoc. Res. Otolaryngol.* 13, 703–713. doi: 10.1007/s10162-012-0332-5

Eckert, M. A., Menon, V., Walczak, A., Ahlstrom, J., Denslow, S., Horwitz, A., et al. (2009). At the heart of the ventral attention system: the right anterior insula. *Hum. Brain Mapp.* 30, 2530–2541. doi: 10.1002/hbm.20688

Eckert, M. A., Walczak, A., Ahlstrom, J., Denslow, S., Horwitz, A., and Dubno, J. R. (2008). Age-related effects on word recognition: reliance on cognitive control systems with structural declines in speech-responsive cortex. *J. Assoc. Res. Otolaryngol.* 9, 252–259. doi: 10.1007/s10162-008-0113-3

Eisner, F., Mcgettigan, C., Faulkner, A., Rosen, S., and Scott, S. K. (2010). Inferior frontal gyrus activation predicts individual differences in perceptual learning of cochlear-implant simulations. *J. Neurosci.* 30, 7179–7186. doi: 10.1523/jneurosci.4040-09.2010

Erb, J., Henry, M. J., Eisner, F., and Obleser, J. (2012). Auditory skills and brain morphology predict individual differences in adaptation to degraded speech. *Neuropsychologia* 50, 2154–2164. doi: 10.1016/j.neuropsychologia.2012.05.013

Erb, J., Henry, M. J., Eisner, F., and Obleser, J. (2013). The brain dynamics of rapid perceptual adaptation to adverse listening conditions. *J. Neurosci.* 33, 10688–10697. doi: 10.1523/jneurosci.4596-12.2013

Fiebach, C. J., Schlesewsky, M., Lohmann, G., Von Cramon, D. Y., and Friederici, A. D. (2005). Revisiting the role of Broca's area in sentence processing: syntactic integration versus syntactic working memory. *Hum. Brain Mapp.* 24, 79–91. doi: 10.1002/hbm.20070

Garrett, D. D., Kovacevic, N., Mcintosh, A. R., and Grady, C. L. (2010). Blood oxygen level-dependent signal variability is more than just noise. *J. Neurosci.* 30, 4914–4921. doi: 10.1523/jneurosci.5166-09.2010

Golomb, J. D., Peelle, J. E., and Wingfield, A. (2007). Effects of stimulus variability and adult aging on adaptation to time-compressed speech. *J. Acoust. Soc. Am.* 121, 1701–1708. doi: 10.1121/1.2436635

Gordon-Salant, S., Yeni-Komshian, G. H., and Fitzgibbons, P. J. (2010). Recognition of accented English in quiet and noise by younger and older listeners. *J. Acoust. Soc. Am.* 128, 3152–3160. doi: 10.1121/1.3495940

Greenwood, D. D. (1990). A cochlear frequency-position function for several species—29 years later. *J. Acoust. Soc. Am.* 87, 2592–2605. doi: 10.1121/1.399052

Hall, D. A., Haggard, M. P., Akeroyd, M. A., Palmer, A. R., Summerfield, A. Q., Elliott, M. R., et al. (1999). "Sparse" temporal sampling in auditory fMRI. *Hum. Brain Mapp.* 7, 213–223. doi: 10.1002/(SICI)1097-0193(1999)7:3<213::AID-HBM5>3.0.CO;2-N

Harris, K. C., Dubno, J. R., Keren, N. I., Ahlstrom, J. B., and Eckert, M. A. (2009). Speech recognition in younger and older adults: a dependency on low-level auditory cortex. *J. Neurosci.* 29, 6078–6087. doi: 10.1523/jneurosci.0412-09.2009

Henry, M. J., Herrmann, B., and Obleser, J. (2013). Selective attention to temporal features on nested time scales. *Cereb. Cortex* doi: 10.1093/cercor/bht240. [Epub ahead of print].

Heuninckx, S., Wenderoth, N., and Swinnen, S. P. (2008). Systems neuroplasticity in the aging brain: recruiting additional neural resources for successful motor performance in elderly persons. *J. Neurosci.* 28, 91–99. doi: 10.1523/jneurosci.3300-07.2008

Jacquemot, C., and Scott, S. K. (2006). What is the relationship between phonological short-term memory and speech processing? *Trends Cogn. Sci.* 10, 480–486. doi: 10.1016/j.tics.2006.09.002

Janse, E., and Adank, P. (2012). Predicting foreign-accent adaptation in older adults. *Q. J. Exp. Psychol. (Hove)* 65, 1563–1585. doi: 10.1080/17470218.2012.658822

Kalikow, D. N., Stevens, K. N., and Elliott, L. L. (1977). Development of a test of speech intelligibility in noise using sentence materials with controlled word predictability. *J. Acoust. Soc. Am.* 61, 1337–1351. doi: 10.1121/1.381436

Li, S. C., and Lindenberger, U. (1999). "Cross-level unification: a computational exploration of the link between deterioration of neurotransmitter systems dedifferentiation of cognitive abilities in old age," in *Cognitive Neuroscience of Memory*, eds L. G. Nilsson and H. J. Markowitsch (Seattle: Hogrefe and Huber), 103–146.

Lindenberger, U., and Ghisletta, P. (2009). Cognitive and sensory declines in old age: gauging the evidence for a common cause. *Psychol. Aging* 24, 1–16. doi: 10.1037/a0014986

Menon, V., and Uddin, L. Q. (2010). Saliency, switching, attention and control: a network model of insula function. *Brain Struct. Funct.* 214, 655–667. doi: 10.1007/s00429-010-0262-0

Obleser, J., Wostmann, M., Hellbernd, N., Wilsch, A., and Maess, B. (2012). Adverse listening conditions and memory load drive a common alpha oscillatory network. *J. Neurosci.* 32, 12376–12383. doi: 10.1523/jneurosci.4908-11.2012

Oldfield, R. C. (1971). The assessment and analysis of handedness: the Edinburgh inventory. *Neuropsychologia* 9, 97–113. doi: 10.1016/0028-3932(71)90067-4

Park, D. C., Polk, T. A., Park, R., Minear, M., Savage, A., and Smith, M. R. (2004). Aging reduces neural specialization in ventral visual cortex. *Proc. Natl. Acad. Sci. U S A* 101, 13091–13095. doi: 10.1073/pnas.0405148101

Peelle, J. E., Gross, J., and Davis, M. H. (2013). Phase-locked responses to speech in human auditory cortex are enhanced during comprehension. *Cereb. Cortex* 23, 1378–1387. doi: 10.1093/cercor/bhs118

Peelle, J. E., Mcmillan, C., Moore, P., Grossman, M., and Wingfield, A. (2004). Dissociable patterns of brain activity during comprehension of rapid and syntactically complex speech: evidence from fMRI. *Brain Lang.* 91, 315–325. doi: 10.1016/j.bandl.2004.05.007

Peelle, J. E., Olafsen, T., Davis, M. H., and Wingfield, A. (2010a). Perceptual learning in speech comprehension governed by power law dynamics. *Poster presentation at the 40th SfN annual meeting, San Diego, US*, November 13–17, 2010.

Peelle, J. E., Troiani, V., Grossman, M., and Wingfield, A. (2011). Hearing loss in older adults affects neural systems supporting speech comprehension. *J. Neurosci.* 31, 12638–12643. doi: 10.1523/jneurosci.2559-11.2011

Peelle, J. E., Troiani, V., Wingfield, A., and Grossman, M. (2010b). Neural processing during older adults' comprehension of spoken sentences: age differences in resource allocation and connectivity. *Cereb. Cortex* 20, 773–782. doi: 10.1093/cercor/bhp142

Peelle, J. E., and Wingfield, A. (2005). Dissociations in perceptual learning revealed by adult age differences in adaptation to time-compressed speech. *J. Exp. Psychol. Hum. Percept. Perform.* 31, 1315–1330. doi: 10.1037/0096-1523.31.6.1315

Pichora-Fuller, M. K. (2003). Cognitive aging and auditory information processing. *Int. J. Audiol.* 42(Suppl. 2), 26–32. doi: 10.3109/14992020309074641

Pichora-Fuller, M. K., Schneider, B. A., and Daneman, M. (1995). How young and old adults listen to and remember speech in noise. *J. Acoust. Soc. Am.* 97, 593–608. doi: 10.1121/1.412282

Pichora-Fuller, M. K., and Souza, P. E. (2003). Effects of aging on auditory processing of speech. *Int. J. Audiol.* 42(Suppl. 2), 11–16. doi: 10.3109/14992020309074638

Piquado, T., Cousins, K. A., Wingfield, A., and Miller, P. (2010). Effects of degraded sensory input on memory for speech: behavioral data and a test of biologically constrained computational models. *Brain Res.* 1365, 48–65. doi: 10.1016/j.brainres.2010.09.070

Pisoni, D. B., and Cleary, M. (2003). Measures of working memory span and verbal rehearsal speed in deaf children after cochlear implantation. *Ear Hear.* 24, 106S–120S. doi: 10.1097/01.aud.0000051692.05140.8e

Priestley, M. B. (1981). *Spectral Analysis and Time Series.* London: Academic Press. p. 375.

Rabbitt, P. M. (1968). Channel-capacity, intelligibility and immediate memory. *Q. J. Exp. Psychol.* 20, 241–248. doi: 10.1080/14640746808400158

Reuter-Lorenz, P., and Cappell, K. A. (2008). Neurocognitive aging and the compensation hypothesis. *Curr. Dir. Psychol. Sci.* 17, 177–182. doi: 10.1111/j.1467-8721.2008.00570.x

Rorden, C., and Brett, M. (2000). Stereotaxic display of brain lesions. *Behav. Neurol.* 12, 191–200.

Rosen, S., Faulkner, A., and Wilkinson, L. (1999). Adaptation by normal listeners to upward spectral shifts of speech: implications for cochlear implants. *J. Acoust. Soc. Am.* 106, 3629–3636. doi: 10.1121/1.428215

Samanez-Larkin, G. R., and D'Esposito, M. (2008). Group comparisons: imaging the aging brain. *Soc. Cogn. Affect. Neurosci.* 3, 290–297. doi: 10.1093/scan/nsn029

Samuel, A. G., and Kraljic, T. (2009). Perceptual learning for speech. *Atten. Percept. Psychophys.* 71, 1207–1218. doi: 10.3758/APP.71.6.120

Schwarz, G. (1978). Estimating the dimension of a model. *Ann. Stat.* 6, 461–464. doi: 10.1214/aos/1176344136

Shannon, R. V., and Galvin, J. J. 3rd., and Baskent, D. (2002). Holes in hearing. *J. Assoc. Res. Otolaryngol.* 3, 185–199. doi: 10.1007/s101620020021

Sharp, D. J., Scott, S. K., Mehta, M. A., and Wise, R. J. (2006). The neural correlates of declining performance with age: evidence for age-related changes in cognitive control. *Cereb. Cortex* 16, 1739–1749. doi: 10.1093/cercor/bhj109

Slotnick, S. D., Moo, L. R., Segal, J. B., and Hart, Jr. J. (2003). Distinct prefrontal cortex activity associated with item memory and source memory for visual shapes. *Brain Res. Cogn. Brain Res.* 17, 75–82. doi: 10.1016/s0926-6410(03)00082-x

Sterzer, P., and Kleinschmidt, A. (2010). Anterior insula activations in perceptual paradigms: often observed but barely understood. *Brain Struct. Funct.* 214, 611–622. doi: 10.1007/s00429-010-0252-2

Von Kriegstein, K., Patterson, R. D., and Griffiths, T. D. (2008). Task-dependent modulation of medial geniculate body is behaviorally relevant for speech recognition. *Curr. Biol.* 18, 1855–1859. doi: 10.1016/j.cub.2008.10.052

Wechsler, D. (1987). *Wechsler Memory Scale - Revised Edition. Manual.* New York: The Psychological Corporation.

7

Diffusion tensor imaging in children with unilateral hearing loss

Tara Rachakonda[1], Joshua S. Shimony[2], Rebecca S. Coalson[2] and Judith E. C. Lieu[1]*

[1] Department of Otolaryngology-Head and Neck Surgery, Washington University School of Medicine, St. Louis, MO, USA
[2] Department of Radiology, Mallinckrodt Institute of Radiology, Washington University School of Medicine, St. Louis, MO, USA
[3] Departments of Neurology and Radiology, Washington University School of Medicine, St. Louis, MO, USA

***Correspondence:**
Judith E. C. Lieu, Department of Otolaryngology-Head and Neck Surgery, Washington University School of Medicine, 660 S. Euclid Ave., Campus Box 8115, St. Louis, MO 63110, USA
e-mail: lieuj@ent.wustl.edu

Objective: Language acquisition was assumed to proceed normally in children with unilateral hearing loss (UHL) since they have one functioning ear. However, children with UHL score poorly on speech-language tests and have higher rates of educational problems compared to normal hearing (NH) peers. Diffusion tensor imaging (DTI) is an imaging modality used to measure microstructural integrity of brain white matter. The purpose of this pilot study was to investigate differences in fractional anisotropy (FA) and mean diffusivity (MD) in hearing- and non-hearing-related structures in the brain between children with UHL and their NH siblings.

Study Design: Prospective observational cohort.

Setting: Academic medical center.

Subjects and Methods: Sixty one children were recruited, tested and imaged. Twenty nine children with severe-to-profound UHL were compared to 20 siblings with NH using IQ and oral language testing, and MRI with DTI. Twelve children had inadequate MRI data. Parents provided demographic data and indicated whether children had a need for an individualized educational program (IEP) or speech therapy (ST). DTI parameters were measured in auditory and non-auditory regions of interest (ROIs). Between-group comparisons were evaluated with non-parametric tests.

Results: Lower FA of left lateral lemniscus was observed for children with UHL compared to their NH siblings, as well as trends toward differences in other auditory and non-auditory regions. Correlation analyses showed associations between several DTI parameters and outcomes in children with UHL. Regression analyses revealed relationships between educational outcome variables and several DTI parameters, which may provide clinically useful information for guidance of speech therapy.

Discussion/Conclusion: Our data suggests that white matter microstructural patterns in several brain regions are preserved despite unilateral rather than bilateral auditory input which contrasts with findings in patients with bilateral hearing loss.

Keywords: hearing loss, unilateral hearing loss, diffusion tensor imaging, children, magnetic resonance imaging

INTRODUCTION

Although unilateral hearing loss (UHL) often goes undetected until children begin school, prevalence rates of UHL in newborns range from 0.04 to 3.4% (Mehl and Thomson, 1998; Widen et al., 2000). Studies have estimated the prevalence of UHL in school-aged children (ages 6–19 years) as high as 5% (Niskar et al., 1998). It was previously assumed that because children with UHL had one functioning ear, speech acquisition and language comprehension skills developed normally. However, several studies have suggested otherwise (Davis et al., 1981; Bess and Tharpe, 1984; Lieu et al., 2010). In one study, when compared with their normal hearing (NH) siblings, children (ages 6–12 years) with UHL had substantially worse oral language scores (Lieu et al., 2010). Other investigators have found evidence of increased rates of behavioral problems, a greater need for intensive educational plans and worse performance in school amongst children with UHL (Bess, 1982; Bess and Tharpe, 1984; Davis et al., 2002).

Presumably, problems with sound localization and the need for a higher signal-to-noise ratio for speech comprehension in children with UHL contribute to their delay in language skills, but they do not explain why some of these children experience behavioral challenges (Bess and Tharpe, 1984; Davis et al., 2002). These difficulties may reflect problems with executive functioning rather than difficulty with auditory processing, similar to children with bilateral hearing loss who may encounter executive functioning difficulties (Figueras et al., 2008; Beer et al., 2011).

Whether "right ear advantage (REA)" exists for speech perception has been controversial (Hugdahl, 2011). Although children with UHL have performed worse on speech-language tests, it is less clear that the side of hearing impairment influences cognitive abilities. According to the REA hypothesis, children with right UHL should have greater difficulties with language skills than those with left UHL. Some have postulated that the right hemisphere preferentially processes spectrally complex sounds (e.g., music), whereas the left hemisphere processes temporally complex sounds (e.g., speech) (Penhune et al., 1996). Older studies point to a higher rate of grade failures and worse verbal test performance in children with right UHL (Bess and Tharpe, 1984; Hartvig et al., 1989; Niedzielski et al., 2006). However, a large case-control study did not find intellectual differences based upon side of hearing impairment (Lieu et al., 2010).

In this study, we sought to find a neuroanatomical basis for educational differences. In a prior investigation in this study cohort, differences in resting state functional connectivity MRI (rs-fcMRI) were found in areas associated with auditory processing, executive function and memory formation between children with UHL and NH controls (Tibbetts et al., 2011). MRI provides a non-invasive means by which to examine the brain for gross anatomical changes, functional changes in activation (fMRI), and microstructural changes (diffusion tensor imaging, DTI) in numerous nervous system pathologies (Rykhlevskaia et al., 2008), and more specifically in hearing loss (Chang et al., 2004; Firszt et al., 2006; Lin et al., 2008; Kim et al., 2009; Propst et al., 2010). DTI measures of microstructural damage in white matter have been associated with behavioral measures in numerous diseases, such as in blindness (Shimony et al., 2006), depression (Shimony et al., 2009), traumatic brain injury (Hulkower et al., 2013), phenylketonuria (Antenor-Dorsey et al., 2013), and numerous other examples. DTI measures the diffusion of water molecules in brain tissues (Shimony et al., 2006). Water in brain tissues diffuses faster parallel to white matter tracts as compared to perpendicular, a property known as anisotropy. Anisotropy has been used to investigate the integrity and course of white matter tracts in the brain. Common DTI parameters include fractional anisotropy (FA), which ranges from 0 for equal diffusion in all directions to 1 for diffusion only along 1 axis, and the mean diffusivity (MD), which measures how easily water diffuses averaged over all directions, also ranging from 0 to 1. Changes in diffusivity or loss of directionality suggest lack of microstructural integrity (Mori and Zhang, 2006; Assaf and Pasternak, 2008; Neil, 2008). Restricted diffusion has been identified in several types of disease processes, including acute demyelination, certain brain tumors and acute ischemia (Mukherjee et al., 2008).

A few studies have used DTI to investigate the neuroanatomic properties of auditory processing regions in patients with hearing loss. These studies focused mainly upon subcortical structures and adults with hearing loss (Chang et al., 2004; Lutz et al., 2007; Lin et al., 2008; Kim et al., 2009; Wu et al., 2009). In light of DTI changes reported in prior studies of hearing loss, the goal of this study was to determine how UHL influences the development of white matter tracts in the brain. Our aims were to compare the microstructural integrity of white matter tracts using DTI in hearing-related and non-hearing-related brain regions between children with UHL and their NH siblings; and to examine relationships between various educational outcome variables and the DTI parameters (FA and MD) of hearing-related regions.

MATERIALS AND METHODS

STUDY PARTICIPANTS

Sixty one participants with severe-to-profound UHL and their NH siblings were enrolled. Participants with UHL were defined as having severe-to profound sensorineural UHL by pure tone audiometry, with pure tone averages (PTA) $\geq$70 dB hearing level (HL) in the affected ear. Participants with NH had PTA $<$ 20 dB HL in both ears. All subjects underwent audiometry, cognitive testing for IQ scores, language testing, and MRI scanning. Imaging data from 12 children had to be excluded from analysis, due to movement artifact ($n = 1$), inability to lie still in the scanner ($n = 1$), inadequate data acquisition ($n = 7$) and inadequate data due to the presence of metallic devices (orthodontic appliances, $n = 2$, and a bone-anchored hearing aid, $n = 1$). Thus, the analysis included 29 children with UHL (13 right UHL, 16 left UHL) and 20 siblings with NH. Children with both acquired and congenital UHL were included. All subjects were cognitively normal per parent report.

This study protocol was approved by the Human Research Protections Office (HRPO) at the Washington University School of Medicine. Informed consent was obtained from all parents of subjects and pediatric assent obtained from all minor participants.

BASELINE VARIABLES

Parents provided demographic, health, and family data. Parents also indicated whether children required speech therapy, special educational accommodations or special services at school, or an individualized educational program (IEP).

MEASURED OUTCOME VARIABLES

Cognitive ability was assessed by the Wechsler Abbreviated Scale of Intelligence (WASI) (Wechsler, 1999).We used standardized performance IQ, verbal IQ, and full scale IQ scores along with vocabulary T-scores as educational outcomes. All scores were standardized to a mean of 100 with a standard deviation (SD) of 15, except for the vocabulary T-score, which is standardized to a mean of 50 and SD of 10. Two standardized language tests were administered to the participants—the Oral and Written Language Scale (OWLS) and the Clinical Evaluation of Language Fundamentals (CELF) (Carrow-Woolfolk, 1995; Semel et al., 2011). Because both language tests use a standardized scale, they were combined as language outcomes for analysis.

MRI SCANNING PROTOCOL AND IMAGE ACQUISITION

Images were obtained on a 3.0 Tesla Siemens Trio, MR scanner (Erlangen, Germany). The imaging protocol included T1-weighted Magnetization Prepared Rapid Acquisition Gradient Echo (MPRAGE) sequence [Time of repetition (TR) /inversion time (TI)/ echo time (TE) = 2400/1000/3.16 ms, voxel size = $1 \times 1 \times 1\ \text{mm}^3$] and a T2-weighted (T2W) fast spin echo (FSE) scan (TR = 4380 ms, TE = 94 ms, $1 \times 1 \times 4$ mm). DTI data ($1.5 \times 1.5 \times 1.5$ mm voxels, TR = 9600 ms, TE = 95 ms), was collected in 25 different directions with b-values linearly distributed between 0 and 1400 s/mm^2.

The images were preprocessed and transformed into modified (Talairach and Tournoux, 1988) space using the following methods. A 9-parameter rigid body alignment registered all frames in all runs and was used for motion correction of each subject. Resampling was done by a 3-dimensional cubic spline interpolation and transformed to a Talairach atlas space using a single common atlas derived from adult and child brains via a warping mechanism (Burgund et al., 2002). After the registration steps, the diffusion data was processed with locally written software using a log linear algorithm into DTI parameter data using the commonly used tensor model (Basser et al., 1994).

REGIONS OF INTERESTS

The 15 regions of interest selected for analysis are listed in **Table 1** and fall into two groups. The first are regions that are known to be involved in auditory processing. The second group are non-auditory regions that are considered important white matter areas that are commonly sampled in DTI studies of the brain.

Auditory regions (**Figures 1A,B**) include: Auditory radiation; Heschl's gyrus (both gray and subcortical white matter); Inferior colliculus; Lateral lemniscus; Superior temporal gyrus (gray matter only).

Non-auditory regions (**Figures 1C–F, 2A–C**) include: Genu and splenium of the corpus callosum; Middle cerebellar peduncle; Globus pallidus; Putamen; Anterior corona radiata; Anterior limb of the internal capsule; Uncinate fasciculus; and Inferior longitudinal fasciculus. These regions are commonly sampled in DTI studies due to their importance in brain function and chosen as "control" regions where no differences would be expected. The latter four were also chosen due to their involvement in executive functioning (Cummings, 1993; Schmahmann et al., 2008).

Regions were located and sampled after the MPRAGE scans were transformed into Tailarach space over three to four slices each by one independent rater under the supervision of an experienced neuroradiologist. ROI location was traced on the MPRAGE anatomy, but guided using coregistered T2-weighted images to avoid cerebrospinal fluid, and FA images to capture fiber centers. The FA and MD values in the ROIs were measured and averaged over consecutive slices for a more accurate measurement than a single slice would give, thus minimizing the risk of type I error. The approximate MNI coordinates for these ROIs are listed in **Table 1** (each subject's regions are slightly different).

Table 1 | MNI coordinates for regions of interest (ROI) used in the study.

	x	*y*	*z*	Average size (mm^3)	Shape
AUDITORY ROIs					
Auditory radiation, left middle	−32	−23	−5	96	Punctate linear
Auditory radiation, right	27	−23	−8	96	Punctate linear
Heschl's gyrus, gray matter left	−41	−21	8	25	Punctate arc
Heschl's gyrus, gray matter right	41	−20	5	23	Punctate arc
Heschl's gyrus, subcortical white matter left	−45	−20	7	22	Oblong
Heschl's gyrus, subcortical white matter right	44	−20	4	20	Oblong
Inferior colliculus, left	−6	−36	−8	26	Oblong
Inferior colliculus, right	2	−35	−8	27	Oblong
Lateral lemniscus, left	−9	−30	−8	34	Oblong
Lateral lemniscus, right	6	−29	−9	50	Oblong
Superior temporal gyrus, left	−68	−42	2	36	Crescent
Superior temporal gyrus, right	66	−41	7	45	Crescent
CONTROL ROIs					
Genu of corpus callosum	−1	21	15	122	Oblong
Splenium of corpus callosum	1	−34	18	188	Oblong
Middle cerebellar peduncle, left	−24	−40	−35	354	Oblong
Middle cerebellar peduncle, right	17	−40	−36	420	Oblong
Globus pallidus, left	−18	1	−24	147	Oblong
Globus pallidus, right	16	1	−3	174	Oblong
Putamen, left	−23	13	−3	147	Oblong
Putamen, right	20	13	−4	147	Oblong
Anterior corona radiata, left	−18	42	−7	122	Oblong
Anterior corona radiata, right	18	44	−8	150	Oblong
Anterior limb of the internal capsule, left	−14	7	6	90	Enlongated oblong
Anterior limb of the internal capsule, right	15	10	5	122	Enlongated oblong
Uncinate fasciculus, left	−20	21	−11	85	Oblong
Uncinate fasciculus, right	16	22	−12	91	Oblong
Inferior longitudinal fasciculus, left	−41	−31	−8	123	Oblong
Inferior longitudinal fasciculus, right	39	−31	−11	170	Oblong

Average size was measured as mm^3.

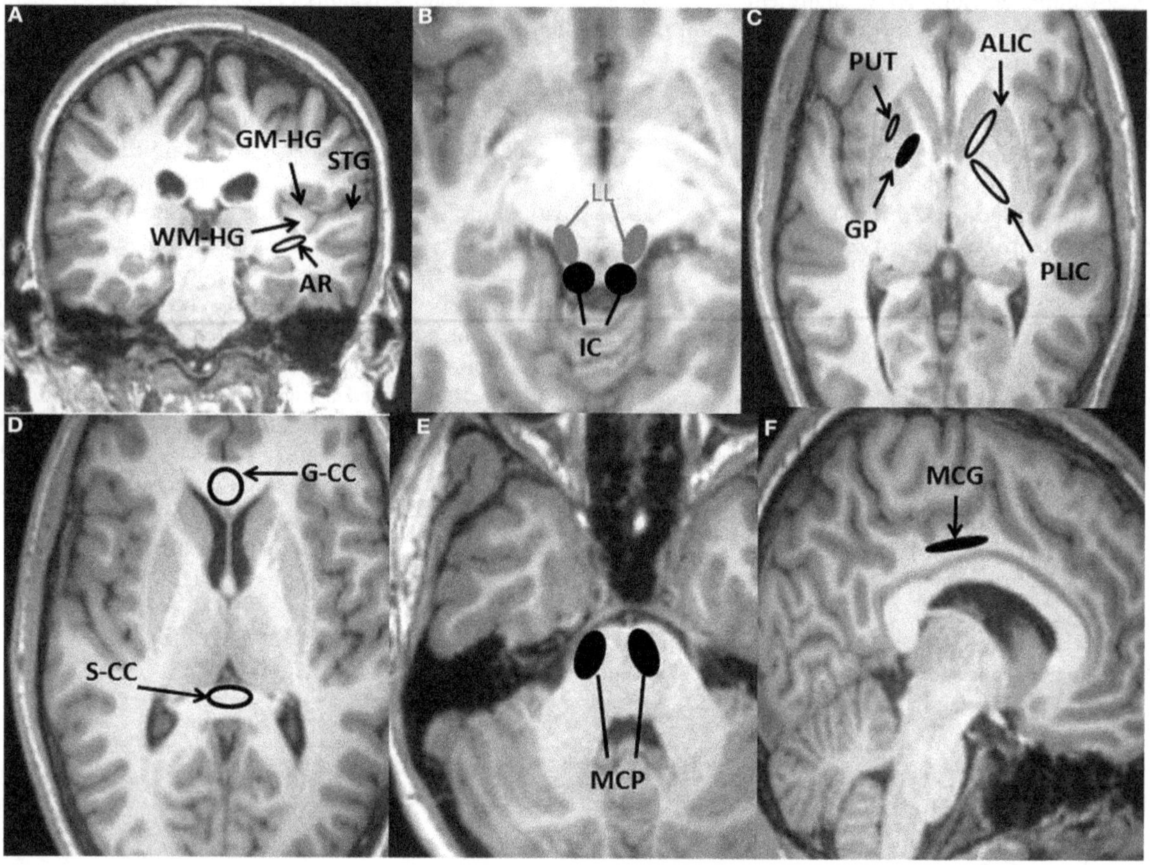

FIGURE 1 | Regions of interest (ROIs) used for DTI measurements placed on anatomical T1-weighted MRI scan. (A) Four auditory ROIs, Gray matter of Heschl's gyrus (GM-HG), White matter of Heschl's gyrus (WM-HG), Superior temporal gyrus (STG), and Auditory radiation (AR). **(B)** Two auditory ROIs, Inferior colliculus (IC), Lateral lemniscus (LL). **(C)** Three non-auditory ROIs, Putamen (PUT), Globus pallidus (GP), Posterior limb of the internal capsule (PLIC), Anterior limb of internal capsule (ALIC). **(D)** Two non-auditory ROIs, Genu of the corpus callosum (G-CC), Splenium of the corpus callosum (S-CC). **(E)** Non-auditory ROI, Middle cerebellar peduncle (MCP). **(F)** Non-auditory ROI, Middle cingulate gyrus (MCG).

STATISTICAL ANALYSIS

Statistical analyses were performed using the Statistical Package for the Social Sciences (SPSS), Version 20.0 (IBM Corp., Armonk, NY, US). Educational performance variables were compared with Mann-Whitney *U*-tests between the UHL and NH groups and between the right and left UHL groups. Pearson's chi-square was used to assess need for speech therapy and/or IEP. We used a Bonferroni correction of $0.05/6 = 0.008$ for a two-sided *alpha* threshold for the six educational outcomes assessed; a *p*-value less than 0.05 was considered a trend.

Kruskal-Wallis tests provided between-group comparisons of DTI parameters. Paired Wilcoxon signed rank-test of DTI parameters between sides (right and left) were performed within each of the groups. Correlations between educational variables and DTI parameters were explored using Spearman's rho coefficient. Due to the concerns of multiple comparisons, we used a Bonferroni correction of $0.05/12 = 0.004$ for a two-sided *alpha* threshold for auditory ROIs (6 ROIs × 2 hemispheres), and $0.05/18 = 0.003$ for non-auditory ROIs (9 ROIs × 2 hemispheres); a *p*-value less than 0.05 was considered a trend.

Because multiple variables can predict outcomes, we used multiple linear or logistic regression modeling to evaluate the role of age and UHL simultaneously with the specific DTI parameters which were statistically significant or trending toward significance in bivariate analysis on the educational outcomes of interest. For the regression analyses, a *p*-value less than 0.05 was considered statistically significant.

RESULTS

Demographic data is presented in **Table 2**. The age of study participants ranged from 7.4 to 17.6 years. There were no significant differences in gender, age, racial composition, handedness or rates of prematurity between the NH and UHL groups. Etiology of hearing loss did not differ significantly between the right UHL and left UHL groups. Age at identification of hearing loss was 3 months to 8 years with a mean of 4.6 years (*SD* 2.8 years); mean duration of UHL was 7.5 years (*SD* 3.3 years), with a range of 2.2–14.2 years.

Though NH subjects performed better on all aspects of the cognitive testing, these differences were not all statistically significant (**Table 3**). No differences in full sum IQ were observed

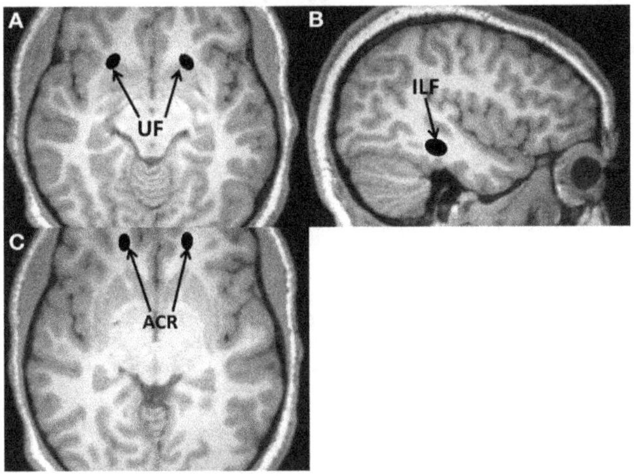

FIGURE 2 | Additional regions of interest (ROIs) used for DTI measurements placed on anatomical T1-weighted MRI scan; all are non-auditory ROIs. **(A)** Uncinate fasciculus (UF); **(B)** Inferior longitudinal fasciculus (ILF); **(C)** Anterior corona radiata (ACR).

between the right and left UHL groups. However, NH individuals trended toward higher scores on the verbal component of the cognitive tests (**Table 3**). In addition, children with UHL had a significantly greater need for IEPs (45%) and speech therapy (41%) than children with NH (5% for both IEPs and speech therapy).

DTI PARAMETERS BETWEEN GROUPS

DTI parameters were compared separately on the left and right side of the brain; for instance, the FA of the right auditory radiation of the UHL group vs. that of the NH group (**Table 4**). FA values trended toward being higher in the NH group than in the UHL group in two auditory regions and two non-auditory regions. The FA of the left lateral lemniscus was significantly higher for NH compared to UHL. The only trends between groups among mean diffusivities were in the MD of the in right subcortical white matter of Heschl's gyrus and left putamen. In general, FA was greater and MD lower in the NH group than in the UHL group, but this did not reach statistical significance in most regions.

We also compared DTI parameters of the right UHL and left UHL groups (**Table 4**). The FA of the left lateral lemniscus and the FA of the left subcortical white matter of Heschl's gyrus trended toward being lower in the left UHL group. The FA of the right centrum semiovale trended toward being higher in the left UHL group.

DTI PARAMETERS BETWEEN SIDES

Paired comparisons between the left and right sides of structures were performed for the UHL and NH groups. In all UHL subjects, the right side FA was greater than the left side FA in both auditory and non-auditory regions, with the exception of the superior temporal gyrus, middle cingulate gyrus, anterior limb of the internal capsule, centrum semiovale and the anterior corona radiata (**Table 5**). Amongst NH subjects, a similar pattern was observed with a few exceptions—superior temporal gyrus, Heschl's gyrus, anterior limb of the internal capsule, middle cingulate gyrus, and the anterior corona radiata. MD results generally corresponded to FA results but in the opposite direction. For both NH and UHL subjects, right sided MD was significantly lower than left sided MD in most structures.

CORRELATIONS

Correlations of educational outcome variables with DTI parameters were performed separately for the following groups: (1) All NH subjects; (2) All UHL subjects; (3) All Right UHL subjects; and (4) All Left UHL subjects.

In general, FA correlated positively and MD negatively with test scores for children with UHL (data not shown). Though there were many trends toward significance in the NH group, there were no significant correlations. In the UHL group, the FA and the MD of several ROIs correlated significantly with several different educational parameters, such as full IQ, verbal IQ, IEP, and speech therapy (**Table 6**). The FA of the left uncinate fasciculus was negatively correlated with Performance and Full IQ, the MD of the right posterior limb of the internal capsule was negatively associated with Verbal IQ, while the FA of the left middle cerebellar peduncle was associated with need for speech therapy. For children with right UHL, the MD of the right middle cerebellar peduncle was highly correlated with Verbal IQ, and the FA of both right and left uncinate fasciculus were highly correlated with both Performance and Full IQ. For children with left UHL, both the MD and FA of the left middle cerebellar peduncle were strongly correlated with speech therapy.

REGRESSION ANALYSES

As DTI parameters have been noted to change with age (Loenneker et al., 2011), we performed multiple linear regression analyses for regions with significant correlations with educational outcome variables as the dependent variable; age, hearing loss status and one DTI parameter (either FA or MD) served as independent variables. As with the correlation analyses, FAs were generally positively related to test scores while MDs were negatively associated with test scores (**Table 7**).

Multiple logistic regression analyses were performed similarly for IEP and speech therapy as the dependent variables. The FAs of the bilateral middle cerebellar peduncles were negatively related to the need for speech therapy (**Table 8**). Hearing loss status was associated with educational outcome variables in several models.

DISCUSSION

Our study is one of the first to apply DTI analysis to children with UHL. Consistent with previous research, children with UHL had significantly worse speech and language scores and required speech therapy and IEPs more often than children with NH (Lieu et al., 2010). Some significant differences were found between DTI parameters of the NH and UHL groups, or between right UHL, left UHL, and NH groups of children. Left-right asymmetries noted in the NH children were retained in the children with UHL.

The main advantage and the most interesting results from our study come from the inclusion of multiple educational outcome

Table 2 | Demographic characteristics of normal hearing (NH) children and children with unilateral hearing loss (UHL).

Characteristic	NH (*n* = 20)	UHL (*n* = 29)	*p*-value	Right UHL (*n* = 13)	Left UHL (*n* = 16)	*P*-value
Male sex, *n* (%)	14 (70)	13 (44.8)	0.082	6 (46.2)	3 (43.8)	0.897
Age in years, mean (*SD*)	12.7 (2.93)	12.2 (2.35)	0.514	11.8 (2.68)	12.5 (2.08)	0.430
Race, *n* (%)			0.805			0.970
Black	3 (15)	6 (20.7)		3 (23.1)	3 (18.8)	
White	15 (75)	18 (62.1)		8 (61.5)	10 (62.5)	
Asian	1 (5.0)	2 (6.9)		1 (7.7)	1 (6.2)	
Other	1 (5.0)	3 (10.3)		1 (7.7)	2 (12.5)	
Ethnicity, *n* (%)			0.401			0.359
Hispanic/latino	0 (0)	1 (3.4)		0 (0)	1 (6.2)	
Not hispanic or latino	20 (100)	28 (96.6)		13 (100)	15 (93.8)	
Handedness, *n* (%)			0.168			0.879
Right-handed	15 (75)	27 (93.1)		12 (92.3)	15 (93.8)	
Left-handed	4 (20.0)	2 (6.9)		1 (7.7)	1 (6.2)	
Both	1 (5.0)	0 (0)		0 (0)	0 (0)	
Hearing loss etiology						
Otitis media	–	2 (6.9)	–	0 (0)	2 (12.5)	0.186
Trauma	–	2 (6.9)	–	1 (7.7)	1 (6.2)	0.879
Meningitis	–	1 (3.4)	–	0 (0)	1 (6.2)	0.359
Congenital	–	5 (17.2)	–	2 (15.4)	3 (18.8)	0.569
Unknown	–	13 (44.8)	–	5 (38.5)	8 (50)	0.534
Other	–	4 (13.8)	–	3 (23.1)	1 (6.20	0.191
Prematurity	3 (15.0)	5 (17.2)	0.835	2 (15.4)	3 (18.8)	0.811

Table 3 | Comparisons between unilateral hearing loss (UHL) group and the normal hearing group (NH) for educational outcome variables, and right unilateral hearing loss (right UHL) and left unilateral hearing loss (left UHL) groups.

Educational outcome	UHL	NH control	*p*-value	Right UHL	Left UHL	*p*-value
IQ SCORES, MEAN (*SD*)						
Full sum	104 (24.5)	110 (14.9)	0.328	101 (23.1)	106 (26.2)	0.577
Performance	100 (18.2)	109 (15.7)	0.082	98.2 (24.7)	101 (11.1)	0.717
Verbal	100 (16.6)	109 (11.9)	0.046*	98 (18.3)	102 (15.4)	0.484
Vocabulary subscale	48 (12.7)	54 (7.4)	0.105	49 (13.9)	48 (12.0)	0.983
NEED FOR SPECIAL SERVICES						
Individualized educational program (*n*, %)	13 (44.8)	1 (5.0)	0.002†	5 (38.5)	8 (50)	0.534
Speech therapy (*n*, %)	12 (41.4)	1 (5.0)	0.005†	4 (30.8)	8 (50)	0.296

**Trend at* $p < 0.05$; †*Significant at* $p < 0.008$ *for multiple comparisons of educational outcomes.*

variables. DTI parameters in several ROIs were significantly correlated with educational outcome variables. Interestingly, the greater the FA of left Heschl's gyrus, the less likely a child needed an IEP, indicating that the greater the organization in this region, the better the educational outcome (**Tables 6, 8**). Notably, IEPs are provided through public schools only when children are diagnosed with an educationally significant problem, such as reading delays or behavioral problems; speech delays are only one diagnosis that would elicit an IEP. In contrast, speech therapy may be pursued privately, especially when a child attends a private school. Heschl's gyrus is tonotopically organized, and monaural deprivation disrupts this organization (Popescu and Polley, 2010). Although this area is anatomically crucial in auditory functioning, the association between test scores and the microstructure of this region requires further confirmation and validation in future studies. As neuroimaging is often an early step in the etiologic work-up of pediatric UHL, acquisition of DTI would be a feasible addition to the protocol and may provide clinically relevant information in regard to special educational needs.

Proposed by Kimura (1963), the dichotic listening paradigm held that the right ear was preferred for listening to speech, due to the predominant representation of a right ear stimulus in the left cerebral hemisphere, where language typically lateralizes (Kimura, 1963). According to a hypothesis of right ear advantage, children with left UHL should enjoy a speech-language advantage, but the evidence is currently inconclusive (Hartvig et al., 1989; Niedzielski et al., 2006; Lieu et al., 2010). The only DTI differences observed between right and left UHL were increased FAs for right UHL in the left lateral lemniscus and the subcortical white matter of the left Heschl's gyrus.

Table 4 | DTI parameters in those with unilateral hearing loss (UHL; $n = 29$) and normal hearing (NH; $n = 20$) participants amongst six auditory regions of interest (ROI) and nine non-auditory ROIs.

	UHL	NH	*p*-value	Right UHL	Left UHL	*p*-value
AUDITORY ROIs						
MD subcortical white matter of Heschl's gyrus, right	0.637	0.591	0.048*	0.643	0.632	0.130
FA lateral lemniscus, left	0.364	0.446	0.001†	0.381	0.351	0.005*
FA subcortical white matter of Heschl's gyrus, left	0.338	0.397	0.013*	0.365	0.315	0.009*
FA lateral lemniscus, right	0.392	0.457	0.025*	0.397	0.351	0.079
NON-AUDITORY ROIs						
MD Putamen, left	0.708	0.686	0.034*	0.715	0.703	0.081
FA anterior limb of the internal capsule, left	0.575	0.607	0.030*	0.571	0.578	0.093
FA centrum semiovale, right	0.468	0.503	0.015*	0.456	0.477	0.030*

Additional columns list values for right unilateral hearing loss (Right UHL; $n = 13$) and left unilateral hearing loss (Left UHL; $n = 16$); adjacent p-value column refers to p-values of Kruskal-Wallis tests between right UHL, left UHL and normal hearing (NH). Only parameters with uncorrected p-values < 0.05 are listed.
**Trend at $p < 0.05$ level; †Significant at $p < 0.004$ for auditory ROIs and <0.003 for non-auditory ROIs.*

Table 5 | Comparison of fractional anisotropy (FA) and mean diffusivity (MD) between right and left hemispheres for unilateral hearing loss (UHL; $n = 29$) and normal hearing (NH; $n = 20$) participants in six auditory and nine non-auditory regions of interest (ROI).

	UHL			NH		
	Right FA mean	**Left FA mean**	***p*-value**	**Right FA mean**	**Left FA mean**	***p*-value**
AUDITORY ROI						
Auditory radiation	0.536	0.490	<0.001†	0.539	0.501	0.037*
Heschl's gyrus	0.187	0.172	0.005*	0.200	0.193	0.296
Subcortical white matter of Heschl's gyrus	0.393	0.338	0.004†	0.449	0.397	<0.001†
NON-AUDITORY ROI						
Posterior limb of the internal capsule	0.704	0.635	<0.001†	0.712	0.641	<0.001†
Middle cerebellar Peduncle	0.691	0.622	<0.001†	0.701	0.646	0.004*
Uncinate fasciculus	0.482	0.431	<0.001†	0.481	0.459	0.135
Middle cingulate gyrus	0.612	0.637	0.071	0.649	0.674	0.025*
Putamen	0.186	0.181	0.364	0.206	0.181	<0.001†
	Right MD mean	**Left MD mean**	***p*-value**	**Right MD mean**	**Left MD mean**	***p*-value**
AUDITORY ROI						
Auditory radiation	0.608	0.667	<0.001†	0.614	0.654	0.040*
Heschl's gyrus	0.738	0.777	0.001†	0.709	0.766	<0.001†
Inferior colliculus	0.728	0.740	0.552	0.657	0.696	0.033*
Lateral lemniscus	0.668	0.724	0.008*	0.617	0.684	0.009†
Subcortical white matter of Heschl's gyrus	0.637	0.722	<0.001†	0.591	0.707	<0.001†
NON-AUDITORY ROI						
Posterior limb of the internal capsule	0.607	0.673	<0.001†	0.594	0.667	<0.001†
Middle cerebellar peduncle	0.595	0.549	0.001†	0.587	0.536	0.001†
Anterior limb of the internal capsule	0.592	0.668	<0.001†	0.579	0.656	<0.001†
Globus pallidus	0.594	0.616	0.020*	0.571	0.594	0.057
Putamen	0.684	0.708	<0.001†	0.676	0.686	0.093
Centrum semiovale	0.655	0.686	0.001†	0.639	0.671	<0.001†
Inferior longitudinal Fasciculus	0.690	0.714	0.039*	0.674	0.698	0.232

Only parameters with uncorrected p-values < 0.05 are listed.
**Trend at $p < 0.05$ level; †Significant at $p < 0.004$ for auditory ROIs and <0.003 for non-auditory ROIs.*

Instead, several DTI regions showed differential strengths in correlation with language and verbal IQ outcomes in children with and without UHL. These discordances suggest that the brains of children with UHL undergo reorganization in the white matter to help compensate for the lack of typical peripheral auditory stimuli to the contralateral hemisphere. Thus, the dichotic listening paradigm may not fit when one ear does not hear.

Table 6 | Spearman rho correlation values between educational outcomes and DTI parameters (fractional anisotropy, FA; mean diffusivity, MD) in auditory and non-auditory regions of interest (ROI) in participants with normal hearing (NH), unilateral hearing loss (UHL), right UHL or left UHL.

	Performance IQ	Full IQ	Verbal IQ	Vocabulary T-score	IEP	Speech-language therapy	Language standard score
AUDITORY ROIs							
NH ($n = 20$)							
No statistically significant correlations							
UHL ($n = 29$)							
FA left Heschl's gyrus	−0.159	0.047	0.367	0.355	−0.522†	−0.167	0.262
Right UHL only ($n = 13$)							
No statistically significant correlations							
Left UHL only ($n = 16$)							
No statistically significant correlations							
NON-AUDITORY ROIs							
NH ($n = 20$)							
No statistically significant correlations							
UHL ($n = 29$)							
MD right posterior limb of the internal capsule	−0.038	−0.171	−0.485†	−0.435*	0.448*	0.343	−0.462*
FA left middle cerebellar peduncle	−0.072	0.275	0.474*	0.342	−0.324	−0.632†	0.270
FA left uncinate fasciculus	−0.569†	−0.554†	−0.358	−0.406*	0.265	0.192	−0.438*
FA left middle cingulate gyrus	0.056	0.156	0.223	0.150	−0.075	−0.460*	0.130
Right UHL only ($n = 13$)							
MD right middle cerebellar peduncle	−0.595	−0.086	−0.905†	−0.795*	0.252	0.504	−0.738*
FA left uncinate fasciculus	−0.819†	−0.841††	−0.451	−0.338	−0.254	0.178	−0.576*
FA right uncinate fasciculus	−0.720†	−0.725†	−0.566*	−0.524	0.380	0.579	−0.736†
Left UHL only ($n = 16$)							
MD left middle cerebellar peduncle	0.147	−0.377	−0.430	−0.328	0.412	0.866††	−0.355
FA left middle cerebellar peduncle	−0.019	0.580*	0.606*	0.455	−0.454	−0.784†	0.517

Statistical significance was considered to be $p < 0.004$ for auditory ROIs and $p < 0.003$ for non-auditory ROIs.

**$p < 0.05$; †$p < 0.01$; ††$p < 0.001$.*

IQ, intelligence quotient; IEP, individualized education plan.

Regardless of hearing status, rightward asymmetries were observed in FA in many auditory structures. In non-auditory structures, asymmetries in DTI parameters were mixed, making interpretation of our results in large structures such as the centrum semiovale and posterior limb of the internal capsule less clear (Bonekamp et al., 2007; Eluvathingal et al., 2007; Liu et al., 2010; Takao et al., 2011). In auditory structures, our findings indicate that despite lack of auditory input from one ear, patterns of microstructural integrity are preserved in children with UHL. These results contrast with stimuli-induced functional MRI findings. When sounds or speech are presented monaurally to a NH individual, there is increased activation in the contralateral primary auditory cortex (Scheffler et al., 1998). Adults with UHL have a more symmetrical fMRI activation, with decreased contralateral primary auditory cortex activation and increased ipsilateral primary auditory cortex activation, when presented with a speech stimulus to the hearing ear (Firszt et al., 2006). While we would have expected more white matter microstructural differences in auditory structures between children with and without UHL, the lack thereof may be due to compensatory plasticity in the face of monaural deprivation, with these structures transmitting signal from the good ear, or being recruited for other brain functions. It is unclear whether UHL affects attentional networks and other aspects of executive functioning. In another study looking at fMRI data in children with and without UHL, children with UHL were found to have less activation of secondary auditory areas compared to NH individuals and failure to activate attentional areas (Propst et al., 2010). In the present cohort, differences in rs-fcMRI were found in areas associated with auditory processing, executive function and memory formation between children with UHL and NH controls (Tibbetts et al., 2011). Since the neuroanatomical microstructure remains intact, it is possible that these underutilized auditory areas have been recruited by other systems in the brain, such as noted by Obretenova et al. (2010), or analogously as has been shown to occur in the occipital cortex of blind subjects (Burton et al., 2012). An early-deaf and early-blind individual who relied on tactile communication modalities was found to have enhanced occipital connectivity as well greater activation of superior temporal and inferior frontal language regions on fMRI relative to a normally sighted and hearing person. This hypothesis could explain the discrepancy in speech-language outcomes between children with

Table 7 | Results of multiple linear regression analyses for all subjects ($n = 49$).

Outcome	Unstandardized coefficient	Standard error	*t*-value	*p*-value
LANGUAGE COMPOSITE SCORE				
Intercept	−3.79	46.14	−0.08	0.94
MD left Putamen	133.0	61.05	2.18	0.035
Age	1.65	0.84	1.96	0.056
UHL	−15.70	4.40	−3.57	0.001
Intercept	61.23	18.81	3.26	0.002
FA right inferior longitudinal fasciculus	55.75	26.24	2.13	0.039
Age	1.12	0.81	1.38	0.175
UHL	−11.66	4.27	−2.73	0.009
FULL IQ				
Intercept	43.56	32.39	1.35	0.188
FA right middle cerebellar peduncle	80.44	35.26	2.28	0.029
Age	0.76	1.33	0.57	0.57
UHL	−7.59	7.01	−1.08	0.286
PERFORMANCE IQ				
Intercept	184.2	22.87	8.05	<0.001
FA left uncinate fasciculus	−129.0	46.54	−2.77	0.008
Age	−1.30	0.89	−1.45	0.153
UHL	−13.20	4.76	−2.77	0.008
VERBAL IQ				
Intercept	44.47	24.20	1.84	0.073
FA splenium of the corpus callosum	62.67	24.03	2.61	0.012
Age	1.14	0.82	1.40	0.168
UHL	−7.90	4.12	−1.92	0.061
Intercept	140.5	21.10	6.66	<0.001
MD right middle cerebellar peduncle	−78.73	30.13	−2.61	0.013
Age	1.16	0.87	1.34	0.189
UHL	−10.24	4.60	−2.23	0.033
Intercept	50.93	20.67	2.47	0.019
FA left middle cerebellar peduncle	61.70	24.21	2.55	0.016
Age	1.43	0.88	1.64	0.112
UHL	−9.31	4.65	−2.00	0.054

Standardized scores for educational outcomes were the dependent variables, and the DTI parameters (FA, Fractional Anisotropy; MD, Mean Diffusivity) for the stated regions of interest, age and hearing status (i.e., unilateral hearing loss, UHL) were entered in the models as predictors. FA, Fractional Anisotropy; MD, Mean Diffusivity.

and without UHL despite the preservation of the microstructure in auditory regions. In contrast to our results here, early blind individuals were noted to have marked differences in the geniculocalcarine tract from normally sighted individuals; however, connections between the visual cortex and the orbital frontal and temporal cortices were preserved in early blind individuals (Shimony et al., 2006).

Contrary to expectations of finding differences in DTI parameters of auditory regions between children with and without UHL, most DTI parameters between the two groups were quite similar. Thus, given the results from prior studies on bilateral hearing loss, UHL seems to affect white matter development differently than bilateral hearing loss. There were no differences between left and right UHL groups. However, our sample size was small, so that our negative findings do not preclude the existence of such differences. We included children with both acquired and congenital hearing loss, which may have influenced our results, although in all cases the hearing loss was at birth or in early childhood. Because most of the children were born before the era of newborn hearing screening, precise onset of UHL could not be determined. However, the severity of UHL and universal lack of patient complaint about hearing indicates that the children were very young and unaware of the hearing loss when it occurred. Sampling ROIs manually may also be perceived as a limitation of this study; however, this is how many of the comparison studies were done, and given the small size of the structures we were sampling, alternative approaches, such as atlas-based approaches, were not feasible.

A few studies have used DTI to examine white matter microstructure in adults with hearing loss. There is a body of evidence indicating that adults with hearing loss have reduced FA in several structures. Chang et al. (2004) examined five ROIs (the lateral lemniscus and inferior colliculus, the trapezoid body, auditory radiation and superior olivary nucleus); reduced FA was observed in subjects with sensorineural hearing loss at all locations bilaterally with the exception of the trapezoid body (Chang et al., 2004). A study of 13 adults with early deafness

Table 8 | Results of multiple logistic regression analyses for all subjects ($n = 49$).

	Unstandardized coefficient	Standard error	Wald statistic	*p*-value
SPEECH THERAPY				
Constant	12.17	4.90	6.17	0.013*
FA left middle cingulate gyrus	−15.16	7.07	4.60	0.032*
Age	−0.05	0.16	0.11	0.740
UHL	−2.28	1.14	4.03	0.045
Constant	−11.75	7.13	2.72	0.099
MD left middle cerebellar peduncle	28.64	12.60	5.16	0.023*
Age	−0.19	0.21	0.80	0.372
UHL	−2.39	1.30	3.40	0.065
Constant	14.30	5.66	6.38	0.012*
FA left middle cerebellar peduncle	−15.51	6.44	5.80	0.016*
Age	−0.22	0.19	1.37	0.242
UHL	−2.49	1.29	3.70	0.054
Constant	13.78	6.23	4.89	0.027*
FA right middle cerebellar peduncle	−12.44	6.02	4.27	0.039*
Age	−0.24	0.20	1.50	0.220
UHL	−2.68	1.29	4.29	0.038*
INDIVIDUALIZED EDUCATIONAL PROGRAM				
Constant	−15.94	10.35	2.37	0.124
MD left Heschl's gyrus	30.07	14.14	4.52	0.033*
Age	−0.37	0.19	4.01	0.045*
UHL	−3.13	1.23	6.47	0.011*
Constant	−30.15	14.4	4.38	0.036*
MD left superior temporal gyrus	46.09	18.62	6.13	0.013*
Age	−0.10	0.21	0.22	0.641
UHL	−4.59	1.72	7.13	0.008†
Constant	13.70	4.55	9.05	0.003†
FA left Heschl's gyrus	−43.75	19.15	5.22	0.022*
Age	−0.24	0.19	1.61	0.204
UHL	−3.55	1.40	6.45	0.011*
Constant	17.65	5.83	9.16	0.002†
FA left superior temporal gyrus	−52.17	20.89	6.24	0.013*
Age	−0.45	0.21	4.64	0.031*
UHL	−3.49	1.36	6.57	0.01*
Constant	−28.51	14.52	3.85	0.050
MD left posterior limb of the internal capsule	51.94	21.27	5.97	0.015*
Age	−0.24	0.20	1.51	0.219
UHL	−3.79	1.43	7.06	0.008†
Constant	−10.73	8.19	1.72	0.190
MD right posterior limb of the internal capsule	27.94	12.79	4.77	0.029*
Age	−0.29	0.19	2.38	0.123
UHL	−2.99	1.21	6.09	0.014*

Standardized scores for educational outcomes were the dependent variables, and the DTI parameters (FA, Fractional Anisotropy; MD, Mean Diffusivity) for the stated regions of interest, age and hearing status (i.e., unilateral hearing loss, UHL) were entered in the models as predictors. $^{*}p < 0.05$; $^{\dagger}p < 0.01$.

revealed decreased FA within the temporal white matter, internal capsule, superior longitudinal fasciculus and the inferior frontal white matter (Kim et al., 2009). In adults with UHL, FA values of the inferior colliculus and the lateral lemniscus were significantly lower on the side contralateral to the hearing loss than those on the ipsilateral side (Lin et al., 2008). The study of Wu et al. looked at 12 subjects with unilateral congenital cochlear nerve deficiency and noted bilateral decrease in FA and increase in MD in the lateral lemniscus and inferior colliculus (Wu et al., 2009). However, the population of this study spanned a wide age distribution (age 8–29 years) and no correction was made for this wide variability in age. Unlike the results of previous studies, our findings indicate that microstructural integrity in children with UHL is not substantially altered from that of children with NH.

The difference in our results could be related to the differences in our cohorts (unilateral vs. bilateral hearing loss in most other studies), to the age of our groups (children vs. adults, or mixed in other studies), and to our statistical methods.

Two studies have used DTI in children with bilateral prelingual deafness to investigate alternations in brain white matter tracts. Children (age 10–18 years) with bilateral prelingual deafness had lower FA values and increased radial diffusivity bilaterally in the superior temporal gyrus, Heschl's gyrus, planum polare, and splenium of the corpus callosum compared to controls with normal hearing (Miao et al., 2013). In addition, the mean radial diffusivity of the right superior temporal gyrus appeared to be correlated with the duration of sign language use. Chang and colleagues used DTI characteristics to compare children who had undergone cochlear implantation but were classified as having "good" or "poor" auditory performance outcomes (Chang et al., 2012). They found higher FA values in Broca's area, genu of the corpus callosum, and auditory tract among the children with "good" auditory performance compared to those with "poor" outcome. Strong correlations were found between FA and auditory performance scores with several brain areas: medial geniculate nucleus, Broca's area, genu of the corpus callosum, and auditory tract. They concluded that preoperative functional imaging prior to placement of cochlear implants might be helpful to understanding clinical outcomes. Although all of the brain areas from these two studies in children are different from the ones identified in adults with hearing loss, most but not all occurred in areas associated with auditory and language processing, and most showed bilateral changes. These findings in children with bilateral prelingual deafness are highly interesting, but they differ from the results of the current study. Whether they apply to the population of children with UHL who have preserved auditory stimulation in one ear would need further investigation.

CONCLUSION

This study detected correlations between educational outcomes and microstructural integrity of brain structures in children with and without UHL that may have clinical relevance in the guidance of speech and language therapy. Our results imply that unilateral auditory input preserves many of the asymmetries in white matter microstructural patterns in children between right and left hemispheres. However, UHL results in functional and behavioral differences on language and educational measures, possibly due to recruitment of certain areas (e.g., middle cerebellar peduncle, superior temporal gyrus, as shown in **Table 8**) for other brain functions.

AUTHOR CONTRIBUTIONS

Judith E. C. Lieu conceived and supervised the project and wrote the paper. Joshua S. Shimony supervised the project and wrote the paper. Tara Rachakonda collected data, performed statistical analyses, and wrote the paper. Rebecca S. Coalson collected data, performed statistical analysis, and revised the paper.

ACKNOWLEDGMENTS

We would like to express our gratitude to Steve Petersen, PhD, and Bradley Schlaggar, MD, PhD, for their support and guidance in this project. Our work would also not be possible without the efforts of Banan Ead. Grants from the American Hearing Research Foundation Wiley H. Harrison Memorial Research Award and the National Institutes of Health (K23 DC006638—JECL) funded this research. Tara Rachakonda was also supported by a training grant (5T32DC000022-2) and a Clinical and Translational science award from Washington University through the NIH/NCRR/NCATS (UL1RR024992). The contents of this publication are solely the responsibility of the authors and do not necessarily represent the official view of the NCRR, NCATS or NIH.

REFERENCES

Antenor-Dorsey, J. A., Hershey, T., Rutlin, J., Shimony, J. S., McKinstry, R. C., Grange, D. K., et al. (2013). White matter integrity and executive abilities in individuals with phenylketonuria. *Mol. Genet. Metab.* 109, 125–131. doi: 10.1016/j.ymgme.2013.03.020

Assaf, Y., and Pasternak, O. (2008). Diffusion tensor imaging (DTI)-based white matter mapping in brain research: a review. *J. Mol. Neurosci.* 34, 51–61. doi: 10.1007/s12031-007-0029-0

Basser, P. J., Mattiello, J., and Lebihan, D. (1994). Estimation of the effective self-diffusion tensor from the NMR spin echo. *J. Magn. Reson. B* 103, 247–254. doi: 10.1006/jmrb.1994.1037

Beer, J., Kronenberger, W. G., and Pisoni, D. B. (2011). Executive function in everyday life: implications for young cochlear implant users. *Cochlear. Implants Int.* 12(Suppl. 1), S89–S91. doi: 10.1179/146701011X13001035752570

Bess, F. H. (1982). Children with unilateral hearing loss. *JARA* 15, 116–130.

Bess, F. H., and Tharpe, A. M. (1984). Unilateral hearing impairment in children. *Pediatrics* 74, 206–216.

Bonekamp, D., Nagae, L. M., Degaonkar, M., Matson, M., Abdalla, W. M., Barker, P. B., et al. (2007). Diffusion tensor imaging in children and adolescents: reproducibility, hemispheric, and age-related differences. *Neuroimage* 34, 733–742. doi: 10.1016/j.neuroimage.2006.09.020

Burgund, E. D., Kang, H. C., Kelly, J. E., Buckner, R. L., Snyder, A. Z., Petersen, S. E., et al. (2002). The feasibility of a common stereotactic space for children and adults in fMRI studies of development. *Neuroimage* 17, 184–200. doi: 10.1006/nimg.2002.1174

Burton, H., Agato, A., and Sinclair, R. J. (2012). Repetition learning of vibrotactile temporal sequences: an fMRI study in blind and sighted individuals. *Brain Res.* 1433, 69–79. doi: 10.1016/j.brainres.2011.11.039

Carrow-Woolfolk, E. (1995). *Oral and Written Language Scales.* Bloomington, MN: Pearson Assessments.

Chang, Y., Lee, H. R., Paik, J. S., Lee, K. Y., and Lee, S. H. (2012). Voxel-wise analysis of diffusion tensor imaging for clinical outcome of cochlear implantation: retrospective study. *Clin. Exp. Otorhinolaryngol.* 5(Suppl. 1), S37–S42. doi: 10.3342/ceo.2012.5.S1.S37

Chang, Y., Lee, S. H., Lee, Y. J., Hwang, M. J., Bae, S. J., Kim, M. N., et al. (2004). Auditory neural pathway evaluation on sensorineural hearing loss using diffusion tensor imaging. *Neuroreport* 15, 1699–1703. doi: 10.1097/01.wnr.0000134584.10207.1a

Cummings, J. L. (1993). Frontal-subcortical circuits and human behavior. *Arch. Neurol.* 50, 873–880. doi: 10.1001/archneur.1993.00540080076020

Davis, A., Reeve, K., Hind, S., and Bamford, J. (2002). "Children with mild and unilateral hearing impairment," in *A Sound Foundation Through Early Amplification 2001. Proceedings of the Second International Conference 2002*, eds R. C. Seewald and J. Gravel (Phonak, AG), 179–186.

Davis, J. M., Shepard, N. T., Stelmachowicz, P. G., and Gorga, M. P. (1981). Characteristics of hearing-impaired children in the public schools: part II–psychoeducational data. *J. Speech Hear Disord.* 46, 130–137.

Eluvathingal, T. J., Hasan, K. M., Kramer, L., Fletcher, J. M., and Ewing-Cobbs, L. (2007). Quantitative diffusion tensor tractography of association and projection fibers in normally developing children and adolescents. *Cereb. Cortex* 17, 2760–2768. doi: 10.1093/cercor/bhm003

Figueras, B., Edwards, L., and Langdon, D. (2008). Executive function and language in deaf children. *J. Deaf Stud. Deaf Educ.* 13, 362–377. doi: 10.1093/deafed/enm067

Firszt, J. B., Ulmer, J. L., and Gaggl, W. (2006). Differential representation of speech sounds in the human cerebral hemispheres. *Anat. Rec. A Discov. Mol. Cell Evol. Biol.* 288, 345–357. doi: 10.1002/ar.a.20295

Hartvig, J. J., Borre, S., and Johansen, P. A. (1989). Unilateral sensorineural hearing loss in children: cognitive abilities with respect to right/left ear differences. *Br. J. Audiol.* 23, 215–220. doi: 10.3109/03005368909076502

Hugdahl, K. (2011). Fifty years of dichotic listening research - still going and going and. *Brain Cogn.* 76, 211–213. doi: 10.1016/j.bandc.2011.03.006

Hulkower, M. B., Poliak, D. B., Rosenbaum, S. B., Zimmerman, M. E., and Lipton, M. L. (2013). A decade of DTI in traumatic brain injury: 10 years and 100 articles later. *AJNR* 34, 2064–2074. doi: 10.3174/ajnr.A3395

Kim, D. J., Park, S. Y., Kim, J., Lee, D. H., and Park, H. J. (2009). Alterations of white matter diffusion anisotropy in early deafness. *Neuroreport* 20, 1032–1036. doi: 10.1097/WNR.0b013e32832e0cdd

Kimura, D. (1963). Speech lateralization in young children as determined by an auditory test. *J. Comp. Physiol. Psychol.* 56, 899–902. doi: 10.1037/h0047762

Lieu, J. E., Tye-Murray, N., Karzon, R. K., and Piccirillo, J. F. (2010). Unilateral hearing loss is associated with worse speech-language scores in children. *Pediatrics* 125, e1348–e1355. doi: 10.1542/peds.2009-2448

Lin, Y., Wang, J., Wu, C., Wai, Y., Yu, J., and Ng, S. (2008). Diffusion tensor imaging of the auditory pathway in sensorineural hearing loss: changes in radial diffusivity and diffusion anisotropy. *J. Magn. Reson. Imaging* 28, 598–603. doi: 10.1002/jmri.21464

Liu, Y., Baleriaux, D., Kavec, M., Metens, T., Absil, J., Denolin, V., et al. (2010). Structural asymmetries in motor and language networks in a population of healthy preterm neonates at term equivalent age: a diffusion tensor imaging and probabilistic tractography study. *Neuroimage* 51, 783–788. doi: 10.1016/j.neuroimage.2010.02.066

Loenneker, T., Klaver, P., Bucher, K., Lichtensteiger, J., Imfeld, A., and Martin, E. (2011). Microstructural development: organizational differences of the fiber architecture between children and adults in dorsal and ventral visual streams. *Hum. Brain Mapp.* 32, 935–946. doi: 10.1002/hbm.21080

Lutz, J., Hemminger, F., Stahl, R., Dietrich, O., Hempel, M., Reiser, M., et al. (2007). Evidence of subcortical and cortical aging of the acoustic pathway: a diffusion tensor imaging (DTI) study. *Acad. Radiol.* 14, 692–700. doi: 10.1016/j.acra.2007.02.014

Mehl, A. L., and Thomson, V. (1998). Newborn hearing screening: the great omission. *Pediatrics* 101:E4. doi: 10.1542/peds.101.1.e4

Miao, W., Li, J., Tang, M., Xian, J., Li, W., Liu, Z., et al. (2013). Altered white matter integrity in adolescents with prelingual deafness: a high-resolution tract-based spatial statistics imaging study. *AJNR* 34, 1264–1270. doi: 10.3174/ajnr.A3370

Mori, S., and Zhang, J. (2006). Principles of diffusion tensor imaging and its applications to basic neuroscience research. *Neuron* 51, 527–539. doi: 10.1016/j.neuron.2006.08.012

Mukherjee, P., Berman, J. I., Chung, S. W., Hess, C. P., and Henry, R. G. (2008). Diffusion tensor MR imaging and fiber tractography: theoretic underpinnings. *AJNR* 29, 632–641. doi: 10.3174/ajnr.A1051

Neil, J. J. (2008). Diffusion imaging concepts for clinicians. *J. Magn. Reson. Imaging* 27, 1–7. doi: 10.1002/jmri.21087

Niedzielski, A., Humeniuk, E., Blaziak, P., and Gwizda, G. (2006). Intellectual efficiency of children with unilateral hearing loss. *Int. J. Pediatr. Otorhinolaryngol.* 70, 1529–1532. doi: 10.1016/j.ijporl.2006.02.011

Niskar, A. S., Kieszak, S. M., Holmes, A., Esteban, E., Rubin, C., and Brody, D. J. (1998). Prevalence of hearing loss among children 6 to 19 years of age: the third national health and nutrition examination survey. *JAMA* 279, 1071–1075. doi: 10.1001/jama.279.14.1071

Obretenova, S., Halko, M. A., Plow, E. B., Pascual-Leone, A., and Merabet, L. B. (2010). Neuroplasticity associated with tactile language communication in a deaf-blind subject. *Front. Hum. Neurosci.* 3:60. doi: 10.3389/neuro.09.060.2009

Penhune, V. B., Zatorre, R. J., Macdonald, J. D., and Evans, A. C. (1996). Interhemispheric anatomical differences in human primary auditory cortex: probabilistic mapping and volume measurement from magnetic resonance scans. *Cereb. Cortex* 6, 661–672. doi: 10.1093/cercor/6.5.661

Popescu, M. V., and Polley, D. B. (2010). Monaural deprivation disrupts development of binaural selectivity in auditory midbrain and cortex. *Neuron* 65, 718–731. doi: 10.1016/j.neuron.2010.02.019

Propst, E. J., Greinwald, J. H., and Schmithorst, V. (2010). Neuroanatomic differences in children with unilateral sensorineural hearing loss detected using functional magnetic resonance imaging. *Arch. Otolaryngol. Head Neck Surg.* 136, 22–26. doi: 10.1001/archoto.2009.208

Rykhlevskaia, E., Gratton, G., and Fabiani, M. (2008). Combining structural and functional neuroimaging data for studying brain connectivity: a review. *Psychophysiology* 45, 173–187. doi: 10.1111/j.1469-8986.2007.00621.x

Scheffler, K., Bilecen, D., Schmid, N., Tschopp, K., and Seelig, J. (1998). Auditory cortical responses in hearing subjects and unilateral deaf patients as detected by functional magnetic resonance imaging. *Cereb. Cortex* 8, 156–163. doi: 10.1093/cercor/8.2.156

Schmahmann, J. D., Smith, E. E., Eichler, F. S., and Filley, C. M. (2008). Cerebral white matter: neuroanatomy, clinical neurology, and neurobehavioral correlates. *Ann. N. Y. Acad. Sci.* 1142, 266–309. doi: 10.1196/annals.1444.017

Semel, E., Wiig, E. H., and Secord, W. A. (2011). *Clinical Evaluation of Language Fundamentalsr—Fourth Edition (CELFr–4).* Available online at: http://psychcorp.pearsonassessments.com/HAIWEB/Cultures/en-us/Productdetail.htm?Pid=015-8037-200 (Accessed July 3, 2012).

Shimony, J. S., Burton, H., Epstein, A. A., McLaren, D. G., Sun, S. W., and Snyder, A. Z. (2006). Diffusion tensor imaging reveals white matter reorganization in early blind humans. *Cereb. Cortex* 16, 1653–1661. doi: 10.1093/cercor/bhj102

Shimony, J. S., Sheline, Y. I., D'Angelo, G., Epstein, A. A., Benzinger, T. L., Mintun, M. A., et al. (2009). Diffuse microstructural abnormalities of normal-appearing white matter in late life depression: a diffusion tensor imaging study. *Biol. Psychiatry* 66, 245–252. doi: 10.1016/j.biopsych.2009.02.032

Takao, H., Hayashi, N., and Ohtomo, K. (2011). White matter asymmetry in healthy individuals: a diffusion tensor imaging study using tract-based spatial statistics. *Neuroscience* 193, 291–299. doi: 10.1016/j.neuroscience.2011.07.041

Talairach, J., and Tournoux, P. (1988). *Co-Planar Stereotaxic Atlas of the Human Brain* (M. Rayport, Trans.). New York, NY: Thieme Medical Publishers, Inc.

Tibbetts, K., Ead, B., Umansky, A., Coalson, R., Schlaggar, B. L., Firszt, J. B., et al. (2011). Interregional brain interactions in children with unilateral hearing loss. *Otolaryngol. Head Neck Surg.* 144, 602–611. doi: 10.1177/0194599810394954

Wechsler, D. (1999). *Wechsler Abbreviated Scale of Intelligence TM (WASI TM).* Bloomington, MN: Pearson Assessment. Available online at: http://www.pearsonassessments.com/HAIWEB/Cultures/en-us/Productdetail.htm?Pid=015-8981-502 (Accessed December 4, 2013).

Widen, J. E., Folsom, R. C., Cone-Wesson, B., Carty, L., Dunnell, J. J., Koebsell, K., et al. (2000). Identification of neonatal hearing impairment: hearing status at 8 to 12 months corrected age using a visual reinforcement audiometry protocol. *Ear Hear* 21, 471–487. doi: 10.1097/00003446-200010000-00011

Wu, C. M., Ng, S. H., Wang, J. J., and Liu, T. C. (2009). Diffusion tensor imaging of the subcortical auditory tract in subjects with congenital cochlear nerve deficiency. *AJNR* 30, 1773–1777. doi: 10.3174/ajnr.A1681

8

Seeing the talker's face supports executive processing of speech in steady state noise

Sushmit Mishra[1]*, Thomas Lunner[1,2,3], Stefan Stenfelt[1,2], Jerker Rönnberg[1] and Mary Rudner[1]

[1] *Linnaeus Centre HEAD, Swedish Institute for Disability Research, Department of Behavioural Sciences and Learning, Linköping University, Linköping, Sweden*
[2] *Department of Clinical and Experimental Medicine, Linköping University, Linköping, Sweden*
[3] *Eriksholm Research Centre, Oticon A/S, Snekkersten, Denmark*

***Correspondence:**
Sushmit Mishra, Linnaeus Centre HEAD, Swedish Institute for Disability Research, Department of Behavioural Sciences and Learning, Linköping University, SE-581 83 Linköping, Sweden
e-mail: sushmit.mishra@liu.se

Listening to speech in noise depletes cognitive resources, affecting speech processing. The present study investigated how remaining resources or cognitive spare capacity (CSC) can be deployed by young adults with normal hearing. We administered a test of CSC (CSCT; Mishra et al., 2013) along with a battery of established cognitive tests to 20 participants with normal hearing. In the CSCT, lists of two-digit numbers were presented with and without visual cues in quiet, as well as in steady-state and speech-like noise at a high intelligibility level. In low load conditions, two numbers were recalled according to instructions inducing executive processing (updating, inhibition) and in high load conditions the participants were additionally instructed to recall one extra number, which was the always the first item in the list. In line with previous findings, results showed that CSC was sensitive to memory load and executive function but generally not related to working memory capacity (WMC). Furthermore, CSCT scores in quiet were lowered by visual cues, probably due to distraction. In steady-state noise, the presence of visual cues improved CSCT scores, probably by enabling better encoding. Contrary to our expectation, CSCT performance was disrupted more in steady-state than speech-like noise, although only without visual cues, possibly because selective attention could be used to ignore the speech-like background and provide an enriched representation of target items in working memory similar to that obtained in quiet. This interpretation is supported by a consistent association between CSCT scores and updating skills.

Keywords: cognitive spare capacity, executive processing, working memory, updating, inhibition, speech processing

INTRODUCTION

Listening in noise challenges explicit cognitive abilities (Rönnberg et al., 2008, 2013). A substantial body of work has shown that once audibility has been accounted for, individual working memory capacity (WMC) accounts for a large part of the variance in the ability to understand speech in noise (Humes, 2007; Akeroyd, 2008). This is not surprising as speech understanding requires encoding of the speech input for temporary storage, inferring meaning and at the same preparing for an appropriate response (Pichora-Fuller and Singh, 2006; Rudner and Lunner, 2013). Because WMC is limited, fewer cognitive resources will remain after processing of a message heard in noise compared to one heard in quiet (Pichora-Fuller, 2007; Lunner et al., 2009). This line of argument has sparked recent interest in measuring cognitive spare capacity (CSC), that is, the cognitive capacity that remains once successful listening has taken place (Rudner et al., 2011a). The concept of CSC is similar to the concept of WMC. However, whereas WMC often refers to a general capacity that is typically measured using a text-based visual task such as the reading span task (Daneman and Carpenter, 1980; Rönnberg et al., 1989), CSC refers specifically to a cognitive reserve that has been depleted by listening under adverse conditions such as against a background of noise or with a hearing impairment. It is likely that different cognitive functions do not tap into a single cognitive resource but have their own dedicated and distinct resources (Mishra et al., 2013). During speech understanding, a cognitive resource that is depleted in the act of speech perception may be compensated for fully or partially by another cognitive process. Hence, a measure of WMC may not provide adequate assessment of CSC. Being able to gauge individual CSC may be an important factor in designing and evaluating interventions for individuals with various communication difficulties. For example, it is likely to assist in appropriate fitting of hearing aids (Rudner et al., 2011a; Mishra et al., 2013).

In a recent publication (Mishra et al., 2013), we evaluated a test of CSC (CSCT) that probes the ability to perform different executive tasks (updating and inhibition) under high and low memory load based on two-digit numbers presented in the auditory modality, with or without a video of the talker's face. We found that CSC, measured using the CSCT, did not correlate with WMC, measured using the reading span task, suggesting that CSC is quantitatively and qualitatively different from WMC.

Rather surprisingly, we found that CSC was reduced when the speaker's face was visible when the to-be-remembered stimuli were presented in quiet conditions. We suggested that when speech is fully audible and there is no competing noise, seeing the talker's face may act as a distraction during performance of the executive tasks. This interpretation is in line with other recent work demonstrating that when the intelligibility of audiovisual (AV) stimuli is equated with that of auditory-only (A-only) stimuli, listening effort gauged using a dual task procedure increases in the AV modality (Fraser et al., 2010; Gosselin and Gagné, 2011). The purpose of the present study was to replicate the findings of Mishra et al. (2013) and to investigate CSC for speech presented in noise.

The Ease of Language Understanding model (ELU; Rönnberg, 2003; Rönnberg et al., 2008, 2013) assumes that in optimal listening conditions, the incoming language signal can be readily matched with lexical and phonological representations stored in Long Term Memory (LTM), making speech understanding implicit. But in the presence of adverse conditions which may include noise or signal degradation (Mattys et al., 2012), a mismatch may occur between the incoming signal and stored representations. In a mismatch situation, explicit or effortful conscious processing is required to infer meaning from the incoming fragments of information. Such processing may include the abilities to achieve linguistic closure and gain access to previous knowledge stored in LTM (Rönnberg et al., 2010; Besser et al., 2013). Also, it has been suggested that individuals may compensate for information lost during signal degradation by directing their attentional capacity towards understanding the signal (Mattys et al., 2012). The use of explicit processing or involvement of attentional capacity for speech perception involves the executive functions of updating and inhibition (Mishra et al., 2010, 2013; Rudner et al., 2011a; Sörqvist and Rönnberg, 2012; Rönnberg et al., 2013). Updating refers to the monitoring and coding of information which is relevant to the task at hand and inhibition involves deliberate, controlled suppression of prepotent responses (Miyake et al., 2000). For example, while listening in modulated noise, the executive function of inhibition is used to suppress distracting noise (Janse, 2012). The involvement of executive functions in the act of listening, especially under adverse listening conditions, may come at the cost of depleted cognitive resources for processing heard material. This means that modulated noise may be more disruptive of performance on the inhibition than the updating task of the CSCT and that individual executive ability may specifically predict the ability to process speech heard in noise (Rudner et al., 2011b).

The ability to perceive speech (Mattys et al., 2012) and to remember speech (Pichora-Fuller et al., 1995; Murphy et al., 2000; Sörqvist and Rönnberg, 2012) is influenced in different ways by different types of noise. It has been regularly observed that speech recognition scores are higher in modulated compared to steady state noise at similar signal-to-noise ratios (SNR) (e.g., Duquesnoy, 1983) at least for younger adults without hearing impairment (George et al., 2006; Zekveld et al., 2013). However, speech recognition in modulated compared to steady state noise is also more likely to be associated with individual cognitive abilities such as WMC (Rönnberg et al., 2010; Besser et al., 2013; Zekveld et al., 2013) and linguistic closure (Zekveld et al., 2007; Besser et al., 2013). It is also likely to be more effortful both in terms of physiological response such as pupil dilation (Koelewijn et al., 2012) and subjective self-ratings, even when performance is better (Rudner et al., 2012). Recently, Janse (2012) showed that listening to speech in speech noise demands inhibition. These findings suggest that better speech recognition in modulated compared to steady state noise is dependent on cognitive resources. This applies in particular to speech noise (Zekveld et al., 2013) and hence CSC may be reduced more by listening to speech in speech-like noise than in steady state noise. Noise has been shown to disrupt recall of spoken items even when intelligibility is fairly high (Murphy et al., 2000). Emerging evidence suggests that speech-like noise, compared to steady state noise, is more disruptive of short-term memory retention of fully audible items in older adults with hearing loss (Ng et al., 2013). Thus, in the present study, we expected lower CSCT scores in noise than in quiet, but higher in steady state than speech-like noise. Because speech recognition in speech-like noise seems to specifically tax inhibition resources, we speculated that listening in speech-like noise might actually reduce the inhibition resources available for performing the CSCT. Thus, we expected speech-like noise to lower CSCT scores more in the inhibition than updating task.

Speech perception in the presence of noise is usually enhanced by observation of the talker's face. Lips, teeth and tongue may provide disambiguating information that is complementary to less well specified auditory information, by helping to determine manner and more importantly place of articulation (Grant et al., 1998). This can provide a substantial benefit in signal to noise ratio (Campbell, 2009) for speech recognition in noise (see also Hygge et al., 1992). The advantage of AV presentation has even been observed when only a graphic representation of the movement of the articulators was shown during speech detection in noise (Tye-Murray et al., 2011). Such visual cues do not provide disambiguating information and thus this finding was interpreted as suggesting that visual cues help the listener to direct their attentional capacities to the incoming signal at the most critical time to encode the target (c.f. Helfer and Freyman, 2005). This causes better signal detection and fewer cognitive demands in anticipating target stimuli in AV compared to A-only presentation (Besle et al., 2004; Moradi et al., 2013). Thus, visual cues help segregate target stimuli from interfering noise. Notwithstanding, it has been found that visual cues reduce performance on executively demanding auditory tasks (Fraser et al., 2010; Gosselin and Gagné, 2011; Mishra et al., 2013).

In a recent article, Yovel and Belin (2013) suggested that despite sensory differences, the neurocognitive mechanisms engaged by perceiving faces and voices are highly similar, facilitating integration of visual and speech information. Indeed, recent investigations of the episodic buffer of working memory (Baddeley, 2000) have shown that contrary to predictions, multimodal integration in working memory is not executively taxing (Rönnberg et al., 2010; Baddeley, 2012). One of the characteristics of the episodic buffer is that it communicates with LTM and exploits the quality of representations stored there (Rönnberg et al., 2013). Moradi et al. (2013) found that the AV speech recognition in the presence of noise for subjects with normal hearing is faster, more accurate and less effortful than A-only speech recognition and inferred that AV presentation taxes cognitive resources to a lesser extent by reducing working memory load. On the basis that AV presentation provides additional complimentary visual cues and helps in anticipating target onset in the presence of noise, we predict that seeing the face of the talker while performing the CSCT in noise will enable participants to form richer representations of the target items that will better survive the executive processing that the task demands. We do not expect visual information to increase the cognitive burden when CSCT is performed in noise. However, in our previous study, CSCT scores in quiet were found to be higher without visual cues in participants with normal hearing (Mishra et al., 2013). This is line with other work showing that visual cues may interfere with performance on executively challenging tasks (Fraser et al., 2010; Gosselin and Gagné, 2011) and may be due to difficulties in prioritizing task-related processing in the presence of low-priority stimuli (Lavie, 2005). In the quiet conditions of the CSCT, the numbers are fully audible and thus visual cues become low-priority stimuli. Thus, the superfluous visual information in the AV modality may act as a distractor when it is not required to segregate the target stimuli from a noise background. Hence, in the present study, we predicted higher CSCT scores in A-only compared to AV modality in quiet and the opposite in noise.

The main purpose of the present study was to investigate how noise influences CSC. In summary, we predicted that noise would disrupt executive processing of intelligible auditory two-digit numbers leading to lower CSCT performance than in quiet. Speech-like noise would be more disruptive than steady-state noise given the same SNR, particularly during the inhibition task. Seeing the talker's face would counteract the noise decrement by helping the listener segregate target from noise and generate richer cognitive representations. However, in quiet conditions, visual cues would act as a distractor and reduce performance.

We have argued that cognitive skills like WMC (Pichora-Fuller and Singh, 2006; Rudner and Lunner, 2013; Rönnberg et al., 2013), executive functions (Mishra et al., 2013), linguistic closure and LTM (Rönnberg et al., 2010) are engaged during the complex processing involved in speech understanding. Moreover, linguistic closure and LTM may play a specific role in solving the updating and inhibition tasks in the CSCT. Even if only part of a two-digit number has been perceived it may provide task-relevant information. For example in an updating task requiring retention of the highest numbers by each speaker, a new list number in the twenties by a particular speaker can be discarded if the retained number by the same speaker is in the thirties or higher. In this particular case it is sufficient to achieve LTM access and linguistic closure for the part of the number that provides the necessary information. To assess the contribution of individual cognitive functions towards CSC and speech intelligibility, we administered a cognitive test battery in the present study along with the CSCT. This battery included, the reading span test (Daneman and Carpenter, 1980; Rönnberg et al., 1989) as a measure of WMC, the Text Reception Threshold test (TRT; Zekveld et al., 2007) as a measure of linguistic closure, the Letter Memory Task (Morris and Jones, 1990; Miyake et al., 2000) as a measure of updating, the Simon task (Simon, 1969; adapted from Pratte et al., 2010) as a measure of inhibition, and delayed recall of the reading span stimuli to measure episodic LTM. We did not predict an overall association between CSCT performance and reading span because reading span measures WMC and not specifically the ability to deploy executive processing resources during listening in noise. However, we did expect an association with TRT and delayed recall of the reading span stimuli because linguistic closure, which TRT measures, and LTM, which delayed recall measures may play key roles in CSC. We predicted that performance on the updating and inhibition tasks of the CSCT would be associated with the respective independent measures of executive function and that individual executive abilities would be more predictive of CSCT performance in noise than in quiet.

METHODS

PARTICIPANTS

Twenty native Swedish speakers with either continuing or completed university education, including 11 females and 9 males, participated in the experiment. They were 19–35 years of age, M = 25.9; SD = 4.4. Hearing thresholds of the participants were within normal limits (better than 25 dB HL) in the frequency range of 125–8 kHz. The participants did not report any psychological or neurological problems. Visual acuity after correction was normal as measured by the Jaeger eye chart (Weatherly, 2002). Ethical approval for the study was obtained from the regional ethical review board, Linköping, Sweden.

MATERIAL

The CSCT stimuli consisted of AV and A-only recordings of the Swedish two-digit numbers 13–99 spoken by a male and a female native Swedish speaker (Mishra et al., 2013). The levels of the numbers were equated for 50% intelligibility in steady state noise using a group of ten young adults with normal hearing. This was accomplished by increasing the SNR in steps of 1 dB for each number until a correct response was given in a procedure similar to that described in Hällgren et al. (2006). For more details of CSCT materials, see Mishra et al. (2013).

NOISE

The stationary noise was a steady-state speech-weighted (SSSW) noise, having the same long term average spectrum as the recorded numbers. The modulated noise was the International Speech Testing Signal (ISTS; Holube et al., 2010). The ISTS noise is designed to be speech-like but unintelligible and is thus composed of concatenated speech segments of around 10 ms duration in six languages (American English, Arabic, Mandarin, French, German and Spanish) spoken by six different female speakers. The stimuli and noises were calibrated for the same root mean square (RMS) levels initially and then the noise levels were changed keeping the speech level constant to obtain individualized SNRs.

INDIVIDUALIZING SNR

The stimulus materials (numbers) in A-only modality and the SSSW noise were used in an adaptive procedure to determine the individualized SNR for presentation of the CSCT. In this adaptive procedure, the first stimulus was presented at an SNR of 5 dB and the participants were instructed to repeat the numbers they heard and were encouraged to guess if they were unsure. For the first run, for each new presented number that was repeated correctly, the noise was increased by steps of 3 dB until the participant's response was incorrect. Thereafter, the step size was changed to 1 dB and 30 numbers were randomly selected and presented consecutively to determine the 84% intelligibility level adaptively in a four-down/one-up procedure (Levitt, 1971). In the second step, the SNR obtained for 84% intelligibility was increased by 0.5 dB to give an approximate intelligibility level of 90% in SSSW noise. This 0.5 dB increment yielded an approximate intelligibility level of 90% in SSSW noise as verified in a piloting study using six participants with normal hearing. The 90% level was chosen so that the participants could perceive most numbers, in order to perform the tasks in CSCT, but requiring effort. To verify the intelligibility at this new SNR, 60 numbers, again randomly selected from the stimulus material, were used. These numbers were presented at the set SNR and the intelligibility with SSSW and ISTS noise was obtained independently. The same individualized SNR levels were applied in the SSSW and ISTS noise during CSCT presentation. The above tests were implemented in MATLAB (Version 2009b).

COGNITIVE SPARE CAPACITY TEST (CSCT)

In the CSCT (Mishra et al., 2013), 48 lists of 13 two-digit numbers (13–99) are presented serially and after each list the participant is requested to report two specified list items, depending on the predetermined criteria. These were designed to elicit updating and inhibition. In the updating task, the participants are asked to recall either the highest (in one version) or the lowest (in the other version) value item spoken by the male and female speaker in the particular list. In the inhibition task, the participants are asked to recall either two odd (in one version) or even (in the other version) value items spoken by a particular speaker. In half the trials, two numbers only are reported; these are low memory load trials. These two numbers are never the first item in the list. In the other half, high memory load trials, the first number in the list is also reported along with the two specified items, i.e., three numbers in total need to be held in working memory but only two of them are subject to processing. The first number (dummy item) in the high memory load trials is not included in the scoring. Thus, all scoring in the CSCT is based on correct report, in any order, of two numbers. These tasks are performed with either AV or A-only stimulus presentation and in the present study presentation took place in quiet (no noise), SSSW noise and ISTS noise.

The CSCT was administered using DMDX software (Forster and Forster, 2003; Mishra et al., 2013). The participants performed all conditions of each of the executive tasks in a balanced order in a single block. Thus, over both task blocks, there were a total of 24 conditions of presentation in the CSCT with two executive tasks, two memory loads, two modalities of presentation and three noise conditions in a 2 × 2 × 2 × 3 design. Two lists per condition were tested. The order of the conditions was pseudo-randomized within the two executive task blocks and balanced across the participants. For the noisy conditions, the noise sound files were played together with the AV and A-only stimulus files in DMDX with noise onset 1 s prior to stimulus onset and offset of at least 1 s after stimulus offset. The lists of numbers were always presented at 65 dB SPL and the level of the noise was varied depending upon the individualized SNR level. Across all the conditions (noisy or quiet), the duration of presentation of each list was 33 s. The time from onset of one stimulus to the onset of the next was 2.5 s. The visual stimuli were presented using a computer with a screen size of 14.1 inches and screen resolution of 1366 × 768 pixels. The video was displayed in 720 × 576 pixels resolution in the center of the screen and the auditory stimuli were presented through Sennheiser HDA 200 headphones.

Before each of the executive task blocks, the participants were provided with written instructions for the particular executive task and the instructions were also elaborated verbally. Before each list, the participant was prompted on the computer screen as to which version of the executive task was to be performed, what the modality was and whether to remember two or three numbers (low or high load). This prompt remained on screen until the participant pressed a button to continue to the test. The order of the noise conditions was pseudo-randomized. At the end of each list, an instruction "Respond now" appeared on the screen and the participant was required to report the target numbers orally. The participants could make corrections in reported numbers and then pressed another button when they were ready to continue. The oral responses of the participants were audio recorded. The participants were specifically instructed to keep looking at the screen during stimulus presentation. This applied even during presentation in the A-only modality where a fixation-cross was provided at center screen. All the participants practiced each task with two lists before doing the actual test.

COGNITIVE TEST BATTERY

Reading span test

In the reading span test (Daneman and Carpenter, 1980; Rönnberg et al., 1989), the participant read series of sentences in Swedish consisting of three words which appeared on the computer screen one at a time. Each word was shown for 800 ms with an interval of 50 ms between words. Each series consisted of three to six sentences presented in increasing series length. Half of the sentences were coherent and half were nonsense. The participants' task was to make a sematic judgment in 1.75 s and respond "yes" (if the sentence was coherent) or "no" (if the sentence was nonsense) before the next sentence appeared. At the end of each series of sentences, the participants were prompted by an instruction on the screen to recall either the first or the last word of all the sentences in the series in the order they appeared on the screen. The participants were provided with written instructions about the test and they did practice with a series of three sentences before the actual testing. There were a total of 54 sentences and the total score obtained on the recall in any order of first and final words was used in the analysis.

Text reception threshold (TRT)

The TRT (Zekveld et al., 2007) test is a visual analogy of a test of speech recognition in noise and measures ability to read partially masked text. A Swedish version of the TRT, using the Hearing In Noise Test (HINT) sentences (Hällgren et al., 2006) was used. The test consisted of presentation of three lists of 20 HINT sentences each, the first list being a practice list. The sentences appeared word by word on the screen in red masked by vertical black bars with the preceding words remained on the screen until the sentence was completed. After presentation of the last word, the sentence remained visible for 3.5 s. The presentation rate of the words in each sentence was equal to the speaking rate in the corresponding speaker file. A one-up-one-down adaptive procedure with a step-size of 6% was applied to target percentage of unmasked text required to read 50% of the sentences entirely correct. The average percentage of unmasked text from the two lists of sentences was used as dependent variable.

Letter memory task

In the letter memory task (Morris and Jones, 1990; Miyake et al., 2000), the participants were presented with sequences of letters and asked to hold the four most recent letters in mind and then prompted to say them at the end of each sequence. Responses were audio-recorded. DMDX software was used to present lists of 5, 7, 9 or 11 consonants serially at the center of the computer screen. Two lists consisting of 7 and 9 letters were presented as practice and the testing consisted of 12 lists. Sequence length of test lists was randomized across trials to ensure that the participant followed the instructed strategy and continuously updated working memory until the end of the trial. The score was the number of consonants correctly recalled irrespective of order.

Simon task

A visual analogue of the go/no go task (Simon, 1969; adapted from Pratte et al., 2010), using red and blue rectangular blocks which appeared on the left or the right of the computer screen successively at intervals of 2 s. The participants were required to respond as quickly as possible by pressing a button on the right hand side of the screen when they saw a red block and when they saw a blue block they pressed a button on the left hand side of the screen. A total of 16 blocks were presented using DMDX without a practice. The participant had to ignore the spatial position in which the block appeared in the task and when the spatial position of the stimulus and correct response key coincided, the trial was termed congruent otherwise incongruent. The difference in reaction time between the incongruent and congruent trials was taken as a measure of inhibition.

Delayed recall of reading span test

Delayed recall of the items presented during the reading span test was used to assess episodic LTM. In this test the participants were asked to recall, without forewarning, words or whole sentences remembered from the reading span test after approximately 60 min. During the 60 min, the participants performed the other tests in the cognitive test battery. The score on delayed recall test was the total number of words correctly recalled by the participant irrespective of the order.

PROCEDURE

The participants, on arriving for the testing, were fully briefed about the study and a consent form was signed. All the participants underwent vision screening and audiometric testing in the audiometric booth. The testing was conducted in two sessions. All auditory testing took place in a sound-treated booth with the participants facing the computer screen. Each session took approximately 90 min. The reading span test was administered followed by the Simon task, the letter memory test and the TRT test in a separate room. Individual SNRs for the CSCT were determined and the delayed recall of the reading span test concluded the first session. In the second session, the CSCT test was conducted. The participants were allowed to take breaks after different tests. Written instructions were provided for all the tests and the participants were given the opportunity to request oral clarification.

DATA ANALYSIS

A repeated measures analysis of variance (ANOVA) on the CSCT scores was conducted. In order to test our a-priori hypotheses, planned comparisons were carried out and the simple main effect observed without a-priori hypothesis was investigated using post-hoc Tukey's Honestly Significant Difference (HSD) test. In order to assess the association between cognitive functions and speech intelligibility and CSCT, Pearson's correlations with the cognitive test battery were computed.

RESULTS

INTELLIGIBILITY

In the noise conditions, the mean SNR for CSCT presentation was −2.17 dB (SD = 0.85). The mean intelligibility level was 93.8% (SD = 3.0) and 92.3% (SD = 2.9) for the SSSW and ISTS noise respectively. There was no statistically significant difference in speech intelligibility performance in SSSW and ISTS noise ($t\ (38) = 1.58, p = 0.12$).

COGNITIVE SPARE CAPACITY TEST (CSCT)

Figure 1 displays the mean scores obtained in the 24 conditions of CSCT. Since there were two lists presented per condition, the maximum score per condition was four. Performance in the inhibition task in the low memory load conditions approached ceiling, and so all analyses of CSCT data were conducted on the rationalized arcsine-transformed scores (Studebaker, 1985) to counteract data skewing. Mean recall of the dummy item in the high memory load conditions, was 22.4 (SD = 1.3) out of 24 possible responses. This demonstrates that the participants carried out the CSCT task in the high memory load conditions according to the instruction.

The repeated measures ANOVA of the CSCT scores revealed main effects of all four factors: executive function, $F(1, 19) = 10.01$, MSE = 0.28, $p < 0.01$, memory load, $F(1, 19) = 28.14$, MSE = 0.23, $p < 0.01$, modality, $F(1, 19) = 4.59$, MSE = 0.10, $p < 0.05$ and noise, $F(2, 38) = 18.25$, MSE = 0.18, $p < 0.01$. The main effect of executive function and memory load showed higher

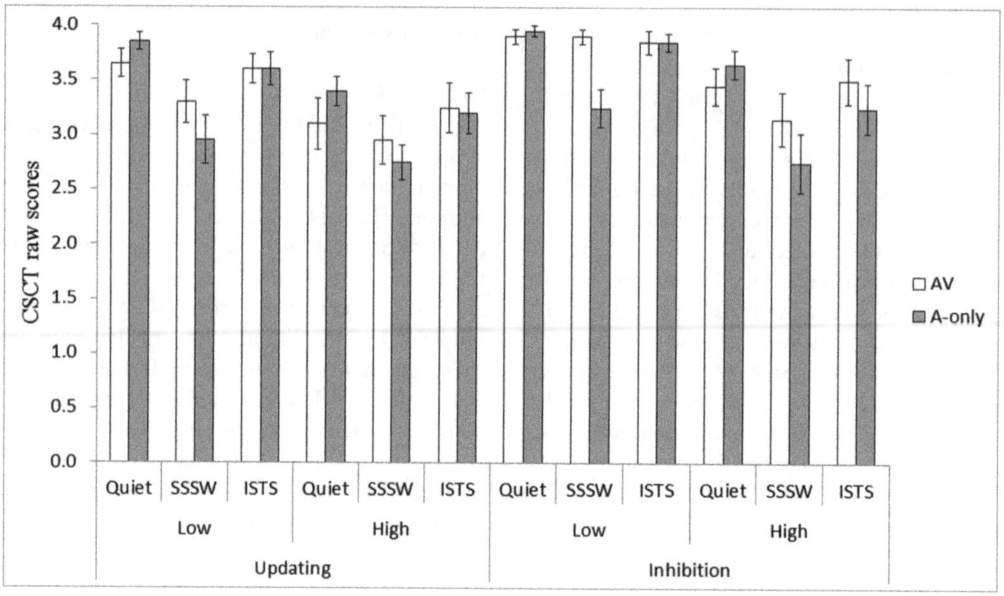

FIGURE 1 | Mean raw CSCT score for the AV (unfilled bars) and A-only (filled bars) modalities of presentation in the high and low memory load conditions of the updating and inhibition tasks in the three noise conditions. Error bars represent standard errors.

CSCT scores in inhibition than updating conditions and in low than high memory load conditions, in line with the predictions. Also, CSCT scores were higher in AV than A-only conditions. In order to identify significant differences in performance between the three levels of noise, pair-wise comparisons with Bonferroni adjustment for multiple comparisons were conducted. They revealed that CSCT scores in quiet and ISTS noise was significantly higher than in SSSW noise ($p < 0.05$) but there was no significant difference between the performance in quiet and ISTS noise ($p = 1.00$), see **Figure 1**.

The two-way interaction between noise and modality was significant, $F(2, 38) = 6.78$, MSE $= 0.14$, $p < 0.01$. We had a hypothesis that performance would be better in the A-only than AV modality in quiet but the opposite in noise. Planned comparisons revealed better performance in A-only compared to AV ($t = 1.86$, $p < 0.05$, one tailed) in quiet, and better performance in AV compared to A-only ($t = 2.52$, $p < 0.05$, one tailed) in SSSW in line with our predictions, see **Figure 2**. However, in ISTS there was no significant difference between performance in AV and A-only conditions ($t = 1.1$, $p > 0.05$, one tailed).

Post-hoc Tukey's HSD tests assessing the two-way interaction revealed that in the A-only modality of presentation, the scores was significantly higher in quiet ($p < 0.01$) and ISTS noise ($p < 0.01$) compared to SSSW noise and also that there was no significant difference between performance in AV modality in SSSW noise and A-only modality in ISTS noise, see **Figure 2**.

We had predicted that modulated noise would disrupt the inhibition task more than the updating task. However, there was no significant interaction between executive function and noise.

COGNITIVE TEST BATTERY

Table 1 shows the mean performance and standard deviation in the cognitive test battery. In the reading span task, the mean performance on semantic judgment was 50.46 (SD $=$ 3.20) out of 54 possible responses, demonstrating that the participants performed that part of the dual task in accordance with instructions.

The correlations between the tests in the cognitive test battery are shown in **Table 2**. The overall pattern of significant correlations without correction for multiple comparisons is shown.

The performance in the reading span test was significantly associated with performance in the letter memory test and the delayed recall of the reading span test. The performance in the TRT was significantly associated with the performance in the reading span and letter memory tests (c.f. Besser et al., 2013).

Table 3 shows the correlations between cognitive tests and the SNR rendering 84% speech intelligibility for SSSW noise and actual speech intelligibility at estimated 90% intelligibility for SSSW and ISTS noise. The speech intelligibility scores in ISTS noise were associated with performance in the Simon task and TRT. Since the TRT score is the average percentage of unmasked text, a higher score in TRT indicates poorer performance. Similarly, in the Simon task, the score is the difference in reaction time between the incongruent and the congruent condition, so a greater difference indicates poorer inhibition ability.

The correlations between CSCT and the battery of cognitive tests are shown in **Table 4**. To gain a detailed picture of the association between CSCT and cognitive function, we looked at the CSCT overall as well as factor-wise. Performance on the letter memory test was associated with CSCT irrespective of how scores were split, except when CSCT was performed in SSSW noise.

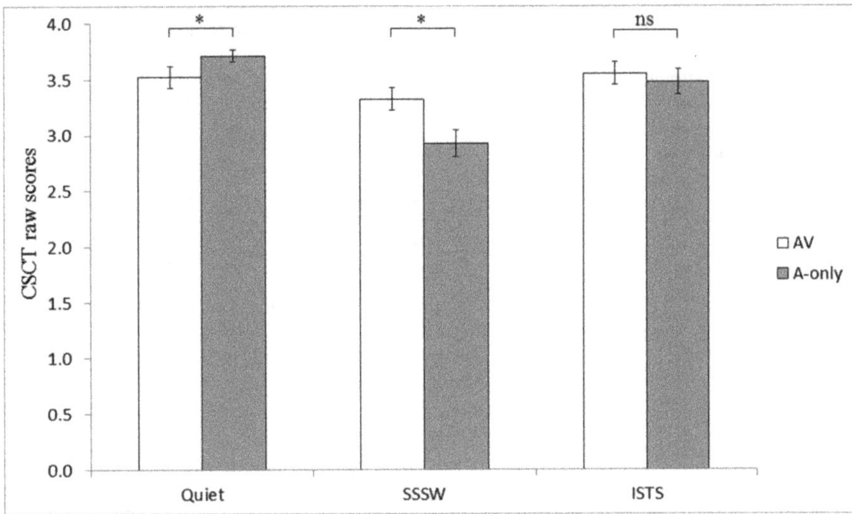

FIGURE 2 | Significant two-way interaction between modality of presentation and noise. Raw scores for AV (unfilled bars) and the A-only modalities of presentation (filled bars) in the three noise conditions of CSCT are represented. Error bars represent standard errors. * Indicates significance at 0.05 level (1-tailed).

Table 1 | Mean performance in the cognitive test battery.

Cognitive test	Mean	Standard deviation
Reading span (total items correctly recalled)	29.7 (of 54 possible)	6.75
Letter memory test (recall of last four letters)	41.7 (of 48 possible)	4.6
Simon task (RT ms difference between incongruent and congruent trials)	83.74	55.23
TRT (Percentage unmasked text)	46.84	3.95
Delayed recall of reading span test (correctly recalled words)	21.7	16.33

Table 2 | Coefficients of correlations (Pearson's *r*) between age and cognitive test scores.

	Age	Reading span	Letter memory test	Simon task	TRT	Delayed recall of reading span test
Age		−0.05	0.42	−0.36	0.04	−0.16
Reading span			0.60**	0.07	−0.55*	0.75**
Letter memory test				−0.01	−0.55*	0.01
Simon task					0.30	0.20
TRT						−0.15

** Correlation is significant at the 0.05 level (2-tailed)*

*** Correlation is significant at the 0.01 level (2-tailed)*

There was no correlation between Simon and CSCT performance. However, TRT was associated with CSCT performance in inhibition conditions. TRT was also associated with performance in A-only modality and high load conditions of CSCT. Performance in reading span was associated with CSCT performance in quiet. Delayed recall of reading span test performance was not associated with performance in CSCT in any of the conditions. The correlation between overall performance in CSCT and TRT tended towards significance (r (20) $= -0.43, p = 0.06$).

DISCUSSION

In the present study, CSC was investigated in young adults with normal hearing. The CSCT was administered in quiet as well as in steady state (SSSW) and speech-like (ISTS) noise at individual speech intelligibility levels approximating 90%. CSCT scores were higher in inhibition conditions compared to updating conditions and when memory load was low compared to when it was high, in line with previous findings (Mishra et al., 2013). SSSW noise reduced CSCT performance as predicted and seeing the talker's face counteracted the noise decrement. However, ISTS noise did not reduce CSCT performance. In quiet conditions, visual cues reduced performance as predicted.

There was no interaction between executive function and noise; hence our prediction that the scores in the inhibition subset of CSCT would be reduced more than in the updating subset in modulated noise was not supported. There was no overall association between CSCT performance and WMC but updating capacity predicted CSCT performance in all conditions.

CSCT PERFORMANCE IN QUIET

As predicted, we found higher CSCT scores in A-only modality compared to AV modality in quiet conditions. It has been argued that integration of visual information from the face of a talker with the speech produced by that talker does not consume cognitive resources (Campbell, 2009; Baddeley, 2012; Moradi et al., 2013; Yovel and Belin, 2013). However, it seems

Table 3 | Coefficients of correlations (Pearson's *r*) between cognitive tests and speech intelligibility.

	SNR at 84% speech intelligibility	Actual speech intelligibility at estimated 90% level in SSSW noise	Actual speech intelligibility at estimated 90% level in ISTS noise
Reading span	0.14	−0.13	0.14
Letter memory test	0.07	0.01	0.29
Simon task	−0.11	−0.19	−0.57**
TRT	−0.38	−0.27	−0.46*
Delayed recall of reading span test	−0.11	−0.36	−0.09

** Correlation is significant at the 0.05 level (2-tailed)*
*** Correlation is significant at the 0.01 level (2-tailed)*

Table 4 | Coefficients of correlations (Pearson's *r*) between collapsed CSCT and cognitive test scores.

CSCT	Reading span	Simon task	Letter memory test	TRT	Delayed recall of reading span test
Overall	0.25	−0.18	0.67**	−0.43	−0.08
Updating	−0.01	−0.24	0.44*	−0.11	−0.15
Inhibition	0.41	−0.06	0.65**	−0.58**	0.12
AV	0.24	−0.18	0.53*	−0.27	0.03
A-only	0.21	−0.14	0.70**	−0.51*	−0.05
Low load	−0.04	−0.23	0.57**	−0.24	−0.32
High load	0.35	−0.12	0.60**	−0.46*	0.15
Quiet	0.44*	0.15	0.73**	−0.37	0.12
SSSW	0.06	−0.20	0.30	−0.24	−0.11
ISTS	0.21	−0.31	0.57**	−0.40	−0.01

** Correlation is significant at the 0.05 level (2-tailed)*
*** Correlation is significant at the 0.01 level (2-tailed)*

that when speech has to be processed executively, superfluous information carried in the visual stream may reduce performance (Fraser et al., 2010; Gosselin and Gagné, 2011; Mishra et al., 2013). This may be because executive load makes it difficult to prioritize task-related processing in the presence of low priority stimuli (Lavie, 2005). In the quiet conditions of the CSCT, the auditory cues alone provide young adults with normal hearing thresholds with sufficient information for performing the executive tasks. Thus, for these individuals, the visual cues may simply compete for cognitive resources without enhancing task performance.

EFFECT OF NOISE AND MODALITY OF PRESENTATION ON CSCT PERFORMANCE

As predicted, CSCT scores were lower in noise than in quiet. However, this applied only to performance in SSSW. Based on the findings of Ng et al. (2013), we expected the CSCT scores to be lower in speech-like noise compared to steady state noise. However, contrary to our expectation, we found that CSCT scores in ISTS noise was significantly higher than in SSSW noise, despite the fact that there was no difference in either SNR or speech intelligibility between the two noise conditions. Also, CSCT performance in ISTS noise did not differ significantly from performance in quiet even in the A-only modality, although it is conceivable that potential differences in CSCT performance in ISTS noise and quiet were concealed by near-ceiling performance. Preserved CSCT performance in ISTS noise may be explained by a selective attention mechanism that comes into play when speech stimuli are presented against a background of speech-like noise (Zion Golumbic et al., 2013); the target speech stimuli are dynamically tracked in the brain but interfering noise is not tracked. This finding suggests that selective attention at higher cortical levels suppresses interfering speech-like noise at the perceptual level and may provide richer representation of the target speech stimuli in memory. In SSSW noise, it is likely that selective attention to the speech stimuli could not be achieved due to the lack of modulation in the interfering noise resulting in a failure to segregate the speech stimuli from the SSSW noise (c.f. Helfer and Freyman, 2005). Pichora-Fuller et al. (1995) have argued that although speech information has been perceived, it may not be adequately encoded in memory for retrieval. In this study, the speech intelligibility performance in SSSW and ISTS noise was similar, but the representation of the target speech stimuli in memory may have been impoverished in SSSW noise due to lack of segregation from noise, but not in ISTS noise. This may have led to lower CSCT scores in SSSW noise than in quiet and ISTS noise.

We also predicted that seeing the face of the talker while performing the CSCT would counteract the negative effects of noise by providing a richer representation of the to-be-remembered items and this is what we found in SSSW noise. Indeed, there was no significant difference in performance in the AV modality between any of the noise conditions including quiet. These findings demonstrate that when noise disrupts executive processing of speech, seeing the face of the talker counteracts the disruptive effect of the noise.

Significant correlations between performance on the Simon task and TRT and speech intelligibility in ISTS demonstrate that listening in ISTS noise is cognitively demanding. The correlation between speech performance in ISTS and performance in the Simon task suggests that inhibition skills may come to the fore to suppress irrelevant information during memory encoding (Janse, 2012) and the association with TRT suggests a role for linguistic closure during speech perception performance in noise when irrelevant cues have to be disregarded (Zekveld et al., 2012, 2013; Besser et al., 2013). However, these demands on cognitive resources while listening in ISTS do not seem to influence CSC as CSCT scores were higher in ISTS compared to SSSW noise. Our interpretation is that while cognitive resources relating to inhibition and linguistic closure are employed for perceiving speech in presence of noise, other higher cognitive processes selectively attenuate the interfering modulated noise such that richer representation of target items in working memory can be achieved. This leads to less load on CSC. This effect may be similar to the benefit afforded by visual cues in terms of generating a richer representation of the items. In the present study, we do not find a significant difference between the performance in SSSW noise in AV modality and ISTS noise in A-only modality. This finding suggests that for young adults with normal hearing, selective attention to speech in the presence of speech-like noise enriches the representation of the target stimuli in working memory in much the same way as the presence of visual cues.

CORRELATIONS BETWEEN CSCT AND THE COGNITIVE TEST BATTERY

Working memory

We have previously reported evidence that CSC is not related to WMC measured using the reading span test (Mishra et al., 2013). The reading span test is a well-established test of verbal WMC (Daneman and Carpenter, 1980; Rönnberg et al., 1989) that has proved to be a potent predictor of the ability to unravel linguistic complexity (Unsworth et al., 2009) and in particular the ability to understand speech under adverse conditions (Akeroyd, 2008; Besser et al., 2013). In particular, it has proved useful as a way of probing the simultaneous storage and processing capacity that characterizes WMC, through the unimpaired modality of vision in persons with hearing impairment (Classon et al., 2013; Ng et al., 2013). Thus, we consider it to be the most suitable measure of general WMC. Although the concept of CSC is related to WMC in the sense that both involve temporary maintenance and processing of information, it is not necessarily the case that CSC can be assessed by simply measuring WMC. This is because general WMC may be depleted in different ways under different sets of listening conditions and reduced ability to deploy one set of processing skills, such as inhibition, may be compensated for fully or partially by other skills, such as updating. Thus, we did not expect CSCT performance to correlate with reading span performance, our measure of WMC in the present study. Indeed, there was no overall correlation, but CSCT performance in quiet conditions did correlate positively and significantly with WMC although not in either of the two noise conditions. On the face of it, it would appear that the quiet conditions in the present study are those that most closely resemble the conditions in the previous study (Mishra et al., 2013). However, there were several methodological differences in the present study compared to Mishra et al. (2013) that may help explain the difference in the pattern of correlations between the two studies. Button-press responses were used in Mishra et al. (2013), whereas voice responses were used in the present study. Button-press responses are more cognitively demanding than vocal responses as they require the synchronization of motor response and visual scanning of buttons. Thus, in our previous study (Mishra et al., 2013) general cognitive resources were probably being engaged for motor planning during the response phase of the task, reducing CSC and leading to a lack of correlation with reading span performance. In the present study, however, CSC in quiet conditions is likely to be more similar to independently measured WMC, which may explain the intercorrelation. Notwithstanding, adjustment for multiple comparisons renders this isolated correlation insignificant.

Executive functions

It is notable that performance in none of the tasks in the cognitive test battery predicted CSCT performance in SSSW noise. This may be because the cognitive skills measured by the test battery in the present study do not contribute towards executive processing of items presented in SSSW noise. However, letter memory performance predicted performance in both quiet and ISTS conditions. In quiet, there is no interfering noise to disrupt representation of the target stimuli in working memory. We have argued that in ISTS noise, good representation in working memory can be achieved by selective attention to speech (Zion Golumbic et al., 2013) whereas this is not the case in the presence of SSSW noise. The association of letter memory performance and CSCT performance in quiet and ISTS noise suggests that updating skills play an important role during processing of encoded representations. This in turn suggests that CSC in young persons with normal hearing thresholds may capitalize on updating ability when cognitive representations are rich.

Because the CSCT taps executive functions, we expected CSCT performance to correlate with the independent tests of executive function (c.f. Mishra et al., 2013). In particular, we expected updating ability to facilitate CSCT performance, especially in updating conditions, and inhibitory ability to facilitate CSCT performance in inhibition conditions. Performance on the letter memory task (Miyake et al., 2000) which was our independent test of updating correlated positively and significantly with performance in both the updating and inhibition conditions of the CSCT. Performance on the Simon task (Simon, 1969; Pratte et al., 2010) which was our independent test of inhibition skill did not correlate with CSCT under any conditions of the CSCT. Performance on letter memory and Simon tasks was not significantly related. In the present study, target items were presented in two different kinds of background noise for two out of three lists in an unpredictable manner. This means that the participants were probably always on the alert, at least at the beginning of each list, to cope with background noise, even when lists were presented in quiet. In other words, cognitive resources, probably inhibition skills, were probably always allocated, even when not specifically needed. This may have meant that participants had fewer inhibition resources available to engage in executive processing of the numbers. We have argued that a cognitive resource that is depleted in the act of speech perception may be compensated for fully or partially by another cognitive function during further processing. The pattern of correlations between CSCT and the cognitive test battery suggests that consistent demands were made on updating skills while inhibition skills had less impact. The explanation may be that during executive processing of numbers, updating skills compensated for the unavailability of inhibition skills engaged in preparing for noise.

Inhibition skills were significantly related to the intelligibility of the stimuli in ISTS noise, which suggests that inhibition skills were required to suppress the irrelevant information present in the ISTS noise during speech perception although they did not enhance memory performance or influence CSC. This may be because the inhibition resources were reduced during perception of numbers in noise and other cognitive skills like linguistic closure and updating were used to perform the inhibition task of CSCT.

Linguistic closure

The association of TRT with the inhibition subset of CSCT suggests that the ability to make use of linguistic closure is related to the processing required to identify and keep in mind auditory two-digit numbers of a certain parity and voice. The common factor may be an underlying ability to generate a coherent response on the basis of diverse pieces of information. The main effects of memory load and modality in CSCT performance revealed that the CSCT scores were lower when memory load was high and when visual cues were absent, suggesting that under these conditions the CSCT task is more difficult. The fact that performance in TRT was associated with CSCT performance in these particular conditions suggests that linguistic closure ability enhances CSCT performance when the task is difficult. This interpretation is supported by evidence that TRT predicts recall of speech heard in noise together with irrelevant visual cues (Zekveld et al., 2012). However, when visual information was available, CSCT performance in the present study was not associated with the TRT performance. This is in line with our prediction that AV integration is not cognitively taxing (Baddeley, 2012; Moradi et al., 2013). Further, we predicted that overall CSCT performance would be associated with performance in TRT and a tendency towards this association was found suggesting that overall performance in CSCT is predicted by an ability to make use of linguistic closure.

Episodic long-term memory

Finally, the delayed recall of the reading span stimuli measuring episodic LTM was not associated with performance in CSCT. Thus, no support was found for an association between episodic LTM and CSC in young adults with normal hearing. Recent work shows that hearing loss is associated with decline in LTM and it has been suggested that the mechanism behind this association is that hearing loss leads to more mismatch due to poor audibility and distortion of the input signal and thus less access to LTM (Rönnberg et al., 2011). Hence, it can be expected that an efficient LTM may facilitate processing of speech in adverse conditions, even though no such evidence was found for the participants with normal hearing in the present study.

COGNITIVE SPARE CAPACITY

Cognitive resources are consumed in the act of listening (Pichora-Fuller, 2009; Rönnberg et al., 2013). Individual WMC capacity is associated with the ability to recognize speech in noise and the reading span task has proved to be a particularly potent predictor (Akeroyd, 2008; Besser et al., 2013). However, because available cognitive resources may be deployed differently under different listening conditions (Pichora-Fuller and Singh, 2006; Pichora-Fuller, 2007), it is important to gain an understanding of CSC which is the cognitive reserve that has been depleted by listening under adverse conditions. This requires an experimental approach. The results of the present study show that the CSCT may be a useful tool in this enterprise. They provide a baseline performance level for CSCT in quiet and in noise for young adults with normal hearing. The next step is to investigate CSCT performance in persons with hearing impairment. In the future, we aim to develop a simplified version of the CSCT which can be used for evaluation of hearing aid fitting and different signal processing strategies used in hearing aids. By using CSCT we will be able to show the influence of signal processing on memory for heard speech. We believe that CSCT performance can provide us with a snap-shot of how hearing-aid signal processing influences cognitive demands in communicative situations (Rudner and Lunner, 2013).

CONCLUSION

The results of the present study replicate the results of Mishra et al. (2013) by showing that CSC in young adults with normal hearing thresholds is sensitive to storage load and executive function but not generally related to WMC and that availability of visual cues may hinder executive processing of speech heard in quiet. They also extend these results by showing that even when speech intelligibility is high, steady-state noise may lower CSCT performance but that this decrement can be restored when the talker's face is visible, probably by aiding segregation of target items and thus enriching their cognitive representation. Speech-like noise did not reduce CSCT performance, which was contrary to our prediction. We suggest that selective attention was used to ignore the speech-like background noise to provide an enriched representation of target items similar to that obtained in quiet. The overall pattern of results suggests that updating skills play a key role in exploiting CSC and may provide high-level compensation when inhibition skills are engaged in low-level processing.

ACKNOWLEDGMENTS

Supported by grant number 2007-0788 to Mary Rudner from the Swedish Council for Working Life and Social Research.

REFERENCES

Akeroyd, M. A. (2008). Are individual differences in speech perception related to individual differences in cognitive ability? A survey of twenty experimental studies with normal and hearing impaired adults. *Int. J. Audiol.* 47(Suppl. 2), S53–S71. doi: 10.1080/14992020802301142

Baddeley, A. (2000). The episodic buffer: a new component of working memory? *Trends Cogn. Sci.* 4, 417–423. doi: 10.1016/s1364-6613(00)01538-2

Baddeley, A. (2012). Working memory: theories, models and controversies. *Annu. Rev. Psychol.* 63, 1–29. doi: 10.1146/annurev-psych-120710-100422

Besle, J., Fort, A., Delpuech, C., and Giard, M. H. (2004). Bimodal speech: early suppressive visual effects in the human auditory cortex. *Eur. J. Neurosci.* 20, 2225–2234. doi: 10.1111/j.1460-9568.2004.03670.x

Besser, J., Koelewijn, T., Zekveld, A. A., Kramer, S. E., and Festen, J. M. (2013). How linguistic closure and verbal working memory relate to speech recognition in noise—a review. *Trends Amplif.* 17, 75–93. doi: 10.1177/1084713813495459

Campbell, R. (2009). "The processing of audiovisual speech: empirical and neural bases," in *The Perception of Speech: From Sound to Meaning*, eds B. C. J. Moore, L. K. Tyler and W. Marslen-Wilson (Oxford, New York: Oxford University Press), 133–150.

Classon, E., Rudner, M., and Rönnberg, J. (2013). Working memory compensates for hearing related phonological processing deficit. *J. Commun. Disord.* 46, 17–29. doi: 10.1016/j.jcomdis.2012.10.001

Daneman, M., and Carpenter, P. A. (1980). Individual differences in working memory and reading. *J. Verbal Learning Verbal Behav.* 19, 450–466. doi: 10.1016/S0022-5371(80)90312-6

Duquesnoy, A. J. (1983). Effect of a single interfering noise or speech source upon the binaural sentence intelligibility of aged persons. *J. Acoust. Soc. Am.* 74, 739–743. doi: 10.1121/1.389859

Forster, K. I., and Forster, J. C. (2003). DMDX:a windows display program with millisecond accuracy. *Behav. Res. Methods Instrum. Comput.* 35, 116–124. doi: 10.3758/BF03195503

Fraser, S., Gagné, J.-P., Alepins, M., and Dubois, P. (2010). Evaluating the effort expended to understand speech in noise using a dual-task paradigm: the effects of providing visual speech-cues. *J. Speech Lang. Hear. Res.* 53, 18–33. doi: 10.1044/1092-4388(2009/08-0140)

George, E. L. J., Festen, J. M., and Houtgast, T. (2006). Factors affecting masking release for speech in modulated noise for normal-hearing and hearing-impaired listeners. *J. Acoust. Soc. Am.* 120, 2295–2311. doi: 10.1121/1.2266530

Gosselin, P. A., and Gagné, J.-P. (2011). Older adults expend more listening effort than young adults recognizing audiovisual speech in noise. *Int. J. Audiol.* 50, 786–792. doi: 10.3109/14992027.2011.599870

Grant, K. W., Walden, B. E., and Seitz, P. F. (1998). Auditory-visual speech recognition by hearing-impaired subjects: consonant recognition, sentence recognition and auditory-visual integration. *J. Acoust. Soc. Am.* 103, 2677–2690. doi: 10.1121/1.422788

Helfer, K. S., and Freyman, R. L. (2005). The role of visual speech cues in reducing energetic and informational masking. *J. Acoust. Soc. Am.* 117, 842–849. doi: 10.1121/1.1836832

Holube, I., Fredelake, S., Vlaming, M., and Kollmeier, B. (2010). Development and analysis of an international speech test signal (ISTS). *Int. J. Audiol.* 49, 891–903. doi: 10.3109/14992027.2010.506889

Humes, L. E. (2007). The contributions of audibility and cognitive factors to the benefit provided by amplified speech to older adults. *J. Am. Acad. Audiol.* 18, 590–603. doi: 10.3766/jaaa.18.7.6

Hygge, S., Rönnberg, J., Larsby, B., and Arlinger, S. (1992). Normal-hearing and hearing-impaired subjects' ability to just follow conversation in competing speech, reversed speech and noise backgrounds. *J. Speech Hear. Res.* 35, 208–215.

Hällgren, M., Larsby, B., and Arlinger, S. (2006). A swedish version of the hearing in noise test (HINT) for measurement of speech recognition. *Int. J. Audiol.* 45, 227–237. doi: 10.1080/14992020500429583

Janse, E. (2012). A non-auditory measure of interference predicts distraction by competing speech in older adults. *Neuropsychol. Dev. Cogn. B Aging Neuropsychol. Cogn.* 19, 741–758. doi: 10.1080/13825585.2011.652590

Koelewijn, T., Zekveld, A. A., Festen, J. M., and Kramer, S. E. (2012). Pupil dilation uncovers extra listening effort in the presence of a single-talker masker. *Ear Hear.* 33, 291–300. doi: 10.1097/aud.0b013e3182310019

Lavie, N. (2005). Distracted and confused?: selective attention under load. *Trends Cogn. Sci.* 9, 75–82. doi: 10.1016/j.tics.2004.12.004

Levitt, H. (1971). Transformed up-down methods in psychoacoustics. *J. Acoust. Soc. Am.* 49, 467–477. doi: 10.1121/1.1912375

Lunner, T., Rudner, M., and Rönnberg, J. (2009). Cognition and hearing aids. *Scand. J. Psychol.* 55, 395–403. doi: 10.1111/j.1467-9450.2009.00742.x

Mattys, S. L., Davis, M. H., Bradlow, A. R., and Scott, S. K. (2012). Speech recognition in adverse conditions: a review. *Lang. Cogn. Process.* 27, 953–978. doi: 10.1080/01690965.2012.705006

Mishra, S., Lunner, T., Stenfelt, S., Rönnberg, J., and Rudner, M. (2013). Visual information can hinder working memory processing of speech. *J. Speech Lang. Hear. Res.* 56, 1120–1132. doi: 10.1044/1092-4388(2012/12-0033)

Mishra, S., Rudner, M., Lunner, T., Stenfelt, S., and Rönnberg, J. (2010). "Speech understanding and cognitive spare capacity," in *Binaural Processing and Spatial Hearing*, eds J. M. Buchholz, T. Dau, J. Christensen-Dalsgaard and T. Poulsen (Elsinore: ISAAR), 305–313.

Miyake, A., Friedman, N. P., Emerson, M. J., Witziki, A. H., Howerter, A., and Wager, T. (2000). The unity and diversity of executive functions and their contribution to complex frontal lobe tasks: a latent variable analysis. *Cogn. Psychol.* 41, 49–100. doi: 10.1006/cogp.1999.0734

Moradi, S., Lidestam, B., and Rönnberg, R. (2013). Gated audiovisual speech identification in silence versus noise: effect on time and accuracy. *Front. Psychol.* 4:359. doi: 10.3389/fpsyg.2013.00359

Morris, N., and Jones, D. M. (1990). Memory updating in working memory: the role of the central executive. *Br. J. Psychol.* 81, 111–121. doi: 10.1111/j.2044-8295.1990.tb02349.x

Murphy, D. R., Craik, F. I. M., Li, K. Z. H., and Schneider, B. A. (2000). Comparing the effects of aging and background noise on short term memory performance. *Psychol. Aging* 15, 323–334. doi: 10.1037/0882-7974.15.2.323

Ng, E. H., Rudner, M., Lunner, T., Pedersen, M. S., and Rönnberg, J. (2013). Effects of noise and working memory capacity on memory processing of speech for hearing aid users. *Int. J. Audiol.* 52, 433–441. doi: 10.3109/14992027.2013.776181

Pichora-Fuller, M. K. (2007). "Audition and cognition: what audiologists need to know about listening," in *Hearing Care for Adults*, eds C. Palmer and R. Seewald (Stäfa: Phonak), 71–85.

Pichora-Fuller, M. K. (2009). How cognition might influence hearing aid design, fitting, and outcomes. *Hear. J.* 62, 32–38. doi: 10.1097/01.HJ.0000364274.44847.dc

Pichora-Fuller, M. K., Schneider, B. A., and Daneman, M. (1995). How young and old adults listen to and remember speech in noise. *J. Acoust. Soc. Am.* 97, 593–608. doi: 10.1121/1.412282

Pichora-Fuller, M. K., and Singh, G. (2006). Effects of age on auditory and cognitive processing: implications for hearing aid fitting and audiologic rehabilitation. *Trends Amplif.* 10, 29–59. doi: 10.1177/108471380601000103

Pratte, M. S., Rouder, J. N., Morey, R. D., and Feng, C. (2010). Exploring the differences in distributional properties between stroop and simon effects using delta plots. *Atten. Percept. Psychophys.* 72, 2013–2025. doi: 10.3758/app.72.7.2013

Rudner, M., Foo, C., Rönnberg, J, and Lunner, T. (2011b). Working memory supports listening in noise for persons with hearing impairment. *J. Am. Acad. Audiol.* 22, 156–167. doi: 10.3766/jaaa.22.3.4

Rudner, M., and Lunner, T. (2013). Cognitive spare capacity as a window on hearing aid benefit. *Semin. Hear.* 34, 297–306. doi: 10.1055/s-0033-1356642

Rudner, M., Lunner, T., Behrens, T., Thoren, E. S., and Rönnberg, J. (2012). Working memory capacity may influence perceived effort during aided speech recognition in noise. *J. Am. Acad. Audiol.* 23, 577–589. doi: 10.3766/jaaa.23.7.7

Rudner, M., Ng, E. H., Ronnberg, N., Mishra, S., Rönnberg, J., Lunner, T., et al. (2011a). Cognitive spare capacity as measure of listening effort. *J. Hear. Sci.* 1, 1–3. doi: 10.4081/audiores.2011.e22

Rönnberg, J. (2003). Cognition in the hearing impaired and deaf as a bridge between signal and dialogue: a framework and a model. *Int. J. Audiol.* 42, S68–S76. doi: 10.3109/14992020309074626

Rönnberg, J., Arlinger, S., Lyxell, B., and Kinnefors, C. (1989). Visual evoked potentials: relation to adult speechreading and cognitive function. *J. Speech Hear. Res.* 32, 725–735.

Rönnberg, J., Danielsson, H., Rudner, M., Arlinger, S., Sternäng, O., Wahlin, A., et al. (2011). Hearing loss is negatively related to episodic and semantic long-term memory but not to short-term memory. *J. Speech Lang. Hear. Res.* 54, 705–726. doi: 10.1044/1092-4388(2010/09-0088)

Rönnberg, J., Lunner, T., Zekveld, A., Sörqvist, P., Danielsson, H., Lyxell, B., et al. (2013). The ease of language understanding (ELU) model: theoretical, empirical and clinical advances. *Front. Syst. Neurosci.* 7:31. doi: 10.3389/fnsys.2013.00031

Rönnberg, J., Rudner, M., and Foo, C. (2010). "The cognitive neuroscience of signed language: applications to a working memory system for sign and speech," in *Memory, Aging and the Brain: A Festschrift in Honour of Lars-Göran Nilsson*, eds L. Bäckman and L. Nyberg (London: Psychology Press), 265–286.

Rönnberg, J., Rudner, M., Foo, C., and Lunner, T. (2008). Cognition counts: a working memory system for ease of language understanding (ELU). *Int. J. Audiol.* 47, S99–S105. doi: 10.1080/14992020802301167

Simon, J. R. (1969). Reactions towards the source of stimulation. *J. Exp. Psychol.* 81, 174–176. doi: 10.1037/h0027448

Studebaker, G. A. (1985). A "rationalized" arcsine transform. *J. Speech Hear. Res.* 28, 455–462.

Sörqvist, P., and Rönnberg, J. (2012). Episodic long-term memory of spoken discourse masked by speech: what role for working memory capacity? *J. Speech Lang. Hear. Res.* 55, 210–218. doi: 10.1044/1092-4388(2011/10-0353)

Tye-Murray, N., Spehar, B., Myerson, J., Sommers, M., and Hale, S. (2011). Cross-modal enhancement of speech detection in young and older adults: does signal content matter? *Ear Hear.* 32, 650–655. doi: 10.1097/aud.0b013e31821a4578

Unsworth, N., Redick, T. S., Heitz, R. P., Broadway, J. M., and Engle, R. W. (2009). Complex working memory span tasks and higher-order cognition: a latent-variable analysis of the relationship between processing and storage. *Memory* 17, 635–654. doi: 10.1080/09658210902998047

Weatherly, S. L. (2002). Back to basics: testing visual acuity with the jaeger eye chart. *Mater. Eval.* 60, 928–929.

Yovel, G., and Belin, P. (2013). A unified coding strategy for processing faces and voices. *Trends Cogn. Sci.* 17, 263–271. doi: 10.1016/j.tics.2013.04.004

Zekveld, A. A., George, E. L. J., Kramer, S. E., Goverts, S. T., and Houtgast, T. (2007). The development of the text reception threshold test: a visual analogue of the speech reception threshold test. *J. Speech Lang. Hear. Res.* 50, 576–584. doi: 10.1044/1092-4388(2007/040)

Zekveld, A. A., Rudner, M., Johnsrude, I. S., Heslenfeld, D. J., and Rönnberg, J. (2012). Behavioral and fMRI evidence that cognitive ability modulates the effect of semantic context on speech intelligibility. *Brain Lang.* 122, 103–113. doi: 10.1016/j.bandl.2012.05.006

Zekveld, A. A., Rudner, M., Johnsrude, I. S., and Rönnberg, J. (2013). The effects of working memory capacity and semantic cues on the intelligibility of speech in noise. *J. Acoust. Soc. Am.* 134, 2225–2234. doi: 10.1121/1.4817926

Zion Golumbic, E. M., Ding, N., Bickel, S., Lakatos, S., Schevon, C. A., McKhann, G. M., et al. (2013). Mechanism underlying selective neuronal tracking of attended speech at a "cocktail party". *Neuron* 77, 980–991. doi: 10.1016/j.neuron.2012.12.037

9

Changes in auditory perceptions and cortex resulting from hearing recovery after extended congenital unilateral hearing loss

Jill B. Firszt[1]*, Ruth M. Reeder[1], Timothy A. Holden[1], Harold Burton[2,3] and Richard A. Chole[1,4]

[1] Department of Otolaryngology-Head and Neck Surgery, Washington University School of Medicine, St. Louis, MO, USA
[2] Department of Anatomy and Neurobiology, Washington University School of Medicine, St. Louis, MO, USA
[3] Department of Radiology, Washington University School of Medicine, St. Louis, MO, USA
[4] Department of Developmental Biology, Washington University School of Medicine, St. Louis, MO, USA

Correspondence:
Jill B. Firszt, Department of Otolaryngology-Head and Neck Surgery, Washington University School of Medicine, 660 South Euclid Avenue, Campus Box 8115, St. Louis, MO 63110, USA
e-mail: firsztj@ent.wustl.edu

Monaural hearing induces auditory system reorganization. Imbalanced input also degrades time-intensity cues for sound localization and signal segregation for listening in noise. While there have been studies of bilateral auditory deprivation and later hearing restoration (e.g., cochlear implants), less is known about unilateral auditory deprivation and subsequent hearing improvement. We investigated effects of long-term congenital unilateral hearing loss on localization, speech understanding, and cortical organization following hearing recovery. Hearing in the congenitally affected ear of a 41 year old female improved significantly after stapedotomy and reconstruction. Pre-operative hearing threshold levels showed unilateral, mixed, moderately-severe to profound hearing loss. The contralateral ear had hearing threshold levels within normal limits. Testing was completed prior to, and 3 and 9 months after surgery. Measurements were of sound localization with intensity-roved stimuli and speech recognition in various noise conditions. We also evoked magnetic resonance signals with monaural stimulation to the unaffected ear. Activation magnitudes were determined in core, belt, and parabelt auditory cortex regions via an interrupted single event design. Hearing improvement following 40 years of congenital unilateral hearing loss resulted in substantially improved sound localization and speech recognition in noise. Auditory cortex also reorganized. Contralateral auditory cortex responses were increased after hearing recovery and the extent of activated cortex was bilateral, including a greater portion of the posterior superior temporal plane. Thus, prolonged predominant monaural stimulation did not prevent auditory system changes consequent to restored binaural hearing. Results support future research of unilateral auditory deprivation effects and plasticity, with consideration for length of deprivation, age at hearing correction and degree and type of hearing loss.

Keywords: unilateral hearing loss, congenital, conductive, stapedotomy, brain imaging, sound localization, speech recognition

INTRODUCTION

Monaural hearing induces auditory system reorganization. This occurs in cases of unilateral sensorineural hearing loss, where there is sensory (inner ear) or neural dysfunction, as well as losses in the conductive pathway between the outer and inner ear. In animals, unilateral conductive hearing loss (UCHL) results in structural and functional changes within the auditory system. For example, on the UCHL side in rats, the size of neurons in the anteroventral cochlear nucleus was smaller (Coleman and O'Connor, 1979) and binaural interactions were absent in the inferior colliculus (Silverman and Clopton, 1977). Likewise in cats, UCHL reduced the inhibition from the ipsilateral ear on neurons in the inferior colliculus when the contralateral ear was deprived of sound (Moore and Irvine, 1981). Additionally, UCHL leads to decreased 2-deoxyglucose uptake bilaterally in the higher auditory medial and lateral superior olive nuclei even in silence, indicating decreased neuronal activity (Tucci et al., 2001). Interestingly, in a number of these studies, bilateral conductive hearing loss had little to no effect on neuronal size or binaural interactions, with normal maintenance of contralateral and ipsilateral projections. Together, these studies suggest that modifications in the balance of afferent activity alter binaural interactions and auditory system structures.

Imbalanced input from UCHL also degrades signal segregation for listening in noise and time-intensity cues for sound localization in humans (Wilmington et al., 1994; Gray et al., 2009). Amongst tasks requiring binaural processing, UCHL participants had lower interaural temporal difference limens, required higher intensities in the affected ear to perceive balanced loudness, had lower speech recognition in noise, and for masking level differences (MLDs), had signal detection affected by lower amplitude noise levels (Hall and Grose, 1993; Wilmington et al., 1994; Gray et al., 2009). Self-assessment questionnaires that probe hearing in different listening environments indicated numerous hearing difficulties in those with congenital UCHL (Priwin et al., 2007). While there have been studies of bilateral sensorineural auditory deprivation and later hearing restoration from implantable devices (e.g., cochlear implants), much less is known about unilateral auditory deprivation from conductive hearing loss and subsequent hearing improvement.

Effects of early abnormal auditory experience and later recovery have been reported in several animal studies. For example, UCHL created by plugging one ear in young owls initially altered localization abilities but abilities then recovered, that is, the owls made use of abnormal cues to accurately localize (Knudsen et al., 1984a,b). After the earplug was removed, these owls again made localization errors but after some weeks they regained accuracy. However, localization performance did not recover when ear plugging occurred in older owls or even in younger owls when the plug remained in place beyond a few weeks. Thus, the ability to recover was affected by the age at which UCHL occurred as well as the age at which hearing was restored. While it is well known that unilateral deprivation of the visual system early in life results in permanent impairment of binocular vision (Hubel and Wiesel, 1970), less is known about the developing auditory system's ability to recover binaural abilities. Undefined in humans is a sensitive period for binaural hearing, where behavior can adapt to abnormal experience and develop accurate abilities, and a critical period, after which the ability to adapt to altered (including restored) hearing is greatly diminished or nonexistent.

Binaural performance improved in some individuals who had UCHL correction when the loss was acquired after maturation (Hausler et al., 1983; Hall and Derlacki, 1986, 1988). Hall and colleagues showed, using measures of MLDs, that reduced binaural abilities may continue after restoration of hearing in adults with otosclerosis (Hall and Derlacki, 1986, 1988; Hall et al., 1990). However, in a later longitudinal study of adults with otosclerosis, MLDs returned to normal in many participants when tested a year after hearing restoration (Hall and Grose, 1993). Otosclerosis is typically diagnosed in young to middle adulthood and the hearing loss is often progressive in nature (and primarily conductive), thus these individuals had several years of normal hearing (NH) prior to hearing loss onset.

Congenital conductive hearing loss may occur for reasons of atresia or middle ear anomalies such as a fused malleus and incus, or fixation of the stapes. Degree of hearing loss and the presence or absence of other inner ear deficits varies with the abnormality, but can result in 60 dB of hearing loss from the conductive aspect alone. Diagnosis of hearing loss and treatment to improve hearing often occurs in childhood. When left untreated into adulthood, individuals will have extended periods of auditory deprivation.

A prior study assessed binaural abilities in patients aged 6–33 years, before and after surgery to correct congenital UCHL (Wilmington et al., 1994). Measures included interaural temporal difference limens, MLDs, sound localization and speech recognition in noise. Post-surgery binaural improvements were significant for some individuals and some tasks but not all; sound localization and speech recognition continued to be difficult especially when noise was towards the NH ear and the restored ear was relied upon for speech understanding. Abnormal auditory experience in early life may affect later binaural abilities; however, the nature and impact of these interactions are not entirely clear.

In the current case study, we investigated the effects of long-term congenital, unilateral mixed (conductive and sensorineural) hearing loss on sound localization, speech understanding, and cortical organization, both before and after the conductive component of the hearing loss was corrected in adulthood.

MATERIALS AND METHODS

Written informed consent was obtained from the participant in accordance with the Declaration of Helsinki and guidelines approved by the Human Research Protection Office at Washington University School of Medicine (WUSM).

PARTICIPANT

The participant (P1) was a 41 year old female who had a history of unilateral hearing loss in the right ear that had been present since early childhood (probably since birth). Family history included a father and paternal grandmother with mixed unilateral hearing loss. P1's father had successful stapes surgery in adulthood as a treatment for otosclerosis induced hearing loss. P1 and her family had believed P1's hearing loss to be sensorineural and non-correctable. A hearing aid was fitted around age 5 but discontinued after a brief trial due to lack of benefit. In adulthood, the participant had a comprehensive audiological evaluation that diagnosed the loss as mixed. P1 consulted an otolaryngologist to discuss treatment options. Audiological air-conduction results (see **Figure 1A**) for the right ear (red triangles) indicated a severe hearing loss at 0.25 and 0.5 kHz, dropping to a profound hearing loss at 1 kHz and rising to a moderate to moderately-severe hearing loss from 3 to 8 kHz. Bone-conduction results (red brackets) identified the loss as mixed with a conductive component (30–70 dB) at all frequencies and an additional sensorineural component from 0.5 to 2 kHz. The difference between the air- and bone-conduction thresholds identifies the conductive component of the participant's hearing loss, that is, the portion of the loss that could potentially be corrected through surgery. Hearing levels were normal in the unaffected left ear (blue symbols) resulting in a large hearing asymmetry between ears. With this level of asymmetry and the mixed nature of the hearing loss in the affected ear, audiological masking approaches become more complicated due to potential cross masking effects. One-third octave narrow bands of masking noise (centered at the test frequency) were presented to the unaffected ear to isolate the affected ear during testing. Testing was completed with TDH-49 headphones with 40–60 dB of interaural attenuation. Although a 15 dB plateau was achieved at each frequency (increases in masking level at the unaffected ear did not increase the patient's response level in the affected ear), high levels of masking noise to the unaffected ear could possibly have been detected by the cochlea of the affected ear via bone

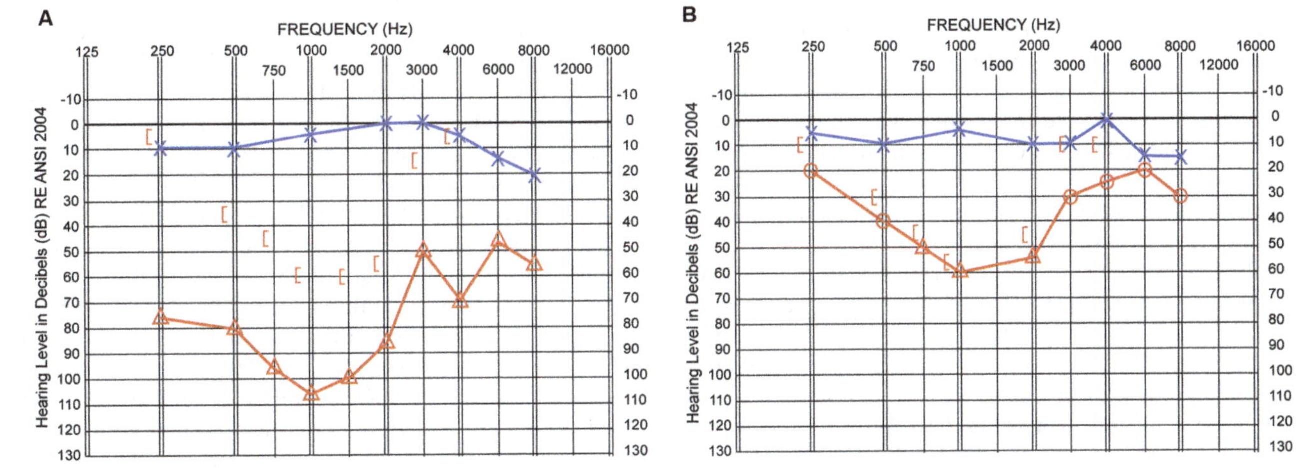

FIGURE 1 | Hearing thresholds in decibels (dB; *y*-axis) are shown as a function of frequency (Hz; *x*-axis). Pre-surgical results in Panel **A** and 3-month post-surgical results in Panel **B**. Air-conduction thresholds via TDH headphones (Panel **A**) or insert earphones (Panel **B**) are indicated with blue Xs for the left ear and red triangles or circles for the right ear. Circles indicate unmasked right ear thresholds and triangles indicate thresholds obtained with masking noise presented to the better hearing left ear. Masked bone-conduction thresholds for the right ear are indicated with red left-facing brackets.

conduction while attempting to identify accurate air-conduction thresholds of the affected ear.

Pre-operative, high resolution CT scanning revealed a slightly thickened stapes footplate with no other abnormalities suggestive of otosclerosis. The participant underwent a laser stapedotomy procedure with prosthetic reconstruction completed under general anesthesia through an aural speculum. This procedure is designed to restore mobility to the middle ear bones for improved sound conduction. A tympanomeatal flap was raised and the middle ear entered. The malleus and incus were mobile and the stapes firmly fixed in the oval window consistent with a congenitally fixed stapes. A CO_2 laser was used to make a stapedotomy in the center of the stapes footplate and a Teflon piston was placed and connected to the incus. The meatal flap was returned into position.

TEST MEASURES

All testing occurred in double-walled sound booths with the participant comfortably seated. All test stimuli were from recordings and individually calibrated for the presentation equipment. Study measures were conducted pre-surgery and 3 and 9 months post-surgery.

Localization was measured with a roving-source Consonant-Vowel-Consonant (CNC) word task (Potts et al., 2009; Firszt et al., 2012a). American English Melbourne CNC words (Skinner et al., 2006) were presented randomly from 15 loudspeakers (10° apart and numbered 1–15) along a horizontal plane and 140° arc at 60 dB SPL (±3 dB). Each test administration included 100 words, presented randomly from each of the 10 active loudspeakers with the carrier "Ready". The participant sat approximately three feet in front of the center loudspeaker, was unaware that five loudspeakers were inactive (#2, 4, 8, 12, 14), and was instructed to face the center loudspeaker between each presentation but was allowed head turns during each carrier-word presentation. Head turns were allowed since it more accurately simulates talker localization in conversational settings. After each presentation, the participant repeated the word and indicated the source speaker number. For localization, a root mean square (RMS) error score was calculated as the mean target-response difference, irrespective of error direction. The task was administered twice and scores from each administration averaged.

Sentence understanding in noise was evaluated with the Hearing In Noise Test (HINT; Nilsson et al., 1994) in the *R*-Space (Revit et al., 2002; Compton-Conley et al., 2004). The *R*-Space consists of eight loudspeakers equally spaced in a 360° array with each loudspeaker 24 inches from the center of the participant's head. All loudspeakers presented a recording of diffuse restaurant noise (60 dB SPL), replicating a challenging real-life listening situation. Two 20 sentence lists were administered and an average signal-to-noise ratio (SNR) for 50% accuracy (SNR-50) obtained. Sentences were presented from the front loudspeaker beginning at a +6 dB SNR and adapted to be easier or more difficult based on the participant's responses. An average of the final 17 SNRs resulted in an SNR-50 for each list.

An adaptive speech reception threshold (SRT) psychoacoustic task resulted in speech thresholds for quiet and nine competing noise conditions (modified from the task described in Litovsky (2005) and Johnstone and Litovsky (2006)). SRT determinations were for test spondees (two-syllable words with equal stress on both syllables) spoken by a male talker and always presented from a loudspeaker facing the front of the seated participant. Testing occurred with noise emanating from one of three loudspeakers each placed 1.5 m from the participant: directly in front, 90° to the right, or 90° to the left. There were three noise types: multi-talker babble (MTB) and two types of single-talker noise (a female talker and a male talker each presenting Harvard IEEE sentences). Initial spondee presentations were at 60 dB SPL for each noise type and source location. A four-alternative forced-choice task, without feedback, determined subsequent presentation levels that continued through four reversals using an adaptive paradigm based on participant responses. Noise conditions varied randomly and were tracked independently, resulting in an SRT (average of the last three reversals) for each noise type and loudspeaker location (e.g., front, left, or right for MTB, female talker, and male talker noise).

A psychoacoustic measure determined the random spectrogram sound (RSS) that was most different from two others during each trial. RSS are noise-like stimuli created with independent control of temporal or spectral sound parameters, but with all stimuli based on summation across the same 6-octave bandwidth (250–16000 Hz) and with matching intensity and durations (Schönwiesner et al., 2005; Burton et al., 2012). Spectral RSS differed by dividing the bandwidth into 3–16 spectral bands and changing between bands at a fixed temporal rate of 3 Hz. Temporal RSS differed by changing between three spectral bands at temporal rates between 8 and 30 Hz. Spectral RSS had greater complexity with more spectral bands and temporal RSS were more complex with higher temporal rates. In a three-interval, three-alternative, forced-choice, "odd-man out" paradigm, one of the stimuli, identified as the "target" differed in complexity from two "standard" stimuli. "Standard" sounds always had the same RSS complexity, but differed in constituent random fields or in amplitude modulations. The manipulated variable was minimum detectable changes (JND) in spectral or temporal complexity.

For spectral RSS, the number of spectral regions of the "standard" was 16, while the spectral regions for the "target" varied. The initial "target" had three spectral regions. After three consecutive correct responses, the "target" spectral regions increased with a "step-size" of three until an error occurred. After the first reversal, the "step-size" decreased to two spectral regions, and after three reversals, the "step-size" decreased to one spectral region. For temporal RSS, the temporal rate of the "standard" was 30 Hz, while the temporal rate varied for the "target" stimuli. The initial "target" temporal rate was 8 Hz. After three consecutive correct responses, the "target" temporal rate increased to 14 Hz. The same 6 Hz "step-size" in temporal rate repeated until an error occurred. After the first reversal, the "step-size" decreased to 3 Hz, and after three reversals, the "step-size" decreased to 1 Hz. After eight reversals, the "mean of target" values of the last four reversals provided an estimate of JNDs for spectral or temporal complexity. Feedback was provided for correct responses and each of four test runs concluded with eight reversals. Each of the JNDs for spectral and temporal RSS complexity was an average of the last four reversals.

A questionnaire also evaluated the participant's perception of listening function. The Speech, Spatial and Qualities of Hearing scale (SSQ; Gatehouse and Noble, 2004) probes three listening domains (14–19 questions each). The Speech domain probes speech recognition in a variety of listening environments and a range of talker visibility. The Spatial domain examines awareness of sound direction, distance and movement. In the Qualities domain, respondents indicate sound naturalness, listening effort and the ability to segregate multiple sounds. Each item is ranked on a scale from 0 (least ability) to 10 (most ability). Individual SSQ items are grouped by processing demands to obtain 10 subscale scores (Gatehouse and Akeroyd, 2006; Dwyer et al., 2013), four subscales within the Speech domain, two within the Spatial domain, and four within the Qualities domain.

Previously described protocols (Burton et al., 2012, 2013) were used to perform functional magnetic resonance imaging (fMRI), preprocess the images, and analyze blood oxygen level-dependent (BOLD) responses to auditory stimulation of the unaffected left ear. BOLD responses to RSS stimuli of 2 s duration were recorded at three times: pre-surgery and at 3 and 9 months post-surgery. Presentation times for RSS stimuli varied during 9-s silent intervals in 11-s volume acquisitions, which enabled capture of BOLD at different stimulus delays with respect to the echo-planar images (EPI) in this interrupted single event design (Belin et al., 1999). Subsequent assembly of BOLD amplitudes relative to baseline (% change in response) at stimulus delays from 2 to 9 s prior to the EPI reconstructed an average BOLD response time course. The average was from 24 trials for each stimulus to EPI delay time. Separately for each imaging session, *F*-tests per voxel evaluated whether the variance of evoked BOLD responses was greater than variance due to baseline noise. *F*-statistics were transformed to equally probable *z*-scores (*F-Z*stats). The significance of *F-Z*stats was determined after multiple comparison corrections based on Monte Carlo simulations (Forman et al., 1995) and with a correction threshold of $z = 4.0$ across 12 face-connected voxels and for $p = 0.05$.

The distribution of volume-based *F-Z*stats from each imaging session was superimposed on coronal slices through the patient's brain. Additionally, BOLD response time courses were extracted from regions of interest for peak *F-Z*stats identified with an automated search (Kerr et al., 2004). After registering the *F-Z*stats to the PALS-B12 surface-based atlas (Van Essen, 2005; Van Essen and Dierker, 2007), the activated auditory cortical fields were evaluated as previously described (Burton et al., 2012). Thus, the analyses evaluated activity in core primary auditory (Te1), planum temporale (Te2), and planum polare (Te3).

RESULTS

Figure 1B shows post-surgical audiometric thresholds as a function of frequency. (Results from the 3-month evaluation are shown. Note that the 9-month results were equivalent.) As expected, thresholds for the NH or left ear (blue symbols) were unchanged compared to pre-surgical results. The red line connects post-surgical air-conduction thresholds (obtained with insert earphones having approximately 75–90 dB interaural attenuation). Open circles indicate unmasked thresholds and open triangles indicate thresholds obtained with the unaffected ear masked. Post-surgical bone-conduction thresholds are indicated by red brackets. Air-conduction thresholds in the right ear improved 35–45 dB through the low and mid frequencies and 5–40 dB in the high frequencies. Surgery successfully eliminated the hearing loss conductive component from 0.5–3 kHz and most of the conductive component at 0.25 and 4 kHz.

Figure 2 shows localization results. For each plot, the location of the loudspeaker source (in degrees azimuth) is indicated along the *x*-axis and of the reported loudspeaker along the *y*-axis. Means and standard deviations of reported loudspeakers are plotted for each source loudspeaker location for pre-surgery

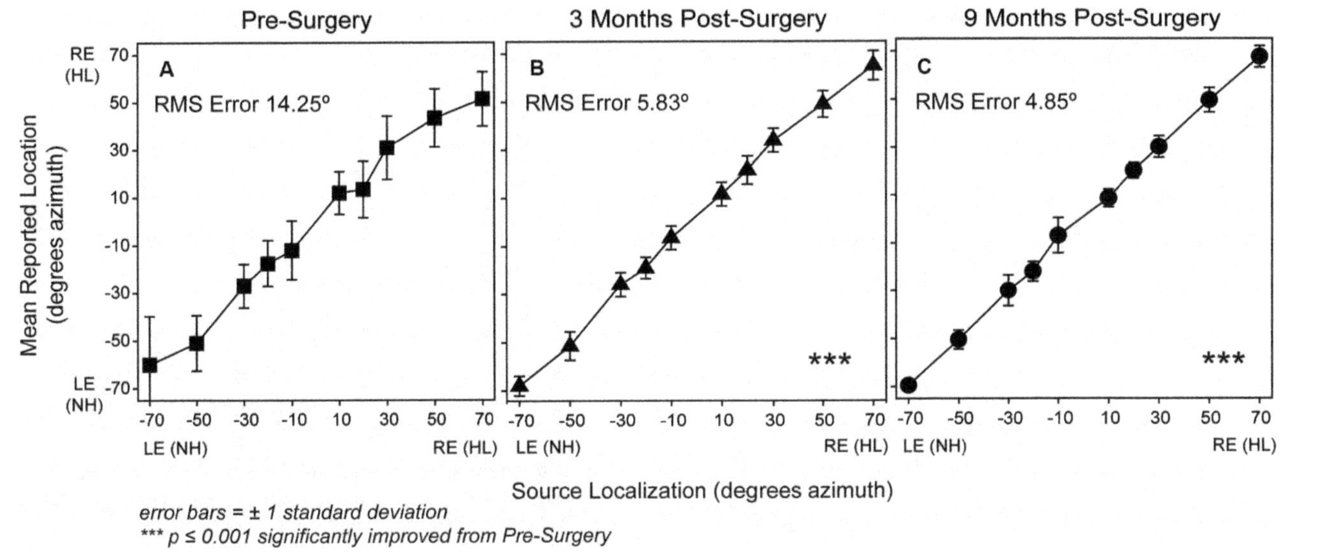

FIGURE 2 | P1's localization responses are plotted for each test interval (Panel A, pre-surgery, square symbols; Panel B, 3 months post-surgery, triangle symbols; Panel C, 9 months post-surgery, circle symbols). The *x*-axis shows the sound-source loudspeaker locations in degrees azimuth that range from −70 degrees toward the NH ear side at axis' left to +70 degrees toward the hearing-impaired ear side at the axis' right. The *y*-axis shows the possible reported response loudspeaker locations in degrees azimuth that range from −70 degrees toward the NH ear side at the bottom of the axis to +70 degrees toward the hearing-impaired ear side at the top of the axis. Symbols indicate mean responses for each active sound-source location and error bars represent ±1 standard deviation. Mean RMS Error in degrees is noted within the plot for each test interval. Asterisks in Panels **B** and **C** indicated significantly improved localization results compared to pre-surgery ($p < 0.001$).

and post-surgery test intervals of 3 and 9 months, respectively in Panels **A** to **C**. Correct identification of all presentations results in a straight diagonal line from the lower left- to the upper right corner. Each panel also includes the RMS error score for that test interval. A robust (Sandwich estimator) regression analysis method (with a Bonferroni adjustment for multiple comparisons) identified a significant effect of test interval [$F(2,594) = 11.97$, $p < 0.003$] and follow-up comparisons indicated significantly improved localization compared to baseline at 3 months [$F(1,549) = 17.26, p < 0.003$] and at 9 months [$F(1,594) = 23.70$, $p < 0.001$]. The improvement at 9 months compared to 3 months was not statistically significant ($p > 0.05$).

Figure 3 displays results for *R*-Space sentence understanding in the presence of restaurant noise. The three test intervals are indicated along the *x*-axis and SNR score along the *y*-axis. Note that for this measure lower scores indicate better performance. Pre-surgery, P1 had 50% accuracy for sentences presented 3.5 dB softer than the surrounding restaurant noise (60 dB SPL). By 9 months post-surgery, P1 was able to understand sentences at even softer levels (4.9 dB softer than the restaurant noise). P1's performance improved (1.4 dB) from pre-surgery to the 9-month test interval. The 95% confidence interval for NH adults and noise from the front is ±1.2 dB (Nilsson et al., 1995).

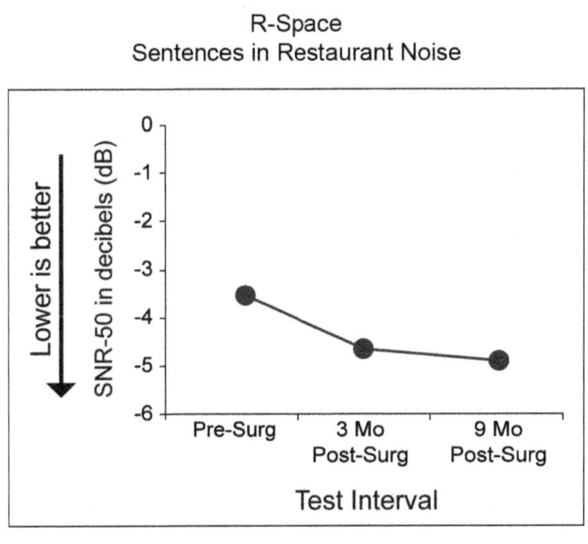

FIGURE 3 | Results of sentence understanding in the R-Space using restaurant noise is shown for the three test intervals (*x*-axis). Black circles indicate P1's SNR-50 scores in dB. Lower SNRs reflect ability to understand sentences in the presence of higher noise levels (e.g., an SNR of −4 dB indicates the restaurant noise was 4 dB louder than the target sentence).

Figure 4 shows performance at the three test intervals for the Adaptive SRT test. A lower score indicates better performance. Panel **A** shows P1's performance in quiet. The softest level that P1 was consistently able to identify target speech from a closed-set of four spondees in quiet did not differ substantially by test interval. Her SRT in quiet ranged from 12.9 dB pre-surgery to 10.3 dB at 3 months post-surgery. This is comparable to performance of a group of 24 NH adults (ages 22–67 years) on this same task (see Figure 6 of Firszt et al., 2012b). Panel **B** shows performance in the presence of the three noise types, female talker (green diamonds), male talker (orange squares) and MTB (purple

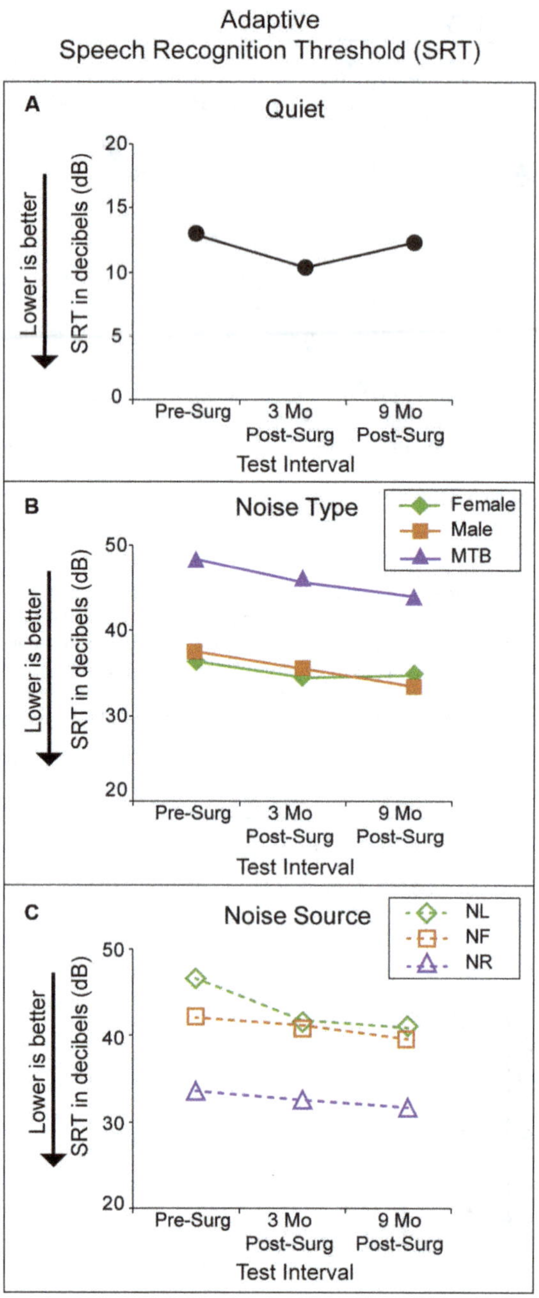

FIGURE 4 | Adaptive SRT scores in dB (*y*-axis) are plotted for each test interval (*x*-axis). Lower SRTs reflect ability to hear speech at softer levels. Panel **A** plots results in quiet (black circles). Panel **B** plots results in noise by noise type (female talker with green diamonds; male talker with orange squares; MTB with purple triangles). Panel **C** plots results in noise by noise source location (noise from the left, or NH ear side with green diamonds; noise from the front with orange squares; noise from the right, or hearing impaired ear side with purple diamonds).

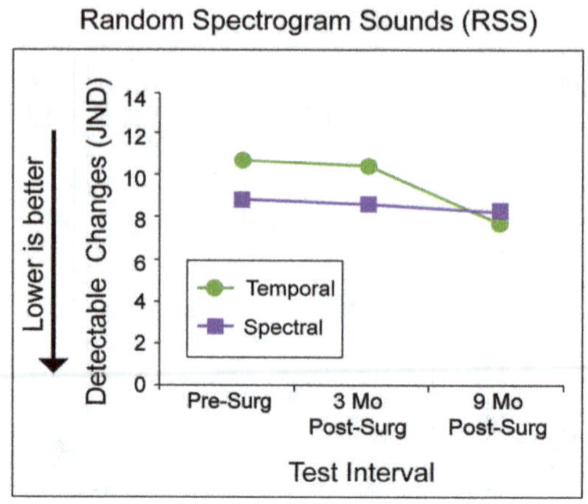

FIGURE 5 | P1's minimum detectable changes (JND; *y*-axis) for temporal (green circles) and spectral complexity (purple squares) are indicated for each test interval (*x*-axis). Lower JNDs reflect better performance.

triangles). Performance was more difficult with MTB than with each single-talker noise type and results were very similar in the presence of female and male talker noise. Performance improved at each successive test interval for each noise type except with female talker noise. Performance with MTB showed the greatest improvement over time (pre-surgery SRT = 48.4 dB, 3-month SRT = 45.6 dB and 9-month SRT = 44.0 dB). Panel **C** shows results by noise location: right side with hearing loss (purple triangles), front (orange squares) and left side with the intact ear (green diamonds). The task was easier with noise from the affected side (right) than noise from the front (orange squares) or from the intact ear side (left). P1's scores for noise from the front were similar to scores for noise from the intact ear side.

Figure 5 shows results from the two psychoacoustic measures with RSS stimuli that differed in spectral or temporal complexity with test interval along the *x*-axis and JND score along the *y*-axis. Performance for detecting differences from a standard of 16 spectral regions in the number of regions (purple squares) included in spectral RSS stimuli (e.g., spectral complexity) was very similar at all three test intervals (JND 8.8 pre-surgery to 8.2 at 9 months). P1's performance detecting differences from a standard temporal rate of 30 Hz in the rates (green circles) of temporal RSS stimuli (e.g., temporal complexity) was similar at pre-surgery (JND 10.8) and at 3 months (JND 10.4). By 9 months P1's JND for RSS temporal complexity differences had improved to 7.8. P1's performance on both tasks is similar to that of a group of 20 NH adults, ages 23–62 years, listening bilaterally across four test runs (**Figure 5**; Firszt et al., 2012b).

Figure 6 shows SSQ questionnaire results describing self-perceived abilities in various listening scenarios by domain and subscale. The rating plots in Panel **A** are from four subscales in the Speech domain: Speech in Quiet (SiQ) as blue circles, Speech in Noise (SiN) as purple triangles, Speech in Speech Contexts (SiSCont) as orange squares, and Multiple Speech Stream Processing and Switching (MultStream) as green diamonds. Mean and SD subscale ratings by a group of 21 NH adults, ages 27–73, were reported by Dwyer et al. (2013). For reference, P1's ratings are compared to that NH group's ratings. P1's SiQ ratings were similar to the NH group's ratings at all three test intervals (9.3 pre-surgery to 10 at 9 months). P1's SiN ratings improved over time (5.1 pre-surgery to 7.3 at

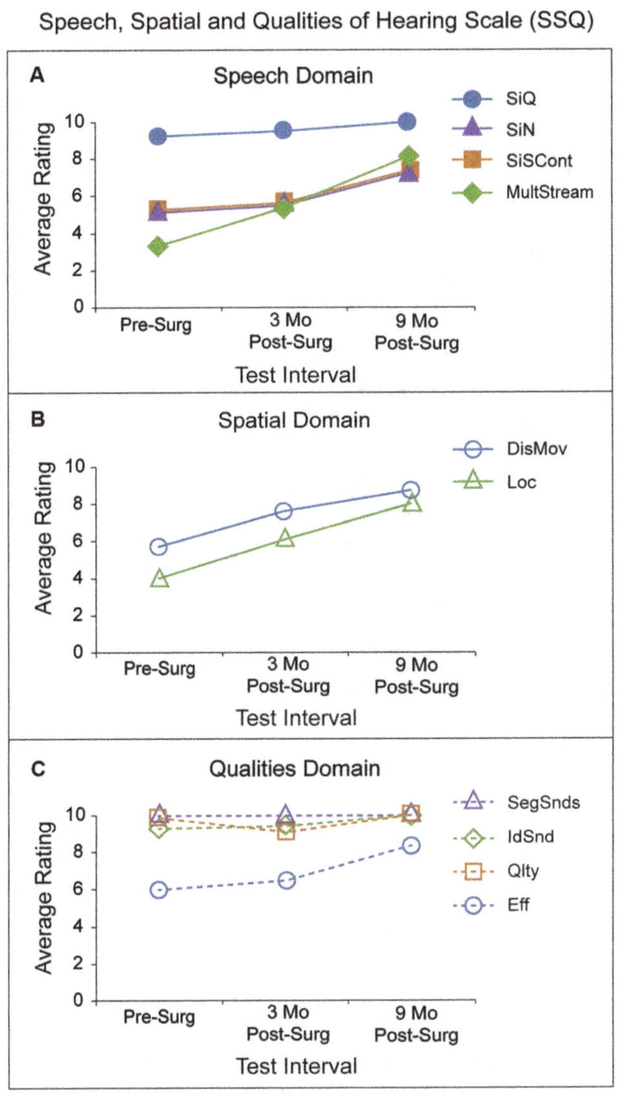

FIGURE 6 | SSQ ratings (*y*-axis) for 10 subscales are divided into three domains and plotted for each test interval (*x*-axis). Panel **A** (Speech Domain) has P1's average ratings for questions assessing four subscale areas: Speech in Quiet (SiQ; blue circles), Speech in Noise (SiN; purple triangles), Speech in Speech Contexts (SiSCont; orange squares), and Multiple Speech Stream Processing and Switching (MultStream; green diamonds). P1's average ratings for questions assessing the two subscales within the Spatial Domain are shown in Panel **B**: Distance and Movement (DisMov; purple circles) and Localization (Loc; green triangles). Average subscale ratings within the Qualities Domain are indicated in Panel **C**: Segregation of Sounds (SegSnds; purple triangles), Identification of Sound and Objects (IdSnd; green diamonds), Sound Quality and Naturalness (Qlty; orange squares) and Listening Effort (Eff; purple circles).

9 months), but were poorer than the NH group. The SiSCont and MultStream ratings improved over time and were similar to the NH group's ratings by 9 months post-surgery (SiSCont 5.3 pre-surgery to 7.4 at 9 months; MultStream 3.3 pre-surgery to 8.2 at 9 months).

The rating plots in Panel **B** are from two subscales in the Spatial domain: Distance and Movement (DisMov) as purple circles and Localization (Loc) as green triangles. P1's ratings for both subscales improved over time and were similar to the NH group ratings by 9 months (DisMov 5.7 pre-surgery to 8.7 at 9 months; Loc 4.0 pre-surgery to 8.0 at 9 months). The rating plots in Panel **C** are from four subscales in the Qualities domain: Segregation of Sounds (SegSnds) as purple triangles, Identification of Sound and Objects (IdSnd) as green diamonds, Sound Quality and Naturalness (Qlty) as orange squares and Listening Effort (Eff) as purple circles. SegSnds, IdSnd and Qlty ratings were all above nine and comparable to the NH group ratings at all three test intervals. Pre-surgery, Eff was poorer than that of the NH group but improved and was similar to that group's ratings by 9 months (6.0 pre-surgery to 8.3 at 9 months). In summary, P1's ratings were poorer than ratings of the NH adults reported by Dwyer et al. (2013) on 6 of 10 subscales prior to surgery. Each of those subscales improved and was more similar to the NH group's ratings by the 9-month test interval except for the SiN subscale.

The top row of **Figure 7** shows an inflated and laterally tilted view of the PALS-B12 atlas that reveals auditory cortex on the superior temporal plane. Drawn onto this plane are cytoarchitectonic borders for three auditory cortical fields (Te1, Te2, and Te3) (Glasser and Van Essen, 2011). The labeled purple spheres (A1, A2, B1 and B2) and comparable locations on the coronal sections indicate the locations of regions of interest strongly activated by the RSS stimuli (i.e., foci with peak *F-Z*stats). The most affected auditory cortical fields were Te1 and Te2. As shown in the left-most column of coronal sections prior to surgery, the extent of significant activation was limited, bilaterally distributed, but slightly more extensive in the left hemisphere (LH), ipsilateral to the stimulated unaffected left ear. The activated zone was larger bilaterally at 3 months post surgery as shown in the middle column of sections. Activity was even more widely distributed by 9 months as shown in the right-most column of sections. Especially prominent at 9 months was a substantial response distribution contralateral to the stimulated left ear that extended over most of the posterior superior temporal plane and spread more than 1 cm from anterior to posterior. The affected contralateral cortex included all Te auditory cortical fields at 9 months post surgery.

The panels in **Figure 8** show response time courses from core (Te1.0 and Te1.1) and posterior belt (Te2) auditory fields. Response amplitudes were largest at 9 months post- surgery, especially in the belt area Te2 ipsilateral to the stimulated left ear and also in the anterior core Te1.0 field, contralateral to the left ear. Amplitudes were more nearly equal bilaterally before and after surgery in the center of primary auditory cortex located in Te1.1 fields of each hemisphere.

DISCUSSION

Corrective surgery for the conductive portion of the hearing loss substantially improved hearing thresholds from 0.25 to 6 kHz. Prior to surgery, P1 could not detect sound in the mid frequencies and perceived loud sounds as soft in the lowest and highest frequencies of the affected right ear. After surgery, air-conduction thresholds were close to P1's bone-conduction thresholds, closing the air-bone gap. Sensorineural threshold levels remained, as expected, and thus hearing levels were essentially in the mild to

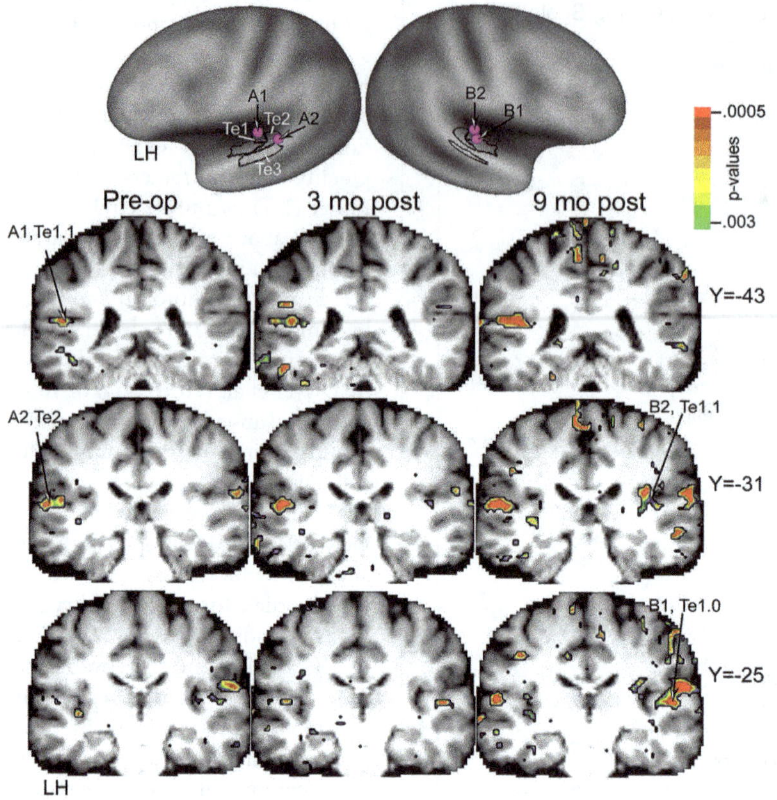

FIGURE 7 | Top row shows superior temporal plane on inflated left and right hemispheres. Black borders indicate the schematic position of auditory cortical fields Te1 to Te3. Labeled purple spheres are placed over cortical surface location of peak *F-Z*stats in activated cortex. Bottom columns of coronal slices through P1's structural brain images at the level of the superior temporal plane coincident with Te1 to Te3 auditory cortex. Left to right columns of identical slices show significantly activated cortex, respectively, at test intervals pre-surgery, 3, and 9 months post-surgery. Sites labeled A1, A2, B1, and B2 indicate corresponding locations on the cortical surface and coronal sections.

moderately-impaired range, reaching 25–35 dB HL at 0.25, 3, 4 and 6 kHz.

Source localization significantly improved following surgery. The largest improvement was between pre-surgery and the 3-month post-surgery test interval with stable performance between the 3 and 9-month test intervals. Wilmington et al. (1994) also showed significant localization improvements pre to post-operatively when measured at 4 and 24 weeks after surgery to correct congenital UCHL in a group of patients' ages 6–33 years; however, only three of the individuals were within the authors' normal confidence interval after hearing correction. Similar to our individual case, there were no significant changes in localization performance over time post-operatively for their study participants; that is between the 4 and 24-week test intervals.

Considering speech recognition in noise, P1's pre-surgical abilities varied by measure as did whether performance improved post-surgery. For example, on the *R*-Space task, P1's ability to understand sentences in the presence of restaurant noise improved between the pre-surgery and 9-month post-surgery test intervals. Noise type and location affected Adaptive SRT results. P1's SRT scores were similar when listening to words in the presence of single talker noise regardless of talker gender. P1's poorest SRTs were in the presence of MTB noise, as were the greatest improvements. With respect to the noise source, it was not surprising that P1 was able to hear the words at softer levels when noise was towards the affected (right) ear, even after surgery, than when the noise was towards the unaffected (left) ear or from the front. These results for the affected and unaffected ear were similar to Wilmington's (1994) results using a speech-in-noise task with low and high context sentences and competing babble (revised SPIN test, Bilger et al., 1984). When noise was toward the atretic ear, the majority of participants were within their NH group's 95% confidence interval, but when noise was toward the NH ear, only three of the 14 participants were within the NH confidence interval. A reported case of corrected long-term UCHL (Anderson, 1985) also had more difficulty understanding speech in speech-shaped noise than 10 NH controls through 5 months post-correction, even at an advantageous SNR (+20 dB). The reduced performance was present for both the affected and unaffected ears. By 14 months post-correction, performance matched that of the NH control group at positive SNRs but continued to be poorer than NH controls at 0 dB SNR, a fairly common SNR in noisy environments.

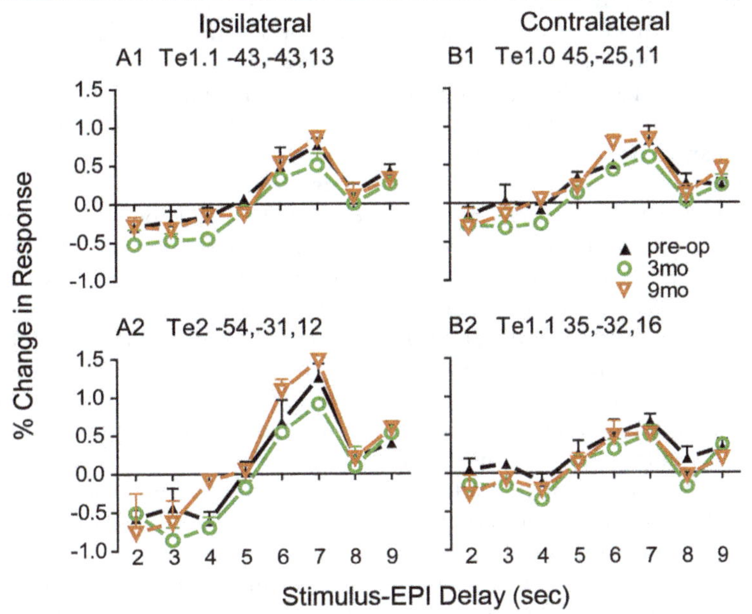

FIGURE 8 | Reconstructed BOLD response time courses based on RSS delays of 2–9 seconds during silent periods immediately before the next volume acquisition. Plotted at each stimulus-EPI delay is the mean and standard error for the per cent change in BOLD amplitude over baseline from trials with no stimulation. BOLD % change response amplitudes extracted from 24 trials per stimulus-EPI delay and averaged across the voxels in spherical ROI with 5 mm radii. A different sphere was centered on the Talairach coordinates listed in each of the four panels. Separately colored connected lines and symbols show time courses for test intervals pre-surgery, 3, and 9 months post-surgery.

For the psychoacoustic task using RSS stimuli, results showed no change in detecting spectral complexity differences after surgical correction of hearing to the right ear. RSS temporal complexity detection did improve at the 9-month test interval, however performance at all test intervals (including pre-operative) was similar to that of NH individuals listening bilaterally (Firszt et al., 2012b). Thus, detection of spectral and temporal cues was not enhanced by unilaterally improved acoustic hearing for this participant. Perhaps this task is less reliant on binaural processing than listening in noise or localizing sound sources. It should be noted that for this task and the speech recognition measures, P1 completed the measures at three test intervals, introducing the possibility of a training effect, whereas the NH group data provided for comparison were from single test sessions.

Results of the SSQ were in general consistent with findings of the behavioral measures. For four of the subscales (SiQ and all of the subscales in the Qualities Domain except Eff), P1's ratings were between 9–10 and similar to ratings of the NH group ($n = 21$) reported by Dwyer et al. (2013). For all other subscales except SiN, ratings were poorer than those of Dwyer's NH group pre-surgery but more similar after 9 months binaural hearing experience. P1 continued to have more difficulty than the NH group, even after 9 months experience with SiN.

The self-assessment results from the SSQ were augmented by comments from P1. According to the participant, 1 week after surgery, all sounds were louder, at times exceptionally loud and even startling; leading to the need to depart from the immediate environment when this occurred and find a location that was quiet. Strategies for dealing with noise that had worked in the past, such as turning the impaired ear towards the noise source, no longer worked and led to confusion. Hearing from behind was a completely new sensation, and also created uncertainty as to where sound was coming from. P1 was involved with music, gave piano and violin lessons, and performed in a band. Sound quality and pitch changes were common during the early post-operative period. It was not always clear "what to make of all this sound".

Three months after surgery, sounds and sources were less confusing, sound was not as loud, and localization and sound quality had improved. P1 reported hearing new sounds that were not previously audible, even though P1 had one NH ear. The ability to hear at greater distances was notable, as was the ability to find and identify sounds in the surroundings without being able to see them. Prior to surgery, P1 often was unaware of a sound until the corresponding source came into view. This changed after surgery, when for example, hearing a person before seeing them was described as something novel. Being in noisy environments was less distracting and the ability to overhear conversation while holding a different conversation was a new experience. P1 commented that while regaining hearing abilities in the right ear, there was a sensation that the left ear (the unaffected ear) was also changing at the same time, and the two ears were "starting to play nice together". The result was hearing in stereo, again a notion that P1 had not realized prior to hearing correction. Finally, P1 reported increased feelings of confidence and reduction of effort to hear and communicate in everyday compared to pre-surgery. When questioned 9 months after surgery, the comments from

P1 were similar to what had been previously reported. Overall, the descriptions mimic a period of over excitation of sound followed by adaptation and shifting to allow both ears to contribute to improved hearing performance using enhanced binaural abilities.

A case study presented by Stange et al. (2001) was of a 62 year old woman with a congenital maximum UCHL who reported hyperacusis (abnormal sensitivity to sound intensity) for more than 2 years following hearing restoration. Both the case reported by Stange et al. (2001) and the current case involved congenital onset and extensive time with UCHL and both reported an increased sensitivity to sound. However in the current case, the sensitivity diminished within the first 3 months following hearing restoration. One possible explanation for the difference may be that P1 continued to have some sensorineural hearing loss after surgery. Prior to surgery, P1 demonstrated a large asymmetry between ears; however hearing thresholds were 50–70 dB HL at 3 kHz and above, providing some high frequency input. Although this hearing was not considered useful based on participant report, some stimulation was present and may have contributed to quicker assimilation of the new auditory information. In this case, extended asymmetry in hearing did not prevent auditory system changes consequent to restored binaural hearing. Also promising was that P1 made significant improvements in binaural abilities despite hearing correction in adulthood at age 41. Gray et al. (2009) reported on combined data from two different studies (participant's age range 6–53 years, mean pre-operative hearing loss about 64 dB) and suggested that after surgery for aural atresia, older (38 years and greater) congenital adults performed more poorly when noise was toward the corrected ear than younger adults. Assessments were made, however, only 1 month after hearing correction and participant ages were not provided.

There was also evidence of neuroplastic reorganization in auditory cortex that especially involved core and belt regions in the current case. The overall extent and amplitudes of contralateral auditory cortex responses increased after hearing recovery, resulting in increased bilateral activation. Vasama et al. (1994) also found enhancements in auditory cortex in six participants with congenital UCHL using magnetoencephalography (MEG). They showed the expected asymmetric larger amplitudes in five patients and shorter latencies in three patients over the hemisphere contralateral to the stimulated NH ear (Vasama et al., 1994). The six patients ranged in age from 7–28 years and had mean hearing threshold levels in the affected ear near 70 dB HL. Only one patient showed larger amplitudes over the ipsilateral hemisphere, a finding similar to reports of cortical responses in patients with profound unilateral sensorineural hearing loss (Khosla et al., 2003; Hanss et al., 2009; Burton et al., 2012, 2013; Maslin et al., 2013). Of note, this individual also had greater hearing loss (about 90 dB HL). A later study compared pre-operative and 2-months post-operative auditory-evoked magnetic fields in seven adults ages 26–51 with UCHL who underwent surgery for otosclerosis or abnormal ossicular chains (Vasama et al., 1998). Duration of hearing loss was 6–14 years and hearing loss in the affected ears was 57 dB HL before surgery and 17 dB afterwards. Based on MEG recordings, all patients showed cortical response changes after surgery and correction of the UCHL. Changes took the form of earlier latencies and increased response strengths contralateral to the stimulated ear, with some ipsilateral changes. Although mean pre-operative values did not differ from NH controls, the post-operative changes differed. This finding parallels that of our present participant, suggesting modification to cortical responses following hearing improvement.

In summary, a re-established balance to binaural activity might explain the trend toward improved performance on measures after the stapedotomy procedure for the studied participant. The SSQ results showed that ratings of the participant's perceived ability were similar to the NH comparison group (Dwyer et al., 2013) by 9 months on all subscales except SiN. It is possible that both the pre-surgery unilateral auditory deprivation and the post-surgery continued asymmetry between ears (due to the sensorineural hearing loss in the affected ear) influenced the speech perception in noise deficits. Persistent sensorineural hearing loss might also explain retained symmetrical activation of auditory cortex as opposed to a normally asymmetrical contralateral activation pattern in NH.

The improvements noted in binaural abilities were clinically promising, because they indicated that auditory system connections could re-activate with elimination of conductive hearing problems despite being physiologically latent well beyond any imagined critical developmental period. Most encouraging was that the restored physiology in native connectivity, even if only partial, had substantial behavioral consequences for the participant. The mechanisms responsible for these changes are unknown. However, they might arise from increased balance to binaural neural firing rates with the reintroduction of crossed inhibition that lead to changes in central gain mechanisms. At the same post-surgery test intervals, the observed enhanced contralateral activity in core and adjacent auditory cortical fields possibly are a manifestation of these changes in central gain. In contrast, sudden sensorineural unilateral hearing loss following surgical resections of acoustic neuromas result in the opposite effect of reduced crossed inhibition from the affected ear together with possible reduced central gain (Burton et al., 2013; Maslin et al., 2013). Together, these results support the need for future research of unilateral auditory deprivation effects and plasticity, with consideration for length of deprivation, age at hearing correction, degree of hearing, and type of hearing loss (conductive versus sensorineural).

ACKNOWLEDGMENTS

The authors acknowledge our participant's time and effort in this study. This work was supported by R01DC009010 from the National Institute on Deafness and Other Communication Disorders.

REFERENCES

Anderson, K. L. (1985). A case study of central processing following long-standing unilateral conductive hearing loss. *J. Aud. Res.* 25, 201–213.

Belin, P., Zatorre, R. J., Hoge, R., Evans, A. C., and Pike, B. (1999). Event-related fMRI of the auditory cortex. *Neuroimage* 10, 417–429. doi: 10.1006/nimg.1999.0480

Bilger, R. C., Nuetzel, J. M., Rabinowitz, W. M., and Rzeczkowski, C. (1984). Standardization of a test of speech perception in noise. *J. Speech Hear. Res.* 27, 32–48.

Burton, H., Firszt, J. B., and Holden, T. (2013). Hearing thresholds and fMRI of auditory cortex following eighth cranial nerve surgery. *Otolaryngol. Head Neck Surg.* 149, 492–499. doi: 10.1177/0194599813495179

Burton, H., Firszt, J. B., Holden, T., Agato, A., and Uchanski, R. M. (2012). Activation lateralization in human core, belt and parabelt auditory fields with unilateral deafness compared to normal hearing. *Brain Res.* 1454, 33–47. doi: 10.1016/j.brainres.2012.02.066

Coleman, J. R., and O'Connor, P. (1979). Effects of monaural and binaural sound deprivation on cell development in the anteroventral cochlear nucleus of rats. *Exp. Neurol.* 64, 553–566. doi: 10.1016/0014-4886(79)90231-0

Compton-Conley, C. L., Neuman, A. C., Killion, M. C., and Levitt, H. (2004). Performance of directional microphones for hearing aids: real-world versus simulation. *J. Am. Acad. Audiol.* 15, 440–455. doi: 10.3766/jaaa.15.6.5

Dwyer, N., Firszt, J. B., and Reeder, R. M. (2013). Effects of unilateral input and mode of hearing in the better ear: self-reported performance using the speech, spatial and qualities of hearing scale. *Ear Hear.* doi: 10.1097/aud.0b013e3182a3648b. [Epub ahead of print].

Firszt, J. B., Holden, L. K., Reeder, R. M., Cowdrey, L., and King, S. (2012a). Cochlear implantation in adults with asymmetric hearing loss. *Ear Hear.* 33, 521–533. doi: 10.1097/aud.0b013e31824b9dfc

Firszt, J. B., Holden, L. K., Reeder, R. M., Waltzman, S., and Arndt, S. (2012b). Auditory abilities after cochlear implantation in adults with unilateral deafness: a pilot study. *Otol. Neurotol.* 33, 1339–1346. doi: 10.1097/mao.0b013e318268d52d

Forman, S. D., Cohen, J. D., Fitzgerald, M., Eddy, W. F., Mintun, M. A., and Noll, D. C. (1995). Improved assessment of significant activation in functional magnetic resonance imaging (fMRI): use of a cluster-size threshold. *Magn. Reson. Med.* 33, 636–647. doi: 10.1002/mrm.1910330508

Gatehouse, S., and Akeroyd, M. (2006). Two-eared listening in dynamic situations. *Int. J. Audiol.* 45(Suppl. 1), 120–124. doi: 10.1080/14992020600783103

Gatehouse, S., and Noble, W. (2004). The speech, spatial and qualities of hearing scale (SSQ). *Int. J. Audiol.* 43, 85–99. doi: 10.1080/14992020400050014

Glasser, M. F., and Van Essen, D. C. (2011). Mapping human cortical areas in vivo based on myelin content as revealed by T1- and T2-weighted MRI. *J. Neurosci.* 31, 11597–11616. doi: 10.1523/jneurosci.2180-11.2011

Gray, L., Kesser, B., and Cole, E. (2009). Understanding speech in noise after correction of congenital unilateral aural atresia: effects of age in the emergence of binaural squelch but not in use of head-shadow. *Int. J. Pediatr. Otorhinolaryngol.* 73, 1281–1287. doi: 10.1016/j.ijporl.2009.05.024

Hall, J. W. 3rd, and Derlacki, E. L. (1986). Effect of conductive hearing loss and middle ear surgery on binaural hearing. *Ann. Otol. Rhinol. Laryngol.* 95, 525–530.

Hall, J. W. 3rd, and Derlacki, E. L. (1988). Binaural hearing after middle ear surgery. Masking-level difference for interaural time and amplitude cues. *Audiology* 27, 89–98. doi: 10.3109/00206098809081579

Hall, J. W. 3rd, and Grose, J. H. (1993). Short-term and long-term effects on the masking level difference following middle ear surgery. *J. Am. Acad. Audiol.* 4, 307–312.

Hall, J. W. 3rd, Grose, J. H., and Pillsbury, H. C. (1990). Predicting binaural hearing after stapedectomy from presurgery results. *Arch. Otolaryngol. Head Neck Surg.* 116, 946–950. doi: 10.1001/archotol.1990.01870080068018

Hanss, J., Veuillet, E., Adjout, K., Besle, J., Collet, L., and Thai-Van, H. (2009). The effect of long-term unilateral deafness on the activation pattern in the auditory cortices of French-native speakers: influence of deafness side. *BMC Neurosci.* 10:23. doi: 10.1186/1471-2202-10-23

Hausler, R., Colburn, S., and Marr, E. (1983). Sound localization in subjects with impaired hearing. Spatial-discrimination and interaural-discrimination tests. *Acta Otolaryngol. Suppl.* 400, 1–62. doi: 10.3109/00016488309105590

Hubel, D. H., and Wiesel, T. N. (1970). The period of susceptibility to the physiological effects of unilateral eye closure in kittens. *J. Physiol.* 206, 419–436.

Johnstone, P. M., and Litovsky, R. Y. (2006). Effect of masker type and age on speech intelligibility and spatial release from masking in children and adults. *J. Acoust. Soc. Am.* 120, 2177–2189. doi: 10.1121/1.2225416

Kerr, D. L., Gusnard, D. A., Snyder, A. Z., and Raichle, M. E. (2004). Effect of practice on reading performance and brain function. *Neuroreport* 15, 607–610. doi: 10.1097/00001756-200403220-00007

Khosla, D., Ponton, C. W., Eggermont, J. J., Kwong, B., Don, M., and Vasama, J. P. (2003). Differential ear effects of profound unilateral deafness on the adult human central auditory system. *J. Assoc. Res. Otolaryngol.* 4, 235–249. doi: 10.1007/s10162-002-3014-x

Knudsen, E. I., Esterly, S. D., and Knudsen, P. F. (1984a). Monaural occlusion alters sound localization during a sensitive period in the barn owl. *J. Neurosci.* 4, 1001–1011.

Knudsen, E. I., Knudsen, P. F., and Esterly, S. D. (1984b). A critical period for the recovery of sound localization accuracy following monaural occlusion in the barn owl. *J. Neurosci.* 4, 1012–1020.

Litovsky, R. Y. (2005). Speech intelligibility and spatial release from masking in young children. *J. Acoust. Soc. Am.* 117, 3091–3099. doi: 10.1121/1.1873913

Maslin, M. R. D., Munro, K. J., and El-Deredy, W. (2013). Evidence for multiple mechanisms of cortical plasticity: a study of humans with late-onset profound unilateral deafness. *Clin. Neurophysiol.* 124, 1414–1421. doi: 10.1016/j.clinph.2012.12.052

Moore, D. R., and Irvine, D. R. F. (1981). Plasticity of binaural interaction in the cat inferior colliculus. *Brain Res.* 208, 198–202. doi: 10.1016/0006-8993(81)90632-6

Nilsson, M., Soli, S. D., and Sullivan, J. A. (1994). Development of the hearing in noise test for the measurement of speech reception thresholds in quiet and in noise. *J. Acoust. Soc. Am.* 95, 1085–1099. doi: 10.1121/1.408469

Nilsson, M., Soli, S. D., and Sumida, A. (1995). *Development of Norms and Percent Intelligibility Functions for the Hint.* Los Angeles: House Ear Institute.

Potts, L. G., Skinner, M. W., Litovsky, R. A., Strube, M. J., and Kuk, F. (2009). Recognition and localization of speech by adult cochlear implant recipients wearing a digital hearing aid in the nonimplanted ear (bimodal hearing). *J. Am. Acad. Audiol.* 20, 353–373. doi: 10.3766/jaaa.20.6.4

Priwin, C., Jonsson, R., Magnusson, L., Hultcrantz, M., and Granstrom, G. (2007). Audiological evaluation and self-assessed hearing problems in subjects with single-sided congenital external ear malformations and associated conductive hearing loss. *Int. J. Audiol.* 46, 162–171. doi: 10.1080/14992020601077984

Revit, L. J., Schulein, R. B., and Julsrom, S. D. (2002). Toward accurate assessment of real-world hearing aid benefit. *Hear. Rev.* 9, 34–38, 51.

Schönwiesner, M., Rubsamen, R., and Von Cramon, D. Y. (2005). Hemispheric asymmetry for spectral and temporal processing in the human antero-lateral auditory belt cortex. *Eur. J. Neurosci.* 22, 1521–1528. doi: 10.1111/j.1460-9568.2005.04315.x

Silverman, M. S., and Clopton, B. M. (1977). Plasticity of binaural interaction. I. Effect of early auditory deprivation. *J. Neurophysiol.* 40, 1266–1274.

Skinner, M. W., Holden, L. K., Fourakis, M. S., Hawks, J. W., Holden, T., Arcaroli, J., et al. (2006). Evaluation of equivalency in two recordings of monosyllabic words. *J. Am. Acad. Audiol.* 17, 350–366. doi: 10.3766/jaaa.17.5.5

Stange, T., Mir-Salim, P. A., and Berghaus, A. (2001). Hyperacusis after tympanoplasty. *HNO* 49, 303–306. doi: 10.1007/s001060050750

Tucci, D. L., Cant, N. B., and Durham, D. (2001). Effects of conductive hearing loss on gerbil central auditory system activity in silence. *Hear. Res.* 155, 124–132. doi: 10.1016/s0378-5955(01)00256-8

Van Essen, D. C. (2005). A population-average, landmark- and surface-based (PALS) atlas of human cerebral cortex. *Neuroimage* 28, 635–662. doi: 10.1016/j.neuroimage.2005.06.058

Van Essen, D. C., and Dierker, D. L. (2007). Surface-based and probabilistic atlases of primate cerebral cortex. *Neuron* 56, 209–225. doi: 10.1016/j.neuron.2007.10.015

Vasama, J. P., Mäkelä, J. P., Parkkonen, L., and Hari, R. (1994). Auditory cortical responses in humans with congenital unilateral conductive hearing loss. *Hear. Res.* 78, 91–97. doi: 10.1016/0378-5955(94)90047-7

Vasama, J. P., Mäkelä, J. P., and Ramsay, H. A. (1998). Modification of auditory pathway functions in patients with hearing improvement after middle ear surgery. *Otolaryngol. Head Neck Surg.* 119, 125–130. doi: 10.1016/s0194-5998(98)70183-4

Wilmington, D., Gray, L., and Jahrsdoerfer, R. (1994). Binaural processing after corrected congenital unilateral conductive hearing loss. *Hear. Res.* 74, 99–114. doi: 10.1016/0378-5955(94)90179-1

10

The effect of mild-to-moderate hearing loss on auditory and emotion processing networks

Fatima T. Husain[1,2,3]*, *Jake R. Carpenter-Thompson*[2,3] and *Sara A. Schmidt*[2,3]

[1] Department of Speech and Hearing Science, University of Illinois at Urbana-Champaign, Champaign, IL, USA
[2] The Neuroscience Program, University of Illinois at Urbana-Champaign, Champaign, IL, USA
[3] Beckman Institute for Advanced Science and Technology, University of Illinois at Urbana-Champaign, Champaign, IL, USA

Correspondence:
Fatima T. Husain, Department of Speech and Hearing Science, University of Illinois at Urbana-Champaign, 901 S. Sixth Street, Champaign, IL 61820, USA
e-mail: husainf@illinois.edu

We investigated the impact of hearing loss (HL) on emotional processing using task- and rest-based functional magnetic resonance imaging. Two age-matched groups of middle-aged participants were recruited: one with bilateral high-frequency HL and a control group with normal hearing (NH). During the task-based portion of the experiment, participants were instructed to rate affective stimuli from the International Affective Digital Sounds (IADS) database as pleasant, unpleasant, or neutral. In the resting state experiment, participants were told to fixate on a "+" sign on a screen for 5 min. The results of both the task-based and resting state studies suggest that NH and HL patients differ in their emotional response. Specifically, in the task-based study, we found slower response to affective but not neutral sounds by the HL group compared to the NH group. This was reflected in the brain activation patterns, with the NH group employing the expected limbic and auditory regions including the left amygdala, left parahippocampus, right middle temporal gyrus and left superior temporal gyrus to a greater extent in processing affective stimuli when compared to the HL group. In the resting state study, we observed no significant differences in connectivity of the auditory network between the groups. In the dorsal attention network (DAN), HL patients exhibited decreased connectivity between seed regions and left insula and left postcentral gyrus compared to controls. The default mode network (DMN) was also altered, showing increased connectivity between seeds and left middle frontal gyrus in the HL group. Further targeted analysis revealed increased intrinsic connectivity between the right middle temporal gyrus and the right precentral gyrus. The results from both studies suggest neuronal reorganization as a consequence of HL, most notably in networks responding to emotional sounds.

Keywords: fMRI, hearing loss, resting-state fMRI, functional connectivity, emotion, IADS

INTRODUCTION

Hearing loss (HL) remains one of the most common chronic conditions affecting older adults (Cruickshanks et al., 1998), with the prevalence rate increasing from between 25 and 40% in adults above 65 years of age to greater than 80% in people older than 85 years (Yueh et al., 2003). In general, mild-to-moderately severe sensorineural HL, which is often untreated, affects about 23–33% of the adult population in the world (Stevens et al., 2013). HL has a significant impact on quality of life and general well-being of an older adult (Mulrow et al., 1990; Carabellese et al., 1993) and may be associated with depression and isolation, especially in those younger than 70 years of age (Gopinath et al., 2009). However, little is known about the consequences of mild-to-moderately severe HL on the neural architecture and functionality of the brain.

The majority of brain imaging studies that have explored HL have done so when HL has occurred in conjunction with tinnitus (e.g., Weisz et al., 2004; Husain et al., 2011b), other disorders (e.g., Yoneda et al., 2012) or in the context of sign language studies when the impairment has been profound (e.g., Petitto et al., 2000; Husain et al., 2009). A few brain imaging studies have investigated the impact of HL on aging (Wong et al., 2010; Peelle et al., 2011); these remain the best sources to understand the neural correlates of HL. These neural correlates are manifested in decrease in gray matter in the frontal cortex (Wong et al., 2010; Peelle et al., 2011) and a decreased response in the superior temporal cortex, thalamus and brainstem in a speech comprehension task (Peelle et al., 2011). Our previous structural MRI study of HL in older adults (conducted as part of a larger study to investigate neural bases of tinnitus and HL) observed gray matter loss in the frontal cortices and disordered white matter tracts leading into and out of the auditory cortex (Husain et al., 2011a). A companion functional study noted increased response of the regions in the frontal and parietal cortices, possibly which related to increased attention processing (Husain et al., 2011b). In the latter fMRI study, participants had mild-to-moderately severe HL with an average age in the mid-fifties and were asked to perform a discrimination task with simple tones and tonal sweeps. When compared to rest trials, task trials resulted in greater response in the temporal, frontal and parietal cortices in the HL group relative to the normal hearing (NH) controls.

In the present study, we investigated the neural correlates of mild-to-moderate sensorineural HL in middle-aged adults without tinnitus or any other chronic physical or mental condition and compared them to age-matched NH controls. We concentrated on extra-auditory networks, specifically the one concerned with emotional processing. The limbic system is typically the main network of emotion processing. It consists primarily of the amygdala, parahippocampus, ventral medial prefrontal cortex, nucleus accumbens, and insula. Recently, studies have begun to map out the regions and connectivity of the auditory emotional network in adults with NH (Blood and Zatorre, 2001; Koelsch et al., 2006; Kumar et al., 2012) and in those with tinnitus (Giraud et al., 1999; Mirz et al., 2000; Seydell-Greenwald et al., 2012; Golm et al., 2013). Using dynamic causal modeling, Kumar et al. (2012) found that the negative valence of a sound modulates the backward connections from the amygdala to the auditory cortex, and the acoustic features of a sound modulate the forward connections from the auditory cortex to the amygdala. It is likely that such acoustic features, processing nodes and their connectivity may be susceptible to changes due to sustained loss of hearing acuity when listening to affective sounds. This may result in delayed processing or misclassification or both of the affective sounds. One of the goals of the present study was to investigate whether loss of hearing acuity affects the acoustic processing of affective sounds and whether this impacts their perception.

HL may also affect the perception of the valence of affective sounds, regardless of the processing of acoustic features. Tinnitus, in particular, has been established to have an altered auditory-limbic system link (Jastreboff, 1990; Rauschecker et al., 2010); behaviorally, there is greater prevalence of depression and anxiety in the tinnitus patient group compared to the general population (Bartels et al., 2008). Not surprisingly then, this disordered link is beginning to be studied in tinnitus. However, HL occurs in about 90% of the individuals with tinnitus (Davis and Rafaie, 2000), and the unique contribution of tinnitus to any changes in emotional processing is unknown. There are other reasons to study emotional processing in HL. As previously noted, prevalence of HL increases with age (Yueh et al., 2003) and may contribute to social isolation (Gopinath et al., 2009). This in turn may impact the emotion processing limbic network, as it has been shown to occur with aging and with tinnitus (Mather and Knight, 2005; Rauschecker et al., 2010; St Jacques et al., 2010; Anticevic et al., 2012). Nevertheless, no brain imaging study has explicitly investigated the emotion processing network in older adults with HL.

We conducted both a task-based and a resting state functional connectivity study of the emotion processing network in middle-aged adults with bilateral sensorineural HL. The task consisted of classification of sounds as being "pleasant," "unpleasant," or "neutral." Our working hypothesis was that a loss of hearing acuity affects behavior, sounds may appear more unpleasant (Franks, 1982; Feldmann and Kumpf, 1988; Leek et al., 2008; Rutledge, 2009; Uys et al., 2012), reaction times may be longer due to effortful listening (Hicks and Tharpe, 2002; Tun et al., 2009). Likewise, the neural network subserving emotion processing may be affected, specifically in the response patterns of the nodes. In order to assess the impact of HL on a baseline, resting state, without the distraction of any task, we measured the functional connectivity of a number of networks, including that connected to the amygdala (a primary node of the limbic system).

Our main focus was on auditory and limbic systems, but these systems interact with intrinsic networks devoted to attention processing and possibly the default mode network (DMN). Intrinsic networks, or resting state networks, are defined as spontaneous, low-frequency oscillations in brain activity that can be organized into coherent networks. In many cases, intrinsic networks mirror task-related networks. For example, the auditory resting state network closely resembles an auditory task network. However, instead of correlations between activated regions in the task-based network, the intrinsic network shows correlations between deactivated brain regions. The DMN is the quintessential resting state network and is unique in that it exhibits deactivation in a task-based state and is active during rest (Raichle et al., 2001). The DMN exhibits a push-pull type of relationship with other networks in the brain (Fox et al., 2005). The dorsal attention network (DAN), for instance, will show activations while the DMN is deactivated (in a task-based state). Its relationship with the DAN and other intrinsic networks warrants study of the DMN. Many disorders, including Alzheimer's disease, schizophrenia, and tinnitus, have been shown to affect the connectivity of the DMN (for reviews see, Greicius, 2008; Husain and Schmidt, 2013). It is also possible that intrinsic connectivity may differ in patients with HL, perhaps relating in particular to limbic areas. Alterations to resting state functional connectivity may result in decreased preparedness to perform a task. In particular, if limbic areas are shown to display irregular connectivity to other brain regions at rest, it may change how individuals process emotional stimuli.

Although we had provisional hypotheses, our study was exploratory because of a lack of brain imaging studies investigating the impact of HL on emotion processing and related extra-auditory networks. In the resting state portion of our study, general hypotheses were made regarding which networks may show altered connectivity, but we did not specify the nodes and the nature of these alterations. We had more constrained expectations about the role of amygdala and auditory processing areas in the emotion-task study, in that we expected reduced engagement of such regions in listeners with HL when processing affective stimuli. In sum, we conducted a comprehensive study, combining both task- and rest-based fMRI using multiple seed regions in order to establish a baseline for future studies.

METHODS

SUBJECTS

Participants were recruited from the Urbana-Champaign area, were scanned under the UIUC IRB 10144 protocol, gave written informed consent, and were monetarily compensated. Subjects belonged to one of two groups: middle-aged adults with bilateral high-frequency sensorineural HL ($n = 12$), or their age- and gender-matched controls with NH ($n = 15$). Three NH subjects were excluded due to excessive motion artifact, and data from only 12 NH participants were included in the final analysis. During recruitment, we excluded subjects that presented with tinnitus or with asymmetric HL at the time of their audiological examination. We defined asymmetric HL to be more than a 15 dB

HL difference between the right and left ear at one or more frequencies, or if the right and left ear differed by 10dB HL at two consecutive frequencies. The Beck Depression Inventory (BDI-II) and the Beck Anxiety Inventory (BAI) were used to assess depression and anxiety levels (Beck and Steer, 1984; Steer et al., 1993, 1999). All subjects scored in the minimal depression range and minimal anxiety range for the BDI-II and BAI, respectively. See **Table 1** for information about subject demographics.

AUDIOMETRIC EVALUATION

A comprehensive audiometric evaluation was performed for each subject. Audiological testing took place inside a sound-attenuating booth and included pure tone testing, word recognition testing, and bone conduction testing. Additional tests included distortion product otoacoustic emissions and tympanometry measurements to eliminate any confounding peripheral hearing pathologies. For pure tone testing, the test frequencies included 0.25, 0.5, 1, 2, 4, 6, and 8 kHz. For all of the test frequencies, each subject in the NH group had pure-tone thresholds of 25dB HL or lower. Participants in the HL group had a pure-tone threshold of 30 dB HL or lower for the test frequencies 0.25–2 kHz, with the exception of two HL subjects who had a slightly elevated threshold of 35 dB HL at 1 kHz. For the test frequencies 4–8 kHz, the HL subjects had pure-tone thresholds between 30 and 70 dB HL, ranging from mild to moderately-severe HL. **Table 1** contains information about the average hearing at testing frequencies for each subject group. None of the HL participants relied on aided hearing.

DATA ACQUISITION

A 3Tesla Siemens Magnetom Allegra head-only scanner was used to acquire all MRI images. A series of two anatomical and two functional images were acquired- the first functional scan was of the emotional task and the second acquired data on resting state; order of acquisition varied across the subjects. Thirty-two low-resolution T2-weighted structural transversal slices ($TR = 7260$ ms, $TE = 98$ ms) were collected for each volume with a 4.0 mm slice thickness and a $0.9 \times 0.9 \times 4.0\,\text{mm}^3$ voxel size [matrix size (per slice), 256×256; flip angle, 150°]. We obtained 160 high resolution magnetization-prepared rapid-acquisition with gradient echo (MPRAGE) sagittal slices for each volume that were 1.2 mm in thickness with a $1.0 \times 1.0 \times 1.2\,\text{mm}^3$ voxel size [$TR = 2300$ ms; $TE = 2.83$ ms; matrix size (per slice), 256×256; flip angle, 9°]. The functional images were acquired using the following parameters: slice thickness, 4 mm; inter-slice gap, 0.4 mm; 32 axial or transverse slices, distance factor, 10%; voxel size, $3.4 \times 3.4 \times 4.0\,\text{mm}^3$; field of view (FoV) read, 220 mm; TR, 9000 ms with 2000 ms acquisition time; TE, 30 ms; matrix size (per slice), 64×64; flip angle, 90°. Functional images were acquired separately for (a) an emotional task and (b) a resting state study.

Table 1 | Subject demographics and clinical characteristics for the subject groups.

Group	NH (Normal hearing)		HL (Hearing loss)	
Group size	12		12	
Age(M ± *SD*)	51.4 ± 9.9		58.2 ± 9.5	
Gender	6 males, 6 females		5 males, 7 females	
BAI(M ± *SD*)	1.25 ± 1.3		2.3 ± 1.7	
BDI-II(M ± *SD*)	1.7 ± 2.3		4.3 ± 4.1	
Average hearing threshold (dB HL, right column) at different testing frequencies (left column) (M ± *SD*)	0.5 kHz	13.5 ± 8.8	0.5 kHz	15.0 ± 8.7
	1 kHz	11.6 ± 7.7	1 kHz	16.7 ± 10.2
	2 kHz	11.0 ± 8.0	2 kHz	24.0 ± 18.7
	4 kHz	14.0 ± 8.1	4 kHz	36.2 ± 19.6
	6 kHz	8.4 ± 9.6	6 kHz	41.1 ± 17.8
	8 kHz	12.1 ± 8.5	8 kHz	47.1 ± 18.7

Pure tone audiogram information at each frequency is averaged across both ears and all subjects. BDI, Beck Depression Inventory; BAI, Beck Anxiety Inventory.

(a) Emotion task

To mitigate the loud noise of the radio frequency gradients generated during image acquisition from interfering with the perception of the stimuli, we used clustered echo-planar imaging (EPI) (Hall et al., 1999; Gaab et al., 2003; Zaehle et al., 2004). Clustered EPI, or sparse sampling, was chosen particularly to improve the listening environment for the subjects with HL. To reduce scanner noise interference with sound perception, we collected one image volume (2 s acquisition time) post stimulus presentation rather than using continuous image acquisition during a period of "relative quiet" when the radio-frequency gradients were switched off and the only source of ambient noise was the scanner pump. The repetition time was 9 s, and within each trial a 6 s stimulus was presented during a 7 s interval of reduced scanner noise. To optimize the scanning procedure to detect neural response from regions within the limbic system, prior to data acquisition, a custom MATLAB (http://www.mathworks.com/products/matlab/) toolbox was used in order to fine-tune the timing of stimulus presentation relative to image acquisition (Dolcos and McCarthy, 2006). Stimuli were selected from the International Affective Digital Sounds (IADS) database and had normative scores for valence and arousal; sounds were rated on a scale of 1–9 (9 very pleasant, 1 very unpleasant for valence and 9 very arousing, 1 not at all arousing for arousal) (Bradley and Lang, 2007). Normative scores were as follows: pleasant (valence: 6.83 ± 0.54, arousal: 6.46 ± 0.56), unpleasant (valence: 2.78 ± 0.58, arousal: 6.9 ± 0.31) and neutral (valence: 4.81 ± 0.43, arousal: 4.85 ± 0.57). The normative valence ratings for P and U sounds are statistically different at $p < 0.00001$, but did not differ in arousal scores. **Supplementary Table 1** contains a complete list of the affective sounds used in the present study. We presented the sounds in the scanner at a maximum comfort level, as indicated by each participant, during the relatively quiet intervals of image acquisition. Prior to data collection, subjects were given both written and verbal instructions. Additionally, subjects were trained using sounds from the IADS database, different from the stimuli chosen in the experiment, to familiarize the participants with the task. During the final experiment, Presentation 14.7 software (www.neurobs.com) on a Windows

XP computer in the fMRI control room was used to deliver sounds and instructions via pneumonic headphones (Resonance Technology, Inc., Northridge, CA.). To complete the task, subjects listened to 90 affective sounds [30 pleasant (P), 30 neutral (N), 30 unpleasant (U)], each 6 s in duration and were instructed to rate the sound as P, N, or U as soon as they felt confident in their rating.

(b) Resting state

To acquire information about the resting state, continuous scanning instead of clustered image acquisition was employed. During the resting scan, which was continuous and lasted approximately 5 min, subjects were instructed to lie still and to look at a fixation cross for the scan duration. One hundred and fifty volumes were collected for each subject. The first four images were discarded prior to preprocessing, leaving 146 volumes for analysis.

PREPROCESSING

Pre-processing was similar for both types of functional scans. Statistical Parametric Mapping 8 (SPM, Welcome Trust Centre for Neuroimaging, http://www.fil.ion.ucl.ac.uk/spm/software/spm8/) software was used to analyze the functional imaging data. The images were first realigned using a rigid body transformation to control for head motion. Next, the low resolution Axial T2 (AxT2) image was registered to the mean fMRI image generated during the first step. The high resolution MPRAGE image was then registered to the AxT2 image. To normalize the functional images to MNI space, the MPRAGE was normalized to match a standard T1 MNI template. The normalized images were then smoothed using a Gaussian kernel of $8 \times 8 \times 8\ mm^3$ full width at half-maximum. To account for artifacts created by head motion, data from 3 NH subjects who displayed excessive motion (defined as at or above ± 1.5 mm translation and $\pm\ 1.5°$ rotation in any direction) were not included for further analysis. We also included regressors of motion as covariates of no-interest in the general linear models created in the different statistical analyses, in order to (partially) remove motion-related artifacts. Further, *t*-tests of root-mean-square estimates of both rotational and translational movement showed that there was no statistical significant difference between the two groups (translational motion mean $\pm$ standard deviation): NH (0.63 ± 0.28); HL (0.67 ± 0.23); rotational motion: NH (0.01 ± 0.005), HL (0.01 ± 0.004).

DATA ANALYSIS

(a) Emotion task

Behavioral data were obtained in the scanner during fMRI data acquisition. We collected individual subject ratings of each sound as P, N, or U along with reaction times. Subject ratings and reaction times were analyzed using separate Two-Way ANOVA tests in SPSS ver. 20 software (statistical package for social sciences, IBM, http://www-01.ibm.com/software/analytics/spss/). Group (NH, HL) and condition (P, N, U) were set as independent fixed factors in a general linear model within SPSS, and significance was set at $p < 0.05$.

For data analysis, trials were coded based upon each individual's subjective rating of the affective sounds. We chose to employ the individual ratings to classify trials as "P," "N," or "U," rather than the norms reported in IADS. Either using the IADS classification or individual rating to analyze data are valid methods of classifying the individual trials for further analysis. The trend in affective neuroscience literature is to move away from the normative classification to the individual classification, particularly when examining special populations where it is expected that emotional responses are altered (e.g., older adults or patient population) (St Jacques et al., 2010). It should be noted that the ratings reported with the IADS were obtained from younger adults with NH (Bradley and Lang, 2007). In the present study, the subject population was older with mean age of 51.4 ± 9.9 for NH adults and 58.2 ± 9.5 for those with HL. Therefore, individual ratings were used rather than the norms for classifying the trials obtained during fMRI scanning. First level fixed effects analysis was performed on each subject's smoothed images to generate P > N and U > N contrast images. Motion parameters were included in the first level model as covariates of no-interest. The contrast images were then included in the flexible factorial analysis and *post-hoc* two-sample *t*-tests at the second level. The P + U > N contrast was computed by performing a *t*-test on the condition vectors for each group separately in the flexible factorial model. The three factor design included group, subject and condition. Group was assumed to be independent and have unequal variance, subject was assumed to be independent and possess equal variance, and condition was assumed to be a dependent factor and to have equal variance. To directly compare the NH and HL groups, we conducted *post-hoc* two-sample *t*-tests within the flexible factorial model. Additionally, we performed a region-of-interest (ROI) analysis using the Wake Forest University (WFU) pickatlas toolbox (http://www.fmri.wfubmc.edu) within SPM8, with regions defined anatomically based on the human MNI atlas within the toolbox. Based on our *a priori* hypothesis about the involvement of auditory and limbic regions in affective sound processing, we created a single anatomically-defined mask via selecting regions including the amygdala, insula, parahippocampus, nucleus accumbens, ventral medial prefrontal cortex, inferior colliculus, medial geniculate body and primary auditory cortex (Brodmann areas 42, 41, 22). ROI analysis was performed on the NH (P + U > N), HL (P + U > N), and between group contrasts, and small volume correction (SVC) was employed. All clusters identified in the results were reported using a significance level set at $p < 0.025$ FWE at either the voxel or cluster level (threshold halved from the standard $p < 0.05$ to account for a two-tailed *t*-test).

(b) Resting state

Preprocessing of the resting state data began with slice time correction for the interleaved, ascending data collection. Following that, the same preprocessing steps used for the emotion task were applied. The Functional Connectivity Toolbox (Conn) (Whitfield-Gabrieli and Nieto-Castanon, 2012) for MATLAB was used for data analysis. The smoothed fMRI data was band-pass filtered from 0.008 to 0.08 kHz. The average BOLD timeseries of the segmented white matter and cerebrospinal fluid as well as the realignment/motion parameters generated during preprocessing were regressed out of the data. Then, seed-to-voxel analysis was performed to analyze the auditory resting state network, the

DMN, and the DAN. Connectivity was assessed using pairs of seed regions for both the DMN and auditory networks; correlations between each seed and the whole brain were measured and averaged across seed pairs. Seed locations are listed in **Table 2**. For the auditory network, seeds were located in the bilateral primary auditory cortices. For the DMN, they were located in the medial prefrontal cortex and the posterior cingulate cortex. The DAN was examined using four seeds in the left and right posterior intraparietal sulci and the left and right frontal eye fields (Burton et al., 2012). All seeds were created using Marsbar (Brett et al., 2002) and were 5 mm in radius. Coordinates of seed regions were the same as those used in (Schmidt et al., 2013). The resting state data used in the present study were partially described in the Schmidt et al. (2013) study, but have been re-analyzed for the purpose of this study. Correlation maps of the whole brain were created for each seed and then averaged over all seeds for a specific network for each subject. These correlations were then z-transformed, group averages were computed, and across-group comparisons were made via two-sample *t*-tests in the Conn toolbox (Whitfield-Gabrieli and Nieto-Castanon, 2012). Results were then exported to SPM8 for display purposes. After whole brain analysis at $p < 0.001$ uncorrected threshold, clusters that were significant at $p < 0.025$ FWE either at voxel or cluster level were selected to account for both tails of the *t*-test, with cluster extent set at 25 voxels.

A seeding analysis designed to examine resting state network connectivity was performed using ROIs determined from published studies as stated earlier, as well as using ROIs identified from the task-based study. The latter ROIs included the left amygdala, left inferior parietal lobule, left superior frontal gyrus, right middle temporal gyrus, and the right superior parietal lobule (**Table 2**). The left amygdala seed was created based on the NH > HL (P + U > N) contrast from the task ROI analysis. The right superior parietal lobule and left inferior parietal lobule were both based on the HL > NH (P + U > N) contrast, and the right middle temporal gyrus and left superior frontal gyrus seeds were based on the NH > HL (P + U > N) contrast from the emotion task results. All of these ROIs were determined from group-level contrasts. Peak maxima were used as the centers for the spherical ROIs, and the mean BOLD timeseries of the voxels in the ROI was generated. Seed specification, data generation and statistical analyses were performed in the manner described earlier for the standard seeds.

Table 2 | Seed regions for the resting state functional connectivity analysis, consisting of seeds for canonical resting state networks and for networks based on local axima from the results of the emotion task study.

Network	Seed region	MNI coordinates *X, Y, Z*
Auditory	Left primary auditory cortex	55, −22, 9
Auditory	Right primary auditory cortex	−41, −27, 6
DMN	Medial prefrontal cortex	8, 59, 19
DMN	Posterior cingulate cortex	−2, −50, 25
DAN	Left posterior intraparietal sulcus	−23, −70, 46
DAN	Right posterior intraparietal sulcus	26, −62, 53
DAN	Left frontal eye field	−25, −11, 54
DAN	Right frontal eye field	27, −11, 54
	Left amygdala	−30, −2, −18
	Left inferior parietal lobule	−44, −36, 26
	Left superior frontal gyrus	−24, 42, 30
	Right middle temporal gyrus	44, −62, 22
	Right superior parietal lobule	30, −62, 44

Coordinates are listed in Montreal Neurological Institute (MNI) coordinates.

RESULTS

BEHAVIORAL DATA

(a) Emotion task

Ratings were obtained in the scanner simultaneous with fMRI data acquisition. There was a statistically significant main effect of group [$F_{(1, 23)} = 69.53$, $p < 0.000001$], main effect of condition [$F_{(1, 23)} = 17.59$, $p < 0.000001$] and interaction between group and condition [$F_{(1, 23)} = 7.79$, $p < 0.000423$] for the reaction time data. The NH group responded significantly slower to the neutral sounds compared to the pleasant and unpleasant sounds (**Figure 1A**). The HL group's reaction time for the three types of sounds did not significantly differ (**Figure 1A**). For between group comparisons, the HL group was significantly slower for both pleasant and unpleasant sounds compared to the NH group (**Figure 1A**). Concerning the type of responses, there was a significant main effect of condition [$F_{(1, 23)} = 7.162$, $p < 0.01$]; however, the main effect of group [$F_{(1, 23)} = 0.118$, $p = 0.733$] and the interactions [$F_{(1, 23)} = 0.109$, $p = 0.897$] did not reach significance. Both groups rated significantly more stimuli as unpleasant compared to pleasant and neutral (determined using *post-hoc* within-group *t*-tests) (**Figure 1B**). Note that the experimental design used an equal number of sounds classified as P, N, and U according to the normative IADS scores (Bradley and Lang, 2007). Due to the observed variation from the normative ratings, we chose to code the trials during analysis according to each individual's rating.

(b) Resting state

No behavioral data were obtained for the resting state study.

fMRI DATA

(a) Emotion task

Within group comparisons: In the NH group, areas of increased activation for the contrast P + U > N were observed in the bilateral middle temporal gyri, right transverse temporal gyrus, left superior temporal gyrus, left post central gyrus, right medial frontal gyrus, left superior frontal gyrus, left middle frontal gyrus, left anterior cingulate and the left insula (**Figure 2, Table 3**). With respect to the HL group, increased response was obtained in the bilateral superior temporal gyri, bilateral transverse temporal gyri, right middle temporal gyrus, right superior frontal gyrus, left middle frontal gyrus, right medial frontal gyrus, right precuneus, left inferior parietal lobule, left precentral gyrus, left lentiform nucleus and corpus callosum for affective sounds compared to neutral sounds (**Figure 2, Table 3**). ROI analysis revealed increased response in bilateral transverse temporal gyri, bilateral

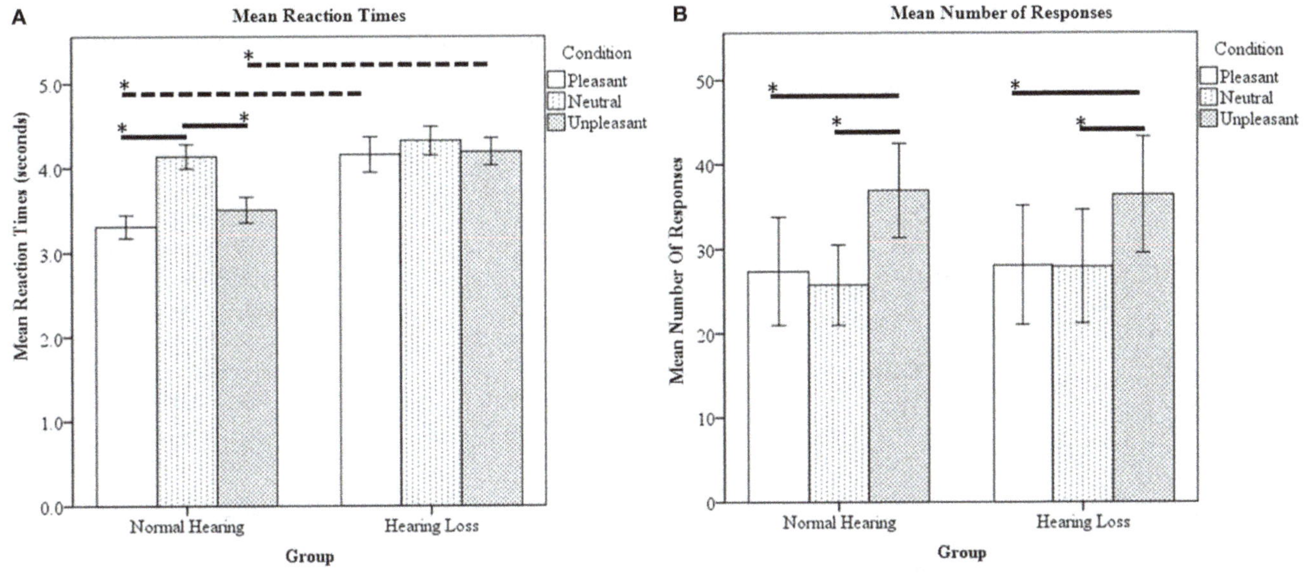

FIGURE 1 | Affective sound categorization task behavioral results. **(A)** Mean reaction time data. For within group comparison, the HL group did not statistically differ between the P, N, and U reaction times. However, the NH group responded significantly slower to the N sounds compared to the P and U stimuli. Compared to the NH group, the HL reaction times were significantly slower for P and U sounds. **(B)** Mean number of responses. The NH and HL groups responded U significantly more than N and P. Statistical significance level $p < 0.05$ indicated by *.

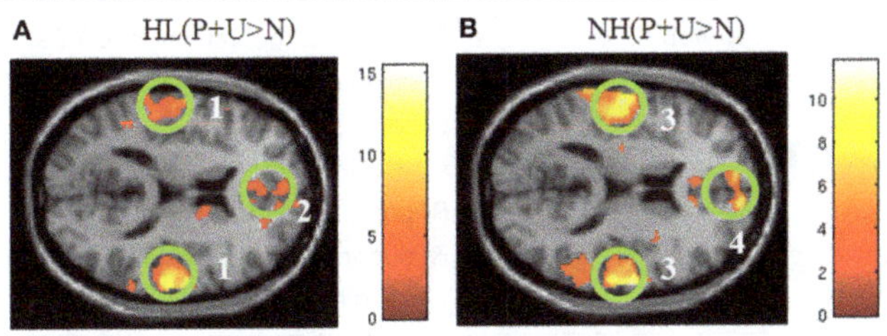

FIGURE 2 | Statistical parametric maps for the effect of affective stimuli (P + U > N) for each group separately (A,B). (A) HL (P + U > N) and **(B)** NH (P + U > N) images illustrate the similar whole brain response patterns from both groups (MNI coordinate $z = +14$). The maps are displayed at $p < 0.001$ uncorrected level for better visualization, but the clusters in the circles are corrected for multiple comparisons ($p < 0.05$ FWE). (1) bilateral middle temporal gyrus, (2) medial frontal gyrus, (3) bilateral middle temporal gyrus, (4) medial frontal gyrus.

superior temporal gyri, bilateral medial frontal gyrus, left insula, right middle temporal gyrus and right parahippocampus for the NH (P + U > N) contrast (**Table 3**). For the HL (P + U > N) comparison, increased response was observed in the bilateral transverse temporal gyri, bilateral superior temporal gyri, bilateral superior frontal gyri, right medial frontal gyrus and left insula (**Table 3**).

Between-group comparisons: For the NH > HL (P + U > N) comparison, we observed heightened response in the left superior frontal gyrus, right middle temporal gyrus, left superior temporal gyrus, and left superior occipital gyrus (**Figure 3**, **Table 4**). Concerning the HL > NH (P + U > N) comparison, elevated response was observed in the right superior parietal lobule, right precuneus, and left inferior parietal lobule (**Figure 3**, **Table 4**).

For the ROI analysis, no suprathreshold voxels were obtained for the HL > NH (P + U > N) contrast. However, for the NH > HL (P + U > N) comparison, increased response was observed in the left amygdala and left parahippocampus (**Figure 3**, **Table 4**).

(b) Resting state

No significant differences were found between groups in the auditory resting state network. With respect to the DMN, a significant difference in the left middle frontal/precentral gyrus was observed in the HL > NH comparison. Analysis of the DAN revealed a significant difference in the left postcentral/precentral gyrus and left insula. These results of the typical intrinsic networks are listed in **Table 5** and displayed in **Figure 4**. For the connectivity analysis with task-based ROIs, no significant differences in connectivity with the left amygdala were seen. Placing a seed in the left inferior parietal lobule also did not reveal significant differences. With the seed in the left superior frontal gyrus, the NH > HL contrast showed significant differences in connectivity with the left middle occipital lobe. The right middle temporal seed showed a stronger correlation with the right precentral gyrus in the HL group compared to the NH group. Finally, no connectivity differences were seen with the seed in the right superior parietal lobule. The results of this analysis are also shown in **Table 5** and **Figure 4**.

DISCUSSION

We used a combined task- and rest-based fMRI study to identify the influence of HL on auditory and emotion processing. Results of the responses collected in the scanner revealed similar ratings for the unpleasant, pleasant, and neutral sounds—both groups tended to rate more sounds as unpleasant relative to the other types of sounds. However, the HL group differed from

Table 3 | Local maxima for the P + U > N contrasts from the emotion task.

Contrast	MNI coordinates *X, Y, Z*	*Z*-score	Cluster (voxels)	Gyrus (brodmann area)
NH group (P + U > N)	62, −10, 12	6.45	3293	R. transverse temporal gyrus (BA 42)
	58, 2, −8	6.42		R. middle temporal gyrus (BA 21)
	56, 6, −18	5.98		R. middle temporal gyrus (BA 21)
	−58, −16, 15	6.06	3974	L. post central gyrus (BA 40)
	−54, −6, 0	5.95		L. superior temporal gyrus (BA 22)
	−66, −28, 4	5.73		L. superior temporal gyrus (BA 22)
	−24, 66, 14	5.59	218	L. superior frontal gyrus (BA 10)
	−32, 62, 16	5.48		L. middle frontal gyrus
	−38, −58, 2	5.57	233	L. middle temporal gyrus (BA 37)
	−40, −34, 20	5.39	10	L. insula (BA 13)
	4, 56, 20	5.38	1765	R. medial frontal gyrus (BA 9)
	10, 60, 16	5.32		R. medial frontal gyrus (BA 10)
	−8, 34, 6	5.12		L. anterior cingulate (BA 32)
HL group (P + U > N)	58, −14, 12	7.21	2289	R. transverse temporal gyrus (BA42)
	60, −22, 14	6.46		R. superior temporal gyrus (BA 42)
	62, −28, 4	5.30		R. superior temporal gyrus (BA 22)
	−42, −36, 22	6.56	2471	L. inferior parietal lobule (BA40)
	−50, −6, 6	5.72		L. precentral gyrus (BA 6)
	−56, −16, 6	5.29		L. superior temporal gyrus (BA 22)
	−62, −10, 12	5.13		L. transverse temporal gyrus (BA42)
	−46, 36, 28	5.64	760	L. middle frontal gyrus (BA46)
	−24, −16, −4	5.64	195	L. lentiform nucleus
	44, −62, 24	5.52	405	R. middle temporal gyrus (BA 39)
	36, −74, 18	5.14		R. middle temporal gyrus (BA 39)
	−8, 32, 6	5.48	1644	Corpus Callosum
	8, 42, −10			R. medial frontal gyrus (BA10)
	24, −50, 52	5.25	63	R. precuneus (BA 7)
	12, 62, 28	5.10	392	R. superior frontal gyrus (BA10)
	−30, 46, 40	5.07	43	L. middle frontal gyrus (BA9)
[ROI] NH group (P + U > N)	62, −10, 12	6.45	534	R. transverse temporal gyrus (BA 42)
	58, 0, −6	6.16		R. superior temporal gyrus (BA 22)
	54, −24, 6	4.90		R. superior temporal gyrus (BA 41)
	52, −34, 2	4.45		R. middle temporal gyrus (BA 22)
	−58, −16, 12	5.94	938	L. transverse temporal gyrus (BA 42)
	−66, −28, 4	5.73		L. superior temporal gyrus (BA 22)
	−50, −22, 16	5.68		L. insula
	−40, −34, 20	5.39		L. insula (BA 13)
	−48, −26, 18	5.38		L. insula (BA 13)
	−54, −20, 6	5.25		L. superior temporal gyrus (BA 41)
	−52, −26, 12	4.69		L. transverse temporal gyrus (BA 41)
	6, 58, 20	5.30	54	R. medial frontal gyrus (BA 10)
	−6, 58, 14	4.52	41	L. medial frontal gyrus (BA 10)
	20, −20, −22	4.31	42	R. parahippocampus (BA 28)
[ROI] HL group (P + U > N)	60, −12, 12	6.72	510	R. transverse temporal gyrus (BA42)
	60, −22, 12	6.18		R. superior temporal gyrus (BA 42)
	56, −10, 8	5.96		R. superior temporal gyrus (BA 22)
	52, −22, 14	5.11		R. insula
	−52, −6, 4	5.60	486	L. superior temporal gyrus (BA 22)
	−42, −34, 20	5.60		L. insula (BA 13)
	−62, −10, 12	5.08		L. transverse temporal gyrus (BA 42)
	−54, −28, 10	4.71		L. superior temporal gyrus (BA 41)

(Continued)

Table 3 | Continued

Contrast	MNI coordinates *X, Y, Z*	*Z*-score	Cluster (voxels)	Gyrus (brodmann area)
	8, 42, −10	5.31	201	R. medial frontal (BA 10)
	12, 62, 28	5.10	13	R. superior frontal gyrus (BA 10)
	−14, 62, 26	4.76	15	L. superior frontal gyrus (BA 10)

The loci are listed for each group separately for the whole-brain analysis and the region-of-interest (ROI) analysis. Reported regions are listed in Montreal Neurological Institute (MNI) coordinates and in terms of Brodmann areas (before determining the Brodmann areas the MNI coordinates were converted to Talairach coordinates). The ROI mask comprised of bilateral regions in the primary auditory cortex, medial geniculate body, inferior colliculus, amygdala, insula, parrahippocampus, nucleus accumbens, and ventral medial prefrontal cortex, defined anatomically. Statistical threshold was set at $p < 0.05$ FWE corrected for multiple comparisons; all clusters noted here were significant at both voxel and cluster level. L, left; R, right.

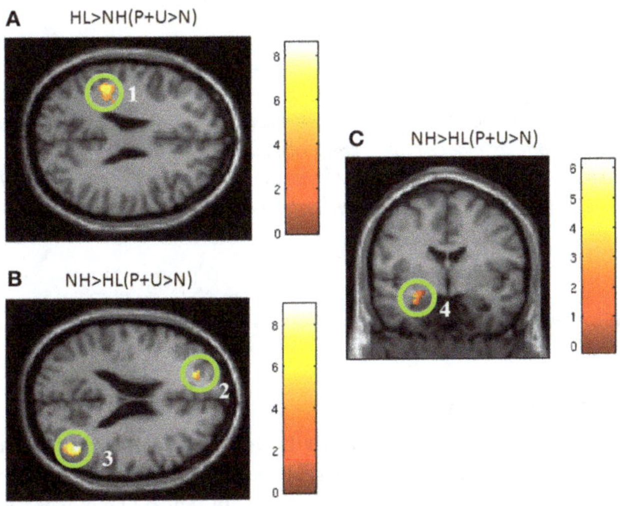

FIGURE 3 | Statistical parametric maps for *post-hoc* two-tailed two sample *t*-tests and region-of-interest analysis (ROI). (A) HL > NH (P + U > N) and **(B)** NH > HL (P + U > N) illustrate the brain regions chosen from the *post-hoc* two sample *t*-tests for the seed analysis (MNI coordinate $z = +26$, $z = +21$, respectively). **(C)** Denotes increased amygdala activation observed for the NH > HL (P + U > N) comparison (MNI coordinate $y = -4$). The maps are displayed at $p < 0.001$ uncorrected level for better visualization, but the clusters in the circles are corrected for multiple comparisons ($p < 0.025$ FWE). (1) left inferior parietal lobule, (2) left superior frontal gyrus, (3) right middle temporal gyrus, (4) left amygdala.

the NH group in their response times, which were significantly slower for the affective sounds. Overlapping patterns of fMRI activation were observed in both groups when processing affective sounds compared to neutral sounds. The main finding for the emotion task was increased activation in the left amygdala/parahippocampal gyrus complex for the NH > HL (P + U > N) comparison, via targeted ROI analysis. The reverse contrast, HL > NH (P + U > N), did not show increased activation within the limbic system, but rather revealed heightened responses in the right superior parietal lobule, right precuneus, and left inferior parietal lobule. Resting-state functional connectivity in the same group of participants focused on the canonical intrinsic networks and on seed regions obtained from the task-based activation patterns. Among the typical intrinsic networks, the default mode and DAN, but not the auditory network, revealed differences between the groups. Using seeds from the local maxima noted in the task-based analysis, decreased connectivity between the frontal cortex and other brain regions was noted, with the exception of stronger connectivity between the middle temporal gyrus and the right precentral gyrus in the HL group compared to the NH group. Our results suggest that HL may alter the emotional processing networks and lead to slower reaction times to affective stimuli.

EMOTION TASK

HL may reduce the engagement of the emotional processing system, either because of disordered processing of acoustic or of valence features. Complex anatomical and functional connections exist between the auditory cortex and the limbic system, primarily with the amygdala (Amaral and Price, 1984; Blood and Zatorre, 2001; Koelsch et al., 2006; Tschacher et al., 2010; Kumar et al., 2012). Forward projections from the auditory cortex to the amygdala have been shown to be modulated by acoustic features, but backward projections appear to be modulated by the valence of sound (Kumar et al., 2012). The forward and backward projections work in concert to interpret incoming affective stimuli (Kumar et al., 2012). Sound deprivation may reduce the amount of acoustic or valence information available for this network. Reduced information may result in a dampened emotional response to affective stimuli, because individuals with HL may not receive all of the acoustic or valence information necessary to cause a robust emotional response. We investigated this hypothesis via whole brain analysis and a targeted ROI analysis of the auditory and limbic areas.

In our study, both positively and negatively valent sounds exhibited greater engagement of the limbic system and faster response times, compared to neutral sounds, in NH individuals. However, this pattern differed in the HL group, with a decreased response in the temporal and frontal cortices (whole brain analysis) and in the amygdala and parahippocampus (ROI analysis), and an increased response in the parietal cortices and precuneus compared to the NH group when processing affective sounds (**Table 4**). Similarly, in behavioral responses, the reaction times for the P and U sounds were significantly slower in the HL group (**Figure 1A**). The behavioral data suggest that the advantageous faster processing of affective sound found in the NH group does not occur in the HL group. The slower responses to pleasant and unpleasant sounds in the HL group may be due to lack of faster, bottom-up engagement of the amygdala and other limbic structures during auditory processing. However, HL does not appear

Table 4 | Local maxima for the P + U > N contrasts from the emotion task for the group comparisons.

Contrast	MNI coordinates *X, Y, Z*	*Z*-score	Cluster (voxels)	Gyrus (brodmann area)
NH > HL (P + U > N)	44, −62, 22	5.77	261	R. middle temporal gyrus (BA 39)
	−34, 2, −18	5.72	133	L. superior temporal gyrus (BA 38)
	−24, 42, 20	5.04	319	L. superior frontal gyrus (BA 10)
	−30, −78, 24	4.45*	272	L. superior occipital gyrus (BA 19)
HL > NH (P + U > N)	18, −64, 44	5.62	402	R. precuneus (BA 7)
	30, −62, 44	4.86		R. superior parietal lobule (BA 7)
	−44, −36, 26	4.68*	288	L. inferior parietal lobule (BA 40)
[ROI] NH > HL (P + U > N)	−30, −2, −18	4.80	57	L. amygdala/parrahippocampus
	−34, 2, −22	4.62		L. parrahippocampus
[ROI] HL > NH (P + U > N)				No significant regions

*The loci are listed for each group separately for the whole-brain analysis and the region-of-interest (ROI) analysis. Reported regions are listed in Montreal Neurological Institute (MNI) coordinates and in terms of Brodmann areas (before determining the Brodmann areas the MNI coordinates were converted to Talairach coordinates). The ROI mask comprised of bilateral regions in the primary auditory cortex, medial geniculate body, inferior colliculus, amygdala, insula, parrahippocampus, nucleus accumbens, and ventral medial prefrontal cortex, defined anatomically. Statistical threshold was set at $p < 0.025$ FWE corrected for multiple comparisons (to account for two-tailed t-test); all clusters noted here were significant at both voxel and cluster level, unless noted with an * which indicates significance only at cluster level. L, left; R, right.*

to affect the response to all sounds, with the reaction times for neutral sounds being nearly identical in the two groups. Instead, the highly valent sounds were most affected, indicating that it is identification of valence information rather than acoustic information that is impacted by HL. Another possible explanation of the differential processing of affective sounds by the HL group could be that there is more energy or information in the high frequency regions in the affective sounds and less so in the neutral sounds. Difficulty of processing high-frequency information in the affective sounds by the HL group led to longer reaction times. In order to maintain ecological validity, we chose not to low-pass filter the sounds to compensate for the HL of the HL group. In a previous study with mild-to-moderate HL (Husain et al., 2011b), we filtered sounds such that there was no energy in frequencies greater than 2 kHz. We found no difference in accuracy or reaction times for a discrimination task between HL and NH groups, nevertheless, the fMRI activation patterns were different (Husain et al., 2011b). In sum, regardless of the actual mechanism, our results suggest that HL may reduce engagement of the amygdala and result in slower reaction to positively and negatively valent sounds.

Another interesting aspect of the behavioral results was the finding that an increased number of sounds were classified as unpleasant, which differed from the published normative data (Bradley and Lang, 2007). There are at least two possible explanations for this finding. First, the normative scores were obtained in a young, NH population; therefore it is not surprising that both sets of older middle-aged participants in our study differed from these ratings, which points to an effect of age. Another possible explanation is that possible discomfort in the scanner may have influenced our participants to be more negative in their ratings. In order to tease apart these explanations and better understand the effect of aging on emotional processing, we intend to conduct a follow-up study with both young and older participants using stimuli from the IADS database.

RESTING STATE DATA

Resting state functional connectivity demonstrated alterations in the frontal cortex in HL patients. Increased connectivity between frontal regions and seed regions for the DAN and DMN was seen in HL patients compared to NH controls. A decreased correlation was seen between the left superior frontal cortex and the left middle occipital gyrus in HL subjects compared to controls. The relationship seen between HL and alterations in frontal connectivity may not just be important at baseline, as engagement of frontal regions was also apparent during the emotion task. The cause of these network alterations is not clear. The alterations could be purely attentional in nature, but they may also be a factor of interactions between emotional and attentional systems. A study including an attentional task without an emotional component may help to clarify this.

Except for activation of the left temporal pole, we did not find evidence to support our expectation that the response of the auditory cortex would differ between the two groups when processing affective sounds. A separate resting-state functional connectivity analysis with seeds in the primary auditory cortices also failed to find significant connectivity differences at rest between the two groups. The lack of significant findings may relate to mild-to-moderate severity of the HL in our study. To date, there have been no studies of resting state functional connectivity in patients with this level of HL. Deafness, however, has been investigated in this context. Intrinsic connectivity has been shown to be impacted by deafness, both within and outside of the temporal cortex (Li et al., 2013). The findings of the (Li et al., 2013) study are similar to those in our own study. Deaf patients showed increased negative correlations between the middle superior temporal sulcus and

Table 5 | Local maxima for results of the resting state functional connectivity analysis.

Network/seed	Contrast	MNI coordinates *X, Y, Z*	*Z*-score	Cluster (voxels)	Gyrus (brodmann area)
AUD	NH > HL				No significant regions
	HL > NH				No significant regions
DMN	NH > HL				No significant regions
	HL > NH	−44, 6, 58	4.38	107	L. middle frontal/precentral gyrus (BA 6)
DAN	NH > HL	−56, −12, 26	5.00	171	L. postcentral gyrus
		−56, −2, 26	4.09		L. precentral gyrus
		−52, −4, 38	3.36		L. postcentral gyrus
		−38, −6, 6	4.36	118	L. insula
		−40, −2, 16	4.00		L. precentral gyrus (BA 6)
		−46, −10, 14	3.43		L. precentral gyrus (BA 6)
	HL > NH				No significant regions
l amyg	NH > HL				No significant regions
	HL > NH				No significant regions
l inf pariet	NH > HL				No significant regions
	HL > NH				No significant regions
l sup front	NH > HL	−18, −96, 8	4.7	167	L. middle occipital gyrus (BA 18)
		−4, −94, 20	4.38		L. cuneus (BA 19)
	HL > NH				No significant regions
r mid temp	NH > HL				No significant regions
	HL > NH	66, −6, 12	4.39	114	R. precentral gyrus (BA 22)
r sup pariet	NH > HL				No significant regions
	HL > NH				No significant regions

The seeds are listed for the canonical resting state networks first, followed by seeds from the task-based study. Reported regions are listed in Montreal Neurological Institute (MNI) coordinates and in terms of Brodmann areas (before determining the Brodmann areas the MNI coordinates were converted to Talairach coordinates). Statistical threshold was set at $p < 0.025$ FWE corrected for multiple comparisons (to account for two-tailed t-test). All regions were significant at the cluster level. Abbreviations: L, left; R, right; amyg, amygdala; inf pariet, inferior parietal; sup front, superior frontal; mid temp, middle temporal; sup pariet; superior parietal.

the left middle occipital and right precentral gyri when compared to NH controls. In our study, the left middle occipital gyrus was shown to be less correlated to the left superior frontal gyrus in the HL group, whereas the right precentral gyrus was more correlated with the right middle temporal gyrus. The presence of altered connectivity in similar regions in both deaf and our mild-to-moderate HL patients warrants further resting state connectivity studies examining varying degrees of HL.

It is important to note that inferences about the directionality of the connections cannot be made from the present functional connectivity analysis. An effective connectivity analysis, perhaps implemented as a structural equation modeling or dynamic causal modeling, would be needed to examine directionality (Horwitz, 2003). Our results suggest only a general alteration in connectivity between two related regions; differences in correlation may not be specifically due to coupling between the seed and a particular region, but may also arise due to the influence of a third region, or changes in noise, etc. (Friston, 1994).

HL is positively correlated with age (Yueh et al., 2003); age is therefore a potential confound in our research. A study examining connectivity in resting state networks (Onoda et al., 2012) noted a significantly decreased correlation between the auditory resting state network and the salience network (which includes the insula, ventrolateral prefrontal cortex (VLPFC), thalamus and cerebellum) with age. In addition, connections between regions of the salience network also weakened with age. The regions of the salience network relate to the processing of emotional stimuli. It is possible that HL within the older population in this study is partially responsible for the observed results. The decreased correlation between regions of the DAN and the insula seen in our study fit well with the results of the aging study. In our own study, however, all participants were matched for age; therefore, we are unable to parse out the effects of age from those of HL. More fMRI studies specifically addressing the effects of HL of varying severity, in different age groups, should be performed to clarify its impact on intrinsic and task-based functional networks. Subject motion in the scanner is another notable confound with the resting state data being particularly sensitive to its influence. Although we excluded data from participants who exhibited excessive head motion, included motion parameters as covariates of no-interest in our statistical models and statistical tests did not show any significant differences between

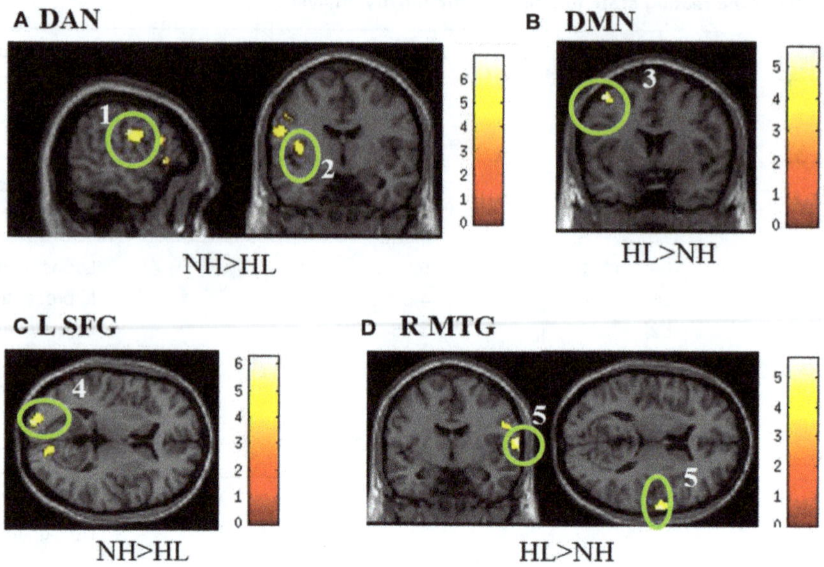

FIGURE 4 | Statistical parametric maps of the two-tailed two sample *t*-tests of the resting state functional connectivity results. (A,B) show the results of the seeding analyses designed to examine the connectivity of the resting state networks, while **(C,D)** show correlations to the task-based seeds. The maps are displayed at $p < 0.001$ uncorrected level for better visualization, but the clusters in the circles are corrected for multiple comparisons ($p < 0.025$ FWE). In **(A)**, the seed regions were located in the bilateral posterior intraparietal sulci and the bilateral frontal eye fields to examine connectivity in the dorsal attention network (DAN). For the default mode network (DMN) in **(B)**, seeds were located in the posterior cingulate and medial prefrontal cortices. **(C,D)** are labeled with the seed regions in the figure. (1) left postcentral gyrus, (2) left insula, (3) left middle frontal/precentral gyrus, (4) left middle occipital, (5). right precentral gyrus. MNI coordinates for the different sub- figures are: **(A)** $x = -56$, $y = 6$, **(B)** $y = 6$, **(C)** $z = -18$ left, **(D)** $y = -6$, $z = 12$. Abbreviations: DAN, dorsal attention network; DMN, default mode network; L SFG, left superior frontal gyrus; R MTG, right middle temporal gyrus.

the groups, it is possible that motion-related artifacts continue to affect our results, as shown by recent publications (Kundu et al., 2012; Van Dijk et al., 2012; Kundu et al., 2013; Power et al., 2014). Future studies with more stringent data acquisition considerations and more advanced analytical methods will need to be conducted to fully account for the possibility of motion artifacts.

CONCLUSION

Our results suggest that HL may affect emotional processing by decreasing amygdalar recruitment, resulting in slower reaction times to highly valent sounds. Although the HL group demonstrated slower response times to affective sounds, there was no difference in sound ratings between the HL and the NH group. Altered engagement of the frontal regions was also demonstrated in both emotion task-based subtraction and resting state functional connectivity analyses. HL is the third most common chronic condition in older adults and is highly comorbid with another hearing disorder, tinnitus. Our results in those with unaided, mild-to-moderately severe HL have implications for auditory rehabilitation for hearing impairment, reducing social isolation in the elderly, and management strategies for tinnitus.

ACKNOWLEDGMENTS

We wish to acknowledge the support of Tinnitus Research Consortium to Fatima T. Husain and of the NeuroEngineering NSF IGERT (Integrative Graduate Education and Research Traineeship) to Jake R. Carpenter-Thompson and Sara A. Schmidt. We are grateful to Kwaku Akrofi and Jaclyn Utz for their assistance in data acquisition.

SUPPLEMENTARY MATERIAL

Supplementary Table 1 | Sounds included in the study. Separated by column are 30 pleasant, 30 unpleasant, and 30 neutral sounds chosen from the IADS database to be included in the study.

REFERENCES

Amaral, D. G., and Price, J. L. (1984). Amygdalo-cortical projections in the monkey (*Macaca fascicularis*). *J. Comp. Neurol.* 230, 465–496. doi: 10.1002/cne.902300402

Anticevic, A., Repovs, G., and Barch, D. M. (2012). Emotion effects on attention, amygdala activation, and functional connectivity in schizophrenia. *Schizophr. Bull.* 38, 967–980. doi: 10.1093/schbul/sbq168

Bartels, H., Middel, B. L., Van Der Laan, B. F., Staal, M. J., and Albers, F. W. (2008). The additive effect of co-occurring anxiety and depression on health status, quality of life and coping strategies in help-seeking tinnitus sufferers. *Ear Hear.* 29, 947–956. doi: 10.1097/AUD.0b013e3181888f83

Beck, A. T., and Steer, R. A. (1984). Internal consistencies of the original and revised Beck Depression Inventory. *J. Clin. Psychol.* 40, 1365–1367. doi: 10.1002/1097-4679(198411)40:6<1365::AID-JCLP2270400615>3.0.CO;2-D

Blood, A. J., and Zatorre, R. J. (2001). Intensely pleasurable responses to music correlate with activity in brain regions implicated in reward and emotion. *Proc. Natl. Acad. Sci. U.S.A.* 98, 11818–11823. doi: 10.1073/pnas.191355898

Bradley, M. M., and Lang, P. J. (2007). *The International Affective Digitized Sounds (IADS-2): Affective Ratings of Sounds and Instruction Manual.* Gainesville, FL: University of Florida, Technical Report: B-3.

Brett, M., Anton, J. L., Valabregue, R., and Poline, J. B. (2002). Region of interest analysis using an SPM toolbox. *NeuroImage* 16, 1140–1141.

Burton, H., Wineland, A., Bhattacharya, M., Nicklaus, J., Garcia, K. S., and Piccirillo, J. F. (2012). Altered networks in bothersome tinnitus: a functional connectivity study. *BMC Neurosci.* 13:3. doi: 10.1186/1471-2202-13-3

Carabellese, C., Appollonio, I., Rozzini, R., Bianchetti, A., Frisoni, G. B., Frattola, L., et al. (1993). Sensory impairment and quality of life in a community elderly population. *J. Am. Geriatr. Soc.* 41, 401–407.

Cruickshanks, K. J., Wiley, T. L., Tweed, T. S., Klein, B. E., Klein, R., Mares-Perlman, J. A., et al. (1998). Prevalence of hearing loss in older adults in Beaver Dam, Wisconsin. The Epidemiology of Hearing Loss Study. *Am. J. Epidemiol.* 148, 879–886. doi: 10.1093/oxfordjournals.aje.a009713

Davis, A., and Rafaie, E. A. (2000). "Epidemiology of tinnitus," in *Tinnitus Handbook*, ed R. S. Tyler (San Diego, CA: Singular), 1–24.

Dolcos, F., and McCarthy, G. (2006). Brain systems mediating cognitive interference by emotional distraction. *J. Neurosci.* 26, 2072–2079. doi: 10.1523/JNEUROSCI.5042-05.2006

Feldmann, H., and Kumpf, W. (1988). [Listening to music in hearing loss with and without a hearing aid]. *Laryngol. Rhinol. Otol. (Stuttg).* 67, 489–497. doi: 10.1055/s-2007-998547

Fox, M. D., Snyder, A. Z., Vincent, J. L., Corbetta, M., Van Essen, D. C., and Raichle, M. E. (2005). The human brain is intrinsically organized into dynamic, anticorrelated functional networks. *Proc. Natl. Acad. Sci. U.S.A.* 102, 9673–9678. doi: 10.1073/pnas.0504136102

Franks, J. R. (1982). Judgments of hearing aid processed music. *Ear Hear.* 3, 18–23. doi: 10.1097/00003446-198201000-00004

Friston, K. J. (1994). Functional and effective connectivity in neuroimaging: a synthesis. *Hum. Brain Mapp.* 2, 56–78. doi: 10.1002/hbm.460020107

Gaab, N., Gaser, C., Zaehle, T., Jancke, L., and Schlaug, G. (2003). Functional anatomy of pitch memory–an fMRI study with sparse temporal sampling. *Neuroimage* 19, 1417–1426. doi: 10.1016/S1053-8119(03)00224-6

Giraud, A. L., Chery-Croze, S., Fischer, G., Fischer, C., Vighetto, A., Gregoire, M. C., et al. (1999). A selective imaging of tinnitus. *Neuroreport* 10, 1–5. doi: 10.1097/00001756-199901180-00001

Golm, D., Schmidt-Samoa, C., Dechent, P., and Kroner-Herwig, B. (2013). Neural correlates of tinnitus related distress: an fMRI-study. *Hear. Res.* 295, 87–99. doi: 10.1016/j.heares.2012.03.003

Gopinath, B., Wang, J. J., Schneider, J., Burlutsky, G., Snowdon, J., McMahon, C. M., et al. (2009). Depressive symptoms in older adults with hearing impairments: the Blue Mountains Study. *J. Am. Geriatr. Soc.* 57, 1306–1308. doi: 10.1111/j.1532-5415.2009.02317.x

Greicius, M. (2008). Resting-state functional connectivity in neuropsychiatric disorders. *Curr. Opin. Neurol.* 21, 424–430. doi: 10.1097/WCO.0b013e328306f2c5

Hall, D. A., Haggard, M. P., Akeroyd, M. A., Palmer, A. R., Summerfield, A. Q., Elliott, M. R., et al. (1999). "Sparse" temporal sampling in auditory fMRI. *Hum. Brain Mapp.* 7, 213–223. doi: 10.1002/(SICI)1097-0193(1999)7:3<213::AID-HBM5>3.0.CO;2-N

Hicks, C. B., and Tharpe, A. M. (2002). Listening effort and fatigue in school-age children with and without hearing loss. *J. Speech Lang. Hear. Res.* 45, 573. doi: 10.1044/1092-4388(2002/046)

Horwitz, B. (2003). The elusive concept of brain connectivity. *Neuroimage* 19, 466–470. doi: 10.1016/S1053-8119(03)00112-5

Husain, F. T., Medina, R. E., Davis, C. W., Szymko-Bennett, Y., Simonyan, K., Pajor, N. M., et al. (2011a). Neuroanatomical changes due to hearing loss and chronic tinnitus: a combined VBM and DTI study. *Brain Res.* 1369, 74–88. doi: 10.1016/j.brainres.2010.10.095

Husain, F. T., Pajor, N. M., Smith, J. F., Kim, H. J., Rudy, S., Zalewski, C., et al. (2011b). Discrimination task reveals differences in neural bases of tinnitus and hearing impairment. *PLoS ONE* 6:e26639. doi: 10.1371/journal.pone.0026639

Husain, F. T., Patkin, D. J., Thai-Van, H., Braun, A. R., and Horwitz, B. (2009). Distinguishing the processing of gestures from signs in deaf individuals: An fMRI study. *Brain Res.* 1276, 140–150. doi: 10.1016/j.brainres.2009.04.034

Husain, F. T., and Schmidt, S. A. (2013). Using resting state functional connectivity to unravel networks of tinnitus. *Hear. Res.* 307, 154–162. doi: 10.1016/j.heares.2013.07.010

Jastreboff, P. J. (1990). Phantom auditory perception (tinnitus): mechanisms of generation and perception. *Neurosci. Res.* 8, 221–254. doi: 10.1016/0168-0102(90)90031-9

Koelsch, S., Fritz, T., Dy, V. C., Muller, K., and Friederici, A. D. (2006). Investigating emotion with music: an fMRI study. *Hum. Brain Mapp.* 27, 239–250. doi: 10.1002/hbm.20180

Kumar, S., Von Kriegstein, K., Friston, K., and Griffiths, T. D. (2012). Features versus feelings: dissociable representations of the acoustic features and valence of aversive sounds. *J. Neurosci.* 32, 14184–14192. doi: 10.1523/JNEUROSCI.1759-12.2012

Kundu, P., Brenowitz, N. D., Voon, V., Worbe, Y., Vertes, P. E., Inati, S. J., et al. (2013). Integrated strategy for improving functional connectivity mapping using multiecho fMRI. *Proc. Natl. Acad. Sci. U.S.A.* 110, 16187–16192. doi: 10.1073/pnas.1301725110

Kundu, P., Inati, S. J., Evans, J. W., Luh, W. M., and Bandettini, P. A. (2012). Differentiating BOLD and non-BOLD signals in fMRI time series using multi-echo EPI. *Neuroimage* 60, 1759–1770. doi: 10.1016/j.neuroimage.2011.12.028

Leek, M. R., Molis, M. R., Kubli, L. R., and Tufts, J. B. (2008). Enjoyment of music by elderly hearing-impaired listeners. *J. Am. Acad. Audiol.* 19, 519–526. doi: 10.3766/jaaa.19.6.7

Li, Y., Booth, J. R., Peng, D., Zang, Y., Li, J., Yan, C., et al. (2013). Altered intra- and inter-regional synchronization of superior temporal cortex in deaf people. *Cereb. Cortex* 23, 1988–1996. doi: 10.1093/cercor/bhs185

Mather, M., and Knight, M. (2005). Goal-directed memory: the role of cognitive control in older adults' emotional memory. *Psychol. Aging* 20, 554–570. doi: 10.1037/0882-7974.20.4.554

Mirz, F., Gjedde, A., Ishizu, K., and Pedersen, C. B. (2000). Cortical networks subserving the perception of tinnitus–a PET study. *Acta Otolaryngol. Suppl.* 543, 241–243. doi: 10.1080/000164800454503

Mulrow, C. D., Aguilar, C., Endicott, J. E., Velez, R., Tuley, M. R., Charlip, W. S., et al. (1990). Association between hearing impairment and the quality of life of elderly individuals. *J. Am. Geriatr. Soc.* 38, 45–50.

Onoda, K., Ishihara, M., and Yamaguchi, S. (2012). Decreased functional connectivity by aging is associated with cognitive decline. *J. Cogn. Neurosci.* 24, 2186–2198. doi: 10.1162/jocn_a_00269

Peelle, J. E., Troiani, V., Grossman, M., and Wingfield, A. (2011). Hearing loss in older adults affects neural systems supporting speech comprehension. *J. Neurosci.* 31, 12638–12643. doi: 10.1523/JNEUROSCI.2559-11.2011

Petitto, L. A., Zatorre, R. J., Gauna, K., Nikelski, E. J., Dostie, D., and Evans, A. C. (2000). Speech-like cerebral activity in profoundly deaf people processing signed languages: implications for the neural basis of human language. *Proc. Natl. Acad. Sci. U.S.A.* 97, 13961–13966. doi: 10.1073/pnas.97.25.13961

Power, J. D., Mitra, A., Laumann, T. O., Snyder, A. Z., Schlaggar, B. L., and Petersen, S. E. (2014). Methods to detect, characterize, and remove motion artifact in resting state fMRI. *Neuroimage* 84, 320–341. doi: 10.1016/j.neuroimage.2013.08.048

Raichle, M. E., Macleod, A. M., Snyder, A. Z., Powers, W. J., Gusnard, D. A., and Shulman, G. L. (2001). A default mode of brain function. *Proc. Natl. Acad. Sci. U.S.A.* 98, 676–682. doi: 10.1073/pnas.98.2.676

Rauschecker, J. P., Leaver, A. M., and Muhlau, M. (2010). Tuning out the noise: limbic-auditory interactions in tinnitus. *Neuron* 66, 819–826. doi: 10.1016/j.neuron.2010.04.032

Rutledge, K. L. (2009). *A Music Listening Questionnaire for Hearing Aid Users.* Unpublished Master's Thesis. University of Canterbury, Christchurch. Available online at: http://hdl.handle.net/10092/3194

Schmidt, S. A., Akrofi, K., Carpenter-Thompson, J. R., and Husain, F. T. (2013). Default mode, dorsal attention and auditory resting state networks exhibit differential functional connectivity in tinnitus and hearing loss. *PLoS ONE* 8:e76488. doi: 10.1371/journal.pone.0076488

Seydell-Greenwald, A., Leaver, A. M., Turesky, T. K., Morgan, S., Kim, H. J., and Rauschecker, J. P. (2012). Functional MRI evidence for a role of ventral prefrontal cortex in tinnitus. *Brain Res.* 1485, 22–39. doi: 10.1016/j.brainres.2012.08.052

Steer, R. A., Clark, D. A., Beck, A. T., and Ranieri, W. F. (1999). Common and specific dimensions of self-reported anxiety and depression: the BDI-II versus the BDI-IA. *Behav. Res. Ther.* 37, 183–190. doi: 10.1016/S0005-7967(98)00087-4

Steer, R. A., Ranieri, W. F., Beck, A. T., and Clark, D. A. (1993). Further evidence for the validity of the Beck Anxiety Inventory with psychiatric outpatients. *J. Anxiety Disord.* 7, 195–205. doi: 10.1016/0887-6185(93)90002-3

Stevens, G., Flaxman, S., Brunskill, E., Mascarenhas, M., Mathers, C. D., Finucane, M., et al. (2013). Global and regional hearing impairment prevalence: an analysis of 42 studies in 29 countries. *Eur. J. Public Health* 23, 146–152. doi: 10.1093/eurpub/ckr176

St Jacques, P., Dolcos, F., and Cabeza, R. (2010). Effects of aging on functional connectivity of the amygdala during negative evaluation: a network analysis of fMRI data. *Neurobiol. Aging* 31, 315–327. doi: 10.1016/j.neurobiolaging.2008.03.012

Tschacher, W., Schildt, M., and Sander, K. (2010). Brain connectivity in listening to affective stimuli: a functional magnetic resonance imaging (fMRI) study and implications for psychotherapy. *Psychother. Res.* 20, 576–588. doi: 10.1080/10503307.2010.493538

Tun, P. A., McCoy, S., and Wingfield, A. (2009). Aging, hearing acuity, and the attentional costs of effortful listening. *Psychol. Aging* 24, 761–766. doi: 10.1037/a0014802

Uys, M., Pottas, L., Vinck, B., and Van Dijk, C. (2012). The influence of non-linear frequency compression on the perception of music by adults with a moderate to sever hearing loss: subjective impressions. *S. Afr. J. Commun. Disord.* 59, 53–67. doi: 10.7196/sajcd.119

Van Dijk, K. R., Sabuncu, M. R., and Buckner, R. L. (2012). The influence of head motion on intrinsic functional connectivity MRI. *Neuroimage* 59, 431–438. doi: 10.1016/j.neuroimage.2011.07.044

Weisz, N., Voss, S., Berg, P., and Elbert, T. (2004). Abnormal auditory mismatch response in tinnitus sufferers with high-frequency hearing loss is associated with subjective distress level. *BMC Neurosci.* 5:8. doi: 10.1186/1471-2202-5-8

Whitfield-Gabrieli, S., and Nieto-Castanon, A. (2012). Conn: a functional connectivity toolbox for correlated and anticorrelated brain networks. *Brain Connect.* 2, 125–141. doi: 10.1089/brain.2012.0073

Wong, P. C., Ettlinger, M., Sheppard, J. P., Gunasekera, G. M., and Dhar, S. (2010). Neuroanatomical characteristics and speech perception in noise in older adults. *Ear Hear.* 31, 471–479. doi: 10.1097/AUD.0b013e3181d709c2

Yoneda, M., Ikawa, M., Arakawa, K., Kudo, T., Kimura, H., Fujibayashi, Y., et al. (2012). *In vivo* functional brain imaging and a therapeutic trial of L-arginine in MELAS patients. *Biochim. Biophys. Acta* 1820, 615–618. doi: 10.1016/j.bbagen.2011.04.018

Yueh, B., Shapiro, N., Maclean, C. H., and Shekelle, P. G. (2003). Screening and management of adult hearing loss in primary care: scientific review. *JAMA* 289, 1976–1985. doi: 10.1001/jama.289.15.1976

Zaehle, T., Wustenberg, T., Meyer, M., and Jancke, L. (2004). Evidence for rapid auditory perception as the foundation of speech processing: a sparse temporal sampling fMRI study. *Eur. J. Neurosci.* 20, 2447–2456. doi: 10.1111/j.1460-9568.2004.03687.x

11

Cochlear neuropathy and the coding of supra-threshold sound

Hari M. Bharadwaj*[1,2], *Sarah Verhulst*[1,3†], *Luke Shaheen*[4,5], *M. Charles Liberman*[3,4,5] and *Barbara G. Shinn-Cunningham*[1,2]

[1] *Center for Computational Neuroscience and Neural Technology, Boston University, Boston, MA, USA*
[2] *Department of Biomedical Engineering, Boston University, Boston, MA, USA*
[3] *Department of Otology and Laryngology, Harvard Medical School, Boston, MA, USA*
[4] *Eaton-Peabody Laboratories, Massachusetts Eye and Ear Infirmary, Boston, MA, USA*
[5] *Harvard-MIT Division of Health Sciences and Technology, Speech and Hearing Bioscience and Technology Program, Cambridge, MA, USA*

Correspondence:
Barbara G. Shinn-Cunningham, Center for Computational Neuroscience and Neural Technology, Boston University, 677 Beacon Street, Boston, MA 02215, USA
e-mail: shinn@cns.bu.edu

†Present address:
Sarah Verhulst, Cluster of Excellence Hearing4all, Department of Medical Physics and Acoustics, Oldenburg University, Oldenburg, Germany

Many listeners with hearing thresholds within the clinically normal range nonetheless complain of difficulty hearing in everyday settings and understanding speech in noise. Converging evidence from human and animal studies points to one potential source of such difficulties: differences in the fidelity with which supra-threshold sound is encoded in the early portions of the auditory pathway. Measures of auditory subcortical steady-state responses (SSSRs) in humans and animals support the idea that the temporal precision of the early auditory representation can be poor even when hearing thresholds are normal. In humans with normal hearing thresholds (NHTs), paradigms that require listeners to make use of the detailed spectro-temporal structure of supra-threshold sound, such as selective attention and discrimination of frequency modulation (FM), reveal individual differences that correlate with subcortical temporal coding precision. Animal studies show that noise exposure and aging can cause a loss of a large percentage of auditory nerve fibers (ANFs) without any significant change in measured audiograms. Here, we argue that cochlear neuropathy may reduce encoding precision of supra-threshold sound, and that this manifests both behaviorally and in SSSRs in humans. Furthermore, recent studies suggest that noise-induced neuropathy may be selective for higher-threshold, lower-spontaneous-rate nerve fibers. Based on our hypothesis, we suggest some approaches that may yield particularly sensitive, objective measures of supra-threshold coding deficits that arise due to neuropathy. Finally, we comment on the potential clinical significance of these ideas and identify areas for future investigation.

Keywords: temporary threshold shift, frequency-following response, auditory steady-state response, individual differences, aging, auditory nerve, noise-induced hearing loss, temporal coding

INTRODUCTION

A significant number of patients seeking audiological treatment have normal hearing thresholds (NHT), but report perceptual difficulties in some situations, especially when trying to communicate in the presence of noise or other competing sounds (e.g., Hind et al., 2011). Such listeners are typically said to have "central auditory processing disorders", more recently known simply as "auditory processing disorders" (CAPD/APD; Catts et al., 1996; Chermak and Musiek, 1997), a catchall diagnosis testifying to how little we know about the underlying causes.

In some ways, the fact that having NHTs does not automatically predict good performance in these conditions is not particularly surprising. Audiometric thresholds measure the lowest intensities that a listener can *detect*. In contrast, the ability to *analyze* the content of sound requires a much more precise sensory representation of acoustic features across a large dynamic range of sound intensities. Specifically, current audiometric screenings test the lowest level of sound listeners can hear at various frequencies, but they do not test whether they can make judgments about the spectral or temporal content of the sound, analogous to seeing an eye doctor and being asked whether you can tell that light is present, without worrying about whether or not you can tell anything about the object the light is coming from.

Consistent with the idea that analysis of supra-threshold sound differs amongst NHT listeners, many APD patients seek help precisely because they notice difficulties in situations requiring *selective auditory attention* (Demanez et al., 2003), which places great demands on the auditory system. Moreover, recent laboratory evidence suggests that the prevalence of NHT listeners with APD-like symptoms may be greater than one might predict based on the number of people seeking audiological treatment. Specifically, in the lab, NHT listeners have vastly different abilities on the types of tasks that typically frustrate APD listeners. One recent study shows that when NHT subjects are asked to report spoken digits from one direction amidst otherwise similar speech, performance ranges from chance levels to nearly 90% correct, with the bottom quartile of listeners falling below 60% correct (Ruggles and Shinn-Cunningham, 2011). Crucially, when subjects made errors, they almost always reported a digit coming from a non-target direction rather than an unspoken digit, suggesting that differences were unlikely due to higher-level deficits involving language such as differences in speech intelligibility. Instead, the errors appeared to be due to failing to select the target stream from amidst the maskers. Yet none of the listeners in the study complained of hearing difficulties, even those at the bottom of the distribution; moreover, none had entertained the idea of seeking audiological treatment.

Differences in higher-order processing clearly contribute to individual differences in complex tasks such as the ability to selectively attend, process speech, or perform other high-level tasks (for instance see Surprenant and Watson, 2001). However, in this opinion paper, we focus on how low-level differences in the precision of spectro-temporal coding may contribute to differences in performance. We argue that poor sensory coding of supra-threshold sound is most likely to be revealed in complex tasks like those requiring selective attention, which helps to explain the constellation of symptoms that lead to APD diagnoses. Selective auditory attention hinges on segregating the source of interest from competing sources (object formation; see Bregman, 1990; Darwin and Carlyon, 1995; Alain and Arnott, 2000; Carlyon, 2004), and then focusing on that source based on its perceptual attributes (object selection; see Shinn-Cunningham, 2008; Shinn-Cunningham and Best, 2008). Both object formation and object selection rely on extracting precise spectro-temporal cues present in natural sound sources, which convey pitch, location, timbre, and other source features. Given this, it makes sense that listeners with poor supra-threshold coding fidelity notice problems in crowded social settings, an ability that depends upon robust coding of supra-threshold sound features.

Here, we argue that the fidelity with which the auditory system encodes supra-threshold sound is especially sensitive to the number of intact auditory nerve fibers (ANFs) encoding the input. In contrast, having NHTs likely depends only on having a relatively small but reliable population of ANFs that respond at low intensities. Indeed, one recent study shows that, in animals, audiometric thresholds can be normal even with only 10–20% of the inner hair cells (IHCs) of the cochlea intact (Lobarinas et al., 2013). Our hypothesis is that the convergence of multiple ANFs, while possibly redundant for detecting sound, is critical for analyzing supra-threshold sound.

In this paper, we first consider how supra-threshold sound content is normally encoded, focusing particularly on temporal coding. We then review animal evidence for *cochlear neuropathy*, a reduction in the number of ANFs responding to supra-threshold sound. We argue that this neuropathy can help explain why some listeners have difficulty performing selective attention and other supra-threshold tasks, despite having NHTs. We discuss evidence that lower-spontaneous rate ANFs (lower-SR ANFs; i.e., those with rates below about 18 spikes/s) may be especially vulnerable to damage. We hypothesize that lower-SR ANFs may play a critical role in coding supra-threshold sound features, particularly under challenging conditions. We then discuss the use of the subcortical steady-state response (SSSR) to quantify temporal coding in the early portions of the auditory pathway, including the challenges inherent in interpreting the SSSR and relating it to single-unit neurophysiology. With the help of simple models of brainstem responses, we suggest measures that may emphasize the effect of neuropathy on the SSSR. Using these ideas, we suggest future experiments to (1) test our hypothesis that cochlear neuropathy contributes to the supra-threshold coding deficits seen in some listeners; and (2) develop sensitive, objective correlates of such deficits that may be useful, clinically.

CODING OF SUPRA-THRESHOLD SOUND

THE DIVERSITY OF AUDITORY NERVE FIBERS

ANFs comprise the sole conduit for information about the acoustic environment, carrying spike trains from the cochlea to the central auditory system. As schematized in **Figure 1A**, each ANF contacts a single IHC via a single synapse. At each synapse, an electron-dense ribbon sits near the pre-synaptic membrane surrounded by a halo of glutamatergic vesicles. Sound in the ear canal leads to cochlear traveling waves that deflect IHC stereocilia, causing the opening of mechanoelectric transduction channels and a graded change in the IHC membrane potential. At the IHC's synaptic pole, this sound-driven receptor potential drives an influx of calcium causing an increased probability of fusion of synaptic vesicles with the IHC membrane in the region of the ribbon. Glutamate released into the synaptic cleft binds to the AMPA-type glutamate receptors at the post-synaptic active zone, causing depolarization and action potentials in the ANF.

Between 10 and 30 ANFs synapse on each IHC, depending on species and cochlear location (**Figure 1B**), and there are roughly 3500 IHCs along the 35 mm cochlear spiral in humans. Thus, all the information we receive about our acoustic world is carried via the roughly 30,000 ANFs emanating from each cochlea. ANFs in the mammalian inner ear can be subdivided into three functional groups. The classification is based on spontaneous discharge rate (SR; i.e., the spike rate in the absence of sound), because it is easy to quantify, but the key functional differences are in the sensitivity to sound. High-SR fibers have the lowest thresholds, low-SR have the highest thresholds, and medium SR thresholds are intermediate between the two (**Figure 2A**). The distribution of SRs is fundamentally bimodal (**Figure 2B**) with roughly 40% in the lower peak (SR < about 18 spikes/second), which includes both low-SR and medium-SR fibers (15% and 25% of all ANFs, respectively) and 60% in the higher peak (Liberman, 1978). In this paper, we shall use the term lower-SR ANFs to refer jointly to the low- and medium-SR groups, which are sometimes distinguished in the literature.

Anatomical studies suggest that all three ANF types can innervate the same IHC, however, lower-SR fibers have thinner axons, fewer mitochondria, and tend to synapse on the modiolar side of the IHC. In contrast, high-SR fibers have thicker axons, more mitochondria, and synapse on the pillar side (Liberman, 1982). There are also systematic differences in the sizes of pre-synaptic ribbons and post-synaptic glutamate-receptor patches (Liberman et al., 2011). All three ANF types send their central axons to the cochlear nucleus (CN), where they branch, sending collaterals to the anteroventral, posteroventral, and dorsal subdivisions. Although branches from all SR types are present in each

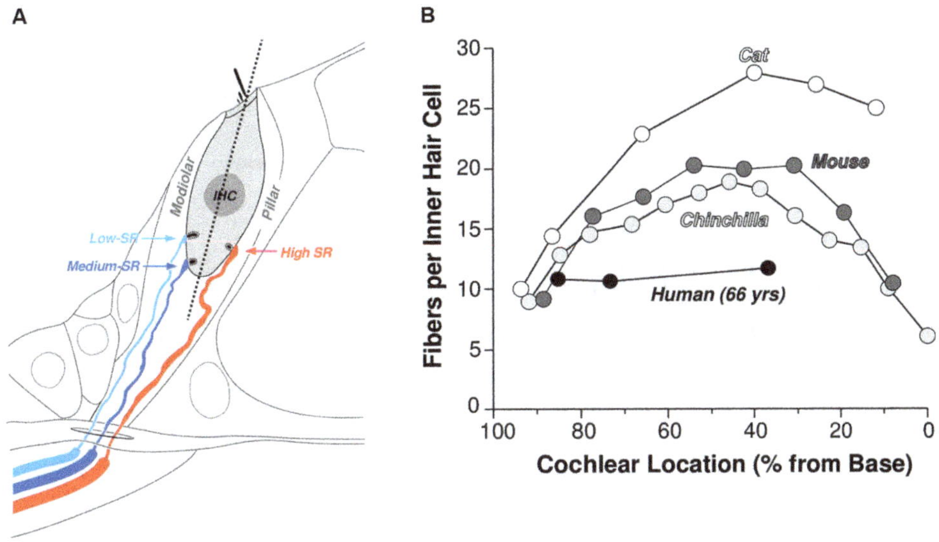

FIGURE 1 | Innervation of the IHCs by terminals of the cochlear nerve. (A) Schematic illustrating the spatial separation of the synaptic contacts of high- (SR > about 18 spikes/s) vs. medium- and low-SR fibers on the pillar vs. modiolar sides of the IHCs, respectively. **(B)** Counts of cochlear nerve terminals per IHCs as a function of cochlear location from four mammalian species: cat (Liberman et al., 1990), mouse (Maison et al., 2013), chinchilla (Bohne et al., 1982) and human (Nadol, 1983).

CN subdivision, low- and medium-SR fibers give rise to more endings than high-SR fibers, especially in the small-cell cap of the anteroventral CN (Ryugo and Rouiller, 1988; Liberman, 1991). Hence, lower-SR fibers may have more downstream influence than suggested by the fact that they make up less than half of the population at the level of the auditory nerve (AN).

The diversity of ANF threshold sensitivity is believed to be important in intensity coding in the auditory system, where level discrimination abilities are near-constant over a range of 100 dB or more (Florentine et al., 1987; Viemeister, 1988). This large dynamic range may be mediated, at least in part, by the differing dynamic ranges of low-, medium-, and high-SR fibers. As represented in **Figure 2C**, high-SR fibers, whose response thresholds are at or near behavioral detection threshold, likely determine the ability to detect sounds in a quiet environment. However, 20–30 dB above threshold, their discharge rate saturates. By virtue of their higher thresholds and extended dynamic ranges, the lower-SR fibers may be particularly important for extending the dynamic range of hearing. Possibly more important is their contribution to hearing in a noisy environment. Activity of high-SR fibers is relatively easy to mask with continuous noise, as schematized in **Figure 2D**. Because they are so sensitive to sound, even near-threshold noise increases the background discharge rate of high-SR fibers. This continuous activation causes synaptic fatigue (i.e., vesicle depletion) and thus also decreases their maximum discharge rate to tone bursts or other transient signals that might be present (Costalupes et al., 1984; Costalupes, 1985). By virtue of their higher thresholds, the lower-SR fibers are more resistant to background noise. Thus with increasing levels of continuous broadband masking noise, lower-SR fibers likely become increasingly important to the encoding of acoustic signals, because they will increasingly show the largest changes in average discharge rate in response to transient supra-threshold stimuli (**Figure 2D**; also see Young and Barta, 1986).

TEMPORAL CODING AND ITS IMPORTANCE FOR AUDITORY PERCEPTION

As a result of cochlear filtering, each ANF is driven by a narrow frequency band of sound energy. Thus, the temporal information encoded by the ANFs can be logically separated into two parts; the temporal fine-structure (TFS), corresponding to the timing of the nearly sinusoidal narrowband carrier fluctuations, and the slower temporal envelope of that carrier, whose temporal fluctuations are limited by the bandwidth of the corresponding cochlear filter. For low-frequency cochlear channels, ANFs convey both TFS and envelope information; neural spikes are phase-locked to the carrier and the instantaneous firing rate follows the envelope. At higher frequencies, ANFs do not phase lock to the TFS; however, responses convey temporal information by phase locking to envelope fluctuations.

Although different perceptual attributes of natural sound are encoded by different spectro-temporal cues, many depend on reliable timing information. For instance, the computation of interaural time differences (ITD), important for spatial perception of sound, requires temporal precision on the order of tens of microseconds (Blauert, 1997). While perceptually, TFS information in low-frequencies is the dominant perceptual cue determining perceived location (at least in anechoic conditions; Wightman and Kistler, 1992), for broadband and high-frequency sounds, ITDs can be conveyed by the envelope alone. Moreover, high-frequency envelope ITDs can be perceived nearly as precisely as low-frequency TFS ITDs (Bernstein and Trahiotis, 2002). In addition, envelopes may play a significant role in space perception in everyday settings such as rooms, where reverberant energy

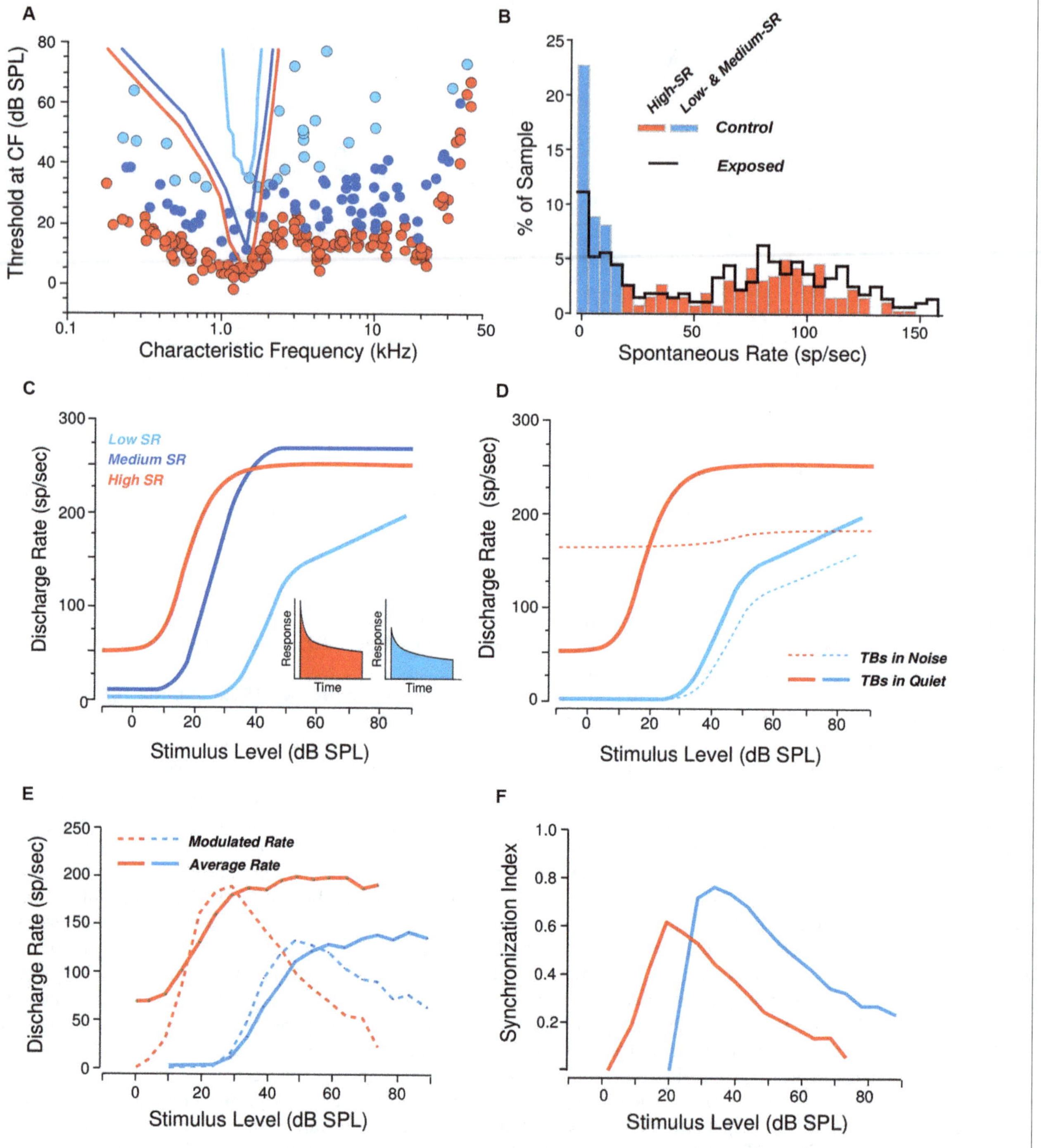

FIGURE 2 | Response differences among cochlear nerve fibers of the three SR groups. (A) Threshold tuning curves of example high- medium- and low-SR fibers (see key in **C**) are superimposed on a scatterplot of thresholds at the characteristic frequency (CF) for all the fibers sampled from one animal. Data from cat (Liberman, 1978). **(B)** Distribution of spontaneous rates in large samples of cochlear nerve fibers before (red and blue bars) vs. after (black line) a noise exposure causing a reversible elevation of thresholds. Data from guinea pig (Furman et al., 2013). **(C, D)** Schematic rate-vs-level functions for high-, medium-, and low-SR fibers to tone bursts (TBs) at the CF, in quiet **(C)** and in continuous background noise at a fixed 0 dB spectrum level **(D)**. Data from cat (Liberman, 1978; Costalupes et al., 1984). The insets in panel **C** show schematic peri-stimulus time histograms of the response to a moderate-level tone burst: onset rates are higher in the high-SR fiber than in the low-SR fiber. **(E, F)** Responses to SAM tones in high- vs. low-SR fibers expressed as average rate and modulated rate **(E)** or average synchrony (**F**; see text for definitions). Responses are to carrier tones at the CF, amplitude modulated (AM) at 100 Hz. Data from cat (Joris and Yin, 1992).

distorts TFS cues (Bharadwaj et al., 2013; Dietz et al., 2013). The coherence of the temporal envelope across channels helps to perceptually bind together different acoustic constituents of an "object" in the auditory scene (Elhilali et al., 2009; Shamma et al., 2011). Coding of pitch and speech formants also may rely, at least in part, on both TFS and envelope temporal information, although the precision needed to convey this information is less than that needed to extract ITDs (see Plack et al., 2005 for a review). On an even slower time scale, speech meaning is conveyed by fluctuations in energy through time. Thus, a range of temporal features in both TFS and envelopes are necessary to enable a listener to parse the cacophonous mixture of sounds in which they commonly find themselves, select a sound source of interest, and analyze its meaning. Importantly, almost all of these tasks, when performed in everyday settings, require analysis of temporal information at supra-threshold sound intensities.

To exacerbate matters, everyday settings typically contain competing sound sources and reverberant energy. Both degrade the temporal structure of the sound reaching a listener's ears, reducing the depth of signal modulations and interfering with the interaural temporal cues in an acoustic signal. If amplitude modulation is weakly coded in a listener with cochlear neuropathy, degradations in the input signal modulations due to competing sound and reverberant energy may render spatial information diffuse and ambiguous, pitch muddy, and speech less intelligible (e.g., see Stellmack et al., 2010; Jørgensen and Dau, 2011). TFS cues convey information important for speech intelligibility in noise (Lorenzi and Moore, 2008). Envelope cues are important for speech-on-speech masking release (Christiansen et al., 2013). Given all of this, a listener with degraded coding of envelope and TFS is most likely to notice perceptual difficulties when trying to understand speech in challenging settings, even if they do not notice any other deficits and have no difficulty in quiet environments. Thus, we hypothesize that differences in the fidelity with which the auditory system encodes supra-threshold TFS and amplitude modulation accounts for some of the inter-subject differences that NHT listeners exhibit in tasks such as understanding speech in noise or directing selective auditory attention (also See Section Human Data Consistent with the Neuropathy Hypothesis). Based on this idea, we argue that a method for measuring supra-threshold temporal coding fidelity may have important clinical applications, enabling quantification of supra-threshold hearing deficits that affect how well listeners operate in everyday environments, but that are not commonly recognized today.

CONSEQUENCES OF COCHLEAR NEUROPATHY FOR TEMPORAL CODING

One consequence of cochlear neuropathy (i.e., a reduction in the number of ANFs conveying sound) will be a reduction in the fidelity of temporal coding of supra-threshold sound. For instance, convergence of multiple, stochastic ANF inputs leads to enhanced temporal precision in the firing pattern of many CN cells (e.g., see Joris et al., 1994; Oertel et al., 2000). Thus, a reduction in the overall number of ANFs will reduce the precision with which both TFS and envelope temporal information are conveyed to higher centers (see also Lopez-Poveda and Barrios, 2013). While the importance of TFS coding for various aspects of sound perception cannot be overstated, we only briefly discuss TFS coding here. We focus primarily on the implications of cochlear neuropathy on the fidelity with which envelope information is conveyed. This focus is motivated particularly by recent data from guinea pigs and mice that suggest that noise-induced neuropathy preferentially damages the higher-threshold, lower-SR cochlear nerve fibers (Furman et al., 2013), rendering envelope coding especially vulnerable, as explained below.

Damage to lower-SR ANFs is likely to be especially detrimental to supra-threshold coding of sound envelopes, as high-SR fibers cannot robustly encode envelope timing cues in sounds at comfortable listening levels. Specifically, the average firing rate of high-SR ANFs (ignoring the temporal pattern of the response) saturates at levels roughly 20–30 dB above threshold, around the sound level of comfortable conversation (see red solid line in **Figure 2E**). In addition, both measures of phase locking to the envelope (namely the modulated rate, which is the magnitude of the frequency domain representation of the post-stimulus time histogram of the ANF response, evaluated at the fundamental frequency of the input signal; see dashed red line in **Figure 2E**) and the synchronization index (also known as the vector strength, calculated as the modulated rate normalized by one half of the average rate; see red line in **Figure 2F**) of high-SR neurons drop off as sound levels approach and exceed comfortable listening levels. This drop off is particularly detrimental for relatively intense sounds with shallow modulation depths, where both the crests and troughs of the envelope of the signal driving the high-SR ANFs fall in the saturation range of intensities, resulting in relatively poor modulation in the temporal response of these fibers (Joris and Yin, 1992). In contrast, lower-SR fibers are more likely to encode these envelope fluctuations because they are likely to be at an operating point where the firing rate (in the steady–state) is still sensitive to fluctuations in the sound level. If noise exposure causes a selective neuropathy that preferentially affects lower-SR fibers, then the ability to analyze envelopes at conversational sound levels is likely to be impaired. Both theoretical simulations and preliminary experimental evidence from envelope following responses (EFRs, described in Section Objective Measures of Subcortical Temporal Coding) recorded in mice and humans are consistent with this reasoning, as discussed in Section Evidence for Cochlear Neuropathy.

OBJECTIVE MEASURES OF SUBCORTICAL TEMPORAL CODING

Many psychophysical studies have been devoted to the development and discussion of behavioral measures to assess temporal coding in both NHT and hearing-impaired listeners (see Moore, 2003; Strelcyk and Dau, 2009). On the other hand, SSSRs provide an objective window into how the subcortical nuclei of the ascending auditory pathway encode temporal information in sound. While behavioral characterizations are important indicators of everyday hearing ability, in order to limit the length and scope of this opinion paper and still provide substantial discussion, here we focus on objective, physiological measures that can quantify the temporal coding precision of supra-threshold sound in the individual listener. Such measures may also be helpful in identifying some of the mechanisms that lead to individual differences in behavioral ability.

SSSRs refer to the scalp-recorded responses originating from subcortical portions of the auditory nervous system. These responses phase lock both to periodicities in the acoustic waveform and to periodicities induced by cochlear processing (Glaser et al., 1976). SSSRs are related to auditory brainstem responses (ABRs; the stereotypical responses to sound onsets and offsets; Jewett et al., 1970); however, whereas ABRs are transient responses to sound onsets and offsets, SSSRs are sustained responses to ongoing sounds that can include responses phase locked to both the fine structure and the cochlear-induced envelopes of broadband sounds. SSSRs have been used extensively in basic neurophysiologic investigation of auditory function and sound encoding (e.g., Kuwada et al., 1986; Aiken and Picton, 2008; Gockel et al., 2011; also see Krishnan, 2006; Chandrasekaran and Kraus, 2010, for reviews). Given the frequency specificity possible with SSSRs, they have also been proposed as a potential tool for objective clinical audiometry (Lins et al., 1996). In addition, SSSRs have been shown to be sensitive to deafferentation in that IHC loss leads to degraded SSSRs, especially at moderate sound levels (Arnold and Burkard, 2002).

While there are many studies of SSSRs, confusingly, different branches of the scientific literature use different names to refer to the same kinds of measurements. Periodic responses to amplitude-modulated sounds originating from both the subcortical and cortical portions of the auditory pathway are often collectively referred to as auditory steady-state responses (ASSRs) (Galambos et al., 1981; Stapells et al., 1984; Rees et al., 1986). However, brainstem SSSRs can be distinguished from responses generated at the cortical level by virtue of their relatively high frequency content; practically speaking, cortical and SSSR responses can be extracted from the same raw scalp recordings by appropriate filtering (e.g., see Krishnan et al., 2012; Bharadwaj and Shinn-Cunningham, 2014). The responses that specifically phase lock to the envelope of amplitude modulated (AM) sounds have been referred to as EFRs or amplitude modulation following responses (AMFRs; Dolphin and Mountain, 1992; Kuwada et al., 2002). In the recent literature, SSSRs are most commonly referred to as frequency following responses (FFRs), a term originally used to denote responses phase locked to pure tones (Marsh et al., 1975). Since the term FFR hints that responses are phase locked to the acoustic frequency content of input sound (i.e., the fine-structure of narrowband or locally narrowband sounds), here we will use the term "SSSR" to describe the sustained responses originating from subcortical portions (at frequencies >80 Hz or so in humans) of the auditory pathway. More specifically, we will focus on EFRs: SSSRs that are locked to the envelope.

While EFRs provide a convenient non-invasive measure of subcortical envelope coding, there are several difficulties in interpreting them. First, they represent neural activity that is the sum of a large population of neurons, filtered by layers of brain tissue, skull, and scalp. Depending on the stimulus parameters, thousands of neurons in each of multiple subcortical nuclei may contribute to the EFR (Kuwada et al., 2002). Neurons from several regions along the tonotopic axis could contribute to the EFR for high-level sounds due to spread of excitation, even for narrow-band sounds. Thus, relating EFR results to physiological responses of single neurons is not straightforward. ANF modulation frequency responses are uniformly low pass; high characteristic frequencies (CFs) fibers (>10 kHz) have cutoff frequencies around 1 kHz in cat (Joris and Yin, 1992). Below 10 kHz, cutoff frequency is dependent on CF, suggesting a limit imposed by an interaction between the content of the input signal and the bandwidths of cochlear filters (Joris and Yin, 1992). As signals ascend the auditory pathway, they are transformed from a temporal to a rate code, with the upper limit of phase locking progressively shifting to lower modulation frequencies (summarized in Figure 9 of Joris et al., 2004; see also Frisina et al., 1990; Joris and Yin, 1992; Krishna and Semple, 2000; Nelson and Carney, 2004). Modulation frequencies in the 70 to 200 Hz range elicit phase-locked responses in a cascade of subcortical auditory structures, from cochlear hair cells to inferior colliculus (IC) neurons, suggesting that many sources can contribute to the EFRs in this frequency range. Luckily, compared to the IC, the more peripheral EFR generators generate relatively weak responses, both because they drive smaller synchronous neural populations and because they are more distant from the measurement site.

Based on single-unit data, reversible inactivation studies, irreversible lesion studies, and studies analyzing EFR group delay, it has been argued that the dominant generators of the EFR move from caudal (AN and CN) to rostral (inferior colliculus or IC) as modulation frequency decreases (Sohmer et al., 1977; Dolphin and Mountain, 1992; Kiren et al., 1994; Herdman et al., 2002; Kuwada et al., 2002). These studies provide evidence that the IC dominates EFRs at modulation frequencies between about 70 and 200 Hz, in all species tested. Changes in the slope of the response phase vs. input modulation frequency can be used to calculate apparent latency of the sources and thereby infer changes in the relative strengths of different neural generators in the mixture (Kuwada et al., 2002); regions where the slope is constant indicate regions where the mixture of generators is constant. Above 200 Hz, the pattern of these changes varies across species, probably due to differing head sizes and shapes. Humans, rabbits, and mice exhibit regions of constant phase slopes out to 500, 700, and 1000 Hz, respectively (Kuwada et al., 2002; Purcell et al., 2004; Pauli-Magnus et al., 2007); in contrast, in gerbils, the phase slopes above 200 Hz are not constant (Dolphin and Mountain, 1992). These differences in phase slopes indicate that the specificity of EFRs is species-dependent. However, in all species it is clear that manipulation of modulation frequency can be used to bias responses towards more rostral or more caudal sources.

Despite these complications, all acoustic information is conveyed to the brain through the ANFs; moreover, deficiencies at the level of the ANF can be expected to have an effect downstream, in higher-order processing centers. Therefore, EFRs originating in the brainstem/mid-brain are likely to reflect the consequences of ANF neuropathy. Indeed, by using different stimuli, it may be possible to emphasize the contribution of different subcortical sources (by changing the modulation frequency of the input) or different portions of the cochlear partition (by changing the acoustic carrier of the signal). In particular, metrics such as the phase-locking value (PLV) can be calculated to quantify the robustness of temporal coding in the EFR, akin to using the vector-strength to assess temporal coding in single-unit physiology studies (Joris et al., 2004).

When analyzing the temporal precision of signals, the PLV has a straightforward interpretation. The details of the PLV computation and its statistical properties are described in a number of previous studies (e.g., see Lachaux et al., 1999; Bokil et al., 2007; Ruggles et al., 2011; Zhu et al., 2013). Briefly, the PLV quantifies the consistency of the response phase across repetitions of the stimulus presentation ("trials"). For a given frequency bin, the response to each trial can be represented as a unit vector (phasor) in the complex plane whose phase equals the response phase. The PLV then equals the magnitude (length) of the vector average of the phasors, averaged across trials (**Figure 3A**). If the response is consistently at or near a fixed phase, then the resulting average has a magnitude near one and the PLV is high (top panel, **Figure 3A**). On the other hand, if the response phase relative to the stimulus is random over the unit circle, the phasors cancel, the resultant vector has a small magnitude, and the PLV is near zero (bottom panel of **Figure 3A**). An example of the PLV spectrum (computed for EFRs from 400 repetitions of a 100 Hz transposed tone at a carrier frequency of 4 kHz and 65 dB SPL) is shown in **Figure 3C**. Strong peaks are evident at the fundamental and harmonic frequencies of the envelope. The PLV thus is one way of assessing the temporal coding fidelity of the EFR, and of subcortical encoding of supra-threshold sound.

EVIDENCE FOR COCHLEAR NEUROPATHY

NEUROPATHY AND SELECTIVE LOSS OF LOWER-SPONTANEOUS DISCHARGE RATE FIBERS IN ANIMALS

Recent studies in both mice and guinea pigs show that noise exposure that causes a *temporary* increase in threshold sensitivity (e.g., initial threshold elevations of as much as 40 dB that completely recover over 3–5 days) nevertheless can cause a rapid loss of 40–50% of the ANF synapses on IHCs as well as a slow death of the ANF cell bodies (spiral ganglion cells) and central axons (Kujawa and Liberman, 2009; Maison et al., 2013). Despite

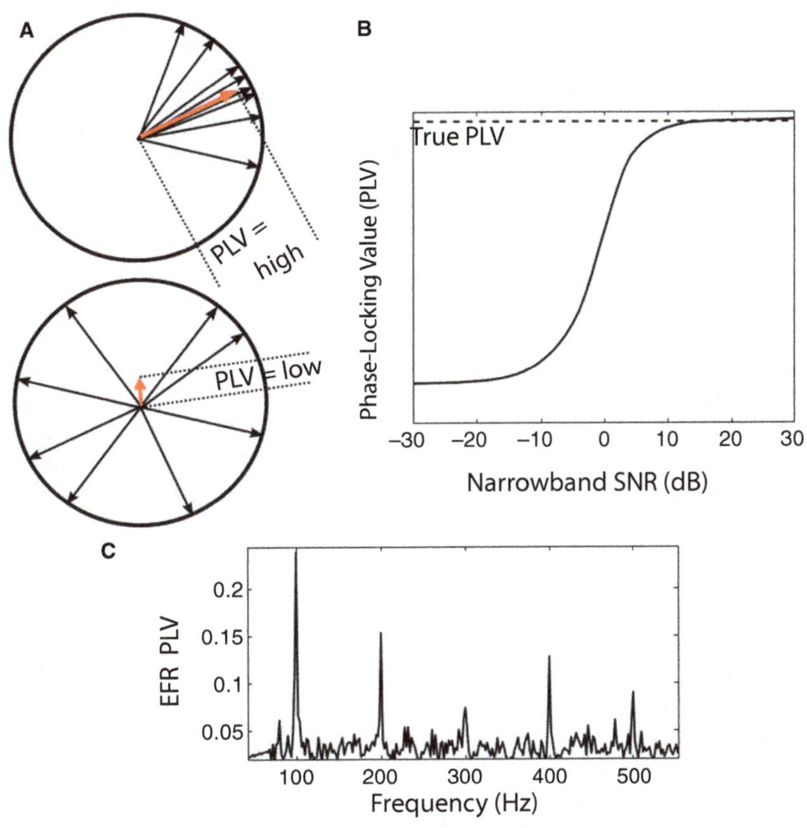

FIGURE 3 | (A) An illustration of the PLV metric computation. The SSSR from each trial is represented by a vector (phasor, shown as a black arrow) with unit magnitude and with phase equal to the EFR phase at the frequency bin of analysis. The vector average of these phasors is computed; the magnitude of the resultant vector (shown as red arrow) yields the PLV. The top panel is an example with high PLV: the phase of the responses varies over a narrow range across trials. The bottom panel is an example with low PLV: response phase relative to stimulus onset is essentially random over the unit circle. **(B)** Relationship between the single-trial SNR of the measurement in the frequency bin of interest and the estimated PLV for a simulated signal in additive noise. At sufficiently high SNR values, the estimated PLV converges to the true PLV (aside from a small sample bias that depends on the number of trials). At lower SNRs, the estimate is biased to be lower than the true value. This is an important consideration when comparing PLVs across sound levels or individuals, since the SNR depends on the magnitude of the true underlying response, the geometry of the generators, and the volume conductor in between. **(C)** Sample PLV spectrum obtained in response to a 100 Hz transposed tone at a carrier frequency of 4 kHz at 65 dB SPL (RMS). Strong peaks are evident in the PLV at multiples of the envelope frequency.

the extent of effects of such exposure on synapses and ganglion cells, it does not typically cause any loss of hair cells. Single-unit recordings in the guinea pig indicate that this noise-induced loss is selective for lower-SR fibers (Furman et al., 2013). Pharmacological studies suggest that this neuropathy is the result of a type of glutamate excitotoxicity, brought on by glutamate overload at particularly active synapses (Pujol et al., 1993). In the central nervous system, glutamate excitotoxicity is mediated by an increase in intracellular calcium concentration (Szydlowska and Tymianski, 2010). Since mitochondria comprise an important intracellular calcium buffering system, the relative paucity of mitochondria in the lower-SR fibers (Liberman, 1980) may contribute to their special vulnerability to glutamate excitotoxicity caused by noise exposure.

In aging mice, there is a steady degeneration of ANFs. Indeed, 30–40% of IHC synapses are lost by roughly 3/4 of the lifespan, an age at which threshold elevation is modest (typically less than 10 dB), but there is no significant loss of hair cells (Sergeyenko et al., 2013). Previous neurophysiological studies of age-related hearing loss in the gerbil suggest that this neurodegeneration is also selective for lower-SR fibers (Schmiedt et al., 1996). Unfortunately, relatively little is known about how aging impacts ANF synapses in humans. The only study that counted IHC synapses in the human inner ear (**Figure 1B**) found relatively low numbers of IHC synapses; however, this low count may reflect a significant degree of age-related neuropathy rather than a species difference, given that the tissue was obtained from a relatively old individual (63 years of age). Indeed, counts of spiral ganglion cells in an age-graded series of human temporal bones show degeneration of 30%, on average, from birth to death, even in cases with no hair cell loss (Makary et al., 2011). The marked delay between synaptic death and spiral ganglion cell death (1–2 years in mouse, and possibly much longer in humans) suggests that the loss of cochlear nerve synapses on IHCs is almost certainly significantly greater than 30%, on average, in the aged human ear.

Considering that only a small number of sensitive, intact ANFs may be needed for detection in quiet (Lobarinas et al., 2013), it seems likely that even considerable neuropathy would not change thresholds for tones in quiet, and thus would not be detected by standard threshold audiometry. This is even more likely the case if the neuropathy is selective for ANFs with higher thresholds, which are not active near perceptual thresholds. It also seems likely that a loss of a large population of high-threshold ANFs could dramatically affect auditory performance on complex tasks that require analysis of supra-threshold sound content, such as those requiring the extraction of precise timing cues or extracting a signal in a noisy environment, as discussed above. Thus, we hypothesize that cochlear neuropathy in general—and possibly selective neuropathy of high threshold fibers in particular—is one of the reasons that aging often is found to degrade human performance on tasks requiring analysis of the content of supra-threshold sound.

HUMAN DATA CONSISTENT WITH THE NEUROPATHY HYPOTHESIS

While there is no human data yet to directly support the neuropathy hypothesis, a series of studies from our lab are consistent with the hypothesis that cochlear neuropathy causes difficulties with coding of supra-threshold sound for humans and accounts for some of the individual variability seen in listeners with normal audiometric thresholds. NHT listeners exhibit marked differences in how well they can utilize precise temporal information to direct selective attention, from near-chance levels to almost perfect performance (Ruggles and Shinn-Cunningham, 2011). As discussed in Section Consequences of Cochlear Neuropathy for Temporal Coding, cochlear neuropathy could result in degraded coding of both TFS and envelope information. In line with this hypothesis, differences in EFR phase locking accounts for some of this inter-subject variability in performance. **Figure 4A** shows the relationship between performance in a spatial attention task in reverberation and the PLV calculated from EFRs obtained separately (data from Ruggles et al., 2011, 2012). Pooled over age groups, listeners with higher EFR phase locking performed better in the selective attention task (Kendall *tau* = 0.42, $p < 0.002$). Though age by itself did not correlate with performance in anechoic conditions, when temporal cues in the acoustic mixture were degraded by adding reverberation, middle-aged listeners showed a bigger drop in performance than younger listeners (Ruggles et al., 2012), as if timing cues are encoded less robustly in middle-aged listeners than in young adults. In addition, as shown in **Figure 4B**, performance also correlated with thresholds for low-rate frequency modulation (FM) detection, a task known to rely on robust temporal coding of TFS (Kendall *tau* = 0.5, $p = 0.001$, data from Ruggles et al., 2011, 2012). Crucially, all listeners in these studies had pure-tone audiometric thresholds of 15 dB HL or better at octave frequencies between 250 Hz and 8 kHz. The small differences in hearing threshold (within the NHT range) that did exist were not correlated with selective attention performance; similarly, reading span test scores (a measure of cognitive ability) were unrelated to performance. These results suggest that both TFS and envelope cues are important in everyday listening under challenging conditions, since individuals with poor TFS and envelope coding (as measured by FM detection thresholds and EFR phase locking respectively) perform poorly in a spatial attention task. (For a complete description of the spatial attention task, the FM detection task and the EFR measures, see Ruggles et al., 2011, 2012).

Several other studies have reported that some listeners with normal thresholds (particularly older participants) perform poorly on certain behavioral tasks, sometimes even on par with hearing-impaired subjects. Yet other studies show that temporal processing of both TFS and envelope degrades with aging and manifests independently of hearing loss (see Fitzgibbons and Gordon-Salant, 2010 for a review). In NHT listeners, sensitivity to ITD varies greatly across the population, with some listeners performing as poorly as older hearing-impaired subjects (see Grose and Mamo, 2010; Strelcyk and Dau, 2009). Recent studies have also demonstrated abnormal speech processing among hearing-impaired listeners even when the frequency content of the speech was limited to regions where thresholds are normal, pointing towards supra-threshold coding deficits (Horwitz et al., 2002; Lorenzi et al., 2009; Léger et al., 2012).

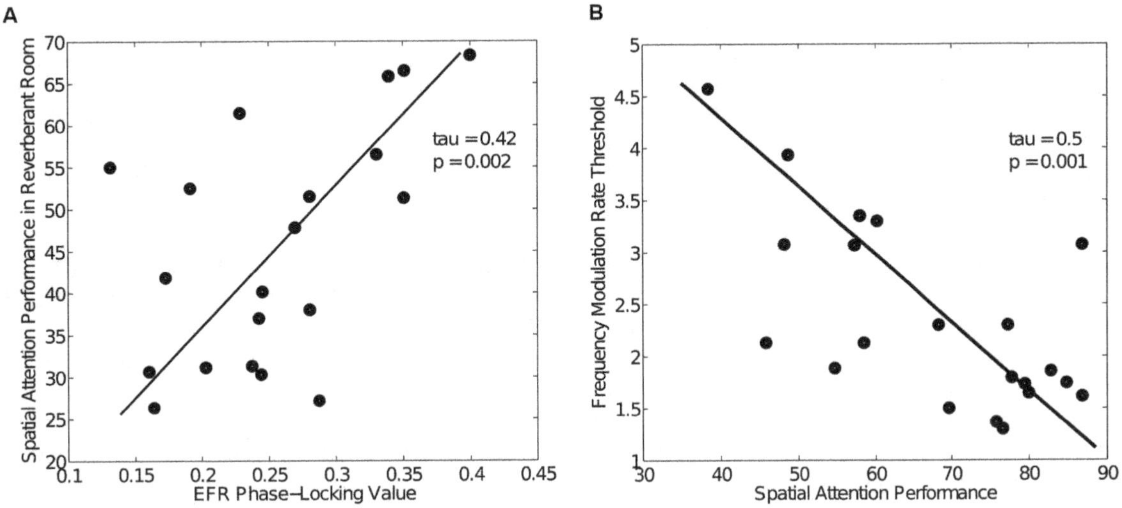

FIGURE 4 | Human behavioral and EFR data (data from Ruggles et al., 2011, 2012) showing large variability in both performance and temporal coding fidelity among NHT participants. (A) Relationship between spatial attention task performance in reverberation and EFR PLV across NHT listeners. Task performance varied from chance levels (30%) to about 70% with a concomitant variation in EFR phase locking. Listeners with good temporal coding of envelopes as measured by the EFR PLV were able to spatially segregate the competing speech streams and performed well. **(B)** Relationship between spatial attention task performance and frequency modulation (FM) detection thresholds (data from Ruggles et al., 2011), a task known to rely on robust encoding of TFS.

Older listeners also have been shown to exhibit deficits specific to envelope processing across a range of tasks, including speech recognition in the presence of modulated noise maskers (Dubno et al., 2003; Gifford et al., 2007) and temporal modulation sensitivity (Purcell et al., 2004; He et al., 2008). Consistent with this, the highest modulation frequency to which EFRs exhibit phase locking decreases with age (Purcell et al., 2004; Leigh-Paffenroth and Fowler, 2006; Grose et al., 2009), supporting the hypothesis that the robustness of supra-threshold modulation coding is reduced with aging. Using measures of both gap detection and word recognition on a sizeable cohort of young and old listeners, Snell and Frisina (2000) concluded that age-related changes in auditory processing occur throughout adulthood. Specifically, they concluded that deficits in temporal acuity may begin decades earlier than age-related changes in word recognition. Though not direct evidence that neuropathy causes these perceptual difficulties, these results are consistent with our hypothesis, especially given animal data suggesting that both aging and noise-exposure degrade ANF responses (especialy lower-SR fibers) and degrade supra-threshold temporal coding without affecting thresholds (Schmiedt et al., 1996; Kujawa and Liberman, 2009; Lin et al., 2011; Furman et al., 2013). If neuropathy underlies deficits in temporal encoding that predict behavioral differences, it may be possible to develop even more sensitive physiological metrics to capture an individual listener's supra-threshold coding fidelity. Section Diagnosing Cochlear Neuropathy is devoted to the discussion of this idea.

DIAGNOSING COCHLEAR NEUROPATHY

The degree of deafferentation in cochlear neuropathy can be studied directly in animals using invasive methods in combination with histological evaluation, or in humans using post-mortem studies (e.g., Halpin and Rauch, 2009; Makary et al., 2011). However, assessment in behaving humans must be non-invasive, and therefore must employ indirect methods. Given that neuropathy should impact supra-threshold temporal coding, individual behavioral assessment of envelope and TFS coding of sound at comfortable listening levels may prove useful in assessing neuropathy. In order to expose supra-threshold deficits and individual differences, selective attention tasks in adverse conditions (e.g., in a noise background or in a complex, crowded scene) may be most effective. However, given that aging and noise exposure cause outer hair cell loss, elevated thresholds, and other (much-studied) effects, assessment of cochlear function is necessary to ensure that supra-threshold deficits are attributable to neuropathy. Measures of brainstem temporal coding, like the ABR and SSSR, may be helpful in assessing neuropathy objectively and passively; exploring these metrics at high sound levels and low modulation depths (which stresses coding of modulations akin to those important when listening in a crowded scene) may be particularly useful (see Section Emphasizing the Contribution of Lower-Spontaneous Discharge Rate Auditory Nerve Fibers to the Envelope Following Responses). In order to develop and interpret effective, sensitive tests using these types of non-invasive physiological measures, quantitative models that provide testable predictions will be vital. In this section, we consider some of these points, with a focus on objective measures.

MEASURING BRAINSTEM CODING: AUDITORY BRAINSTEM RESPONSES VS. SUBCORTICAL STEADY-STATE RESPONSES

In animal work, the preferential loss of higher-threshold (lower-SR fibers) leads to a decrease in the supra-threshold growth of the amplitude of wave I of the ABR, without a change in ABR threshold (Kujawa and Liberman, 2009; Furman et al., 2013). In both noise-exposed mice and noise-exposed guinea pigs, the proportional decrement in the magnitude of wave I at high levels (i.e., 80 dB SPL) closely corresponds to the percentage of loss of auditory-nerve synapses. However, by limiting the analysis to animals without permanent threshold shifts in the noise-exposed ear, these experiments remove the confound that changes in hearing threshold are likely to affect wave I amplitude; by design, the supra-threshold changes in ABR amplitude found in these experiments cannot be due to differences in threshold sensitivity, but instead reflect differences in the number of fibers responding to supra-threshold sound. Even in populations with normal thresholds, inter-subject variability in ABR amplitudes complicates analysis. One past study showed that in age- and gender-matched mice, the variance in normal ABR amplitude measures is relatively low (Kujawa and Liberman, 2009); however, the mice in this study were genetically identical. In age- and gender-matched guinea pigs, the variance in ABR amplitude is significantly higher. In the genetically heterogeneous guinea pigs, neuropathy-related changes in ABR amplitude are revealed clearly only when data are analyzed within subject, measuring the effects of noise exposure by normalizing the post-trauma amplitude responses by the responses from the same ear before exposure (Furman et al., 2013). Of course, such a before-and-after approach is unlikely to prove useful for human clinical testing, except in extraordinarily rare circumstances.

The above studies suggest that the ABR may be useful for assessing neuropathy. However, there are a number of reasons why the electrophysiological responses to an AM carrier tone, i.e., the EFR, might be better suited to the assessment of lower-SR neuropathy than the ABR. For one thing, ABR wave I, generated by tone pips, is proportional to the size of the onset responses in the AN. Since, as schematized in **Figure 2C**, the onset responses of lower-SR fibers are small compared to high-SR fiber onset responses (Taberner and Liberman, 2005; Buran et al., 2010), they make a relatively small contribution to the total onset response, rendering the metric fairly insensitive to the integrity of the lower-SR population. In contrast, the steady-state rates of the three SR groups are of more similar magnitude; a loss of lower-SR fibers should thus cause a greater change in steady-state measures like the SSSR or EFR than transient responses like the ABR. Furthermore, as noted above (see **Figure 2F**), lower-SR ANFs synchronize more tightly to the envelope of an AM tone than their high-SR counterparts, especially at moderate and high sound intensities (Johnson, 1980; Joris and Yin, 1992). Synchronization in response to AM-tones can be assessed both by the modulated rate (the amplitude of the peri-stimulus time histogram at the stimulus modulation frequency) and synchronization index (or vector strength; see Joris et al., 2004 for a discussion about different measures of envelope coding). The synchronization index of lower-SR fibers can be larger than that of high-SR fibers of similar best frequency. Indeed, preliminary results suggest that in noise-exposed mice, amplitude decrements in EFR responses to an amplitude-modulated carrier tone presented at the frequency region of maximum cochlear neuropathy are a more sensitive measure of deficit than decrements in ABR wave I amplitude (Shaheen et al., 2013). Perhaps more importantly, a phase-based analysis like the PLV can be used to analyze EFR strength, which can be a more robust and more easily interpreted metric than amplitude measures of these far-field potentials, which have a weak signal-to-noise ratio (SNR) and depend on factors such as tissue and head geometry.

EMPHASIZING THE CONTRIBUTION OF LOWER- SPONTANEOUS DISCHARGE RATE AUDITORY NERVE FIBERS TO THE ENVELOPE FOLLOWING RESPONSE

As previously discussed (Section Temporal Coding and Its Importance for Auditory Perception), one likely consequence of cochlear neuropathy is a reduction in the fidelity of temporal coding in the brainstem. The idea that cochlear neuropathy may preferentially target lower-SR fibers (Schmiedt et al., 1996; Furman et al., 2013) may be exploited to devise EFR measures that are more likely to capture the effects of neuropathy. Focusing on responses to high-frequency envelopes could prove to be an effective way to assess neuropathy, because envelope fluctuations cannot drive saturated high-SR fibers effectively. Even for "transposed tones" (a modulated high-frequency signal whose envelope mimics the rectified sinusoidal drive of a low-frequency tone operating at low-frequency portions of the cochlea; see van de Par and Kohlrausch, 1997), phase locking of high-SR fibers is reduced at mid to high sound levels (Dreyer and Delgutte, 2006). This effect is likely to be particularly strong for a relatively high-intensity modulated signal with a shallow modulation depth. For such signals, the input intensity of the driving signal will fall within the saturation range of high-SR fibers at all moments; the only fibers that could encode the shallow modulations are the lower-SR fibers. Thus, measures of EFR phase locking to high-frequency, high-intensity, amplitude-modulated signals with shallow modulation may be especially sensitive when assessing lower-SR-fiber status.

Here, we use a simple model of brainstem responses to illustrate why EFRs to shallow amplitude modulations and high sound levels are likely to emphasize the contribution of lower-SR fiber responses to the measurements. Given that EFR responses reflect responses at the level of the brainstem/midbrain, likely the IC, we built a model of IC responses (**Figure 5A**) by combining an established model of the ANF responses (Zilany and Bruce, 2006; Zilany et al., 2009) with previous phenomenological models of amplitude-modulation processing in the IC (Nelson and Carney, 2004). Updated, humanized, ANF model parameters were used for the simulation (Zilany et al., 2014). This model has been shown to predict ANF single-unit envelope response data quite well (Joris and Yin, 1992). Considering that the simulations included stimuli with high sound levels (as in Dau, 2003; Rønne et al., 2012), a tonotopic array of ANFs (and corresponding IC cells) were included to allow for off-frequency contributions. ANFs with 50 CFs uniformly spaced along the basilar membrane according to a place-frequency map were simulated. For each CF, lower- and high-SR fibers were simulated. In order to obtain a population response at the level of the IC, responses to IC cells driven by lower- and high-SR ANFs were averaged with weights

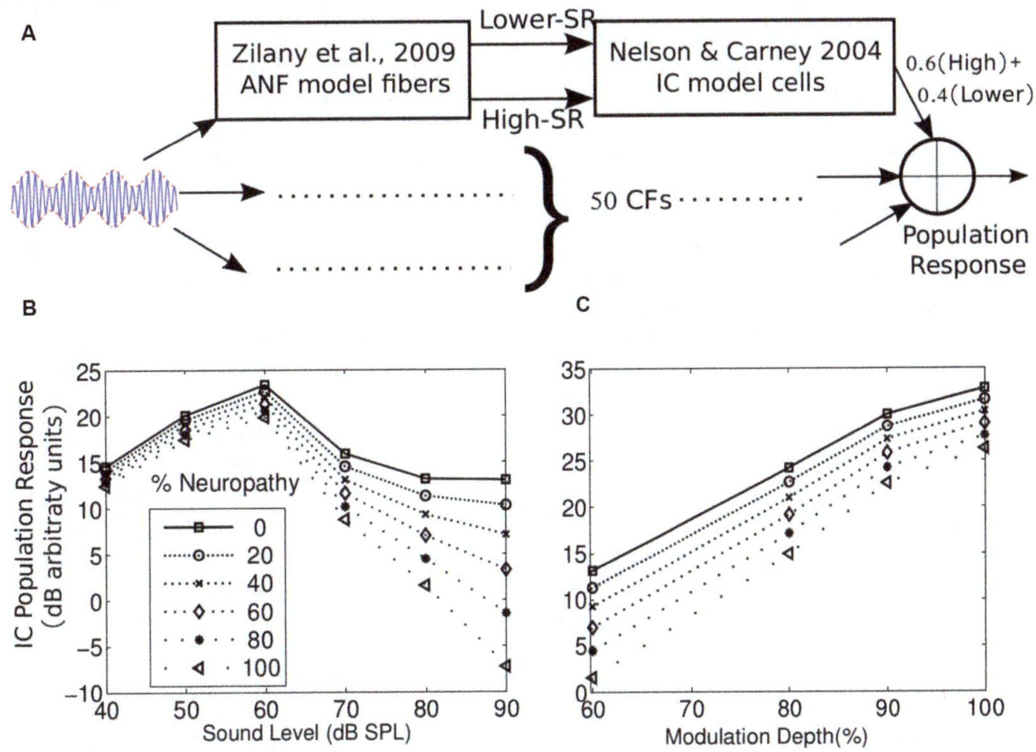

FIGURE 5 | (A) A parsimonious model of the population response of IC cells to envelope fluctuations. The model comprised of ANFs (simulated using the Zilany et al., 2009 model) driving the cochlear nucleus (CN), which in turn drives the IC. CN and IC processing of envelope were simulated using the Nelson and Carney (2004) model. A tonotopic array of 50 CFs was used. High- and lower-SR ANFs were simulated at each CF and the corresponding IC responses were combined with weigths equal to the proportion of each group in the population (60% High- and 40% Lower-SR, Liberman, 1978). Neuropathy was simulated by reducing the weight given to the lower-SR driven response. **(B)** Level curves for the population response with different levels of neuropathy for a 100 Hz SAM tone at 4 kHz, with a 60% modulation depth and added broadband noise with a notch centered around 4 kHz and 800 Hz wide on each side. The SNR was fixed at 20 dB (broadband RMS) at all levels. The differences between the levels of neuropathy are most accentuated in the population response at higher stimulus levels. This also suggests that slopes of the level curve at high levels may reflect the level of neuropathy. **(C)** Population response as a function of modulation depth for different levels of neuropathy for an 80 dB SPL SAM tone in notched noise (SNR = 20 dB broadband RMS). The differences between the levels of neuropathy are more evident for smaller modulation depths. In addition, this suggests that the slope of the population response strength as a function of modulation depth may be sensitive to the level of neuropathy.

proportional to known population ratios (40% Lower-SR fibers and 60% high-SR fibers, see Liberman, 1978). At the level of the IC, the resulting population response is treated as a proxy for the signal driving the EFR. Responses were simulated for a sinusoidally amplitude modulated (SAM) tone with a carrier frequency of 4 kHz and a modulation frequency of 100 Hz. In order to attenuate the contribution of off-frequency neurons to the population response, a broadband noise masker with a notch centered at 4 kHz and extending 800 Hz on either side was added to the SAM tone, as can be done with real EFR measurements in the laboratory. The SNR for the simulations was fixed at 20 dB (broadband root mean square (RMS)). The IC model parameters were set to the values used in Nelson and Carney (2004), which ensured that the 100 Hz modulation frequency was within the band-pass range of the IC cells. Neuropathy was simulated by progressively attenuating the weights given to the IC population driven by lower-SR ANFs, leaving the high-SR population unchanged.

Figure 5 shows the absolute population response magnitude following the 100 Hz modulation in logarithmic units. Results are shown for different amounts of neuropathy, both for different stimulus levels (**Figure 5B**) and for different modulation depths (**Figure 5C**). As seen from the figures, neuropathy has the greatest effect on the population response for stimuli at mid to high sound levels and relatively low modulation depths. This is consistent with the idea that the modulated firing rate of high-SR ANFs is drastically attenuated at moderate to high sound levels and low-modulation depths (Joris and Yin, 1992; Dreyer and Delgutte, 2006). Similar results were obtained (not shown) presenting "transposed" tones to this model as well as when using the Rønne et al. (2012) model, where the EFR is obtained by convolving the ANF population response with a "unitary-response" that is designed to aggregate and approximate all transformations of the ANF population response before being recorded in the EFR. In both model approaches, lower- and high-SR ANF driven IC responses were summed linearly to generate the population response. When the lower- and high-SR ANF responses were mixed non-linearly using a coincidence detection process (i.e., a geometric average instead of an arithmetic average) before being delivered to the IC model, the effects of the lower-SR fiber neuropathy were even larger (not shown).

This analysis supports the idea that EFR responses to shallow amplitude modulation at high levels may provide a sensitive, objective correlate of neuropathy. Apart from emphasizing the contribution of lower-SR ANFs, high sound levels are more likely to reveal differences in the number of intact ANFs even if neuropathy is not specific to lower-SR fibers because larger populations of ANFs are recruited overall. These results are also consistent with the report that the ABR wave I amplitude in noise-exposed mice closely corresponds to the amount of neuropathy when the sound level is high (80 dB, Furman et al., 2013) as well as preliminary data from our lab that suggest that individual differences in the EFR are largest at high stimulus levels (Bharadwaj et al., 2013). In addition, inspection of **Figure 5B, C** suggests that the sizes of the change (i.e., slopes) in the population response with level and with modulation depth both reflect the level of neuropathy. Thus, either of these changes, along with behavioral measures, could be used to assess the ability of the listener to process supra-threshold sound. However, in practice, manipulating modulation depth with the level fixed at a high value may lead to more easily interpreted results than measuring how the EFR changes with overall level (see Section Using Envelope Following Responses to Assess Supra-threshold Coding Fidelity). As explained above, we suggest that individual listeners with normal audiometric thresholds could differ in the number of intact ANFs due to differences in noise exposure, genetic predisposition to hearing damage, and other factors. Given the already-discussed importance of supra-threshold temporal coding for operating in everyday social settings (understanding speech in noise, directing selective auditory attention, etc.), assessment of neuropathy by measurement of EFRs may have a place in audiological practice, especially because such measures are objective and can be recorded passively (making them suitable for use with special populations in which behavioral assessment is not easy).

ISOLATING COCHLEAR NEUROPATHY

As noted above, in order to assess neuropathy, it is critical to rule out or otherwise account for cochlear dysfunction. One of the most basic characteristics of cochlear function is the frequency selectivity of the basilar membrane (BM). BM frequency selectivity is correlated with cochlear gain at low sound levels (Shera et al., 2002, 2010) and typically decreases with hearing impairment. BM frequency selectivity can be estimated psychophysically (Patterson, 1976; Glasberg and Moore, 1990; Oxenham and Shera, 2003); however, it is possible that such measures may include small contributions from extra-cochlear factors (such as neuropathy). Alternatively, distortion product otoacoustic emissions (DPOAEs) in response to fixed-level primaries (DPgrams; e.g., see Lonsbury-Martin and Martin, 2007) can be used to assess cochlear function. Because OAEs are generated within the cochlea as a consequence of outer-hair-cell activity and do not depend on afferent processing, measuring them may be preferable to measuring psychophysical tuning curve measures. Specifically, normal DPgrams can be used to establish that poor supra-threshold coding arises post transduction (e.g., via cochlear neuropathy) rather than from outer-hair-cell loss or other problems with cochlear amplification (an approach taken in the animal studies of Kujawa and Liberman, 2009; Furman et al., 2013). To test that cochlear compression is intact at the frequencies tested, either stimulus-frequency OAEs (SFOAEs; Schairer et al., 2006) or DPOAE growth functions can be used (Kummer et al., 1998; Neely et al., 2003). DPOAE suppression tuning curves (Gorga et al., 2011; Gruhlke et al., 2012) or SFOAE phase gradients at low stimulus levels (Shera et al., 2002) can provide estimates of cochlear filter tuning. Henry and Heinz (2012) recently demonstrated the importance of considering differences in cochlear function in order to interpret differences in measures of temporal coding fidelity properly. As this work shows, establishing that participants have normal cochlear sensitivity by measuring both OAEs and audiometric thresholds is crucial when trying to attribute individual differences in SSSRs and psychoacoustic measures to deficits in supra-threshold coding of sound due to neuropathy.

FUTURE EXPERIMENTS

A growing body of evidence suggests that (1) NHT listeners vary significantly in how well their auditory systems encode supra-threshold sound; and (2) Noise exposure and aging can lead to considerable amounts of neuropathy without affecting audiometric thresholds. We have argued that cochlear neuropathy in general, and selective neuropathy of lower-SR ANFs in particular, may help explain some of the supra-threshold differences in NHT listeners. Although we believe that the diversity of evidence consistent with this hypothesis is compelling, further experiments are necessary to truly establish these ideas and to understand potential implications for audiological practice. Here, we propose a few key areas that we believe merit future investigation.

ACCOUNTING FOR INDIVIDUAL DIFFERENCES IN COCHLEAR FUNCTION

As discussed in Section Isolating Cochlear Neuropathy, experiments seeking to implicate cochlear neuropathy in human perception must account for individual differences in cochlear processing. There are a number of objective metrics of cochlear health including DPOAE and SFOAE growth functions (Kummer et al., 1998; Schairer et al., 2006), DPOAE suppression tuning curves (Gorga et al., 2011; Gruhlke et al., 2012), and SFOAE group delay measurements (Shera et al., 2002; Shera and Bergevin, 2012). However, there are practical concerns that may limit the utility of many of these methods. For instance, using OAE methods to study neuropathy in patients with elevated hearing thresholds may be difficult, as SFOAE amplitudes critically depend on cochlear gain (Shera and Guinan, 1999). DPOAE methods depend more on cochlear compression, rather than cochlear gain (Shera and Guinan, 1999), and thus may prove to be a more robust method for assessing contributions of cochlear function to perception in heterogeneous subject populations (Gruhlke et al., 2012). Experiments are needed to determine what tests best quantify cochlear function, enabling such factors to be teased out when appraising cochlear neuropathy, and developing such tests into clinically useful tools.

DEVELOPING QUANTITATIVE MODELS OF ENVELOPE FOLLOWING RESPONSE GENERATORS

Because any human measurements of EFRs only indirectly reflect the responses of ANFs, quantitative models of the subcortical generators of the measured response are critical for understanding results and using them to quantify supra-threshold envelope coding. Data suggest that EFRs primarily reflect responses from the mid-brain, and are dominated by responses in the IC (Smith et al., 1975; Sohmer et al., 1977; Dolphin and Mountain, 1992; Kiren et al., 1994; Herdman et al., 2002). However, further experiments are needed to assess if current physiological models capture the behavior of real EFRs. When applied to modulated high-frequency sounds, simple models of IC responses predict a graded loss in the population response with cochlear neuropathy (see **Figure 5**), consistent with the idea that the observed heterogeneity of EFR responses in NHT subjects reflects, in part, differences in ANF survival. Instead of modeling individual neurons, others have modeled brainstem responses (ABRs and FFRs) directly using a kernel method (e.g., Dau, 2003; Rønne et al., 2012). In this approach, all subsequent transformations of the AN responses are modeled by a linear system approximation; model AN responses are used to deconvolve click-ABRs to obtain a "unitary response" that aggregates all of the transformations occurring from the nerve through to the electrode (including processing within the midbrain nuclei and any summation and filtering influencing what is recorded on the scalp). Despite the obvious simplifying assumptions of such an approach, model predictions capture many of the observed properties of ABRs and FFRs in response to simple stimuli. A slightly more elaborate model of EFRs that combines both these approaches (taking into account single-unit level phenomena such as in the model in **Figure 5** as well as scalp-recording properties of the measurements as in Dau, 2003), may be considered. For instance, one recent study explored the consequences of cochlear sensitivity and selective cochlear neuropathy on the latency of simulated ABR responses (Verhulst et al., 2013). Further development, testing, and refinement will ensure that results of EFR experiments are interpreted appropriately in the context of these models. Hence, we identify this as a key area for future efforts devoted to interpreting EFR measures.

USING ENVELOPE FOLLOWING RESPONSES TO ASSESS SUPRA-THRESHOLD CODING FIDELITY

A selective loss of lower-SR fibers would likely cause phase locking of the EFR to degrade at high sound levels, in line with the model results presented here (**Figure 5B**). As suggested in **Figure 5**, if neuropathy underlies some supra-threshold deficits, the rate of change of the EFR PLV with sound level (akin to the rate of change of ABR wave I in Furman et al., 2013) would correlate with perceptual abilities on tasks requiring analysis of the envelope of supra-threshold sounds, such as envelope ITD discrimination, spatial selective auditory attention, and related tasks. Preliminary data support this idea (Bharadwaj et al., 2013). Further experiments are needed to corroborate our hypothesis that neuropathy (especially neuropathy that preferentially affects lower-SR fibers) contributes to individual differences in the ability to analyze complex auditory scenes. The use of narrowband stimuli such as transposed tones (van de Par and Kohlrausch, 1997) with off-frequency maskers may allow for a frequency specific assessment of EFR phase locking at different CFs (i.e., at different frequency channels of the auditory pathway). If the neuropathy hypothesis proves correct, this approach may allow for a frequency-specific diagnosis of cochlear neuropathy from non-invasive physiological measures.

Despite the potential of EFRs (especially the EFR-intensity slope) for assessing cochlear neuropathy, there are some limitations. The EFR is a measure of multi-source population activity and produces scalp potentials that are different mixtures of the source activity at different scalp locations. These measures depend on the geometry of the generators, properties of the recording electrodes, the volume conductor in between, the level of unrelated electrical activity from cortex and from muscles, and other subject-specific factors (Hubbard et al., 1971; Okada et al., 1997). All of these parameters cause inter-subject variability in the absolute magnitudes of the measured EFRs. This makes interpretation of the raw EFR magnitude difficult. While phase-based metrics such as the PLV are normalized and have a straightforward interpretation (Zhu et al., 2013), their absolute strength is still influenced by the same factors. Specifically, PLV estimates are biased by the within-band SNR in the raw responses that go into the PLV computation.

This is illustrated in **Figure 3B**, which shows the relationship between estimated and true PLVs for simulated data (signal phase drawn from a von Mises distribution with known concentration and additive noise) as a function of SNR, under the assumptions that the noise phase in any trial is independent of the signal phase (something that can be guaranteed experimentally by jittering the stimulus presentation across trials). In **Figure 3B**, at sufficiently high SNRs, the estimated PLVs converge to the true PLV of the simulated signal, and are insensitive to absolute magnitudes of both signal and noise. However, at intermediate SNR values, the EFR PLV estimates are negatively biased (see Bharadwaj and Shinn-Cunningham, 2014). This has implications when trying to account for individual differences across subjects, whose raw responses may well have different SNRs. Even in within-subject comparisons, if two experimental manipulations produce responses with very different SNRs, the values of the EFR PLVs will have different biases. This is particularly important when assessing the change in PLV as a function of sound level, since high-level sounds are likely to produce stronger responses (higher SNR measurements) than low-level sounds. While an increase in response power at the stimulus modulation frequency is meaningful in itself, it is not easy to dissociate increases in PLV that result from increases in response synchrony (phase consistency) vs. from increases in response level. Minimally, using recordings in the absence of stimuli might serve to provide estimates of background noise and SNR that can then be used to extract metrics to compare fairly across subjects and conditions. How important and robust such corrections will prove depends in no small part on where on the SNR curve a particular experimental measurement falls (**Figure 3B**). Additional experiments are needed to characterize these effects in human listeners across different types of stimuli and experimental procedures.

Another limitation is that physiologically, the change in the basilar membrane excitation pattern with sound level also complicates the interpretation of both EFR and psychophysical results. In particular, when seeking to assess cochlear neuropathy within a specific frequency channel using PLV-level growth curves, effects of the spread of excitation are a confounding factor. Use of off-frequency maskers such as notched noise may ameliorate these effects. However, it has also been reported that at least for mid-frequency stimuli (around 1 kHz), the SSSR at the stimulus component frequency can be attenuated by noise even if the peripheral interaction between the signal and the masking noise is expected to be minimal (Gockel et al., 2012).

Alternately, EFRs can be measured in response to narrow-band stimuli with a fixed peak pressure presented at different modulation depths. For deep modulations, high-SR fibers can entrain to the modulation. At shallow modulation depths with a high sound level (carrier level), even the valleys in the signal will have sufficient energy to keep high-SR fibers saturated; thus, the strength of phase locking to shallow modulations may better reflect the contribution of lower-SR ANFs. By computing how the EFR PLV strength changes as the modulation depth is reduced, the spread-of-excitation confounds associated with manipulating the stimulus level may be avoided. Moreover, the approach of fixing the peak sound pressure and progressively decreasing the modulation depth serves to fix the point of operation on the ANF rate-level curve, so that any reduction in PLV with decreasing modulation depth can be interpreted as being related to a drop in synchrony rather than a change in average rate causing a lower SNR. The model results in **Figure 5C** are consistent with this notion. However, as discussed in Section Developing Quantitative Models of EFR Generators, further work is needed to relate EFR results to physiological responses of single neurons. These issues further underscore the importance of combining electrophysiological, behavioral, and modeling approaches.

SUMMARY AND CONCLUSIONS

Human listeners with normal audiometric thresholds exhibit large differences in their ability to process supra-threshold sound features. These differences can be exposed in the laboratory by challenging behavioral tasks that necessitate the use of temporal information in supra-threshold sound (e.g., segregating and selecting one auditory object out of a complex scene). While some NHT listeners seek audiological help for difficulties of this sort (a population labeled as having APD), a significant percentage of ordinary, NHT listeners recruited for psychophysical studies in the laboratory, none of whom have known hearing problems, show similar deficits under carefully designed, challenging conditions. These observations hint that perceptual problems with supra-threshold sounds are more widespread than is currently appreciated and that there may be a continuum of abilities across NHT listeners, amongst those who seek audiological help and amongst the general population.

Recent animal work shows that noise exposure and aging can result in a loss of significant proportion of ANFs without any permanent shift in detection thresholds. Moreover, this kind of neuropathy appears to preferentially affect lower-SR ANFs. Both physiological responses to AM stimuli in animals and simplistic computational model simulations suggest that lower-SR fiber loss will degrade temporal coding of sound envelopes at comfortable conversational levels, where high-SR fibers are saturated and therefore unable to entrain robustly to envelopes in input sounds.

A number of studies show that individual differences in the perception of supra-threshold sound are correlated with the strength of brainstem responses measured noninvasively on the scalp (especially SSSRs and EFRs driven by signal modulation). While the absolute strength of EFRs correlates with perceptual abilities, sensitivity of such physiological measures may be improved by using stimuli that mimic conditions akin to adverse listening conditions, such as high levels and shallow modulations. In addition, differential measures that consider how EFR phase locking changes with stimulus intensity or modulation depth may be especially sensitive when quantifying supra-threshold hearing status, helping to factor out other subject-specific differences unrelated to neuropathy. Interpretation of such measures requires assessment of cochlear function, as well as development of quantitative models of brainstem responses to establish the correspondence between population responses such as EFRs and single-unit physiology.

There are many challenges in trying to relate behavioral and EFR results to underlying physiological changes such as neuropathy, a number of which are due to gaps in current knowledge. However, converging evidence supports the hypothesis that deficits in supra-threshold coding fidelity are relatively common in the population of NHT listeners, and account for at least part of the important differences in how well these listeners can communicate in difficult everyday social settings. Here, we argue that the neuropathy seen in aging and noise-exposed animals may also be occurring in humans and that it may explain observed supra-threshold individual differences. We have also proposed some objective metrics that, based on our hypothesis, should be sensitive measures of the integrity of ANFs, allowing individual assessment of supra-threshold hearing status, and have discussed some of the limitations of the metrics. Still, there remains a large set of questions to be answered, ranging from what mechanisms cause synaptic loss that preferentially affects lower-SR fibers to what physiological or perceptual tests may be most sensitive for assessing neuropathy. We believe these questions should be addressed immediately, given the potential clinical significance of these ideas.

REFERENCES

Aiken, S. J., and Picton, T. W. (2008). Envelope and spectral frequency-following responses to vowel sounds. *Hear. Res.* 245, 35–47. doi: 10.1016/j.heares.2008.08.004

Alain, C., and Arnott, S. R. (2000). Selectively attending to auditory objects. *Front. Biosci.* 5, D202–D212. doi: 10.2741/alain

Arnold, S., and Burkard, R. (2002). Inner hair cell loss and steady-state potentials from the inferior colliculus and auditory cortex of the chinchilla. *J. Acoust. Soc. Am.* 112, 590–599. doi: 10.1121/1.1494991

Bernstein, L. R., and Trahiotis, C. (2002). Enhancing sensitivity to interaural delays at high frequencies by using "transposed stimuli". *J. Acoust. Soc. Am.* 112, 1026–1036. doi: 10.1121/1.1497620

Bharadwaj, H. M., Masud, M., and Shinn-Cunningham, B. G. (2013). Bottom-up and top-down contributions to individual differences in auditory spatial attention task performance. *Presented at the Abstracts of the Midwinter Meeting of the ARO XXXVI: #887.*

Bharadwaj, H. M., and Shinn-Cunningham, B. G. (2014). Rapid acquisition of auditory subcortical steady state responses using multichannel recordings. *Clin. Neurophysiol.* doi: 10.1016/j.clinph.2014.01.011. [Epub ahead of print].

Blauert, J. (1997). *Spatial Hearing: The Psychophysics of Human Sound Localization.* Cambridge, MA: MIT Press.

Bohne, B. A., Kenworthy, A., and Carr, C. D. (1982). Density of myelinated nerve fibers in the chinchilla cochlea. *J. Acoust. Soc. Am.* 72, 102–107. doi: 10.1121/1.387994

Bokil, H., Purpura, K., Schoffelen, J. M., Thomson, D., and Mitra, P. (2007). Comparing spectra and coherences for groups of unequal size. *J. Neurosci. Methods* 159, 337–345. doi: 10.1016/j.jneumeth.2006.07.011

Bregman, A. S. (1990). *Auditory Scene Analysis: The Perceptual Organization of Sound.* Cambridge, MA: MIT Press.

Buran, B. N., Strenzke, N., Neef, A., Gundelfinger, E. D., Moser, T., and Liberman, M. C. (2010). Onset coding is degraded in auditory nerve fibers from mutant mice lacking synaptic ribbons. *J. Neurosci.* 30, 7587–7597. doi: 10.1523/JNEUROSCI.0389-10.2010

Carlyon, R. P. (2004). How the brain separates sounds. *Trends Cogn. Sci.* 8, 465–471. doi: 10.1016/j.tics.2004.08.008

Catts, H. W., Chermak, G. D., Craig, C. H., Johnston, J. R., Keith, R. W., Musiek, F. E., et al. (1996). Central auditory processing: current status of research and implications for clinical practice. *American Speech-Language-Hearing Association (ASHA) Working Group on Auditory Processing Disorders.* doi: 10.1044/policy.tr1996-00241

Chandrasekaran, B., and Kraus, N. (2010). The scalp-recorded brainstem response to speech: neural origins and plasticity. *Psychophysiology* 47, 236–246. doi: 10.1111/j.1469-8986.2009.00928.x

Chermak, G. D., and Musiek, F. E. (1997). *Central Auditory Processing Disorders: New Perspectives.* San Diego: Singular Publishing Group.

Christiansen, C., MacDonald, E. N., and Dau, T. (2013). Contribution of envelope periodicity to release from speech-on-speech masking. *J. Acoust. Soc. Am.* 134, 2197–2204. doi: 10.1121/1.4816409

Costalupes, J. A. (1985). Representation of tones in noise in the responses of auditory nerve fibers in cats. I. Comparison with detection thresholds. *J. Neurosci.* 5, 3261–3269.

Costalupes, J. A., Young, E. D., and Gibson, D. J. (1984). Effects of continuous noise backgrounds on rate response of auditory nerve fibers in cat. *J. Neurophysiol.* 51, 1326–1344.

Darwin, C. J., and Carlyon, R. P. (1995). "Auditory grouping," in *Hearing*, ed B. C. J. Moore (San Diego, CA: Academic Press), 387–424.

Dau, T. (2003). The importance of cochlear processing for the formation of auditory brainstem and frequency following responses. *J. Acoust. Soc. Am.* 113, 936–950. doi: 10.1121/1.1534833

Demanez, L., Boniver, V., Dony-Closon, B., Lhonneux-Ledoux, F., and Demanez, J. P. (2003). Central auditory processing disorders: some cohorts studies. *Acta Otorhinolaryngol. Belg.* 57, 291–299.

Dietz, M., Marquardt, T., Salminen, N. H., and McAlpine, D. (2013). Emphasis of spatial cues in the temporal fine structure during the rising segments of amplitude-modulated sounds. *Proc. Natl. Acad. Sci. U S A* 110, 15151–15156. doi: 10.1073/pnas.1309712110

Dolphin, W. F., and Mountain, D. C. (1992). The envelope following response: scalp potentials elicited in the Mongolian gerbil using sinusoidally AM acoustic signals. *Hear. Res.* 58, 70–78. doi: 10.1016/0378-5955(92)90010-k

Dreyer, A., and Delgutte, B. (2006). Phase locking of auditory-nerve fibers to the envelopes of high-frequency sounds: implications for sound localization. *J. Neurophysiol.* 96, 2327–2341. doi: 10.1152/jn.00326.2006

Dubno, J. R., Horwitz, A. R., and Ahlstrom, J. B. (2003). Recovery from prior stimulation: masking of speech by interrupted noise for younger and older adults with normal hearing. *J. Acoust. Soc. Am.* 113, 2084–2094. doi: 10.1121/1.1555611

Elhilali, M., Ma, L., Micheyl, C., Oxenham, A. J., and Shamma, S. A. (2009). Temporal coherence in the perceptual organization and cortical representation of auditory scenes. *Neuron* 61, 317–329. doi: 10.1016/j.neuron.2008.12.005

Fitzgibbons, P. J., and Gordon-Salant, S. (2010). "Behavioral studies with aging humans: hearing sensitivity and psychoacoustics," in *The Aging Auditory System*, eds S. Gordon-Salant, R. D. Frisina, A. N. Popper and R. R. Fay (New York: Springer), 111–134.

Florentine, M., Buus, S., and Mason, C. R. (1987). Level discrimination as a function of level for tones from 0.25 to 16 kHz. *J. Acoust. Soc. Am.* 81, 1528–1541. doi: 10.1121/1.394505

Frisina, R. D., Smith, R. L., and Chamberlain, S. C. (1990). Encoding of amplitude modulation in the gerbil cochlear nucleus: I. A hierarchy of enhancement. *Hear. Res.* 44, 99–122. doi: 10.1016/0378-5955(90)90074-y

Furman, A. C., Kujawa, S. G., and Liberman, M. C. (2013). Noise-induced cochlear neuropathy is selective for fibers with low spontaneous rates. *J. Neurophysiol.* 110, 577–586. doi: 10.1152/jn.00164.2013

Galambos, R., Makeig, S., and Talmachoff, P. J. (1981). A 40-Hz auditory potential recorded from the human scalp. *Proc. Natl. Acad. Sci. U S A* 78, 2643–2647. doi: 10.1073/pnas.78.4.2643

Gifford, R. H., Bacon, S. P., and Williams, E. J. (2007). An examination of speech recognition in a modulated background and of forward masking in younger and older listeners. *J. Speech Lang. Hear. Res.* 50, 857–864. doi: 10.1044/1092-4388(2007/060)

Glasberg, B. R., and Moore, B. C. (1990). Derivation of auditory filter shapes from notched-noise data. *Hear. Res.* 47, 103–138. doi: 10.1016/0378-5955(90)90170-t

Glaser, E. M., Suter, C. M., Dasheiff, R., and Goldberg, A. (1976). The human frequency-following response: its behavior during continuous tone and tone burst stimulation. *Electroencephalogr. Clin. Neurophysiol.* 40, 25–32. doi: 10.1016/0013-4694(76)90176-0

Gockel, H. E., Carlyon, R. P., Mehta, A., and Plack, C. J. (2011). The frequency following response (FFR) may reflect pitch-bearing information but is not a direct representation of pitch. *J. Assoc. Res. Otolaryngol.* 12, 767–782. doi: 10.1007/s10162-011-0284-1

Gockel, H. E., Farooq, R., Muhammed, L., Plack, C. J., and Carlyon, R. P. (2012). Differences between psychoacoustic and frequency following response measures of distortion tone level and masking. *J. Acoust. Soc. Am.* 132, 2524–2535. doi: 10.1121/1.4751541

Gorga, M. P., Neely, S. T., Kopun, J., and Tan, H. (2011). Distortion-product otoacoustic emission suppression tuning curves in humans. *J. Acoust. Soc. Am.* 129, 817–827. doi: 10.1121/1.3531864

Grose, J. H., and Mamo, S. K. (2010). Processing of temporal fine structure as a function of age. *Ear Hear.* 31, 755–760. doi: 10.1097/aud.0b013e3181e627e7

Grose, J. H., Mamo, S. K., and Hall III, J. W. (2009). Age effects in temporal envelope processing: speech unmasking and auditory steady state responses. *Ear Hear.* 30, 568–575. doi: 10.1097/aud.0b013e3181ac128f

Gruhlke, A., Birkholz, C., Neely, S. T., Kopun, J., Tan, H., Jesteadt, W., et al. (2012). Distortion-product otoacoustic emission suppression tuning curves in hearing-impaired humans. *J. Acoust. Soc. Am.* 132, 3292–3304. doi: 10.1121/1.4754525

Halpin, C., and Rauch, S. D. (2009). Hearing aids and cochlear damage: the case against fitting the pure tone audiogram. *Otolaryngol. Head Neck Surg.* 140, 629–632. doi: 10.1016/j.otohns.2008.12.020

He, N. J., Mills, J. H., Ahlstrom, J. B., and Dubno, J. R. (2008). Age-related differences in the temporal modulation transfer function with pure-tone carriers. *J. Acoust. Soc. Am.* 124, 3841–3849. doi: 10.1121/1.2998779

Henry, K. S., and Heinz, M. G. (2012). Diminished temporal coding with sensorineural hearing loss emerges in background noise. *Nat. Neurosci.* 15, 1362–1364. doi: 10.1038/nn.3216

Herdman, A. T., Lins, O., Van Roon, P., Stapells, D. R., Scherg, M., and Picton, T. W. (2002). Intracerebral sources of human auditory steady-state responses. *Brain Topogr.* 15, 69–86. doi: 10.1023/A:1021470822922

Hind, S. E., Haines-Bazrafshan, R., Benton, C. L., Brassington, W., Towle, B., and Moore, D. R. (2011). Prevalence of clinical referrals having hearing thresholds within normal limits. *Int. J. Audiol.* 50, 708–716. doi: 10.3109/14992027.2011.582049

Horwitz, A. R., Dubno, J. R., and Ahlstrom, J. B. (2002). Recognition of low-pass-filtered consonants in noise with normal and impaired high-frequency hearing. *J. Acoust. Soc. Am.* 111, 409–416. doi: 10.1121/1.1427357

Hubbard, J. I., Llinas, R., and Quastel, D. M. J. (1971). Electrophysiological analysis of synaptic transmission. *Am. J. Phys. Med. Rehabil.* 50, 303.

Jewett, D. L., Romano, M. N., and Williston, J. S. (1970). Human auditory evoked potentials: possible brain stem components detected on the scalp. *Science* 167, 1517–1518. doi: 10.1126/science.167.3924.1517

Johnson, D. H. (1980). The relationship between spike rate and synchrony in responses of auditory nerve fibers to single tones. *J. Acoust. Soc. Am.* 68, 1115–1122. doi: 10.1121/1.384982

Jørgensen, S., and Dau, T. (2011). Predicting speech intelligibility based on the signal-to-noise envelope power ratio after modulation-frequency selective processing. *J. Acoust. Soc. Am.* 130, 1475–1487. doi: 10.1121/1.3621502

Joris, P. X., and Yin, T. C. (1992). Responses to amplitude-modulated tones in the auditory nerve of the cat. *J. Acoust. Soc. Am.* 91, 215–232. doi: 10.1121/1.402757

Joris, P. X., Carney, L. H., Smith, P. H., and Yin, T. C. (1994). Enhancement of neural synchronization in the anteroventral cochlear nucleus. I. Responses to tones at the characteristic frequency. *J. Neurophysiol.* 71, 1022–1036.

Joris, P. X., Schreiner, C. E., and Rees, A. (2004). Neural processing of amplitude-modulated sounds. *Physiol. Rev.* 84, 541–577. doi: 10.1152/physrev.00029.2003

Kiren, T., Aoyagi, M., Furuse, H., and Koike, Y. (1994). An experimental study on the generator of amplitude-modulation following response. *Acta Otolaryngol. Suppl.* 511, 28–33. doi: 10.3109/00016489409128297

Krishna, B. S., and Semple, M. N. (2000). Auditory temporal processing: responses to sinusoidally amplitude-modulated tones in the inferior colliculus. *J. Neurophysiol.* 84, 255–273.

Krishnan, A. (2006). "Frequency-following response," in *Auditory Evoked Potentials: Basic Principles and Clinical Application*, eds R. F. Burkard, M. Don and J. J. Eggermont (Philadelphia: Lippincott, Williams and Wilkins), 313–333.

Krishnan, A., Bidelman, G. M., Smalt, C. J., Ananthakrishnan, S., and Gandour, J. T. (2012). Relationship between brainstem, cortical and behavioral measures relevant to pitch salience in humans. *Neuropsychologia* 50, 2849–2859. doi: 10.1016/j.neuropsychologia.2012.08.013

Kujawa, S. G., and Liberman, M. C. (2009). Adding insult to injury: cochlear nerve degeneration after "temporary" noise-induced hearing loss. *J. Neurosci.* 29, 14077–14085. doi: 10.1523/jneurosci.2845-09.2009

Kummer, P., Janssen, T., and Arnold, W. (1998). The level and growth behavior of the 2 f1− f2 distortion product otoacoustic emission and its relationship to auditory sensitivity in normal hearing and cochlear hearing loss. *J. Acoust. Soc. Am.* 103, 3431–3444. doi: 10.1121/1.423054

Kuwada, S., Anderson, J. S., Batra, R., Fitzpatrick, D. C., Teissier, N., and D'Angelo, W. R. (2002). Sources of the scalp-recorded amplitude-modulation following response. *J. Am. Acad. Audiol.* 13, 188–204.

Kuwada, S., Batra, R., and Maher, V. L. (1986). Scalp potentials of normal and hearing-impaired subjects in response to sinusoidally amplitude-modulated tones. *Hear. Res.* 21, 179–192. doi: 10.1016/0378-5955(86)90038-9

Lachaux, J. P., Rodriguez, E., Martinerie, J., and Varela, F. J. (1999). Measuring phase synchrony in brain signals. *Hum. Brain Mapp.* 8, 194–208. doi: 10.1002/(sici)1097-0193(1999)8:4<194::aid-hbm4>3.0.co;2-c

Léger, A. C., Moore, B. C., and Lorenzi, C. (2012). Abnormal speech processing in frequency regions where absolute thresholds are normal for listeners with high-frequency hearing loss. *Hear. Res.* 294, 95–103. doi: 10.1016/j.heares.2012.10.002

Leigh-Paffenroth, E. D., and Fowler, C. G. (2006). Amplitude-modulated auditory steady-state responses in younger and older listeners. *J. Am. Acad. Audiol.* 17, 582–597. doi: 10.3766/jaaa.17.8.5

Liberman, M. C., Dodds, L. W., and Pierce, S. (1990). Afferent and efferent innervation of the cat cochlea: quantitative analysis with light and electron microscopy. *J. Comp. Neurol.* 301, 443–460. doi: 10.1002/cne.903010309

Liberman, L. D., Wang, H., and Liberman, M. C. (2011). Opposing gradients of ribbon size and AMPA receptor expression underlie sensitivity differences among cochlear-nerve/hair-cell synapses. *J. Neurosci.* 31, 801–808. doi: 10.1523/jneurosci.3389-10.2011

Liberman, M. C. (1978). Auditory-nerve response from cats raised in a low-noise chamber. *J. Acoust. Soc. Am.* 63, 442–455. doi: 10.1007/springerreference_113985

Liberman, M. C. (1980). Morphological differences among radial afferent fibers in the cat cochlea: an electron-microscopic study of serial sections. *Hear. Res.* 3, 45–63. doi: 10.1016/0378-5955(80)90007-6

Liberman, M. C. (1982). Single-neuron labeling in the cat auditory nerve. *Science* 216, 1239–1241. doi: 10.1126/science.7079757

Liberman, M. C. (1991). Central projections of auditory-nerve fibers of differing spontaneous rate. I. Anteroventral cochlear nucleus. *J. Comp. Neurol.* 313, 240–258.

Lin, H. W., Furman, A. C., Kujawa, S. G., and Liberman, M. C. (2011). Primary neural degeneration in the Guinea pig cochlea after reversible noise-induced threshold shift. *J. Assoc. Res. Otolaryngol.* 12, 605–616. doi: 10.1007/s10162-011-0277-0

Lins, O. G., Picton, T. W., Boucher, B. L., Durieux-Smith, A., Champagne, S. C., Moran, L. M., et al. (1996). Frequency-specific audiometry using steady-state responses. *Ear Hear.* 17, 81–96. doi: 10.1097/00003446-199604000-00001

Lobarinas, E., Salvi, R., and Ding, D. (2013). Insensitivity of the audiogram to carboplatin induced inner hair cell loss in chinchillas. *Hear. Res.* 302, 113–120. doi: 10.1016/j.heares.2013.03.012

Lonsbury-Martin, B. L., and Martin, G. K. (2007). "Distortion-product otoacoustic emissions in populations with normal hearing sensitivity," in *Otoacoustic Emissions Clinical Applications*, eds M. S. Robinette and T. J. Glattke (New York: Thieme Medical Publishers), 107–130.

Lopez-Poveda, E. A., and Barrios, P. (2013). Perception of stochastically undersampled sound waveforms: a model of auditory deafferentation. *Front. Neurosci.* 7:124. doi: 10.3389/fnins.2013.00124

Lorenzi, C., and Moore, B. C. J. (2008). Role of temporal envelope and fine structure cues in speech perception: a review, in *Auditory Signal Processing in Hearing-Impaired Listeners, First International Symposium on Auditory and Audiological Research (ISAAR 2007)*, eds T. Dau, J. M. Buchholz, J. M. Harte and T. U. Christiansen (Denmark: Centertryk).

Lorenzi, C., Debruille, L., Garnier, S., Fleuriot, P., and Moore, B. C. J. (2009). Abnormal processing of temporal fine structure in speech for frequencies where absolute thresholds are normal (L). *J. Acoust. Soc. Am.* 125, 27–30. doi: 10.1121/1.2939125

Maison, S. F., Usubuchi, H., and Liberman, M. C. (2013). Efferent feedback minimizes cochlear neuropathy from moderate noise exposure. *J. Neurosci.* 33, 5542–5552. doi: 10.1523/jneurosci.5027-12.2013

Makary, C. A., Shin, J., Kujawa, S. G., Liberman, M. C., and Merchant, S. N. (2011). Age-related primary cochlear neuronal degeneration in human temporal bones. *J. Assoc. Res. Otolaryngol.* 12, 711–717. doi: 10.1007/s10162-011-0283-2

Marsh, J. T., Brown, W. S., and Smith, J. C. (1975). Far-field recorded frequency-following responses: correlates of low pitch auditory perception in humans responses. *Electroencephalogr. Clin. Neurophysiol.* 38, 113–119. doi: 10.1016/0013-4694(75)90220-5

Moore, B. C. J. (2003). *An Introduction to the Psychology of Hearing.* 5th Edn. San Diego: Academic Press.

Nadol, J. B. Jr. (1983). Serial section reconstruction of the neural poles of hair cells in the human organ of Corti. I. Inner hair cells. *Laryngoscope* 93, 599–614. doi: 10.1288/00005537-198306000-00015

Neely, S. T., Gorga, M. P., and Dorn, P. A. (2003). Cochlear compression estimates from measurements of distortion-product otoacoustic emissions. *J. Acoust. Soc. Am.* 114, 1499–1507. doi: 10.1121/1.1604122

Nelson, P. C., and Carney, L. H. (2004). A phenomenological model of peripheral and central neural responses to amplitude-modulated tones. *J. Acoust. Soc. Am.* 116, 2173–2186. doi: 10.1121/1.1784442

Oertel, D., Bal, R., Gardner, S. M., Smith, P. H., and Joris, P. X. (2000). Detection of synchrony in the activity of auditory nerve fibers by octopus cells of the mammalian cochlear nucleus. *Proc. Natl. Acad. Sci. U S A* 97, 11773–11779. doi: 10.1073/pnas.97.22.11773

Okada, Y. C., Wu, J., and Kyuhou, S. (1997). Genesis of MEG signals in a mammalian CNS structure. *Electroencephalogr. Clin. Neurophysiol.* 103, 474–485. doi: 10.1016/s0013-4694(97)00043-6

Oxenham, A. J., and Shera, C. A. (2003). Estimates of human cochlear tuning at low levels using forward and simultaneous masking. *J. Assoc. Res. Otolaryngol.* 4, 541–554. doi: 10.1007/s10162-002-3058-y

Patterson, R. D. (1976). Auditory filter shapes derived with noise stimuli. *J. Acoust. Soc. Am.* 59, 640–654. doi: 10.1121/1.380914

Pauli-Magnus, D., Hoch, G., Strenzke, N., Anderson, S., Jentsch, T. J., and Moser, T. (2007). Detection and differentiation of sensorineural hearing loss in mice using auditory steady-state responses and transient auditory brainstem responses. *Neuroscience* 149, 673–684. doi: 10.1016/j.neuroscience.2007.08.010

Plack, C. J., Oxenham, A. J., Fay, R. R., and Popper, A. N. (2005). *Pitch Neural Coding and Perception*. (Vol. 24). New York: Springer.

Pujol, R., Puel, J. L., D'aldin, C. G., and Eybalin, M. (1993). Pathophysiology of the glutamatergic synapses in the cochlea. *Acta Otolaryngol.* 113, 330–334. doi: 10.3109/00016489309135819

Purcell, D. W., John, S. M., Schneider, B. A., and Picton, T. W. (2004). Human temporal auditory acuity as assessed by envelope following responses. *J. Acoust. Soc. Am.* 116, 3581–3593. doi: 10.1121/1.1798354

Rees, A., Green, G. G. R., and Kay, R. H. (1986). Steady-state evoked responses to sinusoidally amplitude-modulated sounds recorded in man. *Hear. Res.* 23, 123–133. doi: 10.1016/0378-5955(86)90009-2

Rønne, F. M., Dau, T., Harte, J., and Elberling, C. (2012). Modeling auditory evoked brainstem responses to transient stimuli. *J. Acoust. Soc. Am.* 131, 3903–3913. doi: 10.1121/1.3699171

Ruggles, D., and Shinn-Cunningham, B. (2011). Spatial selective auditory attention in the presence of reverberant energy: individual differences in normal-hearing listeners. *J. Assoc. Res. Otolaryngol.* 12, 395–405. doi: 10.1007/s10162-010-0254-z

Ruggles, D., Bharadwaj, H., and Shinn-Cunningham, B. G. (2011). Normal hearing is not enough to guarantee robust encoding of suprathreshold features important in everyday communication. *Proc. Natl. Acad. Sci. U S A* 108, 15516–15521. doi: 10.1073/pnas.1108912108

Ruggles, D., Bharadwaj, H., and Shinn-Cunningham, B. G. (2012). Why middle-aged listeners have trouble hearing in everyday settings. *Curr. Biol.* 22, 1417–1422. doi: 10.1016/j.cub.2012.05.025

Ryugo, D. K., and Rouiller, E. M. (1988). Central projections of intracellularly labeled auditory nerve fibers in cats: morphometric correlations with physiological properties. *J. Comp. Neurol.* 271, 130–142. doi: 10.1002/cne.902710113

Schairer, K. S., Ellison, J. C., Fitzpatrick, D., and Keefe, D. H. (2006). Use of stimulus-frequency otoacoustic emission latency and level to investigate cochlear mechanics in human ears. *J. Acoust. Soc. Am.* 120, 901–914. doi: 10.1121/1.2214147

Schmiedt, R. A., Mills, J. H., and Boettcher, F. A. (1996). Age-related loss of activity of auditory-nerve fibers. *J. Neurophysiol.* 76, 2799–2803.

Sergeyenko, Y., Lall, K., Liberman, M. C., and Kujawa, S. G. (2013). Age-Related cochlear synaptopathy: an early-onset contributor to auditory functional decline. *J. Neurosci.* 33, 13686–13694. doi: 10.1523/jneurosci.1783-13.2013

Shaheen, L. A., Delgutte, B., and Liberman, M. C. (2013). Using the auditory steady-state response to measure noise-induced auditory nerve degeneration. *Presented at the Abstracts of the Midwinter Meeting of the ARO XXXVI: #649.*

Shamma, S. A., Elhilali, M., and Micheyl, C. (2011). Temporal coherence and attention in auditory scene analysis. *Trends Neurosci.* 34, 114–123. doi: 10.1016/j.tins.2010.11.002

Shera, C. A., and Bergevin, C. (2012). Obtaining reliable phase-gradient delays from otoacoustic emission data. *J. Acoust. Soc. Am.* 132, 927–943. doi: 10.1121/1.4730916

Shera, C. A., and Guinan, J. J. Jr. (1999). Evoked otoacoustic emissions arise by two fundamentally different mechanisms: a taxonomy for mammalian OAEs. *J. Acoust. Soc. Am.* 105, 782–798. doi: 10.1121/1.426948

Shera, C. A., Guinan, J. J. Jr., and Oxenham, A. J. (2010). Otoacoustic estimation of cochlear tuning: validation in the chinchilla. *J. Assoc. Res. Otolaryngol.* 11, 343–365. doi: 10.1007/s10162-010-0217-4

Shera, C. A., Guinan, J. J., and Oxenham, A. J. (2002). Revised estimates of human cochlear tuning from otoacoustic and behavioral measurements. *Proc. Natl. Acad. Sci. U S A* 99, 3318–3323. doi: 10.1073/pnas.032675099

Shinn-Cunningham, B. G. (2008). Object-based auditory and visual attention. *Trends Cogn. Sci.* 12, 182–186. doi: 10.1016/j.tics.2008.02.003

Shinn-Cunningham, B. G., and Best, V. (2008). Selective attention in normal and impaired hearing. *Trends Amplif.* 12, 283–299. doi: 10.1177/1084713808325306

Smith, J. C., Marsh, J. T., and Brown, W. S. (1975). Far-field recorded frequency-following responses: evidence for the locus of brainstem sources. *Electroencephalogr. Clin. Neurophysiol.* 39, 465–472. doi: 10.1016/0013-4694(75)90047-4

Snell, K. B., and Frisina, D. R. (2000). Relationships among age-related differences in gap detection and word recognition. *J. Acoust. Soc. Am.* 107, 1615–1626. doi: 10.1121/1.428446

Sohmer, H., Pratt, H., and Kinarti, R. (1977). Sources of frequency following responses (FFR) in man. *Electroencephalogr. Clin. Neurophysiol.* 42, 656–664. doi: 10.1016/0013-4694(77)90282-6

Stapells, D. R., Linden, D., Suffield, J. B., Hamel, G., and Picton, T. W. (1984). Human auditory steady state potentials. *Ear Hear.* 5, 105–113.

Stellmack, M. A., Byrne, A. J., and Viemeister, N. F. (2010). Extracting binaural information from simultaneous targets and distractors: effects of amplitude modulation and asynchronous envelopes. *J. Acoust. Soc. Am.* 128, 1235–1244. doi: 10.1121/1.3466868

Strelcyk, O., and Dau, T. (2009). Relations between frequency selectivity, temporal fine-structure processing and speech reception in impaired hearing. *J. Acoust. Soc. Am.* 125, 3328–3345. doi: 10.1121/1.3097469

Surprenant, A. M., and Watson, C. S. (2001). Individual differences in the processing of speech and nonspeech sounds by normal-hearing listeners. *J. Acoust. Soc. Am.* 110, 2085–2095. doi: 10.1121/1.1404973

Szydlowska, K., and Tymianski, M. (2010). Calcium, ischemia and excitotoxicity. *Cell Calcium* 47, 122–129. doi: 10.1016/j.ceca.2010.01.003

Taberner, A. M., and Liberman, M. C. (2005). Response properties of single auditory nerve fibers in the mouse. *J. Neurophysiol.* 93, 557–569. doi: 10.1152/jn.00574.2004

van de Par, S., and Kohlrausch, A. (1997). A new approach to comparing binaural masking level differences at low and high frequencies. *J. Acoust. Soc. Am.* 101, 1671–1680. doi: 10.1121/1.418151

Verhulst, S., Bharadwaj, H., Mehraei, G., and Shinn-Cunningham, B. (2013). Understanding hearing impairment through model predictions of brainstem responses. *Proc. Meet. Acoust.* 19, 050182.

Viemeister, N. F. (1988). Intensity coding and the dynamic range problem. *Hear. Res.* 34, 267–274. doi: 10.1016/0378-5955(88)90007-x

Wightman, F. L., and Kistler, D. J. (1992). The dominant role of low-frequency interaural time differences in sound localization. *J. Acoust. Soc. Am.* 91, 1648–1661. doi: 10.1121/1.402445

Young, E. D., and Barta, P. E. (1986). Rate responses of auditory nerve fibers to tones in noise near masked threshold. *J. Acoust. Soc. Am.* 79, 426–442. doi: 10.1121/1.393530

Zhu, L., Bharadwaj, H., Xia, J., and Shinn-Cunningham, B. (2013). A comparison of spectral magnitude and phase-locking value analyses of the frequency-following response to complex tones. *J. Acoust. Soc. Am.* 134, 384–395. doi: 10.1121/1.4807498

Zilany, M. S., and Bruce, I. C. (2006). Modeling auditory-nerve responses for high sound pressure levels in the normal and impaired auditory periphery. *J. Acoust. Soc. Am.* 120, 1446–1466. doi: 10.1121/1.2225512

Zilany, M. S., Bruce, I. C., and Carney, L. H. (2014). Updated parameters and expanded simulation options for a model of the auditory periphery. *J. Acoust. Soc. Am.* 135, 283–286. doi: 10.1121/1.4837815

Zilany, M. S., Bruce, I. C., Nelson, P. C., and Carney, L. H. (2009). A phenomenological model of the synapse between the inner hair cell and auditory nerve: long-term adaptation with power-law dynamics. *J. Acoust. Soc. Am.* 126, 2390–2412. doi: 10.1121/1.3238250

12

Left temporal alpha-band activity reflects single word intelligibility

Robert Becker[1†], Maria Pefkou[2†], Christoph M. Michel[1] and Alexis G. Hervais-Adelman[2*]

[1] *Functional Brain Mapping Lab, Department of Fundamental Neuroscience, University of Geneva, Geneva, Switzerland*
[2] *Brain and Language Lab, Department of Clinical Neuroscience, University of Geneva, Geneva, Switzerland*

Correspondence:
Alexis G. Hervais-Adelman, Brain and Language Lab, Department of Clinical Neuroscience, University of Geneva, 1 Rue Michel-Servet, CH – 1211, Geneva, Switzerland
e-mail: Alexis.Adelman@unige.ch
† These authors have contributed equally to this work.

The electroencephalographic (EEG) correlates of degraded speech perception have been explored in a number of recent studies. However, such investigations have often been inconclusive as to whether observed differences in brain responses between conditions result from different acoustic properties of more or less intelligible stimuli or whether they relate to cognitive processes implicated in comprehending challenging stimuli. In this study we used noise vocoding to spectrally degrade monosyllabic words in order to manipulate their intelligibility. We used spectral rotation to generate incomprehensible control conditions matched in terms of spectral detail. We recorded EEG from 14 volunteers who listened to a series of noise vocoded (NV) and noise-vocoded spectrally-rotated (rNV) words, while they carried out a detection task. We specifically sought components of the EEG response that showed an interaction between spectral rotation and spectral degradation. This reflects those aspects of the brain electrical response that are related to the intelligibility of acoustically degraded monosyllabic words, while controlling for spectral detail. An interaction between spectral complexity and rotation was apparent in both evoked and induced activity. Analyses of event-related potentials showed an interaction effect for a P300-like component at several centro-parietal electrodes. Time-frequency analysis of the EEG signal in the alpha-band revealed a monotonic increase in event-related desynchronization (ERD) for the NV but not the rNV stimuli in the alpha band at a left temporo-central electrode cluster from 420–560 ms reflecting a direct relationship between the strength of alpha-band ERD and intelligibility. By matching NV words with their incomprehensible rNV homologues, we reveal the spatiotemporal pattern of evoked and induced processes involved in degraded speech perception, largely uncontaminated by purely acoustic effects.

Keywords: speech intelligibility, degraded speech, noise-vocoding, alpha oscillations, left inferior temporal cortex

INTRODUCTION

Despite the great acoustic variability of the speech signal, normally-hearing listeners are able to understand speech seemingly effortlessly in day-to-day situations. In order for this to be possible, the human speech perception system must be robust in the face of both natural variability and acoustic degradations. Natural variability can arise from the different realization of speech sounds by different speakers, who can be understood even though they vary in terms of their size and sex (Peterson and Barney, 1952; Smith et al., 2005), accent (Clarke and Garrett, 2004; Clopper and Pisoni, 2004; Evans and Iverson, 2004), and speech rate (Miller and Liberman, 1979), or may suffer from articulation disorders such as dysarthria (Darley et al., 1969; Kent et al., 1989). Beyond signal variations related to the speaker, external factors also have an impact on the quality of speech that is heard, such as transmission through telecommunications systems, in which case it is heavily filtered, the presence of background noise masking part of the speech signal, the presence of echoes, or the presence of multiple talkers simultaneously.

In order to investigate the mechanisms of speech perception, researchers are increasingly turning to paradigms employing artificial acoustic degradations of speech, which allow fine-grained manipulation of the level of intelligibility of a speech signal, rendering the behavioral or neural correlates of speech intelligibility amenable to investigation. Several types of manipulations have been employed, such as interrupted speech (Heinrich et al., 2008; Shahin et al., 2009), masking with noise (Davis and Johnsrude, 2003; Golestani et al., 2013), time-compression (Altmann and Young, 1993; Mehler et al., 1993; Dupoux and Green, 1997; Pallier et al., 1998; Sebastian-Galles et al., 2000), or noise-vocoding (Shannon et al., 1995). We chose to employ the latter of these, as it has been the subject of intensive research both behaviorally (e.g., Davis et al., 2005; Stacey and Summerfield, 2007; Hervais-Adelman et al., 2008, 2011; Dahan and Mead, 2010) and increasingly in neuroimaging experiments (e.g., Scott et al., 2000; Davis and Johnsrude, 2003; Scott et al., 2006; McGettigan et al., 2011; Obleser and Kotz, 2011; Hervais-Adelman et al., 2012; Evans et al., 2013).

An increasing amount of evidence regarding the neural correlates of degraded speech perception is becoming available. Functional magnetic resonance imaging (fMRI) has been extensively used to detect brain regions active while listening to degraded speech (e.g., Scott et al., 2000; Davis and Johnsrude, 2003; Giraud et al., 2004; Davis and Johnsrude, 2007; McGettigan et al., 2011; Hervais-Adelman et al., 2012; Wild et al., 2012a), while electro-encephalography (EEG) and magneto-encephalography (MEG) have been employed to study the timing of degraded speech processing through measures such as evoked response potentials and synchronized brain oscillations (e.g., Obleser and Kotz, 2011; Sohoglu et al., 2012; Peelle et al., 2013). Such experiments also provide insights into the cerebral processes that support speech perception in hearing-impaired listeners.

Neuronal oscillations are an important tool in the study of different brain functions, such as speech perception, as they address the issue of synchronization of neuronal networks within a given brain region as well as between regions, based on data obtained non-invasively and at the temporal scale neuronal activity occurs. Recent studies (reviewed by Weisz and Obleser, 2014) have focused on brain oscillations in auditory processing and speech perception. Among the different "brain rhythms", which differ from each other on the basis of their characteristic frequency (e.g., delta oscillations are of low frequency, 1–3 Hz, while gamma oscillations have a high frequency of 30–80 Hz) and which seem to play a role in speech processing, a major stream of research has focused on the alpha rhythm (the range of 8–13 Hz). Traditionally, alpha rhythm has been considered as being highly related to visual spatial attention (Thut et al., 2006), beginning with the reports of Hans Berger in the late 1920s (Berger, 1929). Berger (1929) observed that opening the eyes lead to clear attenuation of previously visible oscillations in the 10 Hz range over occipital electrodes. Since then, numerous studies have reported findings about the close relationship of alpha rhythm activity and the visual system (e.g., Makeig et al., 2002; Becker et al., 2008; Busch et al., 2009; Mathewson et al., 2009) as well as working memory tasks (Jokisch and Jensen, 2007) to attentional and other cognitive paradigms (for a review, see Klimesch, 1999).

Despite this strong interest in alpha rhythm, much less is known about the relationship of alpha activity and auditory processing. This may be in part owed to the fact that resting alpha is much more prominent in occipital electrodes, likely detecting visual-cortical activity rather than in temporal electrodes. This might be related to the larger volume of the visual cortex compared to the auditory cortex and to the fact that it is impossible to completely deprive a healthy, hearing individual from auditory input but easy to close one's eyes and thereby block visual input (for a review on auditory alpha see Weisz et al., 2011). The first reports of auditory-cortical oscillations in the alpha-band originate from MEG studies, in which the rhythm was initially named "tau" (Tiihonen et al., 1991; Lehtela et al., 1997). Lehtela et al. (1997) demonstrated that the presentation of short (500 ms) noise bursts was followed by decreases in alpha power, localized in the superior temporal lobes, suggesting a role for alpha as a marker of auditory processing similar to that shown in the visual system. Regarding alpha oscillations and speech perception, Krause et al. (1997) reported stronger alpha-band suppression for listening to a comprehensible text passage as when compared to listening to the same passage being played backwards (Krause et al., 1997). Despite their scarcity, such studies point to a functional role of alpha oscillations in processing speech.

In a more recent study, Obleser and Weisz (2012) investigated the role of alpha suppression in speech comprehension using degraded speech. They employed noise-vocoding, a form of artificial degradation which reduces the spectral information in the auditory signal (Shannon et al., 1995), in a graded manner, permitting the generation of stimuli on a continuum from unintelligible to intelligible, by increasing the spectral fidelity of the vocoding. The method is described in Section Stimuli below. Obleser and Weisz (2012) used words at different levels of intelligibility and hypothesized that alpha suppression should be enhanced with intelligibility, reflecting less need for functional inhibition and less effortful speech processing. This idea is compatible with the conception of alpha oscillations as a mechanism of gating or suppressing task-irrelevant high frequency oscillations (Osipova et al., 2008; Jensen and Mazaheri, 2010). In other words, a decrease in alpha power in a task-relevant region would accompany the disinhibition of gamma oscillations in the same region, which are thought to reflect active processing. In general, alpha suppression is accompanied by an increase of oscillations in the gamma band, which reflects engagement/processing as it has been shown by intracranial studies in animals and humans (e.g., Paller et al., 1987; Fries, 2005; Kaiser and Lutzenberger, 2005; Crone et al., 2006; Womelsdorf et al., 2007).

Obleser and Weisz (2012) showed a linear increase in alpha suppression as a function of word intelligibility. They interpret this finding as reflecting the listeners' effort or ability to comprehend degraded speech. The alpha suppression was localized in superior parietal, prefrontal and anterior temporal areas. This may indicate that these brain regions are more active during the task, assuming that a local decrease in alpha power is a marker of activation of the region in question. This idea is backed by early findings of changes in resting-state alpha power as well as by numerous more recent EEG-fMRI studies which reported an inverse relationship between alpha-power and BOLD signal, under rest as well as during stimulation (Laufs et al., 2003; Moosmann et al., 2003; Goncalves et al., 2006; de Munck et al., 2007; Becker et al., 2011). Furthermore, a more recent study showed an even more direct inverse relationship between alpha-power and neuronal firing rate in monkeys (Haegens et al., 2011). The localization of the alpha-suppresion effect reported by Obleser and Weisz (2012) is partially in agreement with previous fMRI studies seeking to identify the brain regions implicated in the processing of degraded but potentially comprehensible speech (Scott et al., 2000; Narain et al., 2003; Giraud et al., 2004; Eisner et al., 2010; Wild et al., 2012a,b), revealing recruitment of brain areas involved in speech processing in general, such as bilateral superior temporal gyrus (STG) and superior temporal sulcus (STS), together with a more left-lateralized inferior-frontal and motor network.

In the present study, our aims were twofold: (1) we aimed to dissociate the EEG signatures of intelligibility and spectral complexity while listening to degraded speech, using a paradigm similar to the one published by Obleser and Weisz (2012). To this end, we asked participants to listen carefully to noise-vocoded (NV) words with different levels of degradation (therefore different levels of spectral complexity), and importantly, to the spectrally rotated version of the same stimuli. Spectrally rotated speech (Blesser, 1972) retains the same amount of spectral complexity as its non-rotated equivalent but it is incomprehensible to the naïve listener [although listeners may adapt to it after extensive training (Green et al., 2013)]. In this way, we had a spectrally-matched control condition for each level of intelligibility in order to rule out the possibility that alpha suppression is purely driven by low-level acoustic properties of the signal. Importantly, we used monosyllabic words, which are very challenging for naïve listeners to understand when degraded, in order to increase task difficulty and limit the use of top-down processes. As lexical and prosodic information facilitate comprehension and perceptual learning of degraded speech (e.g., Davis et al., 2005), by using monosyllabic words our listeners would have to rely almost exclusively on the acoustic information they could extract from the degraded input. The nature of this acoustic input was therefore essential for comprehension, given the lack of other sources of information in the stimuli and (2) by using the approach described above, we wanted to examine both induced and evoked correlates for degraded speech processing, their timing, their topography as well as the putative cerebral sources underlying the observed effects. Although the work presented here employs artificial acoustic degradation to examine the neural underpinnings of degraded speech perception, we hope that the findings will also be relevant to the cerebral processes that help to compensate for degraded auditory input in hearing impaired listeners.

MATERIALS AND METHODS

PARTICIPANTS

Fourteen right-handed native French speakers (two male) participated in the study. Participants self-reported as being right-handed and having no history of hearing or visual impairment. They all gave written informed consent to participate in the study, which was approved by the local ethics committee of the University Hospital of Geneva, and received financial compensation of 40 CHF.

STIMULI

Stimuli were 360 monosyllabic French nouns, among which 36 animal names, selected from the "Lexique 3" database for French words.[1] The animal names were used as targets in the detection task we employed. All words, apart from the animal names, were divided into three groups, matched for spoken wordform frequency ($F_{2,321} = 0.205$, $p = 0.82$; Group 1 mean = 31.94/million, Group 2 mean = 27.43/million and Group 3 mean = 28.37/million). The animal names used had mean frequency = 15.41/million. Stimulus matching was achieved using the Match program.[2]

The words were recorded in a soundproof chamber by a male native French speaker and digitized at a 44.1 kHz sampling rate. Recordings were denoised using the algorithm implemented in Audacity software[3] and trimmed at zero-crossings preceding and succeeding the words. Root mean square (RMS) amplitude of each of the extracted stimuli was set to a fixed level, and the stimuli were then bandpass filtered between 50 and 5000 Hz using a sixth order butterworth filter. Stimuli were then NV using 1, 4, 8 and 16 frequency bands following the procedure described by Shannon et al. (1995). Stimuli were filtered into quasi-logarithmically spaced frequency bands intended to mimic the tonotopic organization of the cochlea (Greenwood, 1990) between 50 and 5000 Hz, using second order butterworth filters and full-wave rectified, producing the amplitude envelope of each band. Each envelope was convolved with noise band-pass filtered into the same frequency range as the source band. The amplitude-modulated carriers were then recombined to produce NV words. The number of frequency bands has been shown to be a crucial factor for the intelligibility of vocoded words, with higher numbers of bands producing more intelligible stimuli (Shannon et al., 1995). The four NV versions of each word were created, producing a continuum from completely unintelligible (1-band noise-vocoded, NV1) to relatively easily comprehensible (16-band noise-vocoded, NV16).

Bandpass-filtered and NV words were also spectrally rotated, in order to create a control condition preserving the same amount of spectral information but rendering the input incomprehensible. Spectral rotation was achieved based on a procedure defined by Blesser (1972) and implemented following the procedure described by Scott et al. (2000). The speech signal was rotated around the midpoint of the frequency range of the bandpass filtered input (i.e., 2.5 kHz) and then pre-emphasized using a finite response (FIR) filter with the same long-term spectral distribution as the original input. Finally, signal was modulated by a sinusoid at 5 kHz. NV1 words were not spectrally rotated, since their spectral profile is that of white noise, i.e., flat, and would not be altered by rotation. Example NV and spectrally-rotated NV stimuli are illustrated in **Figure 1**.

These manipulations yielded four levels of spectral detail, crossed with the factor spectral rotation: band-pass filtered words (BP), NV16 words, 8-band noise-vocoded words (NV8) and 4-band noise-vocoded words (NV4) and their spectrally rotated homologues (rBP, rNV16, rNV8, rNV4), as well as a 1-band NV (NV1, equivalent to signal-correlated noise) control condition.

The experiment was divided into three blocks (see Section Procedure, below), for which stimulus selection proceeded as follows. Words were randomly selected from the pool of 108 non-target stimuli of each stimulus group, and allocated without replacement to one of the four non-rotated conditions (NV4, NV8, NV16, BP). Each selected word was also allocated to the spectrally rotated condition at the same level of spectral detail. Twenty seven words were allocated to each level of degradation per block. Due to the limited number of target stimuli (the 36 animal names) these were randomly allocated without replacement to each of the four levels of degradation, with a new randomization applied for each of the three blocks, thus each target stimulus appeared three times in a non-rotated condition and three times in a rotated

[1] http://www.lexique.org, New et al. (2001)

[2] http://www.mrccbu.cam.ac.uk/~maarten/match.htm, Van Casteren and Davis (2007)

[3] http://audacity.sourceforge.net/

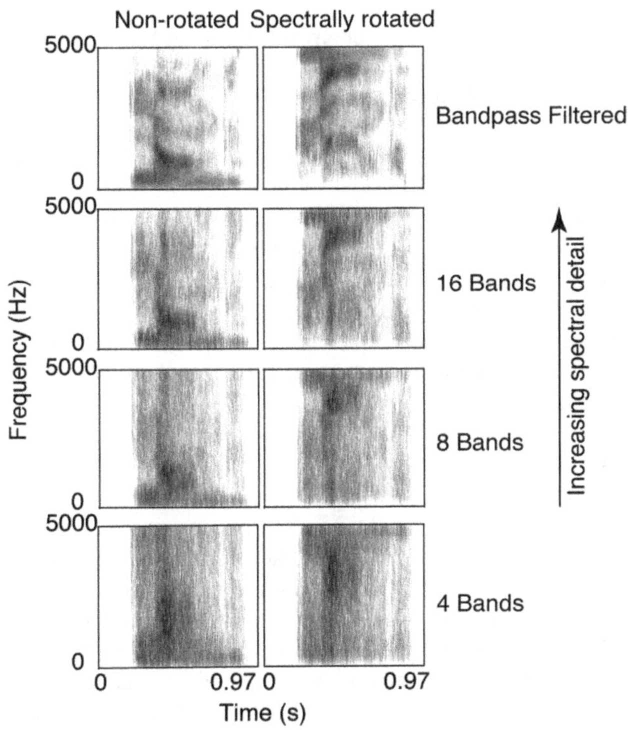

FIGURE 1 | Spectrograms of the French word "langue" (meaning tongue, or language) for the four levels of spectral detail, for spectrally rotated and non-rotated stimuli. Stimuli illustrated with a preceding 200 ms silence.

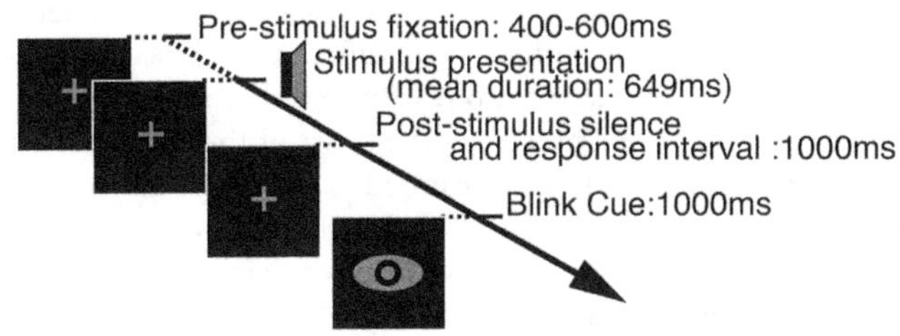

FIGURE 2 | Illustration of a single trial. In the beginning of each trial a fixation cross appeared on the screen for a variable duration of 400–600 ms and remained on the screen as the stimulus was presented. One second of silence was inserted after the stimulus offset, during which participants could make their response, and it was followed by the blink cue whose duration was also fixed at 1 s.

condition over the course of the experiment. For each block, 27 words were randomly selected without replacement from the whole pool of stimuli and allocated to the NV1 condition. There were therefore 81 non-target stimuli per condition and 27 target stimuli in each condition barring NV1, for a total of 279 trials in each of the three blocks.

PROCEDURE

Participants were seated in front of a computer screen, at a distance of approximately 1 m, in a sound-insulated Faraday cage. The overhead light in the booth was turned off while EEG was recorded. Stimuli were delivered through ER4 noise-isolating in-ear headphones (Etymotic Research Inc., Elk Grove Village, Illinois) at a comfortable sound level, adjusted at the beginning of the experiment.

The experiment was divided into three blocks of 12.5 min and 279 trials each. Participants were instructed to listen carefully to the words and respond each time they heard an animal name by pressing a button on a response-box placed on a table in front of them with their right index finger. Brain electrical activity was recorded during the whole period of each block. Short breaks took place after the end of the first two blocks in order to check, and if necessary reduce, the impedances of the electrodes.

Each trial began with the appearance of a fixation cross at the center of the screen. The stimulus was presented after a silent interval whose duration was randomly jittered on a uniform distribution between 400 and 600 ms after the onset of the fixation cross. The fixation cross remained on screen during the presentation of the word so as to encourage fixation and minimize eye movements. 1000 ms after the offset of the stimulus a symbol appeared on-screen for 1000 ms, indicating to participants that they could blink if they wished. By cueing blinks we aimed to ensure that any blinking-related electrical artefacts would not contaminate the recording of EEG responses to the stimuli. The structure of a single trial is illustrated in **Figure 2**.

EEG RECORDING

Brain electrical responses were recorded with a 256-electrode Electrical Geodesics HyrdoCel system (Electrical Geodesics Inc., Eugene, Oregon). Signal was recorded continuously and digitized at a sampling rate of 1000 Hz. By default, the recording system sampled at 20 kHz before applying an analog hardware antialiasing filter with a cut-off frequency of 4 kHz and downsampling the signal to 1000 Hz, and applying a software low-pass Butterworth filter with a cutoff of 400 Hz. The reference electrode was the Cz, situated at the vertex. Electrode impedances were checked at the beginning of the session and after the first and second recording blocks and were under 30 kΩ at the beginning of each block.

DATA ANALYSIS

Behavioral data

We computed and analyzed accuracy scores and response times for correct trials. We also analyzed the number of false alarms per condition.

EEG data preprocessing and artifact removal

EEG data were initially analyzed using custom Matlab (The Mathworks, Natick, MA) scripts and the freely available EEGLAB toolbox (Delorme and Makeig, 2004). Data were re-referenced to average reference and downsampled to 200 Hz (after low-pass filtering to avoid aliasing). For further analyses a set of 204 channels was analyzed (channels covering the cheeks were excluded). The three blocks per subject were concatenated and an Independent Components Analysis (ICA) was computed on the whole dataset using the Infomax routine from the Matlab-based EEGLAB toolbox (Delorme and Makeig, 2004) in order to remove blink artefacts and 50 Hz line-noise. The resulting data were filtered between 0.75 and 40 Hz using a fifth order Butterworth bandpass filter and separated into epochs starting 800 ms before the sound onset and finishing 1000 ms after. A baseline correction was applied by subtracting from each epoch the mean signal computed over 200 ms preceding the onset of the stimulus. The filtered and epoched data were scanned to detect epochs in which the amplitude between 300 ms pre-stimulus onset and the end of the epoch was higher than 75 μV or lower than −75 μV. These epochs were considered outliers and were excluded from further analysis.

Furthermore, only trials with non-target words and no button presses (i.e., false alarms) were kept for further EEG analyses.

Analysis of evoked activity—ERP analysis

Single-trial evoked responses were averaged for each condition separately to examine the component of neural activity being phase-locked to the stimulation event, i.e., to obtain condition-specific event-related potentials (ERPs). Data were analyzed in a time window from −100 to 1000 ms about stimulus onset.

Analysis of induced activity—time-frequency analysis

Using the EEGLAB toolbox, we chose a hanning-tapered short-term fast-fourier-transformation (stFFT) to compute time-frequency representations of our data in the range of the alpha band (8–13 Hz). These time-frequency power fluctuations (referred to as TF_α, in μV^2) were then converted to dB logarithmic scale using the following equation:

$$dB_\alpha = 10 \times \log_{10}(TF_\alpha) \quad (1)$$

and finally averaged across the defined frequency band. As for the ERPs, data were analyzed in a time window from −100 to 1000 ms.

ANOVA

The ERPs as well as the stFFT data were submitted to a repeated-measures ANOVA, including two factors: spectral detail (four levels, 4-bands, 8-bands, 16-bands and band-pass filtered), and spectral rotation (two levels, non-rotated and rotated), and including subject as a random factor. We were specifically interested in the interaction of spectral detail and spectral rotation to identify correlates of degraded word processing, which are not confounded with the factor of spectral detail. ANOVA was performed for each time point and electrode.

Inverse solution modeling

For the ERPs as well as the stFFT results we used the weighted minimum norm (WMN) approach (Lin et al., 2006), which belongs to the family of distributed inverse solution methods. We computed inverse solutions by applying the WMN inverse matrix to the data (5018 solution points, no regularization). The lead field model we employed was a LSMAC model (locally spherical model with anatomical constraints, for details about this approach see Brunet et al., 2011) which then in turn is applied to the MNI brain template (ICBM152) coregistered to EEG electrodes. Standard spatial electrode positions were used in all subjects, co-registered to the template MRI by adjusting the position of the nasion, inion, Cz and pre-auricular landmarks.

For the ERP data, condition and subject specific averages were inverted using the method described above and then subject to the same ANOVA procedure as the surface EEG data. To compute the inverse equivalent of the stFFT surface data in the alpha-band, we filtered the single EEG trials for each condition and subject in the alpha frequency band, inverted them and then averaged the normed (i.e., scalar) values of all single trials (similar to the approach used by de Pasquale et al., 2013). This results in a temporally resolved representation of alpha-band power distributed across 5018 solution points in the inverse space. Afterwards, these WMN inverted averages were subject to the ANOVA procedure as stated above. For visualization, results were projected onto the co-registered MNI brain template using the Cartool toolbox (Brunet et al., 2011).

RESULTS

BEHAVIORAL DATA

Mean accuracy values for the non-rotated potentially intelligible conditions were 26, 66, 80 and 91% for the 4-bands, 8-bands, 16-bands and bandpass-filtered stimuli respectively. Accuracy values entered in a one-way ANOVA with spectral detail as the within-subject factor (four levels: 4-bands, 8-bands, 16-bands and bandpass-filtered), which revealed a significant main effect of spectral detail ($F_{(3,39)} = 339.931, p < 10^{-6}$, partial-$\eta^2 = 0.96$). The mean accuracy value per condition is displayed in **Figure 3A**.

Response times for the intelligible correct trials were also computed and entered in a one-way repeated-measures ANOVA with spectral detail as the within-subjects factor (four levels, as described above). There was a significant main effect of spectral detail ($F_{(3,39)} = 26.531, p < 0.001$, partial-$\eta^2 = 0.67$) with response latencies being faster for intelligible trials and slower for more degraded words. Response time results are displayed in **Figure 3B**. We did not compute accuracy values or response times for the rotated trials, as no response could be categorized as "correct" in the face of incomprehensible stimuli. Those instances where participants did respond must be considered false alarms.

We also analyzed the number of false alarms as we expected more false alarms in the unintelligible or potentially intelligible but difficult conditions. The 1-band NV words were not included in this analysis. Number of false alarms was entered a repeated-measures ANOVA with spectral detail (four-levels, as described above) and spectral rotation (two levels: spectrally rotated and non-rotated) as within-subjects factors. There was a significant main effect of spectral complexity ($F_{(3,19)} = 5.037$, $p = 0.021$, partial-$\eta^2 = 0.279$) and a significant spectral complexity by rotation interaction ($F_{(3,19)} = 8.534$, $p = 0.001$, partial-$\eta^2 = 0.396$). The mean false alarms per condition is displayed in **Figure 3C**.

EVOKED ACTIVITY—ERP ANALYSIS

Average ERPs were entered into a two-way, repeated measures analysis of variance with number of frequency bands (i.e., spectral detail) and rotation as within-subjects factors. ANOVA was performed for each channel and sample point. To correct for multiple comparisons, we employed the approach of controlling the false discovery rate, FDR (Benjamini and Yekutieli, 2001) using a threshold of $p_{(FDR)} < 0.05$. In order to ensure we report robust results, we additionally disregard results involving fewer

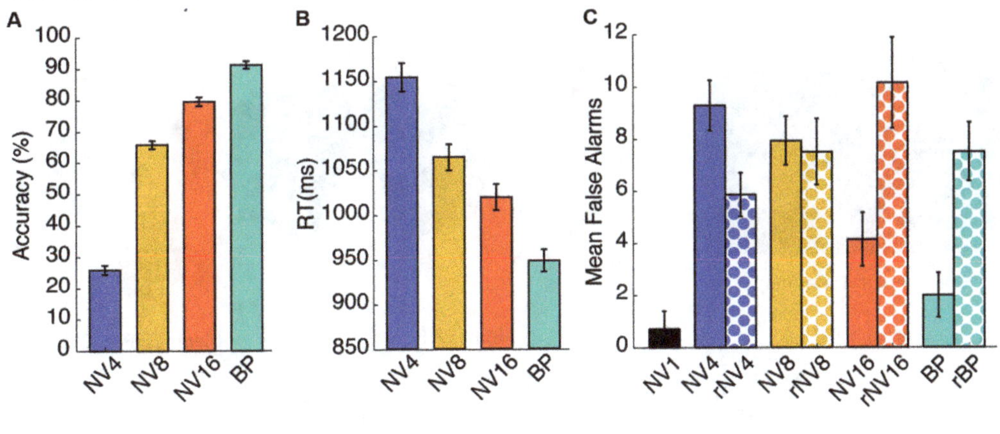

FIGURE 3 | Behavioral results. Panel **(A)** shows the mean accuracy scores for the animal name detection task in each of the non-rotated potentially-comprehensible conditions. Panel **(B)** shows the mean response time for correct responses in the same conditions. Panel **(C)** displays the mean number of false alarms for all conditions. Error bars represent standard error of the mean corrected to be appropriate for repeated-measures comparisons, as described in Loftus and Masson (1994).

than two electrodes or having a duration of less than three consecutive sample points (15 ms). After FDR correction, we found the following main effects, at $p_{(FDR)} < 0.05$, (uncorrected p-values are provided here): There was a significant main effect of rotation, temporally centered around 305 ms, involving up to eight supra-threshold electrodes. At the centroparietal peak electrode 132, $F_{(1,13)} = 57.59$, $p < 3.97{*}10^{-6}$, the effect ranged from 295 to 325 ms. A main effect of spectral detail was found in a set of seven left superior-parietal and right temporal electrodes, in a time-window ranging from 185 to 215 ms post stimulus-onset. At the centroparietal peak electrode 81, $F_{(3,39)} = 16.5$, $p < 4.45{*}10^{-7}$.

The focus of our analysis was the interaction between the number of frequency bands and spectral rotation which was intended to specifically reveal the EEG signatures of listening to degraded words, while controlling for the impact of spectral complexity. We observed a significant spectral detail by rotation interaction located over a set of spatially coherent central parieto-frontal electrodes, in one distinct post-stimulus time-window, from 305–390 ms, peaking at 345 ms (comprising a cluster of up to five supra-threshold electrodes around electrode 186, with maximum $F_{(3,39)} = 21.96$, $p < 1.72{*}10^{-8}$, **Figures 4A, B**). It appears that the effect in this time-window is driven specifically by a significantly greater positivity in response to the bandpass-filtered words in comparison to all other categories of stimuli (see **Figure 4D**). In order to confirm this hypothesis, a post-hoc analysis was carried out, comparing the clear condition with all others, pooled, in a univariate ANOVA, including subject as a random factor. This showed that the clear condition was indeed significantly different from all the others $F_{(1,13)} = 45.303$, $p < 0.001$, partial-$\eta^2 = 0.777$.

INDUCED ACTIVITY—TIME-FREQUENCY ANALYSIS

ANOVA and correction for multiple comparisons was performed as for the ERP analysis reported above. After FDR correction, we found no significant main effects. We found a significant interaction in the alpha-band, at electrodes situated over the left temporal lobe, from 462–633 ms, with the peak of this effect found at 533 ms (comprising a spatially coherent cluster of eight supra-threshold electrodes around left-temporal electrode 75 with maximum $F_{(3,39)} = 12.12$, $p < 9.23{*}10^{-6}$ see **Figures 5A, B**). This spatiotemporally coherent effect was manifest as a decrease in alpha-band power (i.e., alpha suppression) as a function of stimulus clarity for the NV but not rNV conditions (see **Figures 5D, E**). In contrast to the earlier effect revealed in the ERP analysis, this effect showed a graded response, suggesting sensitivity to the difficulty of comprehending words at different levels of degradation. Sidak-corrected post-hoc pairwise comparisons comparing the alpha-band power averaged over the 5 electrodes showing the greatest interaction effect in the period from 462–633 ms for the four potentially-comprehensible conditions partly support this: NV4 > NV16 ($p = 0.021$), NV4 > BP ($p = 0.011$), NV8 shows marginally less alpha power than BP ($p = 0.063$), other comparisons not significant. Although not all pairwise differences between the levels are significant, this is suggestive of increasing alpha-suppression with increasing intelligibility.

INVERSE SOLUTIONS

For visualization of results in the inverse space, we performed identical statistics as those on the surface data, confined to the two temporal windows showing FDR-corrected effects in both the ERP and the induced activity. The results are presented in **Figures 4C, 5C** showing the resulting F-values averaged over the time-window of interest.

For effects on evoked activity, the source of the corresponding effect (i.e., the interaction between spectral complexity and rotation) in the time window from 300–400 ms with a peak at approximately −13, −27, 63 (MNI co-ordinates) principally located in medial precentral gyrus (BA6, extending posteriorly into BA4). This effect is shown in **Figure 4C**.

The source corresponding to the interaction between spectral complexity and rotation in the alpha band (time window 450–650 ms) was localized to the left superior temporal lobe/inferior

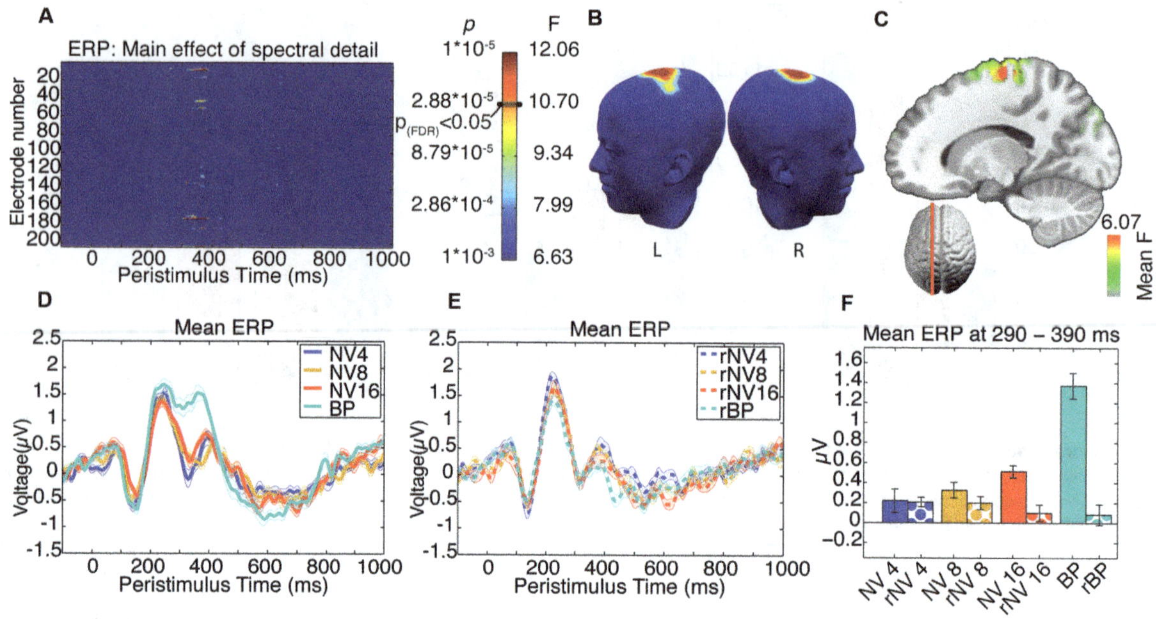

FIGURE 4 | Results of ANOVA of evoked activity. **(A)** Electrode-by-time plot of the interaction of rotation × spectral detail thresholded at $p < 0.001$, revealing the time-window of interest between 305–390 ms. The color bar indicates the corresponding F- and p-values, the threshold for $p_{(FDR)} < 0.05$ is indicated. **(B)** Shows the topography of this effect using the same color scale as in **(A)** at the peak of the effect (345 ms). **(C)** Illustrates the localization of this effect in inverse space, displaying the mean F-statistic averaged over the time-window of interest. **(D)** Average time-course of this effect in a cluster of five contributing electrodes across NV conditions. **(E)** Corresponding time-courses for the rotated conditions, where the effect of spectral detail is absent. **(F)** Mean evoked activity for each condition in the significant time-window, error bars represent standard error of the mean corrected to be appropriate for repeated-measures comparisons, as described in Loftus and Masson (1994).

parietal lobe. The maximum effect was located at −46, −27, 20 (MNI co-ordinates), and spanned the posterior reaches of the left supramarginal gyrus, and covered the superior posterior temporal gyrus. The effect is presented in **Figure 5C**.

DISCUSSION

Behavioral data demonstrate that the rNV conditions were unintelligible to the participants in this study, while the intelligibility of the NV conditions increased as a function of the number of frequency bands used, as previously demonstrated (e.g., Shannon et al., 1995; Davis and Johnsrude, 2003). Although we did not obtain responses for every trial, we are confident that the d' measures established for the target-detection task reflect the mean level of intelligibility of each of the conditions employed.

Our analysis of the EEG data revealed two time-periods in which the brain response is significantly affected by the potential intelligibility of a stimulus. In the earlier one of these, we show an effect in evoked activity that appears to relate to the early identification of clear stimuli as a special category. Its timing and its topography suggest that we may be detecting modulation of the P300 component (for a review of the P300, see Polich, 2007). The P300 is usually apparent as a positivity in the midline parieto-frontal electrodes and is observed in tasks, such as the animal name detection task used here, that require stimulus discrimination. Its appearance has been suggested to be an index of the occurrence of stimulus events sufficiently important to inhibit concurrent processes, and has therefore been associated with attention and memory processes (Polich, 2007). In the present case, it could reflect the fact that deciding whether the stimulus is a target or not is substantially easier when the word is more easily intelligible. Another possibility is that because the clear stimuli are categorically different from all others, this relatively early effect results from an oddball effect (Polich and Margala, 1997). This is also supported by the fact that the probability of a clear stimulus being presented was relatively low, at only 13%. The fact that this evoked effect seems to be rather central than left-lateralized could also be seen to support the view of this component being rather a general cognitive component than one specific to language processing.

We did not find effects in the evoked responses that we can more specifically ascribe to comprehension processes. This may be the result of the inherent difficulty of time-locking EEG responses to specific events during auditory word processing. Although we used the acoustic onset of the stimuli as our marker for the beginning of each epoch, given that we are interested in comprehension processes rather than auditory processes, this may not be the best point. Ideally, we might have used the recognition point determined using (for example) gating (Grosjean, 1980). This issue, of course, applies to all studies of spoken word perception that use measures with a high temporal resolution.

During a second time-window, we showed a significant interaction between spectral rotation and spectral complexity on induced activity—specifically the alpha band, reflecting increased alpha suppression as a function of increasing spectral complexity in the NV (i.e., potentially comprehensible) and not the rNV (always unintelligible) stimuli. This finding is superficially

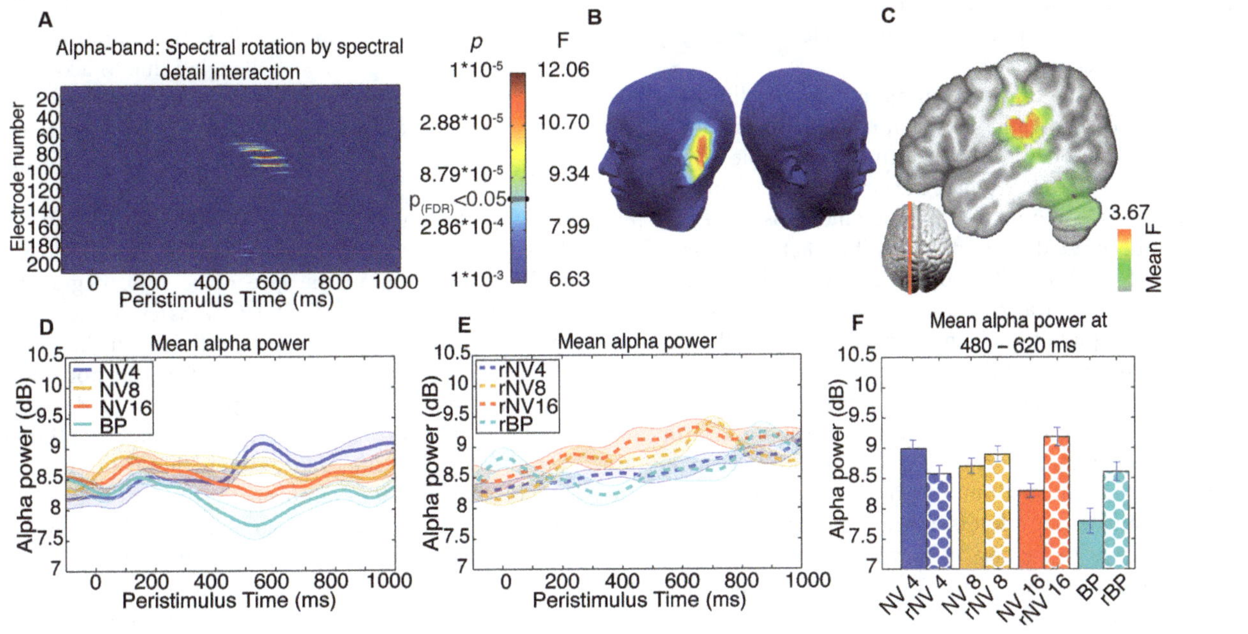

FIGURE 5 | Results of ANOVA of induced activity in the alpha-band. (A) Electrode-by-time plot of the *p*-values for the interaction of rotation × spectral detail with corresponding *F*- and *p*-values, thresholded at $p = 0.001$, revealing the time-window of interest (462–633 ms). The color bar indicates the corresponding *F*- and *p*-values, the threshold for $p_{(FDR)} < 0.05$ is indicated. **(B)** Topography of this effect, using the same color scale as in **(A)** at the peak of the effect (533 ms), indicating a contribution of left-temporal sources. **(C)** Localization of this effect in the inverse space, the main source being in the left supramarginal gyrus extending into left inferior parietal and superior temporal structures, showing the average *F*-statistic over the time-window of interest. **(D)** Average time-course of this effect in a cluster of five contributing electrodes across NV conditions, demonstrating enhanced alpha-band suppression for more intelligible conditions. **(E)** Corresponding time-courses for the spectrally rotated conditions, where the effect of spectral detail is absent. **(F)** Alpha-band activity for each condition in the significant time-window, error bars represent standard error of the mean corrected to be appropriate for repeated-measures comparisons, as described in Loftus and Masson (1994).

similar to that reported by Obleser and Weisz (2012), who demonstrated a connection between alpha-band suppression and intelligibility of stimuli. However, by including the spectrally rotated stimuli as an unintelligible control condition we extended this finding by confirming that the relationship between alpha-suppression and intelligibility is almost certainly the result of brain mechanisms that extract meaning from words, rather than the result of purely acoustic analysis of more vs. less complex auditory input. Furthermore, the effects we find occur earlier than those reported by Obleser and Weisz (2012). This may be the result of our having employed exclusively monosyllabic words rather than the mixture mono-, bi- and trisyllabic words they employed.

As discussed in Section Introduction, the functional role of auditory alpha is unclear, although it is increasingly becoming a focus of attention in the field of speech perception. At present, the relevant evidence seems to indicate that alpha-power suppression is related to comprehension, and it has been suggested that this could relate to the role of alpha-band activity in suppressing higher-frequency oscillations. It may be the case that alpha-band activity reveals an inhibitory process that suppresses processes whose occurrence is indicated by the presence of higher-frequency oscillations (Osipova et al., 2008). Thus, alpha-suppression may reflect the release of inhibition of processing. In the present case, where alpha-suppression reflects the intelligibility of auditory input, it is highly likely that the process indexed by this effect is related to word identification and comprehension. This effect is present in the time range of the N400 complex, which is related to semantic processing (Kutas and Hillyard, 1984).

Increased alpha-suppression for more easily comprehensible words during this time window is consistent with the idea that this effect reveals the on-average greater semantic processing in the easier compared to the harder conditions. However, a less prosaic explanation of this effect would be that the relatively higher alpha power in the more challenging conditions reflects increased functional inhibition related to the demands placed on attention and working memory by the challenge of comprehending acoustically degraded speech. Indeed, several studies have shown that the ability to comprehend degraded speech is influenced by working memory capacity (Ronnberg et al., 2008, 2010; Zekveld et al., 2009, 2011, 2012; Rudner et al., 2011) and selective attention (Shinn-Cunningham and Best, 2008; Wild et al., 2012b). It is possible that this effect is the manifestation of the inhibitory networks that are required to maintain selective attention and working memory processes to support the comprehension of degraded speech. A possibility raised by Obleser and Weisz (2012) is that the increase in alpha-suppression observed in response to less degraded stimuli is not necessarily increased suppression as a function of increased intelligibility, but increasing alpha-power as stimulus intelligibility falls. If this is the case, then the effect may be explained if alpha is considered to be a gating mechanism that inhibits other cognitive processes locally while challenging speech comprehension takes place.

Our data indicate that—in comparison to baseline—there is indeed an increase in alpha-power in response to the most challenging NV condition, indeed suggesting that the role of temporal alpha may be to actively regulate the engagement of downstream cognitive processes (confirmed by one-tailed posthoc t-test, p = 0.017). In the present case, it is possible that suppressing the final stages of word-identification processes (i.e., lexical access or semantic access) is a way of improving word-identification accuracy by enabling additional time for processing of the acoustic input. The possibility that the identification processes are delayed as a function of degradation can be investigated in future studies.

The effect at this time was localized to a region incorporating the left supramarginal gyrus (SMG), left inferior parietal lobule, and the posterior left superior temporal gyrus. This approximate localization situates the effect in a region that has been considered by some authors to be part of Wernicke's region (Geschwind, 1972; Bogen and Bogen, 1976) and has also been associated with sensorimotor integration during speech comprehension (Hickok and Poeppel, 2007). A role for sensorimotor integration during degraded speech comprehension would be consistent with the notion that, when confronted with degraded speech, the speech comprehension system falls back on higher-level (top-down) mechanisms to help resolve the degraded acoustic input. In this case, since very little linguistic information is present in the degraded monosyllabic stimuli, such information could potentially be articulatory in nature (e.g., as suggested by Hervais-Adelman et al., 2012). Nevertheless, beyond implicating this region in degraded speech processing, evidence for its exact role is scant.

The localization of the source of this alpha-suppression effect using a weighted minimum norm estimate was rather different to that shown by Obleser and Weisz (2012) using a beamformer approach. While we show relatively localized sources, they showed more distributed sources incorporating anterior temporal regions, parietal lobes, right dorsolateral prefrontal cortex and left inferior frontal regions.

Another potentially fruitful line of enquiry concerns the link between alpha-suppression and the pulvinar nucleus of the thalamus. Although we do not directly observe any effects in the pulvinar in this study, an investigation by Erb et al. (2012) implicated this structure as being linked to individuals' ability to learn to comprehend NV speech. Activity in the pulvinar nucleus has been suggested as a driver of alpha suppression (Lopes da Silva et al., 1980; Liu et al., 2012), and is also linked to attentional control in vision (e.g., Kastner et al., 2004; Smith et al., 2009) and audition (Wester et al., 2001), while attention has been found to affect the cerebral processing of NV speech (Wild et al., 2012b). Although at this stage this potential link is highly speculative, we would suggest that the thalamo-cortical networks implicated in alpha-band activity are worthwhile targets for investigations of speech comprehension.

Interestingly, we do not find regions in which alpha-suppression shows the opposite response to intelligibility (i.e., alpha is more suppressed when stimuli are harder to understand). This is inconsistent with the fMRI literature, in which many studies have demonstrated the recruitment of additional brain areas when speech perception is challenging due to acoustic degradation compared to when it is clear. For example, several studies have demonstrated that left inferior frontal gyrus regions are engaged when acoustically degraded speech is presented (Davis and Johnsrude, 2003; Giraud et al., 2004; Obleser et al., 2007; Hervais-Adelman et al., 2012; Wild et al., 2012b), others have shown increased recruitment of anterior and posterior temporal lobe structures in the face of acoustic degradation (Scott et al., 2000; Narain et al., 2003; Evans et al., 2013). We would have expected to see such effects reflected in the EEG signature of degraded speech processing. That we do not find effects in this direction in these data is puzzling and demands further investigation. However, generation of alpha oscillations can differ considerably from site to site, even within the visual system. This has been reported for example with regard to originating layers of alpha and even relationship of the measured alpha oscillations to behavioral performance (Bollimunta et al., 2008).

Another interesting detail is that the sites of our observed major effect in the alpha-band and the sites of highest spectral power in the alpha-band do not spatially coincide. As is commonly known, occipital electrodes exhibit much higher resting-state alpha power than the remaining electrodes. The left-temporal cluster identified in our study shows only moderate prestimulus alpha-amplitude. Yet its modulation is highly significant. This demonstrates that while such alpha modulation might be more difficult to identify, it can nonetheless be extracted.

In general, the link between alpha rhythm and language/word processing is relatively sparsely described. While there seems to be some consensus about auditory alpha/tau (see Lehtela et al., 1997), the idea of higher-level language-related alpha oscillations is still quite recent (e.g., Obleser and Weisz, 2012) and highly exciting. Whether this points to an even more universal role of alpha oscillations than previously envisioned remains to be seen and will require further investigations in more diverse experimental settings.

CONCLUSION

Taken together, the data presented above suggest that the auditory system can rapidly differentiate easily-comprehensible speech (approximately 300 ms after stimulus onset), and that potentially-comprehensible degraded speech can begin to be processed differently to incomprehensible speech as early as 480 ms after stimulus onset. We demonstrate that alpha-band power in the left temporal lobe is modulated by stimulus intelligibility. Spatial and temporal features of this effect seem to suggest this effect indexes the ease of access to word meaning. Our paradigm ensures that the alpha-band desynchronization we observe is not simply related to increasing spectral detail in the stimuli, and thus confirms that alpha-band desynchronization at left temporal sites reflects word intelligibility. These findings provide insights into the neural mechanisms of degraded speech perception, and may be taken to suggest that one strategy in compensating for acoustically-degraded input may be to suppress recognition processes that ordinarily take place rapidly and automatically, in order to permit additional processing to be carried out on the degraded signal.

ACKNOWLEDGMENTS

This work was supported by a Marie Curie fellowship to Robert Becker and received funding from the European Union Seventh Framework Programme (FP7/2007-2013) under grant agreement no. 267171. Christoph M. Michel is supported by the Swiss National Science Foundation (Grant No. 310030_132952). Alexis Hervais-Adelman and Maria Pefkou were supported by the Swiss National Science Foundation (Grant No. 320030_122085 awarded to Professor Narly Golestani). The EEG equipment and Cartool software are supported by the Center for Biomedical Imaging (CIBM), Geneva and Lausanne, Switzerland. We would like to thank the reviewers for their careful reading of the manuscript and their helpful comments.

REFERENCES

Altmann, G. T. M., and Young, D. (1993). "Factors affecting adaptation to time-compressed speech," *Paper Presented at the Third European Conference on Speech Communication and Technology*. http://www.isca-speech.org/archive/eurospeech_1993/e93_0333.html

Becker, R., Reinacher, M., Freyer, F., Villringer, A., and Ritter, P. (2011). How ongoing neuronal oscillations account for evoked fMRI variability. *J. Neurosci.* 31, 11016–11027. doi: 10.1523/jneurosci.0210-11.2011

Becker, R., Ritter, P., and Villringer, A. (2008). Influence of ongoing alpha rhythm on the visual evoked potential. *Neuroimage* 39, 707–716. doi: 10.1016/j.neuroimage.2007.09.016

Benjamini, Y., and Yekutieli, D. (2001). The control of the false discovery rate in multiple testing under dependency. *Ann. Stat.* 29, 1165–1188. doi: 10.1214/aos/1013699998

Berger, H. (1929). Über das elektrenkephalogramm des menschen. *Eur. Arch. Psychiatry Clin. Neurosci.* 87, 527–570. doi: 10.1007/BF01797193

Blesser, B. (1972). Speech perception under conditions of spectral transformation. I. Phonetic characteristics. *J. Speech Hear. Res.* 15, 5–41.

Bogen, J. E., and Bogen, G. M. (1976). Wernicke's region—where is it? *Ann. N Y Acad. Sci.* 280, 834–843. doi: 10.1111/j.1749-6632.1976.tb25546.x

Bollimunta, A., Chen, Y., Schroeder, C. E., and Ding, M. (2008). Neuronal mechanisms of cortical alpha oscillations in awake-behaving macaques. *J. Neurosci.* 28, 9976–9988. doi: 10.1523/jneurosci.2699-08.2008

Brunet, D., Murray, M. M., and Michel, C. M. (2011). Spatiotemporal analysis of multichannel EEG: CARTOOL. *Comput. Intell. Neurosci.* 2011:813870. doi: 10.1155/2011/813870

Busch, N. A., Dubois, J., and Vanrullen, R. (2009). The phase of ongoing EEG oscillations predicts visual perception. *J. Neurosci.* 29, 7869–7876. doi: 10.1523/jneurosci.0113-09.2009

Clarke, C. M., and Garrett, M. F. (2004). Rapid adaptation to foreign-accented English. *J. Acoust. Soc. Am.* 116, 3647–3658. doi: 10.1121/1.1815131

Clopper, C. G., and Pisoni, D. B. (2004). Effects of talker variability on perceptual learning of dialects. *Lang. Speech* 47, 207–239. doi: 10.1177/00238309040470030101

Crone, N. E., Sinai, A., and Korzeniewska, A. (2006). High-frequency gamma oscillations and human brain mapping with electrocorticography. *Prog. Brain Res.* 159, 275–295. doi: 10.1016/s0079-6123(06)59019-3

Dahan, D., and Mead, R. L. (2010). Context-conditioned generalization in adaptation to distorted speech. *J. Exp. Psychol. Hum. Percept. Perform.* 36, 704–728. doi: 10.1037/a0017449

Darley, F. L., Aronson, A. E., and Brown, J. R. (1969). Clusters of deviant speech dimensions in the dysarthrias. *J. Speech Hear. Res.* 12, 462–496.

Davis, M. H., and Johnsrude, I. S. (2003). Hierarchical processing in spoken language comprehension. *J. Neurosci.* 23, 3423–3431.

Davis, M. H., and Johnsrude, I. S. (2007). Hearing speech sounds: top-down influences on the interface between audition and speech perception. *Hear. Res.* 229, 132–147. doi: 10.1016/j.heares.2007.01.014

Davis, M. H., Johnsrude, I. S., Hervais-Adelman, A. G., Taylor, K., and Mcgettigan, C. (2005). Lexical information drives perceptual learning of distorted speech: evidence from the comprehension of noise-vocoded sentences. *J. Exp. Psychol. Gen.* 134, 222–241. doi: 10.1037/0096-3445.134.2.222

de Munck, J. C., Goncalves, S. I., Huijboom, L., Kuijer, J. P., Pouwels, P. J., Heethaar, R. M., et al. (2007). The hemodynamic response of the alpha rhythm: an EEG/fMRI study. *Neuroimage* 35, 1142–1151. doi: 10.1016/j.neuroimage.2007.01.022

de Pasquale, F., Sabatini, U., Della Penna, S., Sestieri, C., Caravasso, C. F., Formisano, R., et al. (2013). The connectivity of functional cores reveals different degrees of segregation and integration in the brain at rest. *Neuroimage* 69, 51–61. doi: 10.1016/j.neuroimage.2012.11.051

Delorme, A., and Makeig, S. (2004). EEGLAB: an open source toolbox for analysis of single-trial EEG dynamics including independent component analysis. *J. Neurosci. Methods* 134, 9–21. doi: 10.1016/j.jneumeth.2003.10.009

Dupoux, E., and Green, K. (1997). Perceptual adjustment to highly compressed speech: effects of talker and rate changes. *J. Exp. Psychol. Hum. Percept. Perform.* 23, 914–927. doi: 10.1037/0096-1523.23.3.914

Eisner, F., Mcgettigan, C., Faulkner, A., Rosen, S., and Scott, S. K. (2010). Inferior frontal gyrus activation predicts individual differences in perceptual learning of cochlear-implant simulations. *J. Neurosci.* 30, 7179–7186. doi: 10.1523/jneurosci.4040-09.2010

Erb, J., Henry, M. J., Eisner, F., and Obleser, J. (2012). Auditory skills and brain morphology predict individual differences in adaptation to degraded speech. *Neuropsychologia* 50, 2154–2164. doi: 10.1016/j.neuropsychologia.2012.05.013

Evans, B. G., and Iverson, P. (2004). Vowel normalization for accent: an investigation of best exemplar locations in northern and southern British English sentences. *J. Acoust. Soc. Am.* 115, 352–361. doi: 10.1121/1.1635413

Evans, S., Kyong, J. S., Rosen, S., Golestani, N., Warren, J. E., Mcgettigan, C., et al. (2013). The pathways for intelligible speech: multivariate and univariate perspectives. *Cereb. Cortex* doi: 10.1093/cercor/bht083. [Epub ahead of print].

Fries, P. (2005). A mechanism for cognitive dynamics: neuronal communication through neuronal coherence. *Trends Cogn. Sci.* 9, 474–480. doi: 10.1016/j.tics.2005.08.011

Geschwind, N. (1972). Language and the brain. *Sci. Am.* 226, 76–83. doi: 10.1038/scientificamerican0472-76

Giraud, A. L., Kell, C., Thierfelder, C., Sterzer, P., Russ, M. O., Preibisch, C., et al. (2004). Contributions of sensory input, auditory search and verbal comprehension to cortical activity during speech processing. *Cereb. Cortex* 14, 247–255. doi: 10.1093/cercor/bhg124

Golestani, N., Hervais-Adelman, A., Obleser, J., and Scott, S. K. (2013). Semantic versus perceptual interactions in neural processing of speech-in-noise. *Neuroimage* 79, 52–61. doi: 10.1016/j.neuroimage.2013.04.049

Goncalves, S. I., De Munck, J. C., Pouwels, P. J., Schoonhoven, R., Kuijer, J. P., Maurits, N. M., et al. (2006). Correlating the alpha rhythm to BOLD using simultaneous EEG/fMRI: inter-subject variability. *Neuroimage* 30, 203–213. doi: 10.1016/j.neuroimage.2005.09.062

Green, T., Rosen, S., Faulkner, A., and Paterson, R. (2013). Adaptation to spectrally-rotated speech. *J. Acoust. Soc. Am.* 134, 1369. doi: 10.1121/1.4812759

Greenwood, D. D. (1990). A cochlear frequency-position function for several species—29 years later. *J. Acoust. Soc. Am.* 87, 2592–2605. doi: 10.1121/1.399052

Grosjean, F. (1980). Spoken word recognition processes and the gating paradigm. *Percept. Psychophys.* 28, 267–283. doi: 10.3758/bf03204386

Haegens, S., Nacher, V., Luna, R., Romo, R., and Jensen, O. (2011). Alpha-oscillations in the monkey sensorimotor network influence discrimination performance by rhythmical inhibition of neuronal spiking. *Proc. Natl. Acad. Sci. U S A* 108, 19377–19382. doi: 10.1073/pnas.1117190108

Heinrich, A., Carlyon, R. P., Davis, M. H., and Johnsrude, I. S. (2008). Illusory vowels resulting from perceptual continuity: a functional magnetic resonance imaging study. *J. Cogn. Neurosci.* 20, 1737–1752. doi: 10.1162/jocn.2008.20069

Hervais-Adelman, A., Carlyon, R. P., Johnsrude, I. S., and Davis, M. H. (2012). Brain regions recruited for the effortful comprehension of noise-vocoded words. *Lang. Cogn. Process.* 27, 1145–1166. doi: 10.1080/01690965.2012.662280

Hervais-Adelman, A., Davis, M. H., Johnsrude, I. S., and Carlyon, R. P. (2008). Perceptual learning of noise vocoded words: effects of feedback and lexicality. *J. Exp. Psychol. Hum. Percept. Perform.* 34, 460–474. doi: 10.1037/0096-1523.34.2.460

Hervais-Adelman, A., Davis, M. H., Johnsrude, I. S., Taylor, K. J., and Carlyon, R. P. (2011). Generalization of perceptual learning of vocoded speech. *J. Exp. Psychol. Hum. Percept. Perform.* 37, 283–295. doi: 10.1037/a0020772

Hickok, G., and Poeppel, D. (2007). The cortical organization of speech processing. *Nat. Rev. Neurosci.* 8, 393–402. doi: 10.1038/nrn2113

Jensen, O., and Mazaheri, A. (2010). Shaping functional architecture by oscillatory alpha activity: gating by inhibition. *Front. Hum. Neurosci.* 4:186. doi: 10.3389/fnhum.2010.00186

Jokisch, D., and Jensen, O. (2007). Modulation of gamma and alpha activity during a working memory task engaging the dorsal or ventral stream. *J. Neurosci.* 27, 3244–3251. doi: 10.1523/jneurosci.5399-06.2007

Kaiser, J., and Lutzenberger, W. (2005). Cortical oscillatory activity and the dynamics of auditory memory processing. *Rev. Neurosci.* 16, 239–254. doi: 10.1515/revneuro.2005.16.3.239

Kastner, S., O'connor, D. H., Fukui, M. M., Fehd, H. M., Herwig, U., and Pinsk, M. A. (2004). Functional imaging of the human lateral geniculate nucleus and pulvinar. *J. Neurophysiol.* 91, 438–448. doi: 10.1152/jn.00553.2003

Kent, R. D., Weismer, G., Kent, J. F., and Rosenbek, J. C. (1989). Toward phonetic intelligibility testing in dysarthria. *J. Speech Hear. Disord.* 54, 482–499.

Klimesch, W. (1999). EEG alpha and theta oscillations reflect cognitive and memory performance: a review and analysis. *Brain Res. Brain Res. Rev.* 29, 169–195. doi: 10.1016/s0165-0173(98)00056-3

Krause, C. M., Porn, B., Lang, A. H., and Laine, M. (1997). Relative alpha desynchronization and synchronization during speech perception. *Brain Res. Cogn. Brain Res.* 5, 295–299. doi: 10.1016/s0926-6410(97)00009-8

Kutas, M., and Hillyard, S. A. (1984). Brain potentials during reading reflect word expectancy and semantic association. *Nature* 307, 161–163. doi: 10.1038/307161a0

Laufs, H., Krakow, K., Sterzer, P., Eger, E., Beyerle, A., Salek-Haddadi, A., et al. (2003). Electroencephalographic signatures of attentional and cognitive default modes in spontaneous brain activity fluctuations at rest. *Proc. Natl. Acad. Sci. U S A* 100, 11053–11058. doi: 10.1073/pnas.1831638100

Lehtela, L., Salmelin, R., and Hari, R. (1997). Evidence for reactive magnetic 10-Hz rhythm in the human auditory cortex. *Neurosci. Lett.* 222, 111–114. doi: 10.1016/s0304-3940(97)13361-4

Lin, F.-H., Witzel, T., Ahlfors, S. P., Stufflebeam, S. M., Belliveau, J. W., and Hämäläinen, M. S. (2006). Assessing and improving the spatial accuracy in MEG source localization by depth-weighted minimum-norm estimates. *Neuroimage* 31, 160–171. doi: 10.1016/j.neuroimage.2005.11.054

Liu, Z., De Zwart, J. A., Yao, B., Van Gelderen, P., Kuo, L. W., and Duyn, J. H. (2012). Finding thalamic BOLD correlates to posterior alpha EEG. *Neuroimage* 63, 1060–1069. doi: 10.1016/j.neuroimage.2012.08.025

Loftus, G. R., and Masson, M. E. J. (1994). Using confidence intervals in within-subjects designs. *Psychon. Bull. Rev.* 1, 476–490. doi: 10.3758/bf03210951

Lopes da Silva, F. H., Vos, J. E., Mooibroek, J., and Van Rotterdam, A. (1980). Relative contributions of intracortical and thalamo-cortical processes in the generation of alpha rhythms, revealed by partial coherence analysis. *Electroencephalogr. Clin. Neurophysiol.* 50, 449–456. doi: 10.1016/0013-4694(80)90011-5

Makeig, S., Westerfield, M., Jung, T.-P., Enghoff, S., Townsend, J., Courchesne, E., et al. (2002). Dynamic brain sources of visual evoked responses. *Science* 295, 690–694. doi: 10.1126/science.1066168

Mathewson, K. E., Gratton, G., Fabiani, M., Beck, D. M., and Ro, T. (2009). To see or not to see: prestimulus α phase predicts visual awareness. *J. Neurosci.* 29, 2725–2732. doi: 10.1523/jneurosci.3963-08.2009

McGettigan, C., Warren, J. E., Eisner, F., Marshall, C. R., Shanmugalingam, P., and Scott, S. K. (2011). Neural correlates of sublexical processing in phonological working memory. *J. Cogn. Neurosci.* 23, 961–977. doi: 10.1162/jocn.2010.21491

Mehler, J., Sebastian, N., Altmann, G., Dupoux, E., Christophe, A., and Pallier, C. (1993). Understanding compressed sentences: the role of rhythm and meaning. *Ann. N Y Acad. Sci.* 682, 272–282. doi: 10.1111/j.1749-6632.1993.tb22975.x

Miller, J. L., and Liberman, A. M. (1979). Some effects of later occurring information on the perception of stop consonants and semi-vowels. *Percept. Psychophys.* 25, 457–465. doi: 10.3758/bf03213823

Moosmann, M., Ritter, P., Krastel, I., Brink, A., Thees, S., Blankenburg, F., et al. (2003). Correlates of alpha rhythm in functional magnetic resonance imaging and near infrared spectroscopy. *Neuroimage* 20, 145–158. doi: 10.1016/s1053-8119(03)00344-6

Narain, C., Scott, S. K., Wise, R. J., Rosen, S., Leff, A., Iversen, S. D., et al. (2003). Defining a left-lateralized response specific to intelligible speech using fMRI. *Cereb. Cortex* 13, 1362–1368. doi: 10.1093/cercor/bhg083

New, B., Pallier, C., Ferrand, L., and Matos, R. (2001). Une base de données lexicales du français contemporain sur internet: LEXIQUE. *Annee Psychol.* 101, 447–462. doi: 10.3406/psy.2001.1341

Obleser, J., and Kotz, S. A. (2011). Multiple brain signatures of integration in the comprehension of degraded speech. *Neuroimage* 55, 713–723. doi: 10.1016/j.neuroimage.2010.12.020

Obleser, J., and Weisz, N. (2012). Suppressed alpha oscillations predict intelligibility of speech and its acoustic details. *Cereb. Cortex* 22, 2466–2477. doi: 10.1093/cercor/bhr325

Obleser, J., Zimmermann, J., Van Meter, J., and Rauschecker, J. P. (2007). Multiple stages of auditory speech perception reflected in event-related FMRI. *Cereb. Cortex* 17, 2251–2257. doi: 10.1093/cercor/bhl133

Osipova, D., Hermes, D., and Jensen, O. (2008). Gamma power is phase-locked to posterior alpha activity. *PLoS One* 3:e3990. doi: 10.1371/journal.pone.0003990

Paller, K. A., Kutas, M., and Mayes, A. R. (1987). Neural correlates of encoding in an incidental learning paradigm. *Electroencephalogr. Clin. Neurophysiol.* 67, 360–371. doi: 10.1016/0013-4694(87)90124-6

Pallier, C., Sebastian-Galles, N., Dupoux, E., Christophe, A., and Mehler, J. (1998). Perceptual adjustment to time-compressed speech: a cross-linguistic study. *Mem. Cognit.* 26, 844–851. doi: 10.3758/bf03211403

Peelle, J. E., Gross, J., and Davis, M. H. (2013). Phase-locked responses to speech in human auditory cortex are enhanced during comprehension. *Cereb. Cortex* 23, 1378–1387. doi: 10.1093/cercor/bhs118

Peterson, G. E., and Barney, H. L. (1952). Control methods used in a study of the vowels. *J. Acoust. Soc. Am.* 24, 175–184. doi: 10.1121/1.1906875

Polich, J. (2007). Updating P300: an integrative theory of P3a and P3b. *Clin. Neurophysiol.* 118, 2128–2148. doi: 10.1016/j.clinph.2007.04.019

Polich, J., and Margala, C. (1997). P300 and probability: comparison of oddball and single-stimulus paradigms. *Int. J. Psychophysiol.* 25, 169–176. doi: 10.1016/s0167-8760(96)00742-8

Ronnberg, J., Rudner, M., Foo, C., and Lunner, T. (2008). Cognition counts: a working memory system for ease of language understanding (ELU). *Int. J. Audiol.* 47(Suppl. 2), S99–S105. doi: 10.1080/14992020802301167

Ronnberg, J., Rudner, M., Lunner, T., and Zekveld, A. A. (2010). When cognition kicks in: working memory and speech understanding in noise. *Noise Health* 12, 263–269. doi: 10.4103/1463-1741.70505

Rudner, M., Ronnberg, J., and Lunner, T. (2011). Working memory supports listening in noise for persons with hearing impairment. *J. Am. Acad. Audiol.* 22, 156–167. doi: 10.3766/jaaa.22.3.4

Scott, S. K., Blank, C. C., Rosen, S., and Wise, R. J. S. (2000). Identification of a pathway for intelligible speech in the left temporal lobe. *Brain* 123, 2400–2406. doi: 10.1093/brain/123.12.2400

Scott, S. K., Rosen, S., Lang, H., and Wise, R. J. (2006). Neural correlates of intelligibility in speech investigated with noise vocoded speech—a positron emission tomography study. *J. Acoust. Soc. Am.* 120, 1075–1083. doi: 10.1121/1.2216725

Sebastian-Galles, N., Dupoux, E., Costa, A., and Mehler, J. (2000). Adaptation to time-compressed speech: phonological determinants. *Percept. Psychophys.* 62, 834–842. doi: 10.3758/bf03206926

Shahin, A. J., Bishop, C. W., and Miller, L. M. (2009). Neural mechanisms for illusory filling-in of degraded speech. *Neuroimage* 44, 1133–1143. doi: 10.1016/j.neuroimage.2008.09.045

Shannon, R. V., Zeng, F. G., Kamath, V., Wygonski, J., and Ekelid, M. (1995). Speech recognition with primarily temporal cues. *Science* 270, 303–304. doi: 10.1126/science.270.5234.303

Shinn-Cunningham, B. G., and Best, V. (2008). Selective attention in normal and impaired hearing. *Trends Amplif.* 12, 283–299. doi: 10.1177/1084713808325306

Smith, A. T., Cotton, P. L., Bruno, A., and Moutsiana, C. (2009). Dissociating vision and visual attention in the human pulvinar. *J. Neurophysiol.* 101, 917–925. doi: 10.1152/jn.90963.2008

Smith, D. R., Patterson, R. D., Turner, R., Kawahara, H., and Irino, T. (2005). The processing and perception of size information in speech sounds. *J. Acoust. Soc. Am.* 117, 305–318. doi: 10.1121/1.1828637

Sohoglu, E., Peelle, J. E., Carlyon, R. P., and Davis, M. H. (2012). Predictive top-down integration of prior knowledge during speech perception. *J. Neurosci.* 32, 8443–8453. doi: 10.1523/jneurosci.5069-11.2012

Stacey, P. C., and Summerfield, Q. (2007). Effectiveness of computer-based auditory training in improving the perception of noise-vocoded speech. *J. Acoust. Soc. Am.* 121, 2923–2935. doi: 10.1121/1.2713668

Thut, G., Nietzel, A., Brandt, S. A., and Pascual-Leone, A. (2006). Alpha-band electroencephalographic activity over occipital cortex indexes visuospatial attention bias and predicts visual target detection. *J. Neurosci.* 26, 9494–9502. doi: 10.1523/jneurosci.0875-06.2006

Tiihonen, J., Hari, R., Kajola, M., Karhu, J., Ahlfors, S., and Tissari, S. (1991). Magnetoencephalographic 10-Hz rhythm from the human auditory cortex. *Neurosci. Lett.* 129, 303–305. doi: 10.1016/0304-3940(91)90486-d

Van Casteren, M., and Davis, M. H. (2007). Match: a program to assist in matching the conditions of factorial experiments. *Behav. Res. Methods* 39, 973. doi: 10.3758/bf03192992

Weisz, N., Hartmann, T., Muller, N., Lorenz, I., and Obleser, J. (2011). Alpha rhythms in audition: cognitive and clinical perspectives. *Front. Psychol.* 2:73. doi: 10.3389/fpsyg.2011.00073

Weisz, N., and Obleser, J. (2014). Synchronisation signatures in the listening brain: a perspective from non-invasive neuroelectrophysiology. *Hear. Res.* 307, 16–28. doi: 10.1016/j.heares.2013.07.009

Wester, K., Irvine, D. R., and Hugdahl, K. (2001). Auditory laterality and attentional deficits after thalamic haemorrhage. *J. Neurol.* 248, 676–683. doi: 10.1007/s004150170113

Wild, C. J., Davis, M. H., and Johnsrude, I. S. (2012a). Human auditory cortex is sensitive to the perceived clarity of speech. *Neuroimage* 60, 1490–1502. doi: 10.1016/J.Neuroimage.2012.01.035

Wild, C. J., Yusuf, A., Wilson, D. E., Peelle, J. E., Davis, M. H., and Johnsrude, I. S. (2012b). Effortful listening: the processing of degraded speech depends critically on attention. *J. Neurosci.* 32, 14010–14021. doi: 10.1523/jneurosci.1528-12.2012

Womelsdorf, T., Schoffelen, J. M., Oostenveld, R., Singer, W., Desimone, R., Engel, A. K., et al. (2007). Modulation of neuronal interactions through neuronal synchronization. *Science* 316, 1609–1612. doi: 10.1126/science.1139597

Zekveld, A. A., Kramer, S. E., and Festen, J. M. (2011). Cognitive load during speech perception in noise: the influence of age, hearing loss and cognition on the pupil response. *Ear Hear.* 32, 498–510. doi: 10.1097/aud.0b013e31820512bb

Zekveld, A. A., Kramer, S. E., Kessens, J. M., Vlaming, M. S., and Houtgast, T. (2009). The influence of age, hearing and working memory on the speech comprehension benefit derived from an automatic speech recognition system. *Ear Hear.* 30, 262–272. doi: 10.1097/aud.0b013e3181987063

Zekveld, A. A., Rudner, M., Johnsrude, I. S., Heslenfeld, D. J., and Ronnberg, J. (2012). Behavioral and fMRI evidence that cognitive ability modulates the effect of semantic context on speech intelligibility. *Brain Lang.* 122, 103–113. doi: 10.1016/j.bandl.2012.05.006

13

Noise-induced hearing loss increases the temporal precision of complex envelope coding by auditory-nerve fibers

Kenneth S. Henry[1†], Sushrut Kale[2†] and Michael G. Heinz[1,2*]

[1] *Department of Speech, Language, and Hearing Sciences, Purdue University, West Lafayette, IN, USA*
[2] *Weldon School of Biomedical Engineering, Purdue University, West Lafayette, IN, USA*

Correspondence:
Michael G. Heinz, Department of Speech, Language, and Hearing Sciences, Purdue University, 500 Oval Drive, West Lafayette, IN 47907, USA
e-mail: mheinz@purdue.edu

†Present address:
Kenneth S. Henry, Department of Biomedical Engineering, University of Rochester, Rochester, USA;
Sushrut Kale, Department of Otolaryngology – Head and Neck Surgery, Columbia University, New York, USA

While changes in cochlear frequency tuning are thought to play an important role in the perceptual difficulties of people with sensorineural hearing loss (SNHL), the possible role of temporal processing deficits remains less clear. Our knowledge of temporal envelope coding in the impaired cochlea is limited to two studies that examined auditory-nerve fiber responses to narrowband amplitude modulated stimuli. In the present study, we used Wiener-kernel analyses of auditory-nerve fiber responses to broadband Gaussian noise in anesthetized chinchillas to quantify changes in temporal envelope coding with noise-induced SNHL. Temporal modulation transfer functions (TMTFs) and temporal windows of sensitivity to acoustic stimulation were computed from 2nd-order Wiener kernels and analyzed to estimate the temporal precision, amplitude, and latency of envelope coding. Noise overexposure was associated with slower (less negative) TMTF roll-off with increasing modulation frequency and reduced temporal window duration. The results show that at equal stimulus sensation level, SNHL increases the temporal precision of envelope coding by 20–30%. Furthermore, SNHL increased the amplitude of envelope coding by 50% in fibers with CFs from 1–2 kHz and decreased mean response latency by 0.4 ms. While a previous study of envelope coding demonstrated a similar increase in response amplitude, the present study is the first to show enhanced temporal precision. This new finding may relate to the use of a more complex stimulus with broad frequency bandwidth and a dynamic temporal envelope. Exaggerated neural coding of fast envelope modulations may contribute to perceptual difficulties in people with SNHL by acting as a distraction from more relevant acoustic cues, especially in fluctuating background noise. Finally, the results underscore the value of studying sensory systems with more natural, real-world stimuli.

Keywords: amplitude modulation, auditory nerve, sensorineural hearing loss, temporal envelope, temporal resolution, Wiener-kernel analysis

INTRODUCTION

People with sensorineural hearing loss (SNHL) commonly have difficulty understanding speech under real-world listening conditions, even with amplification from a modern hearing aid (Duquesnoy, 1983; Woods et al., 2010). Research conducted over the last several decades has uncovered changes in cochlear frequency tuning with SNHL that most likely contribute to speech perception problems in these listeners. While the normal-hearing cochlea decomposes broadband signals like speech into a number of sharply tuned "auditory filter" channels for central processing, SNHL causes an increase in the bandwidth of auditory filters that consequently decreases resolution of spectral features by the cochlea (Young, 2012). Furthermore, SNHL causes downward shifts in the best frequency of tuning, particularly in the base of the cochlea, which are also likely to contribute to perceptual impairment (Liberman, 1984; Henry and Heinz, 2013).

In addition to diminished spectral resolution, perceptual difficulties in people with SNHL might also reflect changes in auditory sensitivity to the temporal structure of sound. The effects of SNHL on sensitivity to temporal fine structure and slower varying temporal envelope cues are both topics of active debate and investigation (Lorenzi et al., 2006; Hopkins et al., 2008; Swaminathan and Heinz, 2012). In the current report, we focus on temporal envelope sensitivity. While several studies suggest that SNHL might cause an increase in the perceptual salience of temporal envelope structure that could adversely affect speech perception in fluctuating background noise (through loudness recruitment; Moore and Glasberg, 1993; Moore et al., 1995, 1996), other studies suggest that envelope sensitivity is relatively unaffected by SNHL (Bacon and Gleitman, 1992; Moore et al., 1992; Lorenzi et al., 2006) or even diminished (Bacon and Viemeister, 1985; Formby, 1987; Grant et al., 1998). Physiological data from nonhuman animals have the potential to clarify changes in temporal envelope sensitivity with SNHL.

Our current physiological knowledge of temporal envelope coding in the impaired cochlea is limited (e.g., Kale and Heinz,

2010, 2012). Consistent with enhancement of envelope coding, these studies showed that noise-induced SNHL amplifies phase locking to the temporal envelope of sinusoidally amplitude modulated (SAM) tones and single-formant stimuli in auditory-nerve fibers of anesthetized chinchillas (Kale and Heinz, 2010). Amplified envelope coding was observed over a wide range of modulation frequencies and did not appear to alter the shape of temporal modulation transfer functions (TMTFs) plotting response amplitude as a function of modulation frequency (Kale and Heinz, 2012). Hence, it appears from the SAM-tone data that SNHL may amplify the neural representation of envelope structure in the cochlea without altering the precision with which temporal modulations are encoded, i.e., without extending modulation coding to higher modulation frequencies.

In the present study, we extend this previous physiological work by studying temporal envelope coding using more complex, Gaussian noise stimuli with broad frequency bandwidth and a dynamic temporal envelope. Wiener-kernel analyses of auditory-nerve fiber responses were used to quantify the preferred spectral and temporal stimulus features driving the neuron (van Dijk et al., 1994; Lewis et al., 2002; Recio-Spinoso et al., 2005; Temchin et al., 2005). The 2nd-order Wiener kernel (h_2; **Figure 1A**) is a time domain representation of the spectro-temporal receptive field (STRF; **Figure 1B**) or mean spectrogram in the 10–20 ms time window preceding a spike (the STRF is the 1-dimensional Fourier transform of h_2; Lewis and van Dijk, 2004). Just as STRFs that are compact in frequency indicate sharp frequency tuning (i.e., spikes are driven by a narrow range of acoustic frequencies), STRFs and h_2 that are compact in time indicate high temporal precision, i.e., spikes are driven by acoustic energy falling in a short temporal window.

In previous studies, we used Wiener kernel analyses to quantify the effects of noise-induced SNHL on the frequency tuning of phase-locked responses to the temporal fine structure and envelope of broadband Gaussian noise stimuli (e.g., Henry and Heinz, 2013). Here, we quantify the effects of SNHL on the temporal precision, amplitude, and latency of envelope coding at the level of the auditory nerve in anesthetized chinchillas. The results show that at equal stimulus sensation level, noise-induced SNHL increases the temporal precision of envelope coding by 20–30%. Furthermore, SNHL is associated with a decrease in response latency of 0.4 ms and amplification (~50%) of envelope coding in fibers with CFs from 1–2 kHz.

MATERIALS AND METHODS

ANIMALS

All procedures were performed in chinchillas and approved by the Purdue Animal Care and Use Committee. The neurophysiological data presented here were collected from 10 normal hearing control animals (143 fibers), 6 animals exposed to a 50 Hz band of Gaussian noise with a center frequency of 2 kHz for 4 h at 115 dB SPL (76 fibers), and 5 animals exposed to an octave band of Gaussian noise with a center frequency of 500 Hz for 2 h at 116 dB SPL (46 fibers).

NOISE OVEREXPOSURES

Noise overexposures were performed in a sound-attenuating booth under anesthesia using either a pair of dynamic loudspeakers (Fostex FT28D; for 2 kHz exposures) or single enclosed woofer (Selenium 10PW3; for 500 Hz exposures) suspended 25–30 cm above the animal. Anesthesia was induced with xylazine (1–2 mg/kg subcutaneous) followed after several minutes by ketamine (50–65 mg/kg intraperitoneal). Atropine (0.05 mg/kg intramuscular) was given to control mucous secretions and eye ointment was applied. Animals were held in position with a stereotaxic device, and body temperature was maintained at 37°C using a feedback controlled heating pad (Physitemp TCAT2LV or Harvard Apparatus 50–7220F). Supplemental injections of ketamine (20–30 mg/kg intraperitoneal) were given as needed to maintain an areflexic state.

NEUROPHYSIOLOGICAL RECORDINGS

Neurophysiological data were recorded from auditory-nerve fibers under anesthesia 3 or more weeks after the noise overexposure using standard procedures in our lab (e.g., Kale and Heinz, 2010, 2012). Anesthesia was induced with xylazine and ketamine as described above, but maintained with sodium pentobarbital (~15 mg/kg/2 h intravenous) for neurophysiological recordings. Physiological saline (1–2 ml/2 h intravenous) and lactated ringers (20–30 ml/24 h subcutaneous) were also given, and a tracheotomy performed to facilitate breathing. Animals were positioned in a stereotaxic device in a sound-attenuating booth. The skin and muscles overlying the skull were transected to expose the ear canals and bullae, and both ear canals were dissected to allow insertion of hollow ear bars. The right bulla was vented through 30 cm of polyethylene tubing. A craniotomy was opened in the posterior fossa and the cerebellum partially aspirated and retracted medially to expose the trunk of the auditory nerve bundle. Acoustic stimuli were presented through the right ear bar with a dynamic loudspeaker (Beyerdynamic DT48) and calibrated using a probe microphone placed within a few mm of the tympanum (Etymotic ER7C). Neurophysiological recordings were made using a 10–30 MΩ glass microelectrode advanced into the auditory nerve with a hydraulic microdrive (Kopf 640). Recordings were amplified (Dagan 2400A) and band-pass filtered from 0.03 to 6 kHz (Krohn-Hite 3550). Spikes were identified using a time-amplitude window discriminator (BAK Electronics) and timed with 10-μs resolution.

Single fibers were isolated by listening for spikes on a monitor speaker while advancing the electrode through the auditory nerve during periodic stimulation with broadband noise. When a fiber was encountered, a tuning curve was recorded (**Figure 1D**, black line) using an automated procedure that tracked, as a function of stimulus frequency, the minimum SPL of a 50-ms tone required to evoke at least 1 more spike than a subsequent 50-ms silent period (Chintanpalli and Heinz, 2007). CF (**Figure 1D**, cross) was identified as the frequency of best sensitivity or, in noise-overexposed fibers, as the frequency of the breakpoint in the high frequency slope of the tuning curve because this value provides a robust estimate of CF prior to cochlear damage (Liberman, 1984). The bandwidth of the tuning curve 10 dB above threshold was also quantified (**Figure 1D**, gray line). Next, a sequence of 9 broadband Gaussian noise stimuli were presented repeatedly for up to 10 mins at 10–15 dB above the threshold for the noise stimulus until approximately 20,000 driven spikes were recorded. Due to noise-induced threshold elevation, the SPL of noise stimuli was

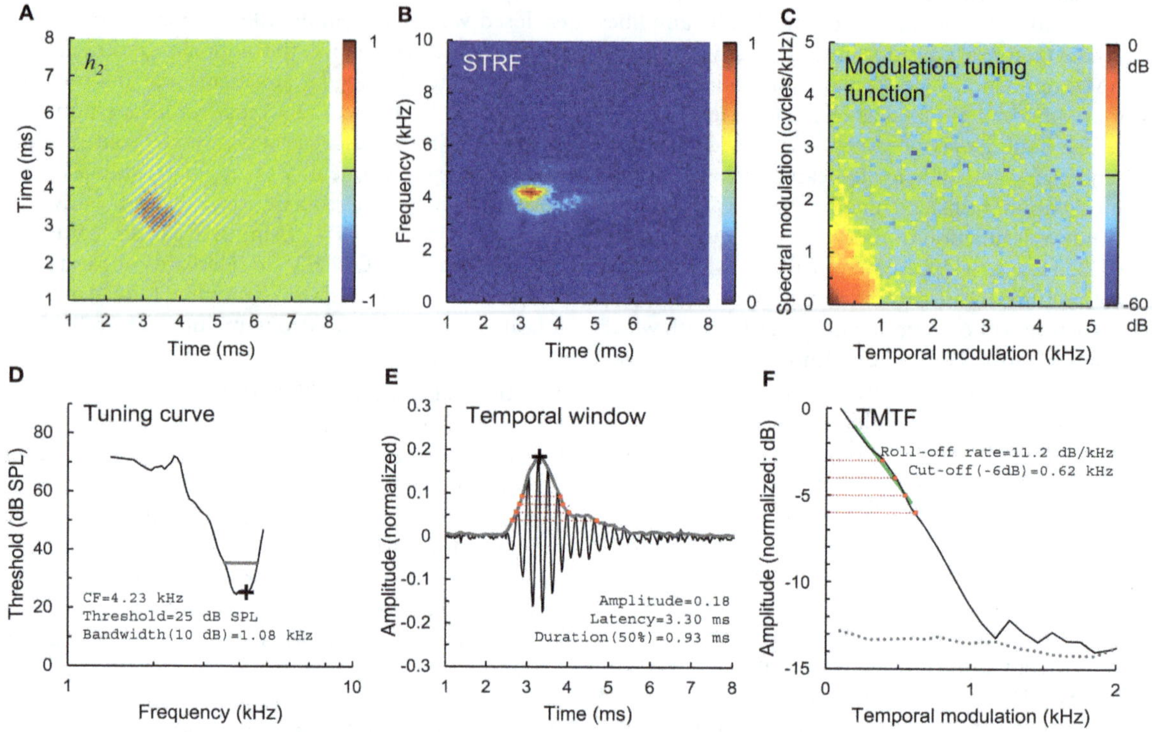

FIGURE 1 | Estimation of temporal envelope coding. (A) 2nd-order Wiener kernel (h_2), computed from 2nd-order cross correlation of a broadband Gaussian noise stimulus and spike train response of a normal-hearing auditory-nerve fiber. Time axes **(A,B,E)** indicate time relative to the occurrence of a spike, and are plotted from a lower limit of 1 ms rather than 0 ms to more clearly show the structure of the kernels. Normalized amplitude color scales **(A–C)** are drawn to the right of each panel. **(B)** Spectro-temporal receptive field (STRF), or mean stimulus spectrogram preceding a spike, calculated from h_2. **(C)** Modulation tuning function, calculated from the STRF. **(D)** Tuning curve showing threshold and CF (black cross) and the 10-dB bandwidth of frequency tuning (gray line). **(E)** Temporal window of sensitivity (gray line), computed as the amplitude envelope of the 1st eigenvector of h_2. Temporal windows were used to calculate the amplitude and latency of envelope coding (black cross) and duration of temporal sensitivity at 50, 40, 30, and 20% of peak amplitude (red dotted lines). **(F)** Temporal modulation transfer function (TMTF, black line), calculated from the modulation tuning function, and TMTF noise floor (gray dotted line). TMTFs were characterized based on roll-off rate (green line) and cut-off modulation frequencies measured 3, 4, 5, and 6 dB down from peak amplitude (red dotted lines).

on average ~20 dB higher in noise-overexposed fibers than in unexposed controls (**Figure 2**). Noise stimuli were 1.7 s in duration with a bandwidth of 16.5 kHz and silent interval between stimuli of 1.2 s.

WIENER-KERNEL COMPUTATIONS

h_2 was computed from 2nd-order cross-correlation between the Gaussian noise stimulus waveform *x(t)* and the response train of $N = \sim 20{,}000$ driven spikes (**Figure 1A**). Only spikes occurring more than 20 ms after stimulus onset and before stimulus offset were included in the cross-correlations, which were calculated with a sampling period of 0.02 ms and maximum time lag τ of 10.2 ms (512 points) or 20.4 ms (1024 points; for fibers with CF < 3 kHz). The basic computations for h_2 have been described previously in detail (van Dijk et al., 1994; Lewis et al., 2002; Recio-Spinoso et al., 2005; Temchin et al., 2005) Briefly, $h_2(\tau_1,\tau_2)$ is calculated as $\frac{N_0}{2A^2}\,[R_2(\tau_1,\ \tau_2) - \phi_{xx}(\tau_2 - \tau_1)]$, where τ_1 and τ_2 are time lags, N_0 is the mean driven spike rate, A is the instantaneous power of the noise, $R_2\,(\tau_1,\ \tau_2) = \frac{1}{N}\sum_{i=1}^{N} x(t_i - \tau_1)x(t_i - \tau_2)$ is the 2nd-order reverse-correlation function, and $\phi_{xx}(\tau)$ is the autocorrelation function of the stimulus. So computed, h_2 is a matrix with units of spikes$\cdot s^{-1} \cdot Pa^{-2}$ that represents the non-linear interaction or "cross-talk" between the responses to two impulses (Recio-Spinoso et al., 2005).

In practice, h_2 can contain bands running parallel to the diagonal (separated in time by ~1/CF), reflecting phase locking to the temporal envelope of the stimulus, and perpendicular to the diagonal, reflecting non-linearity in the phase-locked response to the temporal fine structure. In its 2-dimensional Fourier transform, the envelope component of h_2 falls into the 2nd and 4th quadrants while the fine structure component falls into quadrants 1 and 3 (Recio-Spinoso et al., 2005). Because our primary focus was envelope coding, we removed the fine structure component from h_2 by discarding the contents of the 1st and 3rd quadrants.

QUANTIFYING TEMPORAL ENVELOPE CODING

We quantified the temporal precision of envelope coding using spectral and temporal analysis methods. For the spectral analysis, we computed the STRF as the 1-dimensional Fourier transform of h_2 (**Figure 1B**; Lewis and van Dijk, 2004). Next, the modulation tuning function was calculated at the 2-dimensional Fourier transform of the STRF (**Figure 1C**), and collapsed across spectral

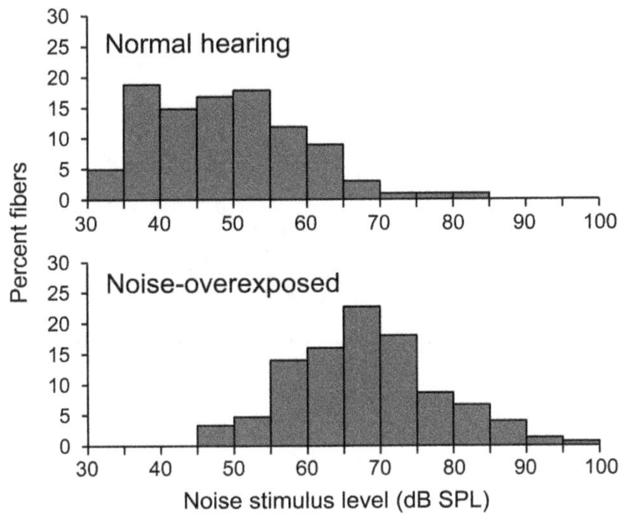

FIGURE 2 | Noise stimulus level. Histograms showing the distribution of noise stimulus levels presented to normal-hearing and noise-overexposed fibers.

modulation frequencies to yield a TMTF (**Figure 1F**, black line; as in Woolley et al., 2005). This TMTF describes the temporal profile of the STRF. TMTFs were quantified based on roll-off rate (**Figure 1F**, green line; measured over the region of the function between peak amplitude and 6 dB below the peak) and cut-off modulation frequencies falling −3, −4, −5, and −6 dB from peak amplitude (red dotted lines). A noise floor for each TMTF (**Figure 1F**, gray dotted line) was generated from portions of the STRF occurring before and after the response (i.e., the first 2 ms and last 3 ms of the STRF in **Figure 1B**) using the same computations. Regions of the TMTF rising less than 3 dB above the noise floor were excluded as not statistically significant. In general, slower (less negative) roll-off rates and greater cut-off modulation frequencies correspond to greater temporal precision of envelope coding.

For the temporal analysis, we calculated the first eigenvector of h_2 as in previous work (**Figure 1E**, black line; Lewis et al., 2002; Recio-Spinoso et al., 2005). The amplitude envelope of this eigenvector (**Figure 1E**, gray line), determined using the Hilbert transform, represents the temporal window to which the fiber responds to acoustic stimulation with an increase in spike rate. For the fiber shown in **Figure 1**, for example, spikes are evoked by acoustic energy falling in a temporal window occurring 2.5–5 ms previously. The noise floor of the temporal window was calculated as the mean amplitude plus 3 standard deviations during the first 2 ms and last 3 ms of the waveform. Portions of the temporal window falling below the noise floor were excluded as not statistically significant. We quantified the duration of the temporal window at amplitude values corresponding to 20, 30, 40, and 50% of peak amplitude (**Figure 1D**, red dotted lines). In general, shorter durations at any given amplitude value reflect greater temporal precision.

Finally, we used the amplitude envelope of h_2 to quantify the amplitude and latency of temporal envelope coding (**Figure 1E**, black cross). To facilitate comparison of data across fibers with varying driven rates and response threshold levels, we normalized h_2 by dividing by N_0A. So normalized, the amplitude values relate to a modulation factor of the mean firing at the average SPL of the noise stimulus.

STATISTICAL ANALYSIS

Statistical analyses were conducted using local regression (LOESS procedure) and mixed models in SAS (MIXED procedure; SAS Institute Inc.). Dependent variables were $\log_{10}$-transformed in all cases except for the analysis of temporal window latency. Local regressions were performed with a smoothing parameter of $\alpha = 0.5$. In general, mixed model analyses were conducted with two continuous independent variables, $\log_{10}(\text{CF})$ and $[\log_{10}(\text{CF})]^2$. $[\log_{10}(\text{CF})]^2$ was dropped from the model when not statistically significant ($P > 0.05$). Categorical independent variables included hearing status (normal vs. noise-overexposed) and spontaneous rate group (low[$\leq$20 spikes/s] or high). Statistical inferences were drawn based on F-tests and T-tests comparing least squares means.

RESULTS

PATTERN OF HEARING LOSS

Acoustic overexposure was associated with increases in both the threshold and 10-dB bandwidth of auditory-nerve fiber tuning curves (**Figure 3**). Threshold elevation and increased tuning bandwidth were most pronounced in fibers with CFs from 1.5 to 4 kHz, but occurred to some extent across the entire CF range studied (0.2–10 kHz).

Patterns of hearing loss were similar between the 2 kHz narrowband and 500 Hz octave band overexposure paradigms (**Figure 3**, red triangles and blue circles, respectively). For example, mean threshold elevation at CFs of 0.5, 1, 2, 4, and 8 kHz were 8, 20, 33, 25, and 25 dB, respectively, for the 2 kHz exposure and 20, 25, 26, 21, and 16 dB, respectively for the 500 Hz exposure. Temporal response patterns were also similar between the overexposed groups, and are therefore described together.

In basal auditory-nerve fibers with CFs > 2.5 kHz, noise overexposure was associated with a decrease in the proportion of fibers with low($\leq$20 spikes/s) spontaneous rates (SR; Chi-square $= 4.79$, $DF = 1$; $P = 0.029$; **Figure 4A**). Furthermore, noise-overexposed basal fibers exhibited an increase in mean driven rate in response to noise stimuli presented at 10–15 dB sensation level [mean difference [$\pm SE = 31.9 \pm 9.8$ spikes/s, $t_{(65)} = 3.25$, $P = 0.002$; **Figure 4B**], suggestive of an increase in the slope of rate-intensity level functions (for broadband noise). More apical fibers with $CFs \leq 2.5$ kHz showed no significant variation with noise overexposure in the proportion of low-SR fibers (Chi-square $= 0.08$, $DF = 1$, $P = 0.77$) or driven firing rate [$t_{(123)} = -0.06$, $P = 0.95$; **Figure 4**].

TEMPORAL MODULATION TRANSFER FUNCTIONS

TMTFs generated from Wiener-kernel analyses of auditory-nerve fiber responses to broadband Gaussian noise invariably exhibited a roll-off in response amplitude with increasing temporal modulation frequency (**Figure 1F**). In general, roll-off rate was slower (i.e., less negative) in fibers with higher CFs

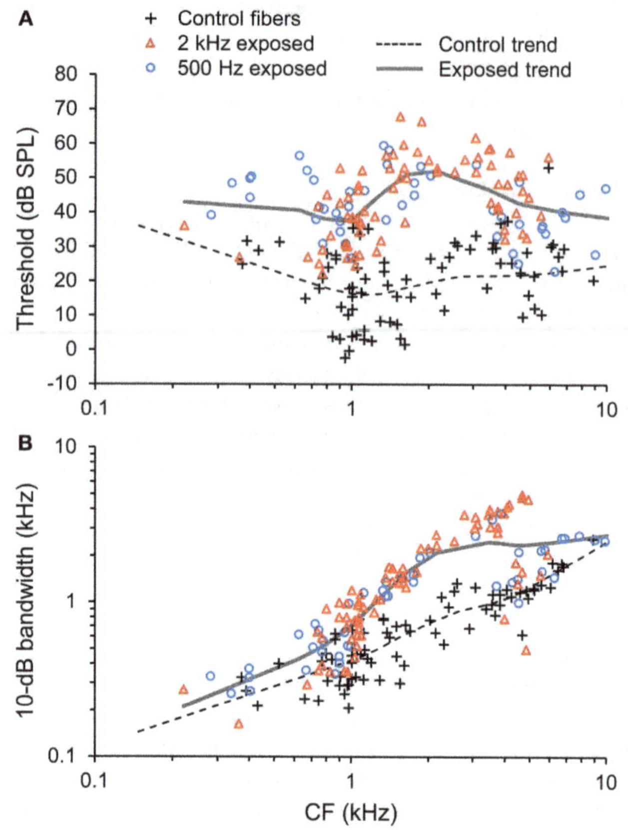

FIGURE 3 | Pattern of noise-induced sensorineural hearing loss (SNHL). **(A)** Tuning curve thresholds and **(B)** and 10-dB bandwidth plotted as a function of CF in normal-hearing control fibers and fibers overexposed to noise. Trend lines are based on local regression analyses. Noise overexposure was associated with threshold elevation and increased tuning bandwidth.

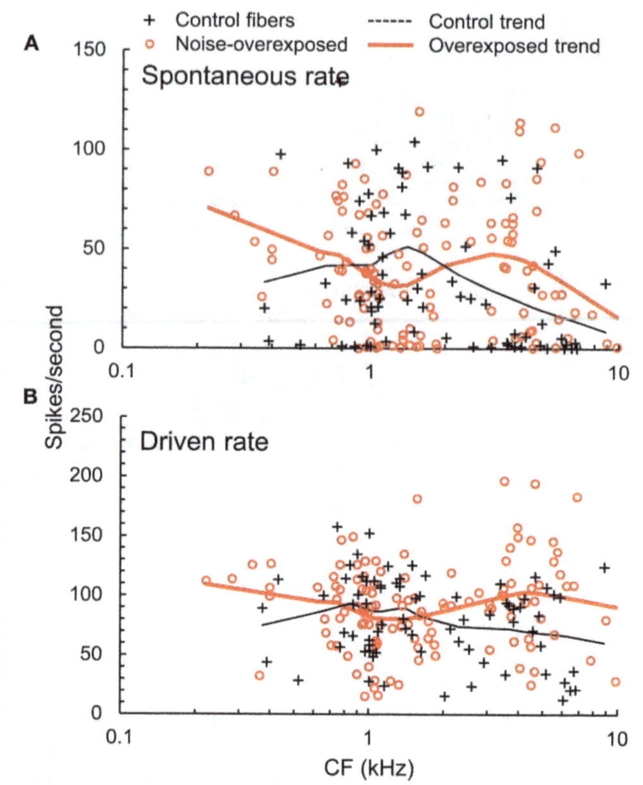

FIGURE 4 | Firing rates. **(A)** Spontaneous rate (SR) and **(B)** driven firing rate plotted as a function of CF in normal hearing and noise-overexposed auditory-nerve fibers. Trend lines are based on local regression analyses. At CFs above 2.5 kHz, noise overexposure was associated with an increase in driven rate and decrease in the proportion of low-SR fibers.

(**Figure 5**), consistent with expectations for the modulation spectra of cochlear-filtered narrowband noises with larger bandwidths (**Figure 3**) (Dau et al., 1999). Notably, the roll-off rate was also slower in noise-overexposed fibers than in normal-hearing control fibers. The mean difference in $\log_{10}$-transformed roll-off rate $\pm SE$ was -0.149 ± 0.033 [$t_{(157)} = -4.45$, $P < 0.001$], which corresponds to a 29% reduction in roll-off rate in noise-overexposed fibers compared to normal-hearing controls. This pattern is consistent with increased temporal precision with SNHL.

Cut-off modulation frequencies were generally greater in noise-overexposed fibers than in normal-hearing control fibers (**Figure 6**). Mean differences ($\pm SE$) in $\log_{10}$-transformed cut-off modulation frequencies measured 3, 4, 5, and 6 dB down the TMTF were 0.0741 ± 0.0249 [$t_{(154)} = 2.98$, $P = 0.003$], 0.0833 ± 0.02509 [$t_{(136)} = 3.32$, $P = 0.001$], 0.0989 ± 0.0248 [$t_{(110)} = 3.99$, $P < 0.001$], and 0.1036 ± 0.0270 [$t_{(82)} = 3.84$, $P < 0.001$], respectively. These results are consistent with the analysis of roll-off rate, and correspond to a 20–25% increase in cut-off modulations with our noise-induced SNHL.

TMTF parameters were generally similar between subpopulations of auditory-nerve fibers with low and high-SRs (**Table 1**; **Figures 5B,C**), except for the −3 dB cut-off modulation frequency, which was moderately greater in the high-SR group (mean difference in $\log_{10}$-transformed cut-off modulation frequency [$\pm SE$]: 0.0532 ± 0.0254; $t_{(152)} = 2.09$, $P = 0.038$).

TEMPORAL WINDOWS

Temporal windows of auditory-nerve fiber sensitivity to acoustic stimulation decreased in duration with increasing CF and moreover, were shorter in noise-overexposed fibers than in normal-hearing controls (**Figure 7**). Mean differences ($\pm SE$) in $\log_{10}$-transformed window duration measured at 50, 40, 30, and 20% of peak amplitude were -0.0982 ± 0.0189 [$t_{(1830)} = -5.20$, $P < 0.001$], -0.0915 ± 0.0185 [$t_{(181)} = -4.94$, $P < 0.001$], -0.0568 ± 0.0199 [$t_{(172)} = -2.86$, $P = 0.005$], and -0.0537 ± 0.0204 [$t_{(153)} = -2.63$, $P = 0.009$], respectively, consistent with the TMTF analyses. On average, noise-induced SNHL decreased the duration of temporal sensitivity by 10–20%, with greater reductions observed for measurements taken closer to peak amplitude (i.e., 40 and 50% of peak amplitude).

Temporal window duration and changes in temporal window duration with noise overexposure were similar between fibers with low and high SRs (**Table 1**).

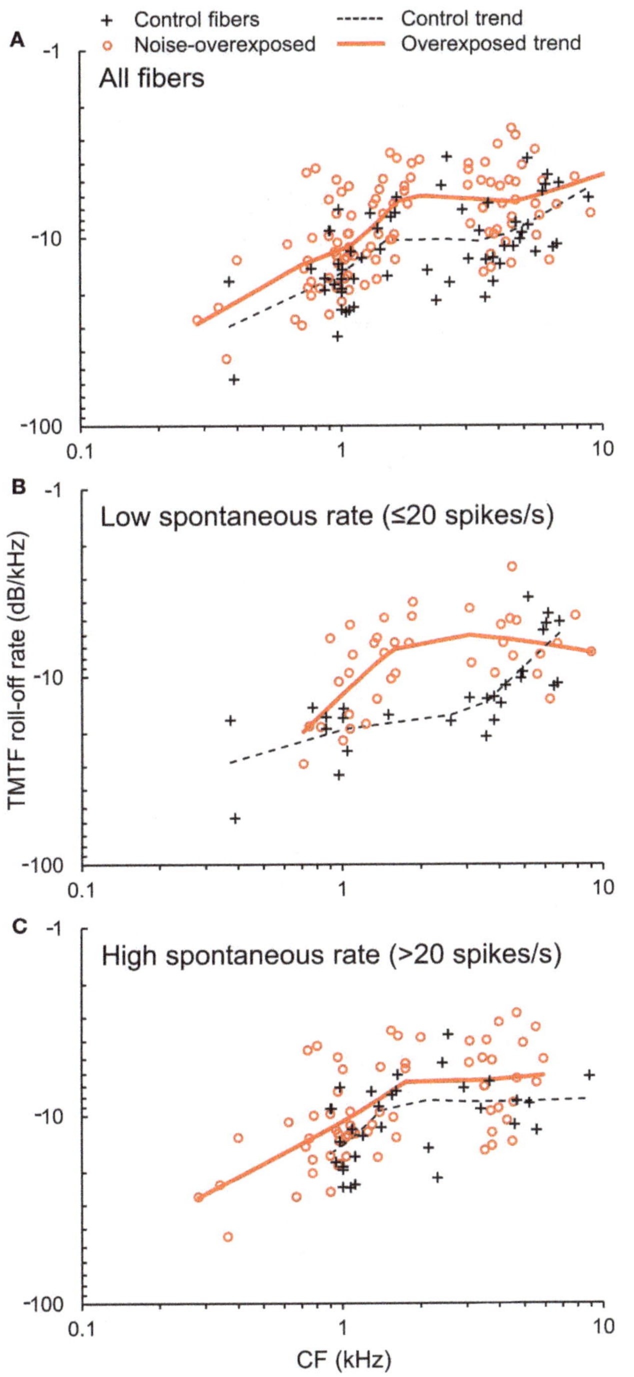

FIGURE 5 | TMTF roll-off rate. (A) The roll-off rate of TMTFs plotted as a function of CF in normal hearing and noise-overexposed auditory-nerve fibers. Data from subpopulations of fibers with low and high spontaneous rate are shown in panels **(B)** and **(C)**. Trend lines are based on local regression analyses. Roll-off rate was 30% slower (less negative) in noise-overexposed fibers than in normal-hearing controls.

AMPLITUDE AND LATENCY OF TEMPORAL ENVELOPE CODING

Noise-induced SNHL was associated with a moderate increase in the amplitude of envelope coding in fibers with CFs between 1 and 2 kHz (**Figure 8A**). The mean ($\pm SE$) increase in $\log_{10}$-transformed amplitude was 0.193 ± 0.044 [$t_{(60)} = 4.38$,

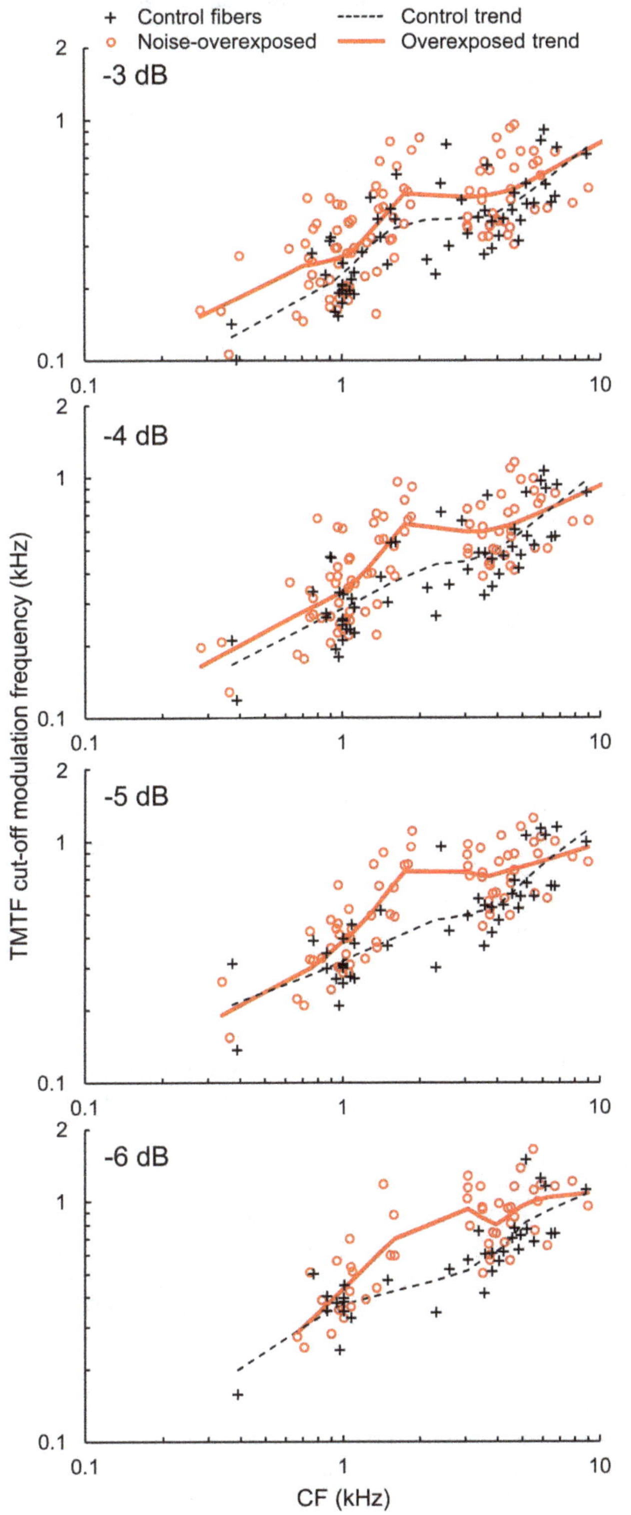

FIGURE 6 | TMTF cut-off modulation frequencies. Cut-off modulation frequencies measured 3, 4, 5, and 6 dB down from the peak of the TMTF plotted as a function of CF in normal hearing and noise-overexposed fibers. Modulation cut-offs in dB are marked at the top left of each panel, and trend lines are based on local regression analyses. Cut-off modulation frequencies were 20–25% greater in noise-overexposed fibers than in normal-hearing controls.

Table 1 | Statistical tests for effects of SR group on temporal precision.

Dependent variable	Effect	*F*-value	*DF*	*P*-value
TMTF slope	SR	2.90	1,155	0.090
	SR*exposure	1.88	1,155	0.17
TMTF -3 dB cutoff	SR	4.32	1,152	0.038
	SR*exposure	0.62	1,152	0.43
TMTF -4 dB cutoff	SR	1.70	1,134	0.19
	SR*exposure	0.55	1,134	0.46
TMTF -5 dB cutoff	SR	0.01	1,108	0.93
	SR*exposure	0.24	1,108	0.62
TMTF -6 dB cutoff	SR	0.02	1,80	0.89
	SR*exposure	0.03	1,80	0.87
Temporal window duration (50% peak amplitude)	SR	0.60	1,181	0.44
	SR*exposure	0.08	1,181	0.77
Temporal window duration (40% peak amplitude)	SR	0.04	1,179	0.85
	SR*exposure	0.10	1,179	0.75
Temporal window duration (30% peak amplitude)	SR	0.13	1,170	0.72
	SR*exposure	0.44	1,170	0.51
Temporal window duration (20% peak amplitude)	SR	0.31	1,151	0.58
	SR*exposure	2.04	1,151	0.16

DF lists the numerator followed by the denominator degrees of freedom.

$P < 0.001$], which corresponds to an increase of 56%. Envelope coding at higher and lower CFs was similar between noise-overexposed fibers and normal-hearing controls [$CF > 2$: $t_{(73)} = -1.91, P = 0.06$; $CF < 1$: $t_{(46)} = -0.57, P = 0.57$].

The latency of envelope coding decreased with increasing CF and notably, was shorter in noise-overexposed fibers than in normal-hearing controls (**Figure 8B**). Across fibers with CFs greater than 0.6 kHz, noise-induced SNHL decreased latency by 0.434 ± 0.061 ms [mean $\pm$ *SE*; $t_{(174)} = -7.08, P < 0.001$].

DISCUSSION

The results of the present study show that noise-induced SNHL increases the temporal precision of envelope coding in auditory nerve fibers by 20–30% at equal stimulus sensation level (i.e., 10–15 dB above threshold). Furthermore, SNHL decreases response latency by 0.4 ms and, in fibers with CFs from 1 to 2 kHz, amplifies the representation of envelope structure by 50%.

The increase in temporal precision with SNHL demonstrated here can most likely be attributed to broader cochlear frequency tuning. Broadly tuned systems have a short impulse response that increases sensitivity to rapid temporal envelope modulations of the input stimulus. Interestingly, tuning curve bandwidths of

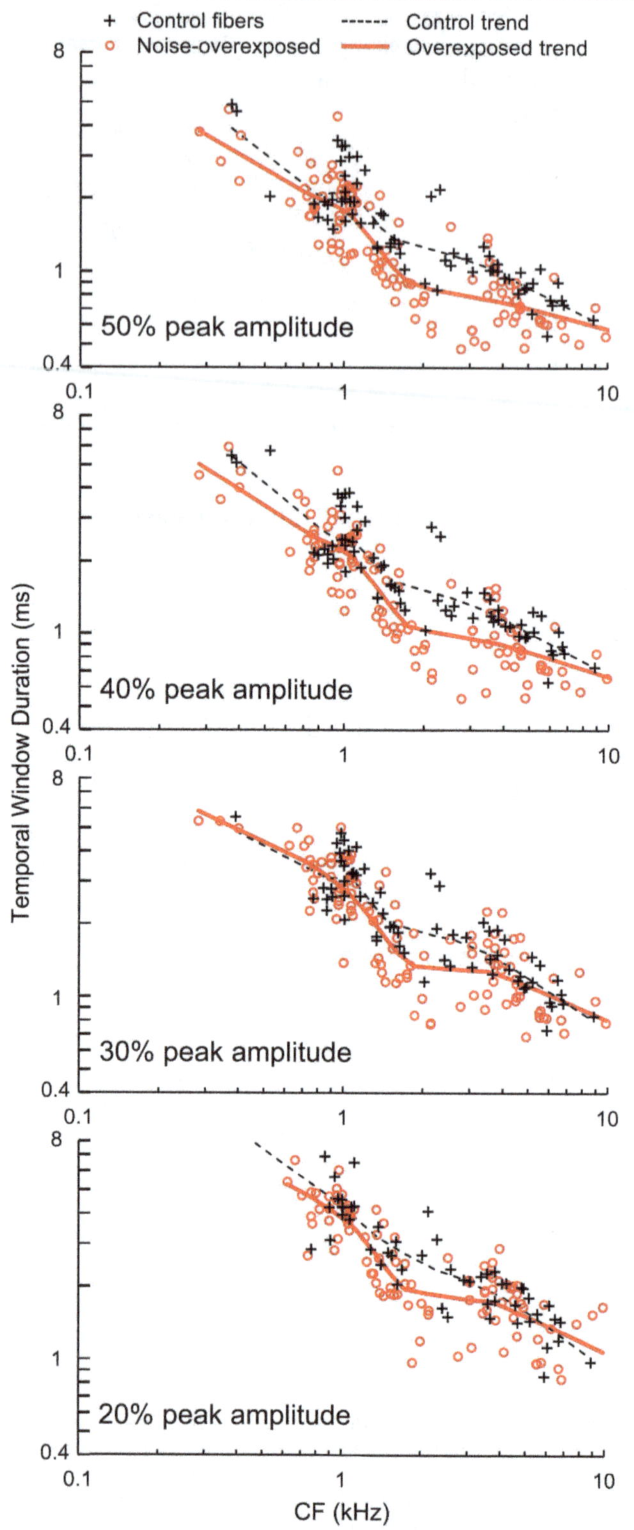

FIGURE 7 | Temporal window duration. Durations of temporal windows measured at 50, 40, 30, and 20% of peak amplitude plotted as a function of CF in normal hearing and noise-overexposed auditory-nerve fibers. Percent of peak amplitude is marked at the bottom left of each panel, and trend lines are based on local regression analyses. Temporal windows were 10–20% shorter in noise-overexposed fibers than in normal-hearing controls.

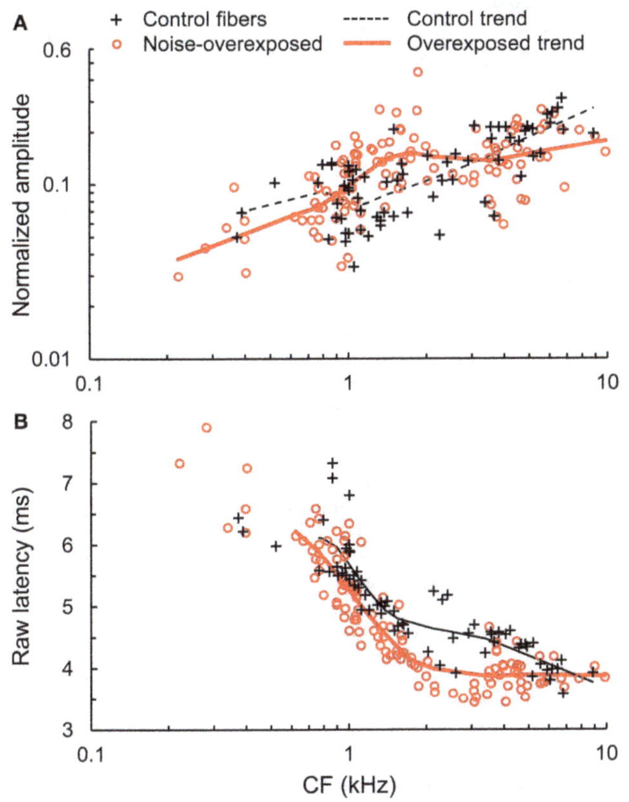

FIGURE 8 | Amplitude and latency of temporal envelope coding. (A) Normalized amplitude and **(B)** raw latency of temporal envelope coding plotted as a function of CF in normal hearing and noise-overexposed auditory-nerve fibers. Trend lines are based on local regression analyses. Latency values include a system delay in addition to neural response latency. Noise overexposure was associated with amplified envelope coding in fibers with CFs from 1 to 2 kHz (~50% amplification) and shorter response latency (by ~0.4 ms) across all CFs.

some noise-overexposed fibers were 100–200% greater than in normal-hearing controls, but temporal precision rarely increased by more than 20–30%. This difference suggests that while broader frequency tuning with SNHL may allow an increase in the temporal precision of envelope coding, temporal precision can only increase to a degree before it becomes constrained by additional limiting factors such as neural refractoriness and adaptation. A similar phenomenon appears to occur in the normal-hearing cochlea of cats, where temporal precision increases with increasing tuning bandwidth up to a CF of approximately 10 kHz, above which temporal precision remains constant despite further increases in tuning bandwidth (Joris and Yin, 1992).

Kale and Heinz (2012) examined the effects of SNHL on the temporal precision of envelope coding using TMTFs generated from auditory-nerve fiber responses to SAM tones. While -3-dB cut-off modulation frequency showed similar CF dependence between SAM tone-based TMTFs and TMTFs from the current study, SAM tone-based TMTFs failed to show a consistent change in temporal precision with SNHL. Wiener kernel-based TMTFs may be more sensitive to the effects of SNHL because, due to the stimulus, fibers are stimulated over their entire frequency tuning bandwidth with a dynamically varying temporal envelope. This task may not only be more challenging, but also more representative of the fiber's behavior during processing of perceptually relevant signals such as speech in fluctuating background noise.

While our results show that temporal precision increases with noise-induced SNHL at equal sensation level, it remains unclear how temporal precision might compare between normal hearing and noise-overexposed auditory-nerve fibers at equal SPL. If temporal precision in the normal-hearing cochlea increases with SPL, as might be expected based on increasing tuning bandwidth with level, temporal precision might converge somewhat between groups at equal SPL. Note, however, that outer hair cell dysfunction causes broader-than-normal frequency tuning up to at least 75 dB SPL (Ruggero and Rich, 1991), suggesting that increased temporal precision with SNHL should persist. Furthermore, previous studies using SAM tone stimuli have shown relatively limited variation in TMTF shape with stimulus level in normal-hearing animals (Joris and Yin, 1992). Greater knowledge of changes in temporal precision with sound level in both normal hearing and impaired cochleae are high priorities for future research.

It should be noted that CF in noise-overexposed fibers was assigned based on the breakpoint in the high-frequency slope of the tuning curve (Liberman, 1984). While we have no reason to suspect that estimates of CF were biased in this group, significant overestimation would be expected to result in a finding of enhanced temporal precision because temporal precision increases with increasing CF (e.g., see **Figures 5–7**).

The decrease observed in the proportion of basal auditory-nerve fibers with low SRs is consistent with previous findings that noise overexposure causes selective degeneration of low-SR fibers. Underrepresentation of low-SR fibers was noted in an earlier study of noise-induced permanent hearing loss in cats (Liberman, 1978). More recent results from a study of guinea pigs suggest that even temporary threshold shifts associated with mild noise overexposure lead to selective degeneration of low-SR fibers (Furman et al., 2013).

While selective loss of low-SR fibers due to SNHL is expected to adversely affect perceptual abilities under real-world listening conditions based on particularly robust coding of signals in noise and high-SPL signals in this group (e.g., Costalupes et al., 1984), underrepresentation of low-SR fibers did not appear to contribute to the differences in temporal precision observed in the present study (see **Table 1**). Differences in temporal precision related to SR might be more prominent at higher SPL. Differences in temporal precision were also not obviously related to mean driven rate. Whereas increases in driven rate were limited to fibers with CFs above 2.5 kHz, changes in temporal precision spanned the entire CF range sampled.

Our finding of amplified envelope coding is consistent with the results of previous physiological work involving SAM tones and single-formant stimuli (Kale and Heinz, 2010). Amplified envelope coding with SNHL may be related to a variety of factors including a reduction in fast-acting cochlear compression with outer hair cell damage. Reduced compression, which has been hypothesized to underlie perceptual "loudness recruitment" or abnormal growth of loudness with increasing SPL, increases the slope of the input-output function of the basilar membrane and therefore leads to larger modulations of basilar membrane velocity (and hence, spike rate) for a given modulation of the stimulus amplitude envelope. Amplified envelope coding with SNHL may also reflect increases in the slope of auditory-nerve fiber rate level functions associated with partial inner hair cell damage (loss of component-1 due to loss of the tallest row of stereocilia; Liberman and Kiang, 1984; Heinz and Young, 2004; Kale and Heinz, 2010; but see **Figure 4**) and changes in auditory-nerve response temporal dynamics (Scheidt et al., 2010).

Taken together with other physiological data (Kale and Heinz, 2010, 2012), these new results help explain previous behavioral findings of enhanced perceptual salience of envelope structure with SNHL. In individuals with unilateral SNHL, more modulation depth must be applied to 1-kHz tones presented to the unimpaired ear than the impaired ear to evoke a sensation of equal modulation depth (Moore et al., 1996).

The 0.4 ms decrease in response latency with noise-induced SNHL found here is consistent with previous results showing reduced response latency to clicks and tone bursts with SNHL, at least at equal sensation level. Noise-overexposure in chinchillas decreases the latency of auditory-nerve fiber onset responses to clicks and tones (Salvi et al., 1979; Scheidt et al., 2010), while kanamycin-induced damage in guinea pigs decreases compound action potential latency (Wang and Dallos, 1972). Similarly, studies employing scalp-recorded auditory evoked potentials have demonstrated reductions in response latency in chinchillas (Henry et al., 2011) and human subjects (Don et al., 1998; Strelcyk et al., 2009). The differences in response latency at equal (high) SPL is not known, but might be smaller in magnitude based on previous findings that the latency of second-order Wiener kernels decreases with increasing level in normal-hearing chinchilla auditory-nerve fibers (Recio-Spinoso et al., 2005).

In conclusion, the changes in envelope coding demonstrated here may contribute to speech perception problems in people with SNHL. Stronger coding of temporal envelope cues and coding of faster envelope modulations may serve as distractions from more relevant cues needed to perceive speech in environments with fluctuating background noise. Several studies have simulated loudness recruitment in normal-hearing listeners to examine the possible effects of enhanced temporal envelope structure on perception of speech in noise. Enhanced envelope structure was shown to increase speech discrimination thresholds by up to 6 dB in steady background noise and by 11–13 dB in single-talker babble (Moore and Glasberg, 1993; Moore et al., 1995). The development of new speech processing strategies aimed at restoring normal-hearing temporal envelope coding in the impaired cochlea may be a promising direction for future research.

AUTHOR CONTRIBUTIONS

Kenneth S. Henry, Sushrut Kale, and Michael G. Heinz designed the experiments and collected data. Kenneth S. Henry analyzed the data and wrote the manuscript with assistance from Sushrut Kale and Michael G. Heinz.

ACKNOWLEDGMENTS

This research was supported by grants F32-DC012236 and R01-DC009838 from the National Institute on Deafness and other Communication Disorders.

REFERENCES

Bacon, S. P., and Gleitman, R. M. (1992). Modulation detection in subjects with relatively flat hearing losses. *J. Speech Hear. Res.* 35, 642–653.

Bacon, S. P., and Viemeister, N. F. (1985). Temporal modulation transfer functions in normal and hearing-impaired listeners. *Audiology* 24, 117–134. doi: 10.3109/00206098509081545

Chintanpalli, A., and Heinz, M. G. (2007). The effect of auditory-nerve response variability on estimates of tuning curves. *J. Acoust. Soc. Am.* 122, EL203–EL209. doi: 10.1121/1.2794880

Costalupes, J. A., Young, E. D., and Gibson, D. J. (1984). Effects of continuous noise backgrounds on rate response of auditory nerve fibers in cat. *J. Neurophysiol.* 51, 1326–1344.

Dau, T., Verhey, J., and Kohlrausch, A. (1999). Intrinsic envelope fluctuations and modulation-detection thresholds for narrow-band noise carriers. *J. Acoust. Soc. Am.* 106, 2752–2760. doi: 10.1121/1.428103

Don, M., Ponton, C. W., Eggermont, J. J., and Kwong, B. (1998). The effects of sensory hearing loss on cochlear filter times estimated from auditory brainstem response latencies. *J. Acoust. Soc. Am.* 104, 2280–2289. doi: 10.1121/1.423741

Duquesnoy, A. J. (1983). Effect of a single interfering noise or speech source upon the binaural sentence intelligibility of aged persons. *J. Acoust. Soc. Am.* 74, 739–743. doi: 10.1121/1.389859

Formby, C. (1987). Modulation threshold functions for chronically impaired Meniere patients. *Audiology* 26, 89–102. doi: 10.3109/00206098709078410

Furman, A. C., Kujawa, S. G., and Liberman, M. C. (2013). Noise-induced cochlear neuropathy is selective for fibers with low spontaneous rats. *J. Neurophysiol.* 110, 577–586. doi: 10.1152/jn.00164.2013

Grant, K. W., Summers, B., and Leek, M. R. (1998). Modulation rate detection and discrimination by normal-hearing and hearing-impaired listeners. *J. Acoust. Soc. Am.* 104, 1051–1060. doi: 10.1121/1.423323

Heinz, M. G., and Young, E. D. (2004). Response growth with sound level in auditory-nerve fibers after noise-induced hearing loss. *J. Neurophysiol.* 91, 784–795. doi: 10.1152/jn.00776.2003

Henry, K. S., and Heinz, M. G. (2013). Effects of sensorineural hearing loss on temporal coding of narrowband and broadband signals in the auditory periphery. *Hear. Res.* 303, 39–47. doi: 10.1016/j.heares.2013.01.014

Henry, K. S., Kale, S., Scheidt, R. E., and Heinz, M. G. (2011). Auditory brainstem responses predict auditory nerve fiber thresholds and frequency selectivity in hearing impaired chinchillas. *Hear. Res.* 280, 236–244. doi: 10.1016/j.heares.2011.06.002

Hopkins, K., Moore, B. C. J., and Stone, M. A. (2008). Effects of moderate cochlear hearing loss on the ability to benefit from temporal fine structure information in speech. *J. Acoust. Soc. Am.* 123, 1140–1153. doi: 10.1121/1.2824018

Joris, P. X., and Yin, T. C. (1992). Responses to amplitude-modulated tones in the auditory nerve of the cat. *J. Acoust. Soc. Am.* 91, 215–232. doi: 10.1121/1.402757

Kale, S., and Heinz, M. G. (2010). Envelope coding in auditory nerve fibers following noise-induced hearing loss. *J. Assoc. Res. Otolaryngol.* 11, 657–673. doi: 10.1007/s10162-010-0223-6

Kale, S., and Heinz, M. G. (2012). Temporal modulation transfer functions measured from auditory-nerve responses following sensorineural hearing loss. *Hear. Res.* 286, 64–75. doi: 10.1016/j.heares.2012.02.004

Lewis, E. R., Henry, K. R., and Yamada, W. M. (2002). Tuning and timing in the gerbil ear: Wiener-kernel analysis. *Hear. Res.* 174, 206–221. doi: 10.1016/S0378-5955(02)00695-0

Lewis, E. R., and van Dijk, P. (2004). New variations on the derivation of spectro-temporal receptive fields for primary auditory afferent axons. *Hear. Res.* 189, 120–136. doi: 10.1016/S0378-5955(03)00406-4

Liberman, M. C. (1978). Auditory-nerve response from cats raised in a low-noise chamber. *J. Acoust. Soc. Am.* 63, 442–455. doi: 10.1121/1.381736

Liberman, M. C. (1984). Single-neuron labeling and chronic cochlear pathology. I. threshold shift and characteristic-frequency shift. *Hear. Res.* 16, 33–41. doi: 10.1016/0378-5955(84)90023-6

Liberman, M. C., and Kiang, N. Y. S. (1984). Single-neuron labeling and chronic cochlear pathology. IV. Stereocilia damage and alterations in rate- and phase-level functions. *Hear. Res.* 16, 75–90. doi: 10.1016/0378-5955(84)90026-1

Lorenzi, C., Gilbert, G., Carn, H., Garnier, S., and Moore, B. C. J. (2006). Speech perception problems of the hearing impaired reflect inability to use temporal fine structure. *Proc. Natl. Acad. Sci. U.S.A.* 103, 18866–18869. doi: 10.1073/pnas.0607364103

Moore, B. C. J., and Glasberg, B. R. (1993). Simulation of the effects of loudness recruitment and threshold elevation on the intelligibility of speech in quiet and in a background of speech. *J. Acoust. Soc. Am.* 94, 2050–2062. doi: 10.1121/1.407478

Moore, B. C. J., Glasberg, B. R., and Vickers, D. A. (1995). Simulation of the effects of loudness recruitment on the intelligibility of speech in noise. *Br. J. Audiol.* 29, 131–143. doi: 10.3109/03005369509086590

Moore, B. C. J., Shailer, M. J., and Schooneveldt, G. P. (1992). Temporal modulation transfer functions for band-limited noise in subjects with cochlear hearing loss. *Br. J. Audiol.* 26, 229–237 doi: 10.3109/03005369209076641

Moore, B. C. J., Wojtczak, M., and Vickers, D. A. (1996). Effect of loudness recruitment on the perception of amplitude modulation. *J. Acoust. Soc. Am.* 100, 481–489. doi: 10.1121/1.415861

Recio-Spinoso, A., Temchin, A. N., van Dijk, P., Fan, Y., and Ruggero, M. A. (2005). Wiener-kernel analysis of responses to noise of chinchilla auditory-nerve fibers. *J. Neurophsyiol.* 93, 3615–3634. doi: 10.1152/jn.00882.2004

Ruggero, M. A., and Rich, N. C. (1991). Furosemide alters Organ of Corti mechanics: evidence for feedback of outer hair cells upon the basilar membrane. *J. Neurosci.* 11, 1057–1067.

Salvi, R. J., Henderson, D., and Hamernik, R. P. (1979). Single auditory-nerve fiber and action potential latencies in normal and noise-treated chinchillas. *Hear. Res.* 1, 237–251. doi: 10.1016/0378-5955(79)90017-0

Scheidt, R. E., Kale, S., and Heinz, M. G. (2010). Noise-induced hearing loss alters the temporal dynamics of auditory-nerve responses. *Hear. Res.* 269, 23–33. doi: 10.1016/j.heares.2010.07.009

Strelcyk, O., Christoforidis, D., and Dau, T. (2009). Relation between derived-band auditory brainstem response latencies and behavioral frequency selectivity. *J. Acoust. Soc. Am.* 126, 1878–1888. doi: 10.1121/1.3203310

Swaminathan, J., and Heinz, M. G. (2012). Psychophysiological analyses demonstrate the importance of neural envelope coding for speech perception in noise. *J. Neurosci.* 32, 1747–1756. doi: 10.1523/JNEUROSCI.4493-11.2012

Temchin, A. N., Recio-Spinoso, A., van Dijk, P., and Ruggero, M. A. (2005). Wiener kernels of chinchilla auditory-nerve fibers: verification using responses to tones, clicks, and noise and comparison with basilar membrane vibrations. *J. Neurophysiol.* 93, 3635–3648. doi: 10.1152/jn.00885.2004

van Dijk, P., Wit, H. P., Segenhout, J. M., and Tubis, A. (1994). Wiener-kernel analysis of inner ear function in the American bullfrog. *J. Acoust. Soc. Am.* 95, 904–919. doi: 10.1121/1.410009

Wang, C. Y., and Dallos, P. (1972). Latency of whole-nerve action potentials: influence of hair-cell normalcy. *J. Acoust. Soc. Am.* 52, 1678–1686. doi: 10.1121/1.1913302

Woods, D. L., Yund, E. W., and Herron, T. J. (2010). Measuring consonant identification in nonsense syllables, words, and sentences. *J. Rehabil. Res. Dev.* 47, 243–260 doi: 10.1682/JRRD.2009.04.0040

Woolley, S. M. N., Fremouw, T. E., Hsu, A., and Theunissen, F. E. (2005). Tuning for spectro-temporal modulations as a mechanism for auditory discrimination of natural sounds. *Nat. Neurosci.* 8, 1371–1379. doi: 10.1038/nn1536

Young, E. D. (2012). "Neural coding of sound with cochlear damage," in *Noise-Induced Hearing Loss: Scientific Advances*, eds D. Henderson and C. G. LePrell (New York, NY: Springer), 87–135. doi: 10.1007/978-1-4419-9523-0_6

14

Neural correlates of moderate hearing loss: time course of response changes in the primary auditory cortex of awake guinea-pigs

Chloé Huetz, Maud Guedin and Jean-Marc Edeline*

Centre de Neurosciences Paris-Sud, CNRS, UMR 8195, Université Paris-Sud, Orsay, France

Correspondence:
Jean-Marc Edeline, Centre de Neuroscience de Paris-Sud, CNRS, UMR 8195, Université Paris-Sud, Bâtiment 446, Orsay 91405, France
e-mail: jean-marc.edeline@u-psud.fr

Over the last decade, the consequences of acoustic trauma on the functional properties of auditory cortex neurons have received growing attention. Changes in spontaneous and evoked activity, shifts of characteristic frequency (CF), and map reorganizations have extensively been described in anesthetized animals (e.g., Noreña and Eggermont, 2003, 2005). Here, we examined how the functional properties of cortical cells are modified after partial hearing loss in awake guinea pigs. Single unit activity was chronically recorded in awake, restrained, guinea pigs from 3 days before up to 15 days after an acoustic trauma induced by a 5 kHz 110 dB tone delivered for 1 h. Auditory brainstem responses (ABRs) audiograms indicated that these parameters produced a mean ABR threshold shift of 20 dB SPL at, and one octave above, the trauma frequency. When tested with pure tones, cortical cells showed on average a 25 dB increase in threshold at CF the day following the trauma. Over days, this increase progressively stabilized at only 10 dB above control value indicating a progressive recovery of cortical thresholds, probably reflecting a progressive shift from temporary threshold shift (TTS) to permanent threshold shift (PTS). There was an increase in response latency and in response variability the day following the trauma but these parameters returned to control values within 3 days. When tested with conspecific vocalizations, cortical neurons also displayed an increase in response latency and in response duration the day after the acoustic trauma, but there was no effect on the average firing rate elicited by the vocalization. These findings suggest that, in cases of moderate hearing loss, the temporal precision of neuronal responses to natural stimuli is impaired despite the fact the firing rate showed little or no changes.

Keywords: acoustic trauma, vocalization, animal, spike timing, tuning curve, single unit recording

INTRODUCTION

Over the last decade, an increasing number of studies have described the reorganizations occurring in the adult auditory system after partial hearing loss performed either by traumatic noise or by partial lesions of the cochlea (e.g., Robertson and Irvine, 1989; Kamke et al., 2003; Noreña and Eggermont, 2003, 2005; Rosen et al., 2012). At the thalamocortical level, electrophysiological studies have documented that exposure to loud, traumatic sounds generating partial hearing loss produced alterations in frequency tuning (Rajan, 1998, 2001; Kimura and Eggermont, 1999; Noreña and Eggermont, 2003; Scholl and Wehr, 2008; Gourévitch and Edeline, 2011) and tonotopic map reorganizations (Noreña and Eggermont, 2005). These changes in functional properties may result both from physiological modifications already occurring at subcortical levels (Wang et al., 1996, 2002; Kamke et al., 2003; Vale et al., 2003) and/or from morphological alterations of cortical cells such as modifications in dendritic morphology and in dendritic spine numbers (Fetoni et al., 2013).

In all but three cases (Sun et al., 2008; Noreña et al., 2010; Rosen et al., 2012), the electrophysiological experiments performed so far after hearing loss have assessed the functional properties of auditory cortex neurons under general anesthesia a few hours (Kimura and Eggermont, 1999; Noreña and Eggermont, 2003) to a few days (Rajan, 1998, 2001) or months (Robertson and Irvine, 1989; Gourévitch and Edeline, 2011) after hearing loss. The apparent discrepancy between all these results might be simply due to the use of different delays between the beginning of hearing loss and the time at which the recordings are collected. More precisely, if neuronal activity is collected shortly after hearing loss, it will reveal a neuronal correlate of temporary threshold shift (TTS), whereas recording neural activity months after hearing loss will reveal a correlate of permanent threshold shift (PTS) with a potential contribution of functional reorganizations occurring at the cortical and subcortical levels.

In the present study, we aimed at following the time course of cortical changes from day to day after an acoustic trauma. Single neuron activity was recorded from micro-electrodes chronically implanted in the primary auditory cortex of awake guinea pigs and the responses of cortical neurons were tested from 3 days before to 15 days after the acoustic trauma. On a subset of cells, we also recorded responses to conspecific vocalizations before and up to 3 days after the acoustic trauma.

MATERIALS AND METHODS

SUBJECTS AND SURGERY

Experiments were performed on 10 adult (3–6 month old, 5 males, 5 females) pigmented guinea pigs (390–650 g) with a national authorization N°91–271 to conduct animal research and protocol specifically approved by the CNRS and Paris-Sud University (CEEA, Ethic committee N°59). The animals were housed in a colony room and were grouped by four or five animals in large plastic cages (75 × 55 × 25 cm; Tecniplast, Buguggiate, Italy) with large wire mesh doors (55 × 20 cm). All animals frequently emitted vocalizations during social interactions with the other animals of the same cage and loudly vocalized during animal care and feeding. We did not notice obvious changes in behavior or in amount of emitted vocalizations before vs. after the acoustic trauma.

Initially, the animals underwent a sterile surgery under anesthesia (atropine 0.08 mg/kg, diazepam 8 mg/kg, pentobarbital 20 mg/kg; see Evans, 1979). Three silverball electrodes were inserted between the bone and dura: one was used as a reference during the recording sessions; the other two, placed over the frontal and parietal cortices, served to monitor the cortical electroencephalogram (EEG) during the subsequent recording sessions. A large opening was made in the temporal bone and very small slits (200 μm) were made in the dura matter under microscopic control. A diagram of the vasculature pattern was drawn and the primary field (AI) location was estimated based on those observed in our previous studies (Edeline and Weinberger, 1993; Manunta and Edeline, 1999; Edeline et al., 2001; Huetz et al., 2009). A coarse mapping of the cortical surface was made to confirm the location of AI: neuronal clusters were recorded with low impedance (<1 MW) electrodes until a progression from low to high frequency was observed in the caudo-rostral direction (Wallace et al., 2000; Gaucher et al., 2012). An array of 5 tungsten electrodes (~1.0 MΩ at 1 kHz, spaced 200–300 μm in the rostro-caudal axis) was slowly inserted in the auditory cortex under electrophysiological control. Starting from 600 μm below the pia, responses to pure tone frequencies were tested at regular depths to optimize the strength of evoked responses; the final placement depth of the electrodes ranged from 800 to 1250 μm which correspond to cortical layers III/IV (Wallace and Palmer, 2008).

A dental acrylic cement pedestal, including two cylindrical threaded tubes, was built to allow for atraumatic fixation of the animal's head during the subsequent recording sessions. An antiseptic ointment (Cidermex, neomycine sulfate, Rhone-Poulenc Rorer) was liberally applied to the wound around the pedestal. An injection of non-steroidal anti-inflammatory (Tolfedine 0.1 mg/kg) was given at the end of the surgery and the 2 following days. All surgical procedures were performed in compliance with the guidelines determined by the National (JO 887-848) and European (86/609/EEC) legislations on animal experimentation, which are similar to those described in the *Guidelines for the Use of Animals in Neuroscience Research of the Society of Neuroscience.* Regular inspections of our laboratory by accredited veterinarians designated by the CNRS and Paris-Sud University confirmed that care was taken to maximize the animals' health and comfort throughout the different phases of the experiment.

RECORDING PROCEDURES

Three days after surgery, each animal was adapted to restrained conditions in an acoustically isolated chamber (IAC, model AC2) for several days. The animal was placed in a hammock with the head fixed for increasing periods of time (from 10–20 min to 1–2 h per day). The animal was also accustomed to hearing sequences of pure tone bursts as well as different vocalizations used subsequently to test the neuronal responses. At least 4 days of adaptation of restrained conditions were allowed before the collection of neuronal recordings.

The recording procedures were the same as in previous studies (Edeline et al., 2000, 2001; Huetz et al., 2009). The signal from the electrode was amplified (gain 10000; bandpass 0.6–10 kHz,) then multiplexed in an audio monitor and a voltage window discriminator. The action potentials waveform and the corresponding TTL pulses generated by the discriminator were digitized (50 kHz sampling rate, Superscope, GW Instruments), visualized on-line and stored for off-line analyses. The pulses were sent to the acquisition board (PClab, PCL 720) of a laboratory microcomputer, which registered them with a 50 μs resolution and provided on-line displays of the neuronal responses. For each animal, the signal from each electrode was tested daily and the data collection only started when, under 1–3 electrodes, action potential waveforms can be unambiguously attributed to a single neuron.

AUDIOMETRY AND EXPOSURE TO THE TRAUMATIC SOUND

Auditory brainstem responses (ABRs) were recorded as previously described (Gourévitch et al., 2009; Gourévitch and Edeline, 2011). Briefly, ABR were recorded via subcutaneous electrodes (SC25, Neuro-Services); using a Centor-USB interface and software (DeltaMed, France). The signal was filtered (0.2–3.2 kHz, sampling rate 100 kHz), waveforms were averaged (500–1000 waveforms depending on the stimulus intensity) and stored for off-line analyses on a computer. An artifact rejection procedure was used during averaging, the rejection criterion being ±40 μV. The stored waveforms were examined and the threshold was defined as the lowest level (dB re:20 μPa) at which a clear waveform could be observed. Intensity levels were always below 90 dB in order to avoid inducing additional hearing loss on traumatized animals.

Hearing loss was realized by a single 1 h exposure to a loud sound. The animals, placed individually in a wire mesh cage (23 × 23 × 15 cm), were exposed to a traumatic tone (pure tone of 5 kHz at 110 dB SPL) in an acoustically isolated chamber (IAC model AC2). The pure tone was generated by the wave generator (Hewlett-Packard, model HP 8903B), amplified (Prism-Audio, model LA-150M) and sent to two piezoelectric tweeters (Motorola, model KSN 1005) located on each side of the cage. The sound delivery system was calibrated to obtain 110 ± 10 dB at various locations in the cage using a calibrated type I precision sound level meter (B&K model 2235). A videocamera, installed in the acoustic chamber, allowed visualizing the animal during exposure and checking that there was no preferred orientation of the animal regarding the two speakers. During the 5 first minutes of exposure, freezing behavior was observed most of the animals ($n = 8$), then the animals moved toward a corner of the cage and stayed there for the rest of the exposure. In two other cases, the animal explored the cage and moved during the 5 first minutes then stayed at the same location in the cage. During the rest of the 1 h exposure, we did not observed particular signs of stress, panic, or abnormal behavior. The amount of excretion (urine and feces) found in the cage at the end of the 1 h exposure session was not different from what is usually found when guinea pigs are placed for 2 h in a new environment (Manunta and Edeline, 1999; Tith and Edeline, unpublished data).

AUDITORY STIMULI AND EXPERIMENTAL PROTOCOL

All the cells included in the present study exhibited reliable tuning curves when tested with pure tone frequencies. The sound generating system to deliver pure tone frequencies was the same as that previously described, (Edeline et al., 2001; Manunta and Edeline, 2004; Huetz et al., 2009). Pure tones (100 ms, rise/fall time 5 ms) were generated by a remotely controlled wave analyzer (Hewlett-Packard model HP 8903B) and attenuated by a passive programmable attenuator (Wavetek, P557, maximal attenuation 127 dB), both controlled via an IEEE bus. Stimuli were delivered through a calibrated earphone (Beyer DT48) placed close to the ear canal. The system was calibrated using a sound level calibrator and a condenser microphone/preamplifier (Bruel and Kjaer models 4133 and 2639T) placed at the same distance from the speaker as the animal's ear (<5 mm). The whole sound delivery system (HP 8903B, attenuators, and speaker) was calibrated from 0.1 to 35 kHz and could deliver tones of 80 dB up to 20 kHz and of 70 dB up to 35 kHz. Harmonic distortion products were measured to be down about 50 dB from the fundamental. The EEG (bandpass 1–90 Hz) was displayed on a polygraph (Grass, model 79D) to make sure that the animal was awake during the entire recording session (the data collection was stopped when large voltage EEG signals characteristic of slow-wave sleep were present).

When the recordings were stable enough and the animal quiet enough after completion of the tuning curve determination, three typical guinea pig vocalizations (Berryman, 1976; Harper, 1976) used in our previous studies (Philibert et al., 2005; Huetz et al., 2009) were presented in their natural and time-reversed versions. These vocalizations were collected from five adult male guinea pigs recorded either in pairs or individually in a sound attenuated room. Calls were recorded using a Sennheiser MD46 microphone connected to a microcomputer and digitized using SoundEdit software (44 kHz sampling rate). The relationships between these calls and the animal behavioral repertoire have been previously described (Berryman, 1976; Harper, 1976). A "chirp" is a brief call (0.7–15 kHz, <100 ms) that is believed to be a low-intensity distress call or a warning signal. A "chutter" consists of a chain of five components (0.5–3.5 kHz, 150–250 ms separated from each other by 140–175 ms) emitted during discomfort. A "whistle" is a two-part call (250–400 ms, with the first part from 1–3 kHz and the second part rising steeply to 8–20 kHz) emitted when animals are isolated or in response to stimuli associated with caretaking. The time-reversed versions of the stimuli were generated by reversing the natural calls in the time domain, i.e., playing the call backward. Each call was presented at a peak intensity of 70 dB sound pressure level. The synchronization between the vocalizations' onset and the spike trains was made by a synchronization pulse triggered when the vocalization intensity crossed a voltage threshold. Therefore, the neuronal recordings to different vocalizations were not synchronized with the real onset of each vocalization but rather with a fixed sound pressure level reached by the vocalization. The natural and time-reversed versions of the three calls were presented in random order, with each call repeated 20 times with a 2-s period of silence between each vocalization. The whole protocol, i.e., testing the frequency tuning with pure tones and the responses to the four vocalizations (natural and time-reversed) lasted approximately 60 min. The EEG was displayed on a polygraph and a computer to make sure that the animal was awake during the entire recording session. The animals did not vocalize during the recording sessions. Neuronal activity was recorded during recording sessions separated by 24 h from 3 days before up to 15 days after the trauma. In all cases, the recording session was stopped each time the spike waveform became unstable. Systematic off-line examination of the digitized waveforms confirmed that spike trains of unambiguously isolated single units were recorded.

HISTOLOGICAL ANALYSES

After the last recording session, the animals received a lethal dose of pentobarbital (200 mg/kg), and small electrolytic lesions were made by passing anodal current (10 μA, 10 s) through the recording electrodes. The animals were perfused transcardially with 0.9% saline (200 ml) followed by 2000 ml of fixative (4% paraformaldehyde in 0.1 M phosphate buffer, pH 7.4). The brains were subsequently placed in a 30% sucrose solution for 3–4 days; then coronal sections were cut on a freezing microtome (50 μm thickness) and counterstained with cresyl violet. The analysis of histological material was always done blind of the electrophysiological results. The sections were examined under several microscopic magnifications to find the electrode tracks corresponding to the implanted tungsten electrodes. Determinations of the relative thickness of cortical layers in the guinea-pig Auditory Cortex (ACx) (Wallace and Palmer, 2008) were used to assign each recording to a cortical layer.

DATA ANALYSIS

For each cell, the frequency tuning was quantified from threshold up to 80 or 70 dB by 10 dB steps. At each intensity, the best frequency was determined as the frequency eliciting the largest evoked responses. The breadth of tuning was quantified by the $Q_{20\,dB}$ (but the $Q_{10\,dB}$ and the $Q_{40\,dB}$ were computed as well). The latency of the tone-evoked responses was computed at each intensity used to test the frequency tuning curve. At a given intensity, the responses obtained for all the tested frequencies were considered, and the latency of the first spike after tone onset was computed (1-ms precision). For each cell, at each intensity, the variability of the latency was quantified by the standard deviation of the mean latency value.

For each cell, the responses to the vocalizations were analyzed in terms of evoked firing rate and spike timing reliability. Since the three tested vocalizations had different lengths (from 90 ms for the "chirp," up to 1740 ms for the "chutter"), only the first 90 ms were analyzed to allow pooling of the responses to different vocalizations. The spike timing reliability was computed using the *CorrCoef* as in previous studies (Gaucher et al., 2013a). It corresponds to the normalized covariance between each pair of spike trains recorded at presentation of this vocalization and was calculated as follows:

$$CorrCoef = \frac{1}{N(N-1)} \sum_{i=1}^{N-1} \sum_{j=i+1}^{N} \frac{\sigma x_i x_j}{\sigma x_i \sigma x_j}$$

where N is the number of trials and $\sigma x_i x_j$ is the normalized covariance at zero lag between spike trains x_i and x_j where i and j are the trial numbers. Spike trains x_i and x_j were previously convolved with a 10 ms half-width Gaussian window.

Onset PSTHs were constructed by summing up all the trials of all cells recorded on each day before and after the hearing loss. These PSTHs were constructed only for the onset response, i.e., for the first 90 ms after the beginning of each vocalization. They were made for the days on which a sufficient number of recordings was available (from day −3 to day +3). They were first computed for each vocalization, but as the main result was similar for all vocalizations, the figures show averaged onset PSTH over all vocalizations.

In the following text and figures, days before and after trauma are labeled D−X or D+X (X being the number of days before −, or after + the acoustic trauma).

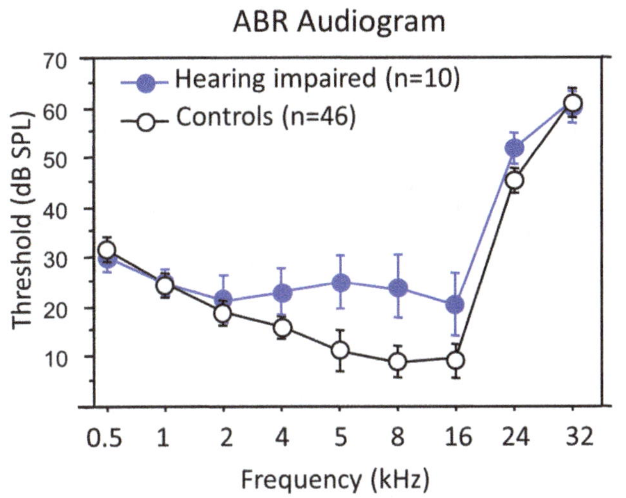

FIGURE 1 | Average audiogram of hearing impaired animals as compared to control animals. Blue dots represent the averaged threshold of the ABR audiogram of the animals ($n = 10$) included in this study, and the error bars indicate the standard error of the mean. White dots are computed from a database of ABRs obtained in control guinea pigs ($n = 46$) of similar age and weight.

RESULTS

EVALUATION OF THE HEARING DEFICIT BY ABR

Since we did not record the ABRs of our animals ($n = 10$) before and after the acoustic trauma, hearing loss evaluation is only based on ABRs obtained a few weeks (between 4 and 8 weeks) after the last recording session. We compared the ABRs obtained from our hearing impaired animals with a large database of ABRs obtained (with exactly the same equipment) in control guinea pigs ($n = 46$) of the same age (4.7 ± 0.6 months) and weight (585 ± 113 g) than the ones used here. The control animals had typical ABR audiograms similar to those previously published (Gourévitch et al., 2009; Gourévitch and Edeline, 2011). Compared to control animals, the animals used in the present experiment had a consistent hearing deficit (15–20 dB on average) in the 4–8 kHz range (**Figure 1**). Statistical analyses confirmed that there was no hearing deficit in the low frequency range (unpaired t-tests, $p > 0.10$ at 0.5, 1 and 2 kHz), a clear and significant hearing deficit in the mid frequency range ($p < 0.01$ for 4, 5, and 8 kHz). The hearing loss was modest but still significant at 16 kHz ($p = 0.047$); it was not for 24 and 32 kHz ($p > 0.08$ in both cases). Thus, the long-term effects of the exposure were mostly an increased threshold of 15 dB at, and one octave above, the trauma frequency. Most likely, these changes should be considered as a PTS since they were obtained 1.5–2.5 months after the acoustic trauma.

CONSEQUENCES OF THE TUNING CURVES PARAMETERS

Thirty-two cortical sites were studied in eight animals from 3 days before to 15 days after the acoustic trauma (for two animals none of the electrodes gave satisfactory signal-to-noise ratio to record clear single unit activity over the 2 weeks of recording). On each recording session, special cares were taken to make sure that the discharges of a single unit were actually recorded. From 1 day to the next, it was not possible to determine whether or not the same neuron was recorded and, rather than claiming that the same cells were recorded over time, we prefer to consider that it was the same cortical site from which cells were sampled across the 3 weeks of the protocol.

On a given recording session, the neuronal responses were determined at 3–7 intensities (from 80 or 70 dB to threshold) thus allowing quantifications of functional parameters. The scattergrams presented on **Figure 2** display the characteristic frequency (CF) derived at each cortical site before trauma vs. after trauma. Comparing the CF obtained 3 days vs. 1 day before the acoustic trauma (**Figure 2A**) indicates that there was a relative good match between the CF values, which suggests that there was a decent amount of stability of the CF in control conditions. During all the following recording sessions after the trauma, the general tendency was the same: cortical sites with initial CF above 8 kHz displayed lower CF after the trauma (dots below the diagonal lines in **Figures 2B–F**). Statistical analyses indicated that there was no change in CF value between two recording sessions before the acoustic trauma ($p > 0.32$), whereas there was a significant decrease of the CF values from the first (D+1) to the last (D+15) recording session after the trauma (paired t-test, $p < 0.05$ in all cases). This effect is illustrated on **Figure 3**: For two different cortical sites, the tuning curves clearly display a shift of at least one octave in the low frequency range. Note that there was a partial recovery of the threshold between the first day and the third day after the trauma. Also, as shown in **Figure 4**, there was no correlation between the threshold shifts and the shifts in CF values: even at D+15, cells within the same frequency band can display either large increase in threshold or a small decrease in threshold.

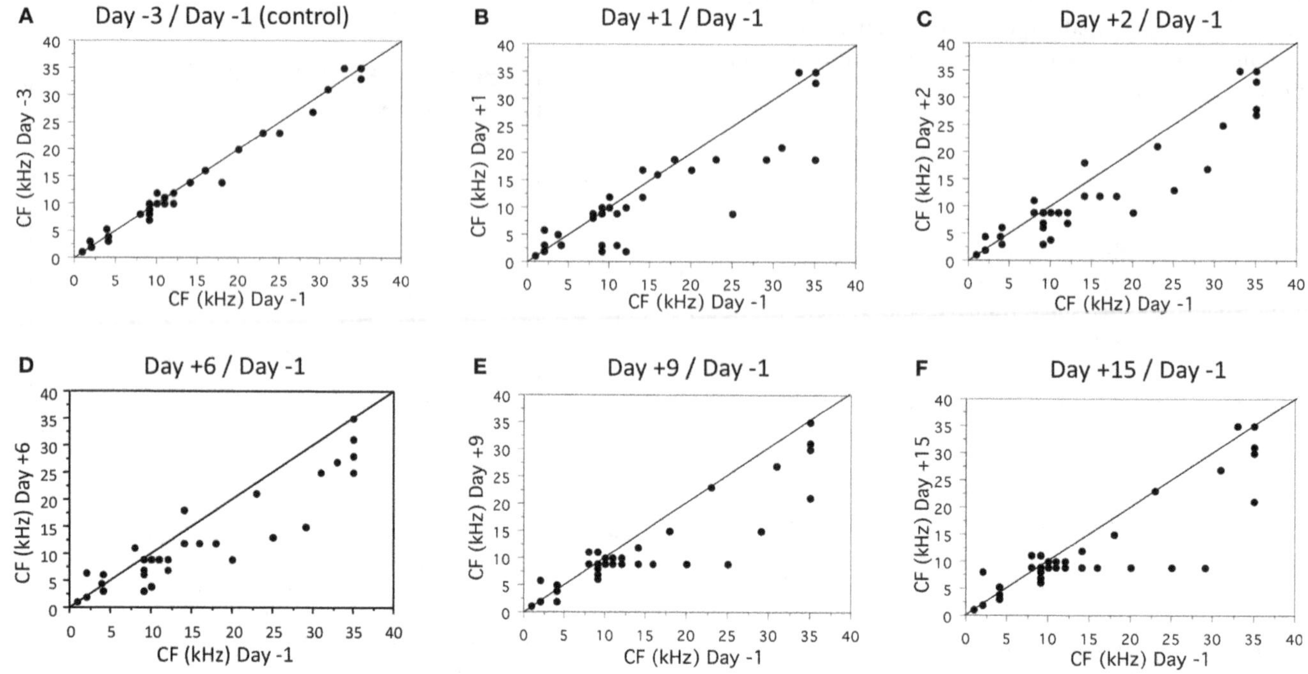

FIGURE 2 | Time course of Characteristic Frequency shifts from 1 day to 15 days after the trauma. Each scatterplots represent the Characteristic Frequency (CF) of the recorded neurons on the day of interest (y-axis) against a control value computed the day before the trauma (x-axis). The day of interest (y-axis) corresponds to 3 days before trauma **(A)**, and 1 day **(B)**, 2 days **(C)**, 6 days **(D)**, 9 days **(E)**, and 15 days **(F)** after trauma. Dots below the diagonal black lines correspond to neurons for which the CF was decreased after the trauma.

Based on the tuning curves obtained at each cortical site before and after the trauma, the group data clearly pointed out that there was an increase in cortical threshold. **Figure 5A** shows the evolution of the mean threshold value from 3 days up to 15 days after the acoustic trauma. There was a 20 dB increase (from 39.6 to 61.4 dB, $p < 0.01$) in threshold when comparing the day preceding the trauma and the day following the trauma. In the following days, this increase in threshold was less pronounced (10 dB on average) but the mean threshold remained significantly higher than before trauma ($p < 0.05$ at 9 and 15 days post-trauma). It tended to stabilize after the trauma since there was not threshold difference at 9 and 15 days post-trauma ($p > 0.20$).

As shown in **Figure 5B**, the quantification of the tuning width by the $Q_{20\,dB}$ revealed neither systematic tuning curve enlargement nor systematic shrinkage after the acoustic trauma (all p-values > 0.18). Quantification of the $Q_{10\,dB}$ or the $Q_{40\,dB}$ did not reveal effect that could have been masked by the arbitrary choice of quantifying the tuning curve at a particular intensity ($p > 0.15$ in all cases). Analyzing the tuning width according to the CF frequency did not reveal more effects: There were no statistical differences in tuning width for cells with low CF (<5 kHz), middle CF ($5 < CF < 10$ kHz) and high frequency CF (>10 kHz).

In contrast, quantification of the latency of the tone evoked responses revealed a marked effect (**Figure 5C**): At the highest intensity tested (70 or 80 dB), there was a large and significant ($p < 0.01$) increase in response latency the first day following the acoustic trauma (from 27.2 to 32.5 ms). This increase in latency was no longer present the subsequent days ($p > 0.25$ in all cases). Similarly, the variability of the response latency was increased the first day after the acoustic trauma ($p < 0.05$, **Figure 5D**) but not the following days ($p > 0.27$ in all cases). In fact, subsequent analyses revealed that this increase in response latency and latency variability was present for the cells exhibiting a CF above 5 kHz before the trauma ($p < 0.01$) but was less pronounced for the cells exhibiting lower CF ($p = 0.07$). Note that this increase in latency and latency variability was still significant ($p < 0.05$) when the responses obtained at all the tested intensities (80–20 dB) were pooled together.

To summarize, the quantification of the tuning curves indicated that there was a 20 dB increase in cortical threshold in the 24 h following the acoustic trauma accompanied by a 5 ms mean increase in response latency and in variability of response latency. Although attenuated, the increase in cortical auditory threshold was still present up to 15 days post-trauma, but the changes in latency and latency variability could no longer be detected after the first day post-trauma. Whatever the frequency band that was considered (below the trauma frequency, within 1.5 octave above, or more than 1.5 octave above it), there was no correlation between the ABR threshold shift and the cortical threshold shift (lowest p-value, $p = 0.23$). This lack of relationship was previously reported (see Figure 4 in Gourévitch and Edeline, 2011).

ALTERATIONS OF THE RESPONSES TO CONSPECIFIC VOCALIZATIONS

Each time the animal was still quiet after the completion of the tuning curve determination, a set of previously used conspecific vocalizations (Philibert et al., 2005; Huetz et al., 2009) was presented at 70 dB SPL (peak amplitude) in their normal and

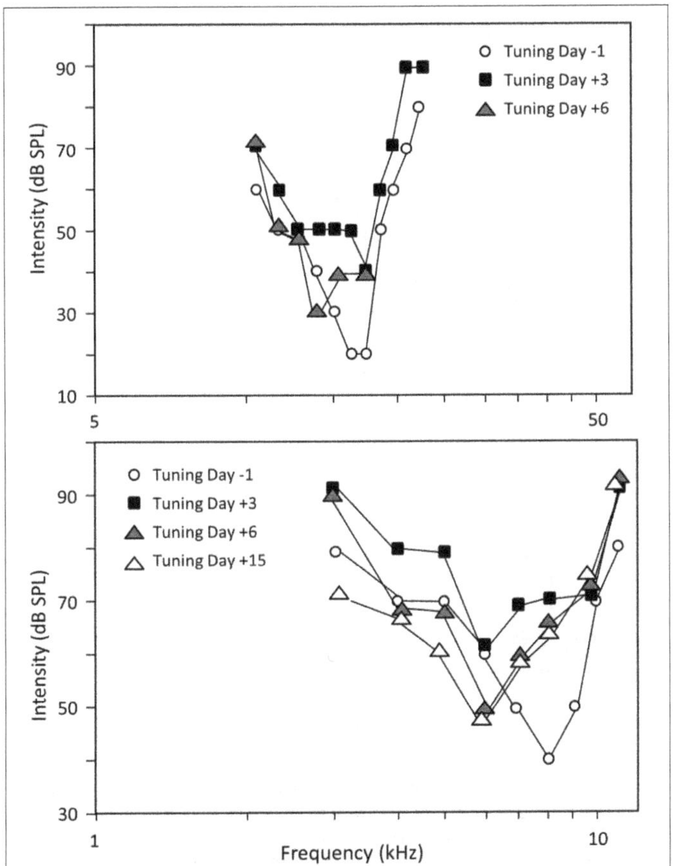

FIGURE 3 | Frequency shifts of two cortical tuning curves. Frequency tuning curves of two individual neurons (top and bottom). For each neuron, the tuning curve is represented the day before the trauma (white circles), 3 days (black square) and 6 days (gray triangle) after the trauma. The decrease in threshold value at CF from D+3 to D+6 might reflect a putative transition between TTS and PTS.

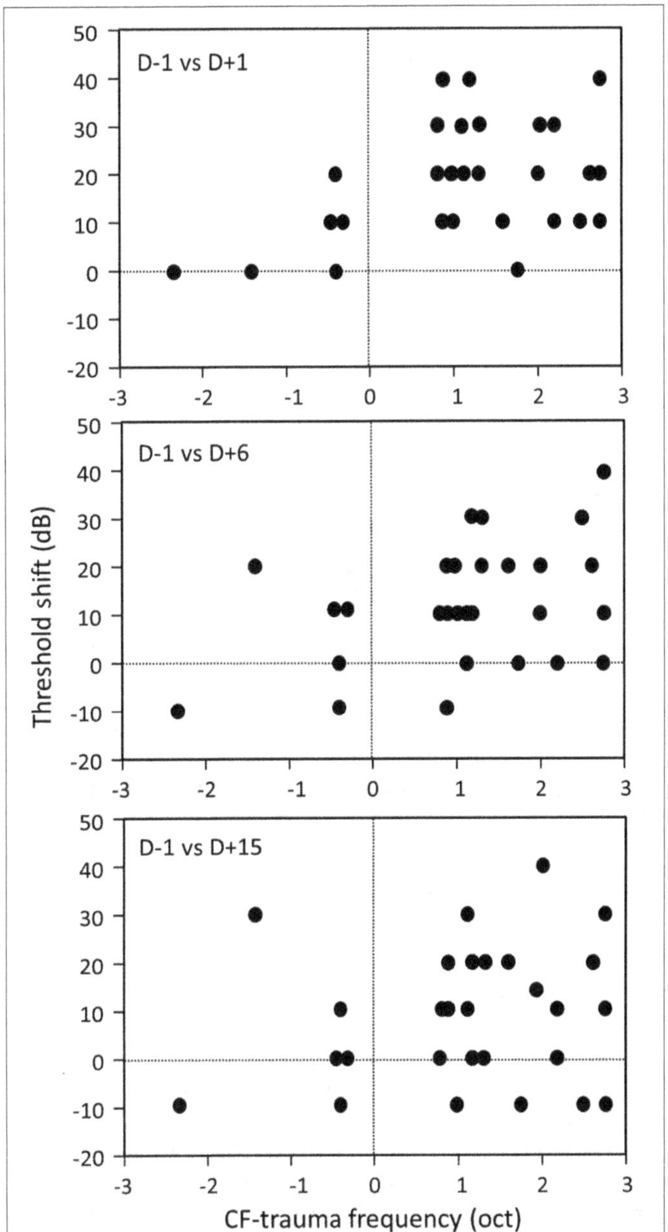

FIGURE 4 | Lack of correlation between ABR threshold shifts and CF distance from trauma frequency. Each scatterplot represents the ABR threshold shift as a function of the frequency shift (e.g., CF—trauma frequency) of each neuron 1 day (top), 3 days (middle), and 6 days (bottom) after the trauma.

time-reversed versions. Based upon previous studies (review in Huetz et al., 2011; Gaucher et al., 2013b), two parameters were quantified to assess the effect of hearing loss on the responses to communication sounds, the firing rate and the spike timing reliability of the responses. On average, we could not detect significant change in evoked firing rate during the presentation of the vocalizations at 70 dB. **Figure 6A** displays the evoked firing rate for the 3 days before and the 3 days after the acoustic trauma: There was a slight increase in evoked response the 2 first days after the trauma, and a non-significant decrease on the third day. None of these variations were significant as they were in the range of the pre-trauma response fluctuations. Similarly, we could not detect significant effect on the spontaneous firing rate. Even if an ANOVA across days was significant ($F = 7.14, p < 0.01$), the difference between D−1 (3.1 spikes/s) and D+1 (3.9 spikes/s) was smaller than the difference between D-2 (4.7 spikes/s) and D−1. Thus, day-to-day fluctuations in spontaneous firing rate before the acoustic trauma might have prevented to detect significant effects after the acoustic trauma.

The *CorrCoef* index, i.e., the index quantifying the spike timing reliability of evoked responses, did not indicate significant changes (**Figure 6B**). There was a small decrease in spike timing reliability on the 2 first days after the acoustic trauma, but, as for the firing rate, this change was in the range of the pre-trauma fluctuations (ANOVA, $F = 1.82$, $p = 0.10$). For the cells with CF above 5 kHz, we did not detect significant changes in terms of evoked firing rate. However, for these cells the *CorrCoef* index showed a significant decrease on the first day after the trauma compared to the day before trauma (ANOVA, $F = 2.34$, $p = 0.04$, paired t-test between D−1 and D+1, $p = 0.007$) suggesting that the acoustic trauma transiently

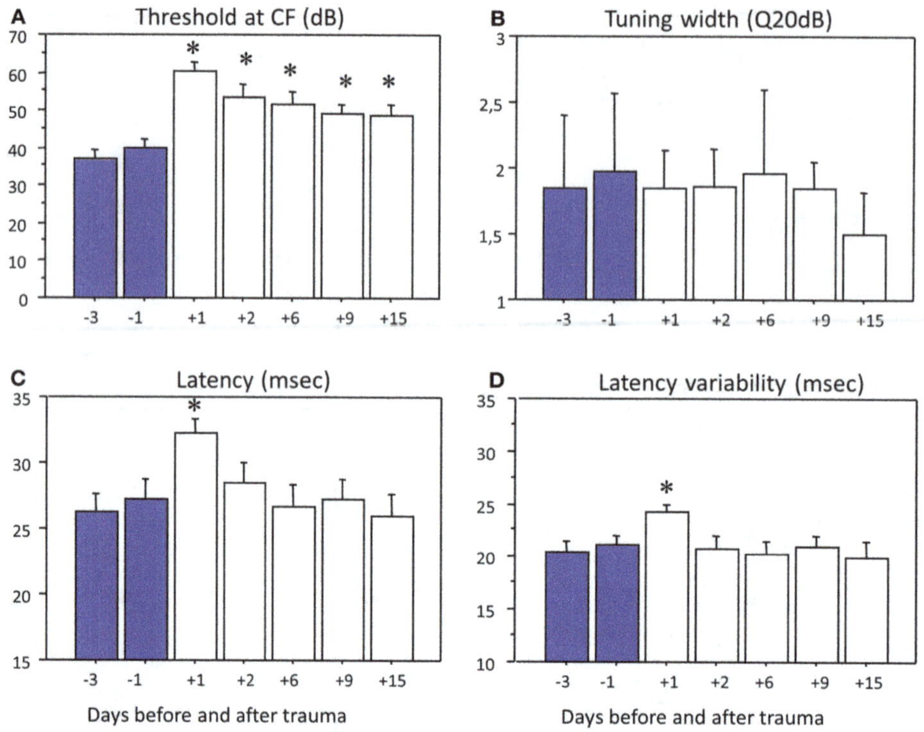

FIGURE 5 | Impact of hearing loss on the tuning curve parameters. The histograms display the averaged values of the threshold at CF **(A)**, tuning width **(B)**, latency **(C)**, and latency variability **(D)** across days before and after trauma (from 3 days before to 15 days after the trauma). Values before trauma are indicated in blue, whereas values after trauma are in white. The error bars show the standard error of the mean. The decrease in threshold value at CF from D+1 to D+9 might reflect a dissipation of the TTS effect and the stabilization of threshold value at CF between D+9 and D+15 could suggest that a PTS is reached. Stars correspond to statistically significant difference ($p < 0.05$) from control level at Day-1.

impacts the spike timing reliability of middle and high CF cells (**Figure 6C**).

Interestingly, analyzing the average latency obtained from the onset responses to the different vocalizations indicated clear effects. **Figure 7A** shows average onset PSTHs obtained when pooling the response to the different vocalizations across all the recorded cells. Over the 3 first days before the trauma (blue curves), the latency was relatively stable with a mean latency of 10 ms[1]. During the 3 days after the acoustic trauma (red curves), the latency was increased to a value of 11 ms: Although small in absolute value, this increase in latency was systematic as attested by the shifts of the onset PSTHs. This increase was more pronounced the first day following the trauma then the response latency progressively moved back to control values. The overall shape of the response was also modified. The onset response was reduced and the response duration was increased, suggesting a lack of synchronization of the response at the onset of the vocalizations. Moreover, analyzing the duration of the onset response (by taking a threshold at 0.15 spikes/s which correspond to the baseline level plus 2 standard deviations) revealed that the trauma strongly increased the variability and/or the duration of the onset response: before the trauma, the responses returned to the background firing rate (0.15 spikes/s) after 9 ms, whereas the first day after the trauma, the onset response lasted for 19 ms.

To investigate how the acoustic trauma affects the responses of cells with different CFs, we split the population into three groups according to the cell's CF: the "low CF" group (CF < 5 kHz, $n = 6$) for which the CF was below the trauma frequency, the middle frequency CF (5 kHz < CF < 10 kHz) for which the CF was in one octave above the trauma frequency and high CF (CF > 10 kHz) for which the CF was more than one octave above the trauma frequency. **Figure 7B** shows the onset PSTHs computed for these three groups the day before and the day after the trauma. Before the trauma, we observed that the higher the CF, the longer the latency and the smaller the onset response. This effect probably results from the fact that there was little energy in the vocalization in the high frequencies, so the strength of the inputs was probably very weak for the neurons with high CF. This pattern was conserved the day following the trauma, but in the three groups, the response latencies was increased after the acoustic trauma (compare the different blue curves with the red-yellow curves). More importantly, for the low CF neurons, only the latency was shifted without any effect on the strength of the onset response. For the two other groups, the trauma not only induced a shift in latency but also a slight decrease of the strength of the onset response.

[1]Note that this value corresponds to the latency of the neuronal response as measured from the time at which the vocalizations reached a fixed threshold in terms of SPL level (the same for all vocalizations; see Methods).

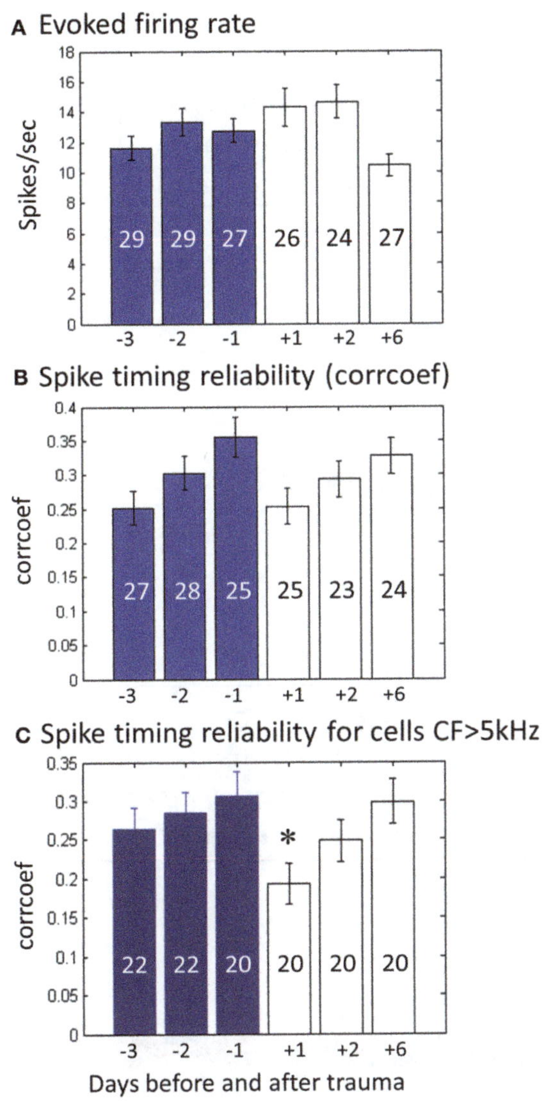

FIGURE 6 | Impact of hearing loss on the responses to vocalizations. (A) Histogram of the average firing rate during the first 90 ms of the responses to the different vocalizations from 3 days before trauma (blue) to 3 days after (white). The number of neurons in each recording day is indicated within each bar. **(B)** Same for the spike timing reliability as computed from the *CorrCoef* (see Methods) for all recorded neurons. The *CorrCoef* is an index of the trial-to-trial reliability of the response. **(C)** Same as **(B)**, but only for neurons which CF is above the trauma frequency (CF > 5 kHz). Stars correspond to statistically significant difference ($p < 0.05$) from control level at Day-1.

DISCUSSION

We show here that an acoustic trauma, producing moderate but permanent hearing loss triggers both transient (D+1) and long-lasting (D+15) events in the responses of auditory cortex neurons. When tested with pure tones, auditory cortex neurons displayed 24 h after the trauma an increase in threshold, accompanied by an increase in latency and latency variability. Only a modest increase in threshold persisted a few days after. When tested with conspecific vocalizations, the responses of cortical neurons displayed a decrease in spike-timing reliability especially for the cells with CF above the trauma frequency, and there was a significant shift in response latency and response duration. These effects clearly suggest that moderate hearing loss impacts on several temporal parameters of neuronal responses in the auditory cortex of awake animals. The immediate effects differ from those observed 15 days later probably reflecting the difference between TTS and PTS.

METHODOLOGICAL CONSIDERATIONS

An obvious pitfall of our experiment is that the ABRs were only recorded at the end of the experiment. Therefore, the hearing loss was assessed by comparing the post-trauma ABRs with a large database of ABR obtained from control animals of the same age and weight. Another consequence was that we could not follow the time course of the ABRs changes in parallel with the changes in cortical responses. However, testing the ABR daily would have required to anesthetize the animals daily (or every other days), which was a risk we did not want to take given that (i) the animals were implanted with chronic micro-electrodes and (ii) they were already adapted to restrained conditions. Despite these limitations, there is clear evidence for hearing loss within one octave at, and above, the trauma frequency. This loss is weaker than in previous studies (Gourévitch et al., 2009; Gourévitch and Edeline, 2011) because of the shorter time of exposure. The increase in cortical thresholds observed here is modest, but it should be kept in mind that even with much larger ABR threshold shifts (about 40 dB), cortical threshold shifts were found to be 5–20 dB (Noreña and Eggermont, 2003; Noreña et al., 2003).

Other limitations are (i) that the size of our population is quite small compared with previous studies performed in anesthetized conditions, and (ii) that we cannot claim that the same neurons were tested before and after trauma. Nonetheless, we sampled the same cortical sites before and after trauma, as it was the case when multiunit recordings were compared before and after trauma (Eggermont and Komiya, 2000; Noreña and Eggermont, 2003; Noreña et al., 2003), which led us to consider that comparison with previous studies is possible.

COMPARISON WITH OTHER STUDIES TESTING AUDITORY CORTEX RECEPTIVE FIELDS AFTER HEARING LOSS

Over the last two decades, several studies have provided compelling evidence for cortical reorganizations after hearing loss (review in Pienkowski and Eggermont, 2011). The origins of hearing loss can be quite diverse ranging from a physical lesion of the cochlea (Robertson and Irvine, 1989; Rajan et al., 1993; Rajan and Irvine, 1996), to intense noise exposure (Eggermont and Komiya, 2000; Noreña and Eggermont, 2003, 2005; Tomita et al., 2004), ototoxic drugs (Harrison et al., 1991; Schwaber et al., 1993), or to genetic pathology (Willott et al., 1993). When the consequences of hearing loss were assessed weeks/months after injury or acoustic trauma, large-scale reorganizations of cortical maps were reported (Robertson and Irvine, 1989; Rajan et al., 1993; Rajan and Irvine, 1996; Eggermont and Komiya, 2000; Noreña and Eggermont, 2005). In contrast, when immediate changes were evaluated, the authors mainly focused on alterations of frequency tuning curves, spontaneous and evoked firing rates (Noreña and Eggermont, 2003; Noreña et al., 2003). Results obtained here in awake animals within a few days after acoustic trauma share some similarities with some of the immediate

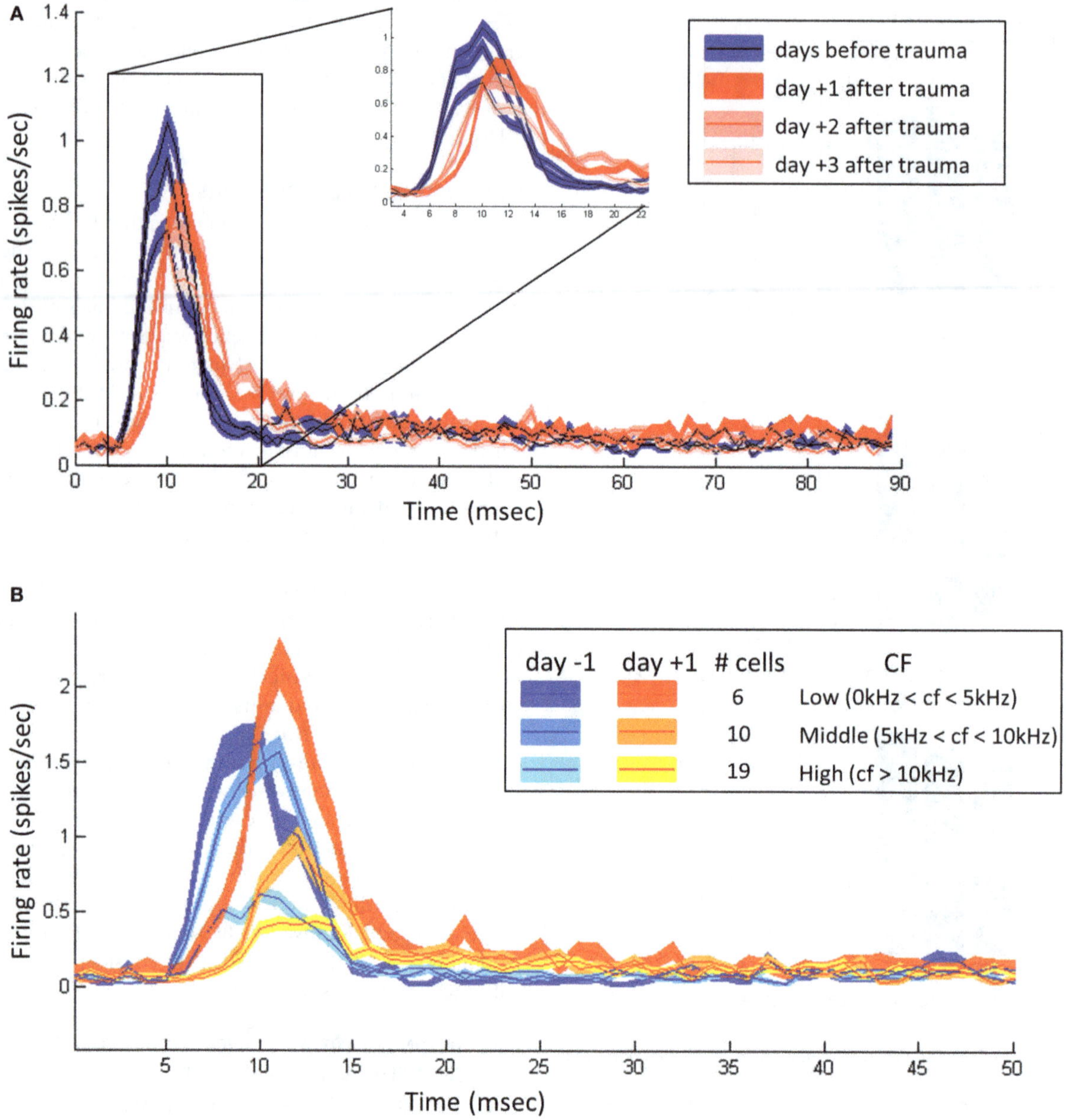

FIGURE 7 | Impact of hearing loss on the latency and duration of the responses to vocalizations. (A) Onset Post Stimulus Time Histograms (PSTHs) computed from the responses to the three vocalizations and their time-reversed versions. The blue curves represent the onset PSTHs recorded the 3 days before the trauma (control). The reds curve represent the onset PTSH computed 1 day (deep red), 2 days (light red), and 3 days (lightest red) after the trauma. **(B)** Onset PSTHs computed for three groups of cells (low, middle and high CF) 1 day before and 1 day after the trauma. The inset indicates the color corresponding to each group.

effects following a trauma. For example, the shifts of CF toward lower values for cells having their original CF above the trauma frequency is similar to what was reported in the cat auditory cortex after a trauma at the same frequency as here (Noreña and Eggermont, 2003; Noreña et al., 2003). However, several other changes described in previous studies were not observed in the present data. For example, we could not detected systematic changes in evoked (**Figure 6**) or in spontaneous activity after acoustic trauma. In fact, as explained in the Results section, day-to-day fluctuations in evoked and spontaneous activity (either due to differences in the cell types recorded from 1 day to the next by a given electrode, or to other uncontrolled factors) may have masked potential increase in spontaneous and evoked firing rates. In addition, we should keep in mind that based on cortical evoked potentials recorded in awake animals, there was no increase in evoked potentials amplitude 1 day after an acoustic trauma despite the fact that increases were detected 4 h after trauma (Sun et al., 2008).

Also, we could not detect any effect on the width of tuning curves as reported in some studies (Noreña et al., 2003). This is not totally surprising given that, as shown by Scholl and Wehr (2008), a complex disruption of the excitation/inhibition balance occurs immediately after the acoustic trauma, which selectively increases and decreases the strength of inhibition at different positions within the receptive field. In addition, besides the small size of the neuronal population we have studied, it is possible that the lack of effect on the frequency tuning stems from differences between anesthetized and unanesthetized conditions. Changes in the excitation/inhibition balance converging onto a particular cell are obviously important for controlling the shape of the frequency and intensity tuning but, in awake animals, these effects can be masked by the state of vigilance, the animals' attention and/or the concentrations of neuromodulators at the vicinity of the recorded cells (review in Edeline, 2003, 2012). Despite the fact that the EEG was collected to make sure the recording sessions took place in waking conditions, it was neither possible to evaluate the animals' attention to the different stimuli nor to evaluate its level of arousal or alertness.

Conflicting results were previously described on the latency changes observed immediately after an acoustic trauma. On the one hand, Noreña and colleagues show examples of shorter latencies and shorter response durations in the cat auditory cortex within the 2–4 h following trauma (see the example in Figure 12 in Noreña et al., 2003). On the other hand, in the rat auditory cortex, Scholl and Wehr (2008) showed that membrane potential responses were delayed and prolonged throughout the receptive field in the tens of minutes following the trauma. The methodological differences explaining this discrepancy remain unknown. However, when auditory cortex neurons were tested 2–5 months after the acoustic trauma, the mean response latency was 5 ms longer in traumatized cats than in normal cats (Eggermont and Komiya, 2000). In any case, this suggests that the time at which cortical neurons are tested after an acoustic trauma is potentially a crucial factor. This urges for additional studies during which the time course of cortical changes will be evaluated. Several mechanisms, having different time courses, can underlie our results: the effects on the response latency were transient whereas the effects on the cortical thresholds, although attenuated, were long lasting, potentially reflecting that TTS and PTS have different consequences on the responses of auditory cortex neurons.

Whether or not the cortical alterations reported here reflect residual responses or a central (thalamo-cortical) plasticity is a challenging question. When testing the different levels of the auditory system after hearing loss, evidence for responses having the properties of residual responses come from studies performed at the cochlear nucleus (Rajan and Irvine, 1998) and inferior colliculs levels (Irvine et al., 2003), whereas the map changes reported at the cortical and thalamic level were considered as real reorganizations (Robertson and Irvine, 1989; Rajan et al., 1993; Kamke et al., 2003). As shown in **Figure 3**, some of our recording sites recovered CFs with threshold close from the pre-trauma level which suggests that the changes described here result from plastic changes and not from residual responses.

RESPONSES TO NATURAL STIMULI AFTER ACOUSTIC TRAUMA

Many previous studies have stressed that the discrimination performance of auditory cortex neurons are better when based on the temporal organization of spike trains rather than when based on the average firing rate (e.g., see Schnupp et al., 2006; Huetz et al., 2009; Gaucher et al., 2013a). At presentation of conspecific vocalizations, we found here that there was no significant change in firing rate but a decrease of the *CorrCoef* (for the cells with CF > 5 kHz), an index quantifying the spike-timing reliability (**Figure 6**). This means that at the level of individual cells, the trial-to-trial reliability of evoked responses is impaired after the trauma. The latency shift, and more importantly, the increase in response duration (**Figure 7**) observed from the onset PSTH indicate that the synchronization of cortical cells is also impaired by the trauma. Altogether, these results point out that important aspects of neuronal responses to communication sounds are modified after hearing loss. A puzzling result is the fact that the responses latency was only increased the day after trauma when tested with pure tones, whereas it was increased for several days when tested with communication sounds, suggesting that more pronounced effects can be detected with natural stimuli. Potentially, one explanation is that each pure tone activates relatively small sets of afferents converging on the recorded cell, whereas the onset of vocalizations recruits a much larger proportion of afferents converging on this cell. This is consistent with the fact that acoustic trauma induces an important loss of inhibition far away from the receptive field of the cell (Scholl and Wehr, 2008). In addition, because the response of cortical neurons to communication sounds does not depend only on the spectral content of these sounds (see Figure 1 in Gaucher et al., 2013b), one can consider that communication sounds can reveal effects that are undetectable with the test of classical tuning curves.

Often, alterations observed after hearing loss at the cortical level are interpreted as resulting from intracortical reorganizations. Based on recent results, it is unlikely that the effects described here result from an attenuation of intracortical inhibition. When reducing intracortical inhibition by pharmacological treatments, it was found that the trial-to-trial reliability and phasic inhibition were enhanced at presentation of communication sounds (Gaucher et al., 2013a). Therefore, the effects described here cannot be simply explained by a local alteration of cortical inhibition. Most likely, some of the alterations observed at the cortical level can stem from effects already occurring at subcortical levels. For example, after an acoustic trauma, the acute loss of the IHC ribbon synapses connected to high-threshold, low spontaneous firing rate, auditory nerve fibers may lead to decrease the synchronization of auditory nerve fiber responses. At the central level, a down-regulation of inhibition can be detected days or weeks after a noise-induced hearing loss: the level of GAD-65/67 (the enzyme responsible for the conversion of glutamate into GABA) and the levels of $GABA_A$ receptor subunit $\alpha 1$ were found to be lowered both in inferior colliculus and auditory cortex, respectively (Wang et al., 2002; Browne et al., 2012; Kou et al., 2013).

CONCLUSIONS

So far, very few studies have studied the consequences of hearing loss in non-anesthetized animals. Recording evoked potentials in auditory cortex 24 h after an acoustic trauma, Sun et al. (2008) did not detect increase in evoked potential amplitude despite transient increases 4 h after the trauma. The cortical recordings in performed in awake gerbils by Rosen et al. (2012) after developmental hearing loss is the only one making the link between behavior and neuronal deficits. These authors examined behavioral and neural detection thresholds for sinusoidally amplitude modulated (SAM) stimuli. In animals with bilateral conductive hearing loss, behavioral SAM detection for slow modulation (<5 Hz), but not for fast modulation (100 Hz) was impaired in hearing impaired animals. Auditory cortex neurons displayed limited impairments for static stimuli but respond poorly to slow, but not to fast, SAM tones. Comparisons between psychometric and neurometric curves (based on firing rate) indicated similar impairment at the behavioral and neural levels (Rosen et al., 2012).

To the best of our knowledge, the present study is the first one describing the consequences of partial hearing loss on the responses to communication sounds. By analyzing the responses to conspecific vocalizations we found significant alterations of parameters related with the temporal synchronization of neuronal responses. For several reasons, analyzing the cortical responses to communication sounds can be a good model for understanding how speech stimuli are processed by cortical neurons. Many studies in human now suggest that very subtle hearing loss, or sometime undetectable hearing loss, can lead to abnormal speech processing (e.g., Léger et al., 2012). This study could be a starting point to link more tightly the deficit in speech intelligibility observed in human and the alterations in cortical responses after modest hearing loss.

ACKNOWLEDGMENTS

This work was supported by grants from the National Research Agency (ANR program Neuro2006, ANR-11-BSH2-004-01 HEARFIN) and from the Fédération pour la Recherche sur le Cerveau (FRC) to Jean-Marc Edeline. Special thanks to Nathalie Samson and Pascale Leblanc-Veyrac for taking care of the guinea-pig colony.

REFERENCES

Berryman, J. C. (1976). Guinea-pig vocalizations: their structure, causation and function. *Z. Tierpsychol.* 41, 80–106. doi: 10.1111/j.1439-0310.1976.tb00471.x

Browne, C. J., Morley, J. W., and Parsons, C. H. (2012). Tracking the expression of excitatory and inhibitory neurotransmission-related proteins and neuroplasticity markers after noise induced hearing loss. *PLoS ONE* 7:e33272. doi: 10.1371/journal.pone.0033272

Edeline, J. M. (2003). The thalamo-cortical auditory receptive fields: regulation by the states of vigilance, learning and the neuromodulatory systems. *Exp. Brain Res.* 153, 554–572. doi: 10.1007/s00221-003-1608-0

Edeline, J. M. (2012). Beyond traditional approaches to understanding the functional role of neuromodulators in sensory cortices. *Front. Behav. Neurosci.* 6:45. doi: 10.3389/fnbeh.2012.00045

Edeline, J. M., Dutrieux, G., Manunta, Y., and Hennevin, E. (2001). Diversity of receptive field changes in auditory cortex during natural sleep. *Eur. J. Neurosci.* 14, 1865–1880. doi: 10.1046/j.0953-816x.2001.01821.x

Edeline, J. M., Manunta, Y., and Hennevin, E. (2000). Auditory thalamus neurons during sleep: changes in frequency selectivity, threshold and receptive field size. *J. Neurophysiol.* 84, 934–953.

Edeline, J. M., and Weinberger, N. M. (1993). Receptive field plasticity in the auditory cortex during frequency discrimination training: selective retuning independent of task difficulty. *Behav. Neurosci.* 107, 82–103. doi: 10.1037/0735-7044.107.1.82

Eggermont, J. J., and Komiya, H. (2000). Moderate noise trauma in juvenile cats results in profound cortical topographic map changes in adulthood. *Hear. Res.* 142, 89–101. doi: 10.1016/S0378-5955(00)00024-1

Evans, E. F. (1979). Neuroleptanesthesia for the guinea pig. *Arch. Otolaryngol.* 105, 185–186. doi: 10.1001/archotol.1979.00790160019004

Fetoni, A. R., De Bartolo, P., Eramo, S. L., Rolesi, R., Paciello, F., Bergamini, C., et al. (2013). Noise-induced hearing loss (NIHL) as a target of oxidative stress-mediated damage: cochlear and cortical responses after an increase in antioxidant defense. *J. Neurosci.* 33, 4011–4023. doi: 10.1523/JNEUROSCI.2282-12.2013

Gaucher, Q., Edeline, J. M., and Gourévitch, B. (2012). How different are the local field potentials and spiking activities? Insights from multi-electrodes arrays. *J. Physiol. Paris* 106, 93–103. doi: 10.1016/j.jphysparis.2011.09.006

Gaucher, Q., Huetz, C., Gourévitch, B., and Edeline, J. M. (2013a). Cortical inhibition reduces information redundancy at presentation of communication sounds in the primary auditory cortex. *J. Neurosci.* 33, 10713–10728. doi: 10.1523/JNEUROSCI.0079-13.2013

Gaucher, Q., Huetz C., Gourévitch, B., Laudanski, J., Occelli, F., and Edeline, J. M. (2013b). How do auditory cortex neurons represent communication sounds? *Hear. Res.* 305, 102–112. doi: 10.1016/j.heares.2013.03.011

Gourévitch, B., Doisy, T., Avillac, M., and Edeline, J. M. (2009). Follow-up of latency and threshold shifts of auditory brainstem responses after single and interrupted acoustic trauma in guinea pig. *Brain Res.* 1304, 66–79. doi: 10.1016/j.brainres.2009.09.041

Gourévitch, B., and Edeline, J. M. (2011). Age-related changes in the guinea pig auditory cortex: relationship with peripheral changes and comparison with tone-induced hearing loss. *Eur. J. Neurosci.* 34, 1953–1965. doi: 10.1111/j.1460-9568.2011.07905.x

Harper, L. V. (1976). "Behavior," in *The Biology of the Guinea-Pig*, eds J. E. Wagner and P. J. Manning (New York, NY: Academic), 31–51. doi: 10.1016/B978-0-12-730050-4.50010-7

Harrison, R. V., Nagasawa, A., Smith, D. W., Stanton, S., and Mount, R. J. (1991). Reorganization of auditory cortex after neonatal high frequency cochlear hearing loss. *Hear. Res.* 54, 11–19. doi: 10.1016/0378-5955(91)90131-R

Huetz, C., Gourévitch, B., and Edeline, J. M. (2011). Neural codes in the thalamocortical auditory system: from artificial stimuli to communication sounds. *Hear. Res.* 271, 147–158. doi: 10.1016/j.heares.2010.01.010

Huetz, C., Philibert, B., and Edeline, J. M. (2009). A spike-timing code for discriminating conspecific vocalizations in the thalamocortical system of anesthetized and awake guinea pigs. *J. Neurosci.* 29, 334–350. doi: 10.1523/JNEUROSCI.3269-08.2009

Irvine, D. R., Rajan, R., and Smith, S. (2003). Effects of restricted cochlear lesions in adult cats on the frequency organization of the inferior colliculus. *J. Comp. Neurol.* 467, 354–374. doi: 10.1002/cne.10921

Kamke, M. R., Brown, M., and Irvine, D. R. (2003). Plasticity in the tonotopic organization of the medial geniculate body in adult cats following restricted unilateral cochlear lesions. *J. Comp. Neurol.* 459, 355–367. doi: 10.1002/cne.10586

Kimura, M., and Eggermont, J. J. (1999). Effects of acute pure tone induced hearing loss on response properties in three auditory cortical fields in cat. *Hear. Res.* 135, 146–162. doi: 10.1016/S0378-5955(99)00104-5

Kou, Z. Z., Qu, J., Zhang, D. L., Li, H., and Li, Y. Q. (2013). Noise-induced hearing loss is correlated with alterations in the expression of GABAB receptors and PKC gamma in the murine cochlear nucleus complex. *Front. Neuroanat.* 7:25. doi: 10.3389/fnana.2013.00025

Léger, A. C., Moore, B. C. J., and Lorenzi, C. (2012). Abnormal speech processing in frequency regions where absolute thresholds are normal for listeners with high-frequency hearing loss. *Hear. Res.* 294, 95–103. doi: 10.1016/j.heares.2012.10.002

Manunta, Y., and Edeline, J. M. (1999). Effects of noradrenaline on frequency tuning of auditory cortex neurons during wakefulness and slow-wave sleep. *Eur. J. Neurosci.* 11, 2134–2150. doi: 10.1046/j.1460-9568.1999.00633.x

Manunta, Y., and Edeline, J. M. (2004). Noradrenergic induction of selective plasticity in the frequency tuning of auditory cortex neurons. *J. Neurophysiol.* 92, 1445–1463. doi: 10.1152/jn.00079.2004

Noreña, A. J., and Eggermont, J. J. (2003). Changes in spontaneous neural activity immediately after an acoustic trauma: implications for neural correlates of tinnitus. *Hear. Res.* 183, 137–153. doi: 10.1016/S0378-5955(03)00225-9

Noreña, A. J., and Eggermont, J. J. (2005). Enriched acoustic environment after noise trauma reduces hearing loss and prevents cortical map reorganization. *J. Neurosci.* 25, 699–705. doi: 10.1523/JNEUROSCI.2226-04.2005

Noreña, A. J., Moffat, G., Blanc, J. L., Pezard, L., and Cazals, Y. (2010). Neural changes in the auditory cortex of awake guinea pigs after two tinnitus inducers: salicylate and acoustic trauma. *Neuroscience* 166, 1194–1209. doi: 10.1016/j.neuroscience.2009.12.063

Noreña, A. J., Tomita, M., and Eggermont, J. J. (2003). Neural changes in cat auditory cortex after a transient pure-tone trauma. *J. Neurophysiol.* 90, 2387–2401. doi: 10.1152/jn.00139.2003

Philibert, B., Laudanski, J., and Edeline, J. M. (2005). Auditory thalamus responses to guinea-pig vocalizations: a comparison between rat and guinea-pig. *Hear. Res.* 209, 97–103. doi: 10.1016/j.heares.2005.07.004

Pienkowski, M., and Eggermont, J. J. (2011). Cortical tonotopic map plasticity and behavior. *Neurosci. Biobehav. Rev.* 35, 2117–2128. doi: 10.1016/j.neubiorev.2011.02.002

Rajan, R. (1998). Receptor organ damage causes loss of cortical surround inhibition without topographic map plasticity. *Nat. Neurosci.* 1, 138–143. doi: 10.1038/388

Rajan, R. (2001). Plasticity of excitation and inhibition in the receptive field of primary auditory cortical neurons after limited receptor organ damage. *Cereb. Cortex.* 11, 171–182. doi: 10.1093/cercor/11.2.171

Rajan, R., and Irvine, D. R. (1996). "Features of and boundary conditions for lesion-induced reorganization of adult auditory cortical maps," in *Auditory System Plasticity and Regeneration,* eds R. J. Salvi, D. Henderson, F. Fiorino, and V. Colletti (New York, NY: Thema), 224–237.

Rajan, R., and Irvine, D. R. (1998). Neuronal responses across cortical field A1 in plasticity induced by peripheral auditory organ damage. *Audiol. Neurootol.* 3, 123–144. doi: 10.1159/000013786

Rajan, R., Irvine, D. R., Wise, L. Z., and Heil, P. (1993). Effect of unilateral partial cochlear lesions in adult cats on the representation of lesioned and unlesioned cochleas in primary auditory cortex. *J. Comp. Neurol.* 338, 17–49. doi: 10.1002/cne.903380104

Robertson, D., and Irvine, D. R. (1989). Plasticity of frequency organization in auditory cortex of guinea pigs with partial unilateral deafness. *J. Comp. Neurol.* 282, 456–471. doi: 10.1002/cne.902820311

Rosen, M. J., Sarro, E. C., Kelly, J. B., and Sanes, D. H. (2012). Diminished behavioral and neural sensitivity to sound modulation is associated with moderate developmental hearing loss. *PLoS ONE* 7:e41514. doi: 10.1371/journal.pone.0041514

Schnupp, J. W., Hall, T. M., Kokelaar, R. F., and Ahmed, B. (2006). Plasticity of temporal pattern codes for vocalization stimuli in primary auditory cortex. *J. Neurosci.* 26, 4785–4795. doi: 10.1523/JNEUROSCI.4330-05.2006

Scholl, B., and Wehr, M. (2008). Disruption of balanced cortical excitation and inhibition by acoustic trauma. *J. Neurophysiol.* 100, 646–656. doi: 10.1152/jn.90406.2008

Schwaber, M. K., Garraghty, P. E., and Kaas, J. H. (1993). Neuroplasticity of the adult primate auditory cortex following cochlear hearing loss. *Am. J. Otol.* 14, 252–258.

Sun, W., Zhang, L., Lu, J., Yang, G., Laundrie, E., and Salvi, R. (2008). Noise exposure-induced enhancement of auditory cortex response and changes in gene expression. *Neuroscience* 156, 374–380. doi: 10.1016/j.neuroscience.2008.07.040

Tomita, M., Noreña, A. J., and Eggermont, J. J. (2004). Effects of an acute acoustic trauma on the representation of a voice onset time continuum in cat primary auditory cortex. *Hear. Res.* 193, 39–50. doi: 10.1016/j.heares.2004.03.002

Vale, C., Schoorlemmer, J., and Sanes, D. H. (2003). Deafness disrupts chloride transporter function and inhibitory synaptic transmission. *J. Neurosci.* 23, 7516–7524.

Wallace, M. N., and Palmer, A. R. (2008). Laminar differences in the response properties of cells in the primary auditory cortex. *Exp. Brain Res.* 184, 179–191. doi: 10.1007/s00221-007-1092-z

Wallace, M. N., Rutkowski, R. G., and Palmer, A. R. (2000). Identification and localisation of auditory areas in guinea pig cortex. *Exp. Brain Res.* 132, 445–456. doi: 10.1007/s002210000362

Wang, J., Ding, D., and Salvi, R. J. (2002). Functional reorganization in chinchilla inferior colliculus associated with chronic and acute cochlear damage. *Hear. Res.* 168, 238–249. doi: 10.1016/S0378-5955(02)00360-X

Wang, J., Salvi, R. J., and Powers, N. (1996). Plasticity of response properties of inferior colliculus neurons following acute cochlear damage. *J. Neurophysiol.* 75, 171–183.

Willott, J. F., Aitkin, L. M., and McFadden, S. L. (1993). Plasticity of auditory cortex associated with sensorineural hearing loss in adult C57BL / 6J mice. *J. Comp. Neurol.* 329, 402–411. doi: 10.1002/cne.903290310

15

Developmental plasticity of spatial hearing following asymmetric hearing loss: context-dependent cue integration and its clinical implications

Peter Keating * and Andrew J. King *

Department of Physiology, Anatomy and Genetics, University of Oxford, Oxford, UK

***Correspondence:**
Peter Keating and Andrew J. King, Department of Physiology, Anatomy and Genetics, University of Oxford, Parks Road, Oxford OX1 3PT, UK
e-mail: peter.keating@dpag.ox.ac.uk; andrew.king@dpag.ox.ac.uk

Under normal hearing conditions, comparisons of the sounds reaching each ear are critical for accurate sound localization. Asymmetric hearing loss should therefore degrade spatial hearing and has become an important experimental tool for probing the plasticity of the auditory system, both during development and adulthood. In clinical populations, hearing loss affecting one ear more than the other is commonly associated with otitis media with effusion, a disorder experienced by approximately 80% of children before the age of two. Asymmetric hearing may also arise in other clinical situations, such as after unilateral cochlear implantation. Here, we consider the role played by spatial cue integration in sound localization under normal acoustical conditions. We then review evidence for adaptive changes in spatial hearing following a developmental hearing loss in one ear, and show that adaptation may be achieved either by learning a new relationship between the altered cues and directions in space or by changing the way different cues are integrated in the brain. We next consider developmental plasticity as a source of vulnerability, describing maladaptive effects of asymmetric hearing loss that persist even when normal hearing is provided. We also examine the extent to which the consequences of asymmetric hearing loss depend upon its timing and duration. Although much of the experimental literature has focused on the effects of a stable unilateral hearing loss, some of the most common hearing impairments experienced by children tend to fluctuate over time. We therefore propose that there is a need to bridge this gap by investigating the effects of recurring hearing loss during development, and outline recent steps in this direction. We conclude by arguing that this work points toward a more nuanced view of developmental plasticity, in which plasticity may be selectively expressed in response to specific sensory contexts, and consider the clinical implications of this.

Keywords: auditory localization, binaural, monaural, conductive hearing loss, adaptation, learning, cortex, midbrain

INTRODUCTION

The ability to hear is of critical importance for a wide variety of species. Indeed, in many naturalistic situations, auditory input provides the only source of information about distant events. However, whilst the identity of a sound source is clearly important, its location also plays a critical role in guiding behavior. In noisy and reverberant acoustic environments, spatial hearing can additionally help to separate different sound sources, thereby enabling their subsequent identification (Yost, 1997; Kidd et al., 2005). For these reasons, numerous species have developed and refined the ability to localize sounds in space.

Unlike the visual and somatosensory systems, however, the auditory system does not contain an implicit map of space at the level of the receptor surface. Instead, the receptors that transduce sound are arranged along the cochlea according to their tuning for sound frequency. The brain must therefore actively construct a representation of auditory space by transforming and processing the acoustical inputs provided to each ear. In doing so, the brain takes advantage of the fact that specific aspects of the acoustical input tend to depend on the position of the sound source relative to that of the listener (Blauert, 1997). The challenge faced by the brain is therefore to interpret and combine the information provided by these different spatial cues in order to create a coherent representation of auditory space.

In many cases, the most effective way to localize sounds will depend on the precise properties of the acoustical environment. While this varies with the nature of the sound sources themselves and the acoustical conditions in which they are encountered, developmental changes in the relative dimensions of the ears and in the neural circuits that process sound will also cause the acoustical environment to change. In order to maintain stable representations of space, the auditory system must therefore adapt to these changes by processing auditory spatial cues dynamically in ways that are appropriate to the prevailing sensory conditions. To understand these adaptive mechanisms, one popular approach that has been used is to manipulate the acoustical input experimentally and study its consequences on the perception and processing of sound. Although the sounds reaching the ears can be altered in a variety of ways, important insights into developmental plasticity have been gained by introducing a hearing loss to one ear (Clopton and Silverman, 1977; Silverman and Clopton, 1977; Clements and Kelly, 1978; Moore and Irvine, 1981; Brugge et al., 1985; Popescu and Polley, 2010; Keating et al., 2013a; Polley et al., 2013). In this way, asymmetric hearing loss has become an important model system for understanding basic principles of neural development, complementing studies of monocular deprivation in the visual system (Daw, 2009).

However, whilst monaural occlusion provides a powerful method for studying basic aspects of developmental plasticity, the developmental effects of asymmetric hearing loss are also clinically important. This is because periods of unilateral hearing loss are extremely common during development. For example, otitis media with effusion, colloquially referred to as "glue ear," is experienced by approximately 80% of children before the age of 3, and is often associated with a temporary hearing loss in one ear (Engel et al., 1999; Whitton and Polley, 2011). In rarer cases, children may also experience a congenital hearing loss in one ear (Wilmington et al., 1994; Gray et al., 2009). Similarly, in situations where children with bilateral deafness receive a cochlear implant in only one ear, the auditory system may be exposed to long periods of unilateral stimulation. This can result in marked changes in auditory pathway circuitry, with important implications for the restoration of normal functions if the second ear is subsequently implanted (Gordon et al., 2013; Illg et al., 2013; Kral et al., 2013). From both a fundamental and clinical perspective, it is therefore extremely important to understand the developmental consequences of asymmetric hearing loss.

In this review, we briefly outline auditory spatial processing under normal acoustical conditions, highlighting the importance of integrating the information provided by the different cues to sound source location. We then review evidence for adaptive changes in spatial hearing following a developmental hearing loss in one ear, and argue that adaptation may be achieved either by learning to use altered cues correctly or by learning to change the way cues are integrated. Having outlined the positive aspects of developmental plasticity, we next consider this plasticity as a source of vulnerability, describing evidence for effects of asymmetric hearing loss that persist and become maladaptive when normal hearing is restored. We then ask whether the consequences of asymmetric hearing loss are mediated by its timing and duration, and suggest that spatial hearing may be particularly vulnerable to prolonged periods of imbalanced hearing early in development.

Although much of the experimental literature has focused on the effects of a stable hearing loss in one ear, some of the most common forms of hearing loss experienced by children tend to fluctuate over time (Hogan et al., 1997; Whitton and Polley, 2011). We therefore propose that there is a need to bridge this gap by investigating the effects of recurring hearing loss during development, and outline recent steps in this direction. In addition to its clinical relevance, we suggest that this approach may also provide a useful experimental tool for understanding how the brain learns the importance of sensory context in complex environments. We then conclude by arguing that this work points toward a more nuanced view of developmental plasticity following asymmetric hearing loss, in which plasticity may be selectively expressed in response to specific hearing conditions.

AUDITORY SPATIAL PROCESSING UNDER NORMAL ACOUSTICAL CONDITIONS

AUDITORY SPATIAL CUES

In individuals with normal hearing, the location of a sound can be inferred from a variety of different cues. However, whilst a complete description of sound source location requires information about both distance and direction, relatively little is known about the neural mechanisms underlying distance perception (Zahorik et al., 2005; Kopčo et al., 2012). For this reason, this review will focus on how the direction of a sound source is computed. In this respect, it has long been known that sounds originating on one side of space tend to be more attenuated in the ear contralateral to the source (**Figure 1A**). This acoustical shadowing effect of the head produces an interaural level difference (ILD) that varies systematically with sound source direction (Blauert, 1997). Similarly, due to differences in path length between a sound source and the two ears, the acoustic waveform of a sound will often arrive at one ear slightly before the other (**Figure 1A**). This produces an interaural time difference (ITD) that also varies systematically with the angular direction of the source relative to the head (Blauert, 1997).

Because ITDs and ILDs both require a comparison of the input provided to the two ears, these cues are collectively referred to as binaural spatial cues. In many instances, however, the relative usefulness of these binaural cues depends on sound frequency (Strutt, 1907; Middlebrooks and Green, 1991; Blauert, 1997; Macpherson and Middlebrooks, 2002). For example, since low-frequency sound waves can diffract around the head, ILD cues tend to be relatively small at low frequencies, which limits the usefulness of these cues. This means that ILDs tend to be used primarily for localizing high-frequency sounds.

Conversely, for simple periodic sounds, ITDs become spatially ambiguous as the sound frequency is increased, as it becomes harder to tell at which ear the sound is leading and at which it is lagging (Schnupp et al., 2011). Moreover, ITDs can only be calculated in situations where information is preserved in the auditory system about the temporal structure of the auditory waveform, a feat that many species find difficult to achieve at higher frequencies. This is because auditory nerve fibers represent temporal structure by locking their activity to specific phases of the stimulus waveform. In many species, phase locking begins to decline at frequencies greater than 1 kHz (Sumner and Palmer, 2012), which produces a corresponding reduction in ITD sensitivity at these higher frequencies (Brughera et al., 2013). In such cases, any residual sensitivity to ITDs therefore depends on the envelope of a sound (Henning, 1974; Bernstein and Trahiotis, 2002), rather than its fine temporal structure. The frequency dependence of ILD and ITD sensitivity provides the basis for the duplex theory of sound localization (Strutt, 1907), which applies to humans as well as to at least some other mammalian species (Wakeford and Robinson, 1974; Brown et al., 1978; Houben and Gourevitch, 1979; Keating et al., 2013b).

In addition to these binaural cues, spatial information may also be inferred from the relative intensities of different frequency components present at one ear. This is because, at least in mammals, the filtering properties of the head and external ears serve to shape the spectrum of a sound in a direction-dependent

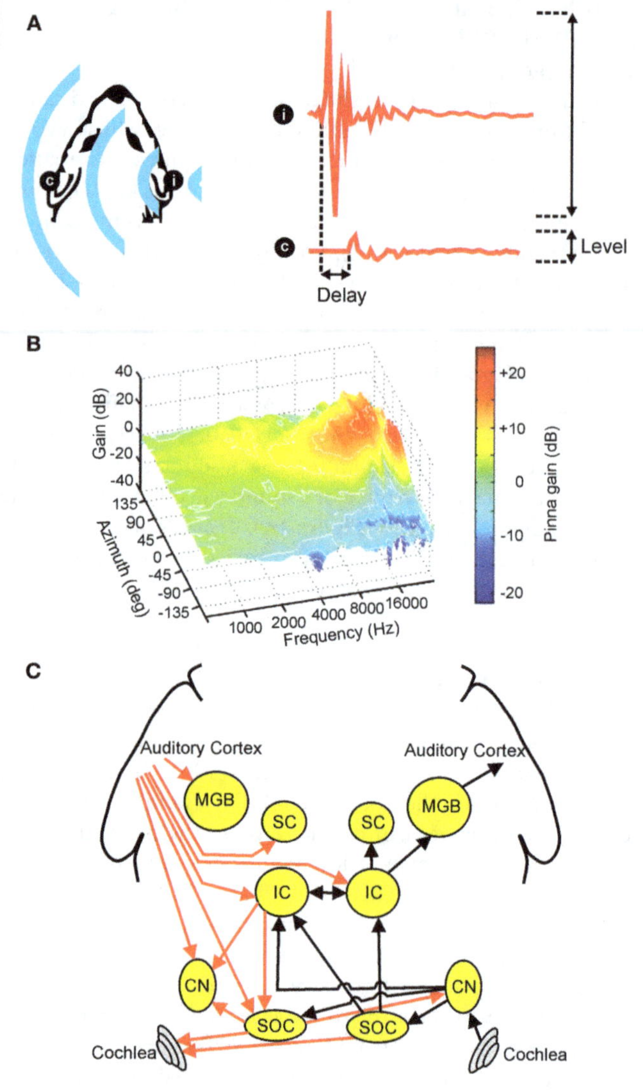

FIGURE 1 | Overview of auditory spatial processing. (A) Sample acoustic waveforms are shown for the ipsilateral (i) and contralateral (c) ears following presentation of sound from a source located to one side of the head. The incoming sound is typically delayed and attenuated in the contralateral ear, producing interaural time differences (ITDs) and interaural level differences (ILDs), respectively. These cues are referred to as binaural spatial cues as they depend on comparisons between the two ears. **(B)** Gain is plotted for an adult ferret ear as a function of sound frequency and azimuth. Because the filtering effects of the head and ears depend on the direction of a sound source, the observed spectra vary with respect to azimuth (and elevation), producing spectral shape cues to sound location. **(C)** Simplified schematic of the mammalian auditory pathway showing the principal ascending (black) and descending (red) projections between the cochlea, cochlear nuclei (CN), superior olivary complex (SOC), inferior colliculus (IC), superior colliculus (SC), medial geniculate body (MGB), and auditory cortex. For clarity, each of these projections is shown for one side of the brain only. **(B)** adapted with permission from King et al. (2001).

way (**Figure 1B**). Commonly referred to as spectral cues, these monaural spatial cues are most pronounced at high frequencies, and are thought to be critical for distinguishing between locations that produce identical ITD and ILD values (Musicant and Butler, 1984; Musicant et al., 1990; Carlile et al., 2005). For this reason, spectral cues are thought to play an important role in determining whether sounds are located in the front or rear hemifields. In many mammalian species, including humans, spectral cues are also critical for determining the elevation of a sound (Parsons et al., 1999; Carlile et al., 2005; Tollin et al., 2013). Although the acoustical properties of spectral cues make them equally suitable for determining the lateral angle of sounds in the horizontal plane, these cues typically contribute very little to this process, with ITDs and ILDs instead dominating the perceived azimuth under normal listening conditions (Macpherson and Middlebrooks, 2002).

IMPORTANCE OF CUE INTEGRATION

The findings outlined in the previous section illustrate that the importance of different spatial cues can vary depending on the properties of the sound and the region of space in which it needs to be localized. Consequently, under a particular set of hearing conditions, different cues tend not to contribute equally to judgments of sound location. Determining the weight that should be given to each cue therefore represents a key aspect of sensory processing. Individually, monaural and binaural spatial cues typically provide only partial, and even potentially contradictory, information about stimulus location. This can occur because neural representations are often noisy and imprecise and the nature of these coding errors may be independent for different cues, thereby giving rise to cue conflict. In addition, whereas monaural spectral cues are influenced by the spectrum of a sound (Wightman and Kistler, 1997), binaural cues are much more robust with respect to the source spectrum. In certain situations, the auditory system may therefore misattribute the spectral properties of a sound to the filtering effects of the head and ears (Hofman and Van Opstal, 2002; Keating et al., 2013a), with the result that monaural and binaural cues may indicate that the sound originated from different directions. Over time, the reliability of each cue can also change. The challenge faced by the brain is therefore to determine the best way of combining these different cues to provide a coherent representation of the external world.

This need for cue integration, however, is not unique to the auditory system. Different sensory systems, for example, often provide complementary information about the location of a particular target object or event. By taking into account the information provided by each system, it is therefore possible to achieve a better estimate of object location than would be possible using either system in isolation (Knill and Pouget, 2004; Alais et al., 2010).

Previous studies have shown that this kind of cue integration may be described by a process that takes the weighted average of individual cues, with the weights given to each being proportional to the relative reliability of that cue. It can also be shown that this simple process is statistically optimal under certain conditions (Ernst and Banks, 2002; Alais and Burr, 2004). Although there has been much recent emphasis on multisensory cue integration, models of cue integration have also been applied to the combination of depth cues within the visual system (Jacobs, 1999), as well as the combination of speech cues within the auditory system (Clayards et al., 2008). It is therefore likely that similar models may apply to the integration of auditory spatial cues (Van Wanrooij and Van Opstal, 2007; Keating et al., 2013a).

NEURAL BASIS OF SPATIAL HEARING

Although the auditory system must ultimately combine the information provided by different spatial cues, monaural and binaural cues are initially processed separately prior to integration at higher levels of the neuroaxis. In mammals, for example, acoustical inputs are transduced into neural signals by cochlear hair cells before being passed via the auditory nerve to the cochlear nuclei, and it is within the dorsal cochlear nuclei that processing of monaural spectral cues is subsequently thought to occur (Young et al., 1992). Projections originating in the ventral divisions of the cochlear nuclei target the superior olive bilaterally (**Figure 1C**), allowing input from the two ears to converge for the first time. The nature of this convergence is such, however, that the processing of different binaural cues remains segregated to a large extent, with the lateral superior olive (LSO) involved primarily in ILD processing and the medial superior olive (MSO) more associated with the processing of ITDs (Yin, 2002).

Projections from these brainstem nuclei then ascend to the midbrain, where they are thought to target partially overlapping populations of neurons in the central nucleus of the inferior colliculus (ICc) (Loftus et al., 2010). From here, auditory signals are transmitted via the medial geniculate nucleus of the thalamus to the auditory cortex (**Figure 1C**), which has been shown by inactivation studies to play a critical role in sound localization (Heffner and Heffner, 1990; Malhotra et al., 2004; Nodal et al., 2012). Although cortical cells presumably integrate the information provided by different auditory spatial cues, there is currently very little evidence to suggest that a topographic map of auditory space is constructed at the level of the cortex (Recanzone and Sutter, 2008; Razak, 2011) or indeed at any subcortical level of the primary auditory pathway in mammals [reviewed in Grothe et al., 2010]. A crude map of auditory space has, however, been described in the nucleus of the brachium of the inferior colliculus (nBIC) (Schnupp and King, 1997), which receives a major source of input from the ICc. The nBIC projects topographically to the superior colliculus (SC), where a more refined map of auditory space is found that shows the same topographic order observed for the representation of other sensory modalities (Palmer and King, 1982; King and Hutchings, 1987). Whilst the precise neural architecture invariably differs across species, broadly similar organizational principles apply to the avian brain, with the optic tectum and the external nucleus of the inferior colliculus (ICx) both showing maps of auditory space in the absence of any topographical representation in the forebrain (Cohen and Knudsen, 1999). However, in contrast to mammals, topographic representations of ITDs and ILDs have been found in the brainstem nuclei where these cues are first computed (Singheiser et al., 2012).

DEVELOPMENTAL PLASTICITY OF SPATIAL HEARING FOLLOWING ASYMMETRIC HEARING LOSS

TYPES OF HEARING LOSS

In attempting to understand developmental plasticity in the auditory system, numerous studies have investigated the effects of early hearing loss. Although hearing loss can be produced in a number of different ways, these can be broadly categorized as being either sensorineural or conductive in nature, each of which has distinct advantages from an experimental perspective. For example, experimental induction of sensorineural hearing loss, which can be achieved via cochlear ablation (Moore and Kowalchuk, 1988), tends to completely abolish both the transduction of sound as well as any spontaneous activity at the site of the lesion (Tucci et al., 1987). Although this form of hearing loss can completely eliminate binaural spatial cues, it is typically irreversible, making it very difficult to determine what happens to the behavioral and neurophysiological representation of the affected ear unless cochlear implants are used. It is also less appropriate as a model for the types of hearing loss that are typically experienced by children during development (Moore and King, 2004; Tollin, 2010; Whitton and Polley, 2011).

In contrast, conductive hearing loss is typically incomplete, producing only a partial attenuation of acoustic input to the affected ear (Moore et al., 1989; Gravel and Wallace, 2000; Kumpik et al., 2010; Lupo et al., 2010). Conductive hearing loss is also often fully reversible and represents an excellent model for the types of hearing loss that are most commonly experienced during development. This is particularly true of otitis media with effusion (Gravel and Wallace, 2000; Whitton and Polley, 2011), which is associated with an accumulation of fluid in the middle ear. In many cases, this prevents the normal transmission of sound by the middle ear, thereby producing a conductive hearing loss.

Although otitis media with effusion can occur either unilaterally or bilaterally (Hogan et al., 1997; Engel et al., 1999), a situation common to many other forms of hearing loss, experimental studies have shown that the effects of a unilateral hearing loss are typically more dramatic than those observed following a bilateral hearing loss (Silverman and Clopton, 1977; Clements and Kelly, 1978; Moore, 2002; Moore and King, 2004; Keuroghlian and Knudsen, 2007; Tollin, 2010; Whitton and Polley, 2011). In addition to its prominence as an experimental model, unilateral hearing loss therefore represents a major source of vulnerability in clinical populations.

From an experimental perspective, a partial hearing loss in one ear can be reversibly induced either by surgical ligation of the ear canal (Silverman and Clopton, 1977; Moore and Irvine, 1981; Brugge et al., 1985; Popescu and Polley, 2010) or by occluding the ear canal with a material that attenuates sound (Knudsen, 1985; Gold and Knudsen, 1999; Kacelnik et al., 2006; Kumpik et al., 2010; Polley et al., 2013). In addition to reducing the input amplitude, these manipulations tend to delay the transmission of sound to the affected ear. Monaural deprivation therefore has a profound effect on both the ITDs and ILDs available to the listener (Moore et al., 1989; Hartley and Moore, 2003; Kumpik et al., 2010; Lupo et al., 2010), which is likely to be shared by the effects of otitis media with effusion in children (Gravel and Wallace, 2000).

Unilateral hearing loss therefore alters the usefulness of auditory spatial cues as well as the precise relationship between specific cue values and spatial location, but leaves any monaural spatial cues available to the intact ear unchanged. The methods used to induce hearing loss also tend to act as low-pass filters, attenuating higher frequencies to a greater extent than lower frequencies (Moore et al., 1989; Kumpik et al., 2010; Lupo et al., 2010; Polley et al., 2013). Consequently, ILDs will typically be altered in a frequency-dependent manner. Although this frequency-dependent attenuation can have profound effects on tonotopic representations in the brain (Popescu and Polley, 2010), this review will focus on its impact on spatial hearing.

CUE REMAPPING

In principle, spatial hearing could adapt to a unilateral hearing loss in two distinct ways. First, in situations where the affected ear retains some acoustical sensitivity, the auditory system could utilize the cues that have been altered by hearing loss. In particular, this would require the brain to acquire new mappings between specific locations and the values of individual spatial cues (**Figure 2A**). In other words, the auditory system could adapt by learning to reinterpret the spatial meaning of particular acoustical inputs. Prior to the onset of hearing loss, for example, a sound located directly in front of an observer is likely to produce an ILD of zero, since the sound will be of equal intensity at each ear. However, if the sound transmitted to one ear is attenuated due to hearing loss, sounds located in front of the observer will no longer produce an ILD of zero. Instead, an ILD of zero may be produced by sounds originating from more peripheral locations ipsilateral to the hearing loss. In such circumstances, the auditory system could therefore adapt by adjusting the ILD sensitivity of neurons to compensate for the imbalance in inputs between the ears.

Thus, far, the clearest evidence for cue remapping has been obtained by studies of partial unilateral hearing loss in the developing barn owl. In particular, sound localization behavior in this species readily adapts to a unilateral hearing loss introduced early in development (Knudsen et al., 1984a). At a neural level, this adaptation is paralleled by shifts in ILD and ITD tuning, thereby changing the location of the receptive fields in ways that compensate for the effects of hearing loss (**Figures 2B,C**). For example, compensatory shifts in ITD sensitivity emerge at the level of ICx (Gold and Knudsen, 2000b) and, in turn, are observed in the optic tectum (Gold and Knudsen, 2001), thalamus (Miller and Knudsen, 2003) and forebrain (Miller and Knudsen, 2001). Similarly, adaptive shifts in ILD sensitivity initially appear in the brainstem nucleus that is the first site of ILD processing in the barn owl (Mogdans and Knudsen, 1994), prior to subsequent elaboration at the level of the ICx (Mogdans and Knudsen, 1993), optic tectum (Mogdans and Knudsen, 1992), and forebrain (Miller and Knudsen, 2001).

There are, however, key differences in the way in which barn owls and mammals localize sound, which likely reflect the independent evolution of mechanisms for sound localization in different groups of vertebrates (Grothe et al., 2010). Consequently, we should not necessarily expect the way the brain responds to unilateral hearing loss to be the same in birds and mammals. Indeed, in contrast to the experiments carried out in barn owls, very little evidence has been obtained for cue remapping in mammals. Thus, cats and rats reared with a partial unilateral hearing loss similar to that used in barn owl studies do not show compensatory shifts in the neural sensitivity to binaural spatial cues, either in the inferior colliculus (IC) (Clopton and Silverman, 1977; Silverman and Clopton, 1977; Moore and Irvine, 1981; Popescu and Polley, 2010) or the primary auditory cortex (Brugge et al., 1985; Popescu and Polley, 2010). Although it is conceivable that compensatory changes occur at higher levels of processing, these results highlight the possibility that cue remapping may not occur under all circumstances when a unilateral hearing loss is experienced.

Although there is currently very little evidence in mammals for experience–dependent adjustments in binaural cue sensitivity equivalent to those seen in barn owls, this does not necessarily mean that mammals are incapable of adapting in this manner to the altered cues produced by a unilateral hearing loss. In situations where normal hearing cannot be restored, it is therefore important to ask whether it might be possible to devise targeted intervention strategies that promote adaptive adjustments in ILD or ITD sensitivity. The mechanisms of plasticity revealed by research in barn owls therefore illustrate the potential for adaptive changes in the encoding of binaural spatial cues, even if the immediate clinical implications of this work remain unclear.

CUE REWEIGHTING

A compensatory adjustment in neural sensitivity represents one viable mechanism for adapting to changes in auditory spatial cues, but this could also be achieved by the auditory system becoming more dependent on other cues that remain unchanged. In the specific case of unilateral hearing loss, this would require the auditory system to ignore the affected binaural spatial cues and instead rely more on the monaural spatial cues available to the intact ear. For individuals with a complete loss of hearing in one ear, this may be the only way in which a recovery in sound localization accuracy can be achieved. Indeed, behavioral evidence in at least some unilaterally deaf humans supports the idea that monaural spectral cues might be used to localize sounds in the horizontal plane (Slattery and Middlebrooks, 1994; Van Wanrooij and Van Opstal, 2004). Similarly, in cases of partial hearing loss, binaural cues are eliminated when the sound level is insufficiently high to be transmitted to the affected ear, which appears to enable humans to use spectral cues at these lower sound levels (Van Wanrooij and Van Opstal, 2007).

In such cases, however, it is unclear whether this amounts to cue reweighting, since these individuals do not have access to binaural spatial cues. Nevertheless, in situations where altered binaural cues remain available, it is clear that spatial hearing can adapt to a partial unilateral hearing loss by relying to a greater extent on the spectral cues provided to the intact ear. This has been demonstrated in both ferrets and humans with a unilateral hearing loss experienced either during adulthood (Kacelnik et al., 2006; Kumpik et al., 2010; Agterberg et al., 2012) or development (Newton, 1983; Keating et al., 2013a).

At a neuroanatomical level, developmental studies of unilateral hearing loss in mammals have demonstrated a relative weakening of the pathways that convey input from the affected ear, which include reduced connectivity, reductions in the size and number of neurons as well as changes in dendritic morphology (Tollin, 2010). Changes consistent with a weakening of these pathways have been observed in a variety of brain regions, including the cochlear nucleus (Coleman and O'Connor, 1979; Webster and

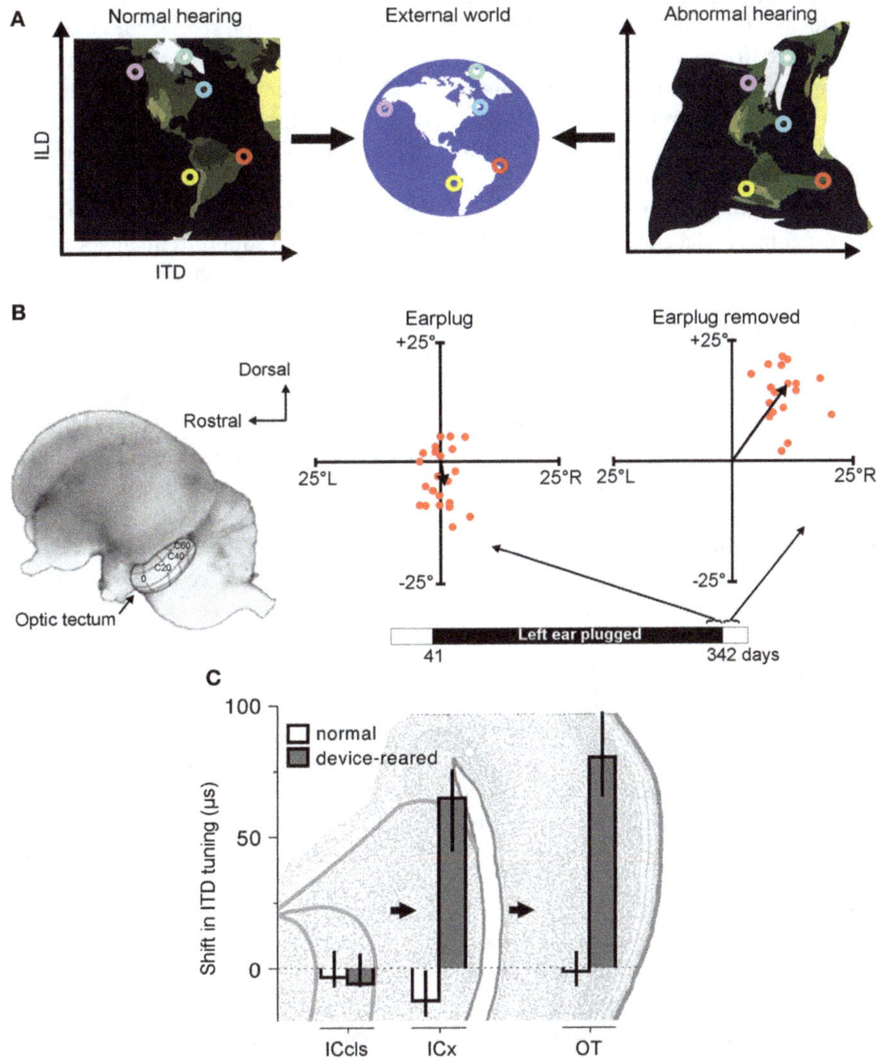

FIGURE 2 | Adaptation to abnormal cues can be achieved by remapping the relationship between cue values and sound-source location. **(A)** Under normal listening conditions (left), specific combinations of cue values correspond to particular locations in the external world. Small circles of the same color represent particular cue combinations and their corresponding locations in the external world. Under abnormal listening conditions, such as when one ear is occluded by an earplug, these relationships are distorted and altered (right). In order to use these abnormal cues for accurate sound localization, the brain must therefore learn that the same locations now correspond to different cue combinations. **(B)** At present, robust neurophysiological evidence for cue remapping has only been observed in barn owls reared with one ear occluded. Electrophysiological recordings from neurons in the optic tectum of these animals show that compensatory shifts take place in the neurons' auditory spatial tuning. Tectal neurons respond most strongly to visual and auditory stimuli presented from overlapping locations, with their receptive fields arranged systematically to produce topographically-aligned maps of visual and auditory space (represented by the contour lines superimposed on the optic tectum in the picture of the owl's brain). Recordings from the rostral region of the tectum in an owl that was reared with the left ear occluded until 342 days after hatching revealed little difference between the visual and auditory receptive field centers when the earplug was still in place ("Earplug"). Misalignment in elevation is plotted on the ordinate, with misalignment in azimuth plotted on the abscissa. When the ear was occluded, the data points cluster around the origin, demonstrating that auditory and visual receptive fields are broadly in register. Following earplug removal, however, the receptive fields became systematically misaligned in both azimuth and elevation, indicating that the neurons were tuned to binaural cue values that no longer corresponded to their preferred visual location. **(C)** Site of auditory plasticity in the ascending auditory pathway of the barn owl. Frequency-dependent shifts in ITD tuning are plotted for barn owls reared either with normal hearing or with a passive filtering device in one ear that delays and attenuates sound. Positive values indicate shifts in ITD tuning that compensate for the effects of the device. Bars and lines show medians and interquartile ranges. Data are shown for the optic tectum (OT), external nucleus of the inferior colliculus (ICx) and the lateral shell of the central nucleus of the inferior colliculus (ICcls). Shifts in ITD tuning emerge at the level of the ICx. Modified with permission from Knudsen (1985) and Gold and Knudsen (2000b).

Webster, 1979; Blatchley et al., 1983; Webster, 1983b; Moore and Kowalchuk, 1988), superior olive (Webster and Webster, 1979; Webster, 1983a; Sanes et al., 1992; Russell and Moore, 1999) and IC (Webster, 1983a,b), although the precise nature of these changes varies across different brain regions and different types of hearing loss. Studies of unilateral conductive hearing loss have shown that the neurophysiological representation of the developmentally occluded ear is similarly weakened, with neurons in the IC (Clopton and Silverman, 1977; Silverman and Clopton, 1977; Popescu and Polley, 2010) and auditory cortex (Brugge et al., 1985; Popescu and Polley, 2010) becoming relatively more driven by acoustical input provided to the intact ear. Although these studies were unable to measure the relative weight given to different spatial cues, a change in the relative efficacy with which each ear can activate central auditory neurons is precisely what would be expected if the auditory system were to become more dependent upon the monaural spatial cues provided by the intact ear.

In a recent study, we therefore set out to test this cue reweighting hypothesis explicitly (**Figure 3**) (Keating et al., 2013a). We found that ferrets reared with a hearing loss in one ear were able to localize sounds accurately when tested as adults, despite wearing an earplug in the developmentally occluded ear (**Figure 3A**). Moreover, these behavioral experiments revealed that they did so by relying more on the monaural spectral cues provided to the intact ear (**Figures 3D–F**). At a neurophysiological level, this was paralleled by a corresponding reweighting of auditory spatial cues in the primary auditory cortex, with neurons carrying relatively less information about binaural spatial cues and relatively more information about the spectral cues that were unaffected by the hearing loss (**Figure 3C**). Thus, the animals were able to adapt to a unilateral hearing loss during the postnatal period when the auditory system is particularly plastic by giving greater weight to the spatial cues that remain unchanged. In conjunction with previous work in humans (Newton, 1983), these results therefore show that cue reweighting represents a viable strategy for adapting to developmental changes in sensory input.

CHOICE OF ADAPTIVE STRATEGY

These studies demonstrate that the developing auditory system possesses the capacity to adapt to a partial unilateral hearing loss in one of two distinct ways. Whereas barn owls can adjust their sensitivity to the altered binaural cues (Keuroghlian and Knudsen, 2007) (**Figure 2**), mammals can accommodate the imbalance in inputs between the ears by becoming more dependent on the monaural spatial cues that remain intact (Newton, 1983; Keating et al., 2013a) (**Figure 3**). At present, however, it is unclear what determines which of these strategies is adopted. Perhaps the most obvious answer is that species differences may play an important role. Given that the barn owl possesses highly-specialized neural machinery for processing sound source location, the possibility of differences between species is certainly plausible.

The barn owl, for example, is capable of using fine-structure ITDs over the full range of frequencies to which it is sensitive, a truly remarkable feat that is made possible by phase-locking to much higher sound frequencies than is the case in mammals (Köppl, 1997). The acoustical properties of the head and ears also mean that this species respectively uses ITDs and ILDs for localizing sound sources in azimuth and elevation (Moiseff and Konishi, 1981; Moiseff, 1989). In this respect, barn owls differ considerably from mammals, which primarily use both ITDs and ILDs for determining the azimuth of a sound (Macpherson and Middlebrooks, 2002). Moreover, as discussed in an earlier section, there are differences in the way in which ITDs are encoded between these species (Harper and McAlpine, 2004). For these reasons, it is therefore possible that barn owls are capable of remapping binaural spatial cues onto abnormal spatial locations, whereas developing mammals are not.

On the other hand, barn owls may adapt to the altered binaural cues simply because this is the only viable strategy for adapting to a unilateral hearing loss in this species. In our experiments in ferrets that were monaurally deprived during development, we found that adaptive reweighting of auditory spatial cues is specific to the high sound frequencies (above approximately 16 kHz; **Figure 3D**) where spectral cues in this species are likely to be most informative (Keating et al., 2013a). Because their upper frequency limit of hearing is only approximately 10 kHz, it is possible that barn owls may not have access to the high-frequency spectral cues that would enable adaptation via cue reweighting, and may instead be forced to map altered binaural spatial cues onto their correct sound locations in order to adapt to a unilateral hearing loss. However, the frequency range over which the auditory periphery generates useful monaural spatial cues varies with the dimensions of the head and external ears. For example, studies in adult humans, where these structures are relatively large, have shown that subjects can learn to use abnormal spectral features available at much lower frequencies to make elevation judgments (Van Wanrooij and Van Opstal, 2005). Confirmation of whether barn owls are capable of experience-dependent cue reweighting will therefore require determining whether the spectral cues generated by the facial ruff in this species (Hausmann et al., 2009) contribute more to sound localization in birds that have adapted to a unilateral hearing loss.

Although these different viewpoints provide alternative, and perhaps complementary, explanations for the apparent differences between species, they remain speculative. As such, they serve to highlight important limitations in our understanding of the fundamental mechanisms underlying developmental plasticity. Under certain circumstances, for example, it is possible that both remapping and reweighting strategies could be utilized for adaptation in the same species. This would be consistent with the results of sound localization measurements in human listeners with acquired conductive hearing loss in one ear (Agterberg et al., 2012), although other work indicates that subjects with normal hearing can adapt to a temporary unilateral hearing loss without learning to use abnormal binaural spatial cues (Kumpik et al., 2010). Nevertheless, there is evidence that adult humans may be able to adapt to altered ILDs and ITDs following some acoustical manipulations (Javer and Schwarz, 1995; Shinn-Cunningham et al., 1998), so further research is needed, particularly at a neurophysiological level, to determine the relative contributions of spatial cue remapping and reweighting to the ability of the auditory system to accommodate the changes in input associated with hearing loss.

Factors likely to influence which adaptation strategy is used include the experience of the individual prior to the onset of hearing loss and the extent to which hearing is restored in the affected ear. It is conceivable, for example, that the ability to use binaural spatial cues, whether normal or abnormal, depends on normal binaural hearing during development (Seidl and Grothe, 2005; Grothe et al., 2010; Litovsky et al., 2010; Agterberg et al., 2012). Consequently, in the case of partial unilateral hearing loss,

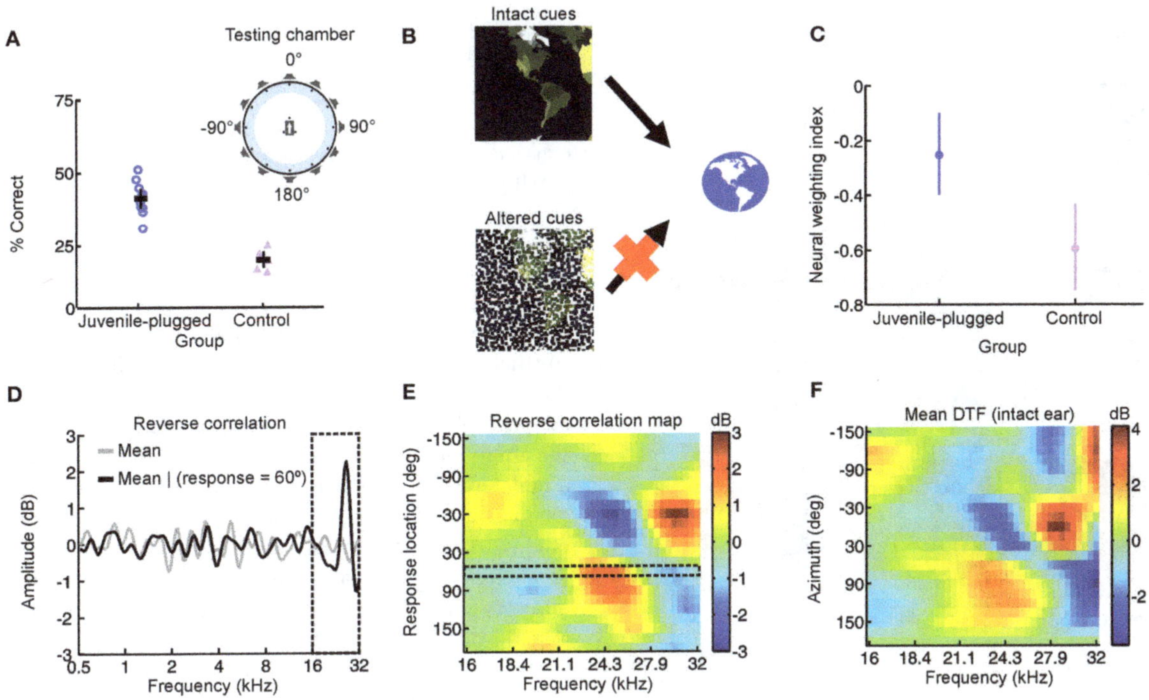

FIGURE 3 | Adapting to a unilateral hearing loss by changing the dependence of the auditory system on different spatial cues. **(A)** Performance on an approach-to-target sound localization task is shown for normally-reared, control ferrets fitted with an earplug in one ear for the first time, as well as ferrets reared with a unilateral earplug (juvenile-plugged) and tested with an earplug in the developmentally-occluded ear. The animals initiated a trial by waiting on a central platform and approached the source of a sound presented from one of 12 loudspeakers positioned at equal intervals around the periphery, as illustrated in the accompanying schematic (top right). Juvenile-plugged animals performed the task with much greater accuracy than controls. **(B)** When spatial cues are altered or degraded by hearing loss, the auditory system can adapt by becoming less dependent on the abnormal cues and more dependent on the cues that remain intact. **(C)** Cue reweighting in primary auditory cortex. Neural weighting index is shown for neurons in the primary auditory cortex of juvenile-plugged ferrets while a virtual earplug was experienced in the developmentally-occluded ear. Stimuli were presented over earphones so that individual cues could be manipulated independently, which enabled a weighting index to be constructed. Higher values indicate that relatively more weight was given to the spatial cues provided by the intact ear. Data are also shown for normally-reared, control animals experiencing a virtual earplug in one ear. Neural weighting index values are higher in juvenile-plugged animals than controls, indicating greater reliance on the unchanged spectral cues provided by the intact ear. **(D–F)** Behavioral reweighting of auditory spatial cues revealed using reverse correlation. If approach to target localization responses are determined by the spectral cues provided by the intact ear, it is possible to recover these cues using reverse correlation. Juvenile-plugged ferrets performed the task in **(A)**, but the stimulus spectra were randomized across trials. The mean stimulus spectrum across all trials was very close to zero (gray line). However, on the subset of trials on which behavioral responses were made to a particular location (60° in the example shown), the mean stimulus spectrum deviated considerably from zero, with distinct spectral features emerging at frequencies >16 kHz **(D)**. Repeating this analysis for each response location produced a reverse correlation map **(E)**, which closely resembled the directional transfer function (DTF) of the intact (right) ear **(F)**. These results indicate that localization behavior in juvenile-plugged animals is guided by spectral features that resemble those produced by the directional filtering properties of the intact ear. This was not the case in controls, indicating that the juvenile-plugged animals had developed a greater dependence on, and therefore adapted to the unilateral hearing loss by giving greater weight to, the spectral cues that are unaffected by an earplug. Modified with permission from Keating et al. (2013a).

unravelling the factors that determine the nature of the adaptive mechanism represents a key goal for future work, with implications that are of interest from both a clinical and fundamental perspective.

NEURAL BASIS OF CUE REWEIGHTING

As previously discussed, the capacity of ferrets to adapt to a conductive hearing loss in one ear during postnatal development relies on their greater use of monaural spectral cues provided by the contralateral ear, with equivalent cue reweighting being displayed by auditory cortical neurons in these animals (Keating et al., 2013a). It is presently unclear, however, whether this reflects plasticity at the level of the cortex itself or at lower levels of processing. In mammals, for example, it is known that a unilateral hearing loss produces changes in the binaural tuning properties of IC neurons (Clopton and Silverman, 1977; Silverman and Clopton, 1977; Moore and Irvine, 1981; Popescu and Polley, 2010) (**Figures 4D,F**). Since IC neurons can combine the information provided by different auditory spatial cues (Chase and Young, 2005), it is possible that changes in cue integration are implemented at the level of the IC. More generally, this is consistent with the idea that the IC may be an important site of plasticity due to its role as a major site of convergence for many auditory pathways (Yu et al., 2007).

On the other hand, some measures of spatial processing by IC neurons are immune to the effects of a unilateral hearing loss, despite undergoing changes at higher levels of processing (Popescu and Polley, 2010) (**Figures 4C,E**). Moreover, plasticity

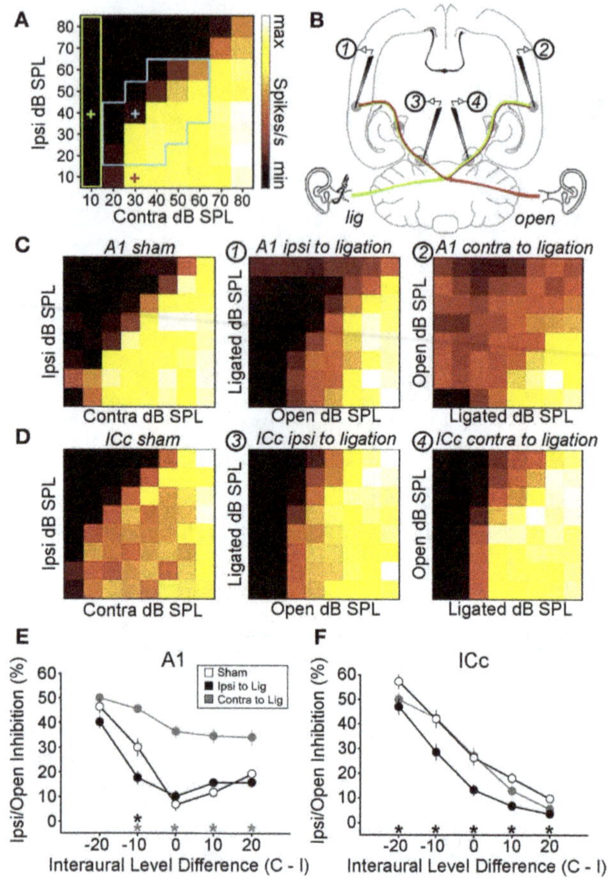

FIGURE 4 | Maladaptive effects of asymmetric hearing loss during development. (A) Example of a binaural interaction matrix recorded from a unit in the central nucleus of the inferior colliculus (ICc) in a normally reared rat. Contralateral sound level is plotted against ipsilateral level, with color denoting the number of spikes fired for each combination. Firing rates typically increase as the contralateral level is increased, but are suppressed when the ipsilateral level exceeds that in the contralateral ear. For each interaural level combination enclosed by the blue box, binaural suppression was quantified by comparing it with the linear sum of its monaural intercepts (e.g., blue cross relative to the sum of the red and green crosses). **(B)** To investigate the developmental effects of monaural deprivation, rats were reared with a hearing loss in one ear that was induced by ligation of the ear canal, which was reversed prior to electrophysiological experiments. Bilateral recordings were then performed in the ICc and primary auditory cortex (A1) of these animals and compared with data from sham-operated controls reared with normal hearing. **(C,D)** Examples of binaural interaction matrices from A1 **(C)** and ICc **(D)** in sham operated controls (left), and in ligated animals. For ligated animals, data are shown for the hemisphere ipsilateral (middle) and contralateral (right) to the ligated ear. Color scales and axis labels are identical to (A). **(E,F)** Ipsilaterally mediated suppression expressed as a function of ILD for A1 **(E)** and ICc **(F)** recordings. Data are shown for sham operated controls (open symbols) as well as ligated animals, both contralateral (gray) and ipsilateral (black) to the ligated ear. Asterisks denote significant differences between ligated animals and controls, with asterisk grayscale indicating the hemisphere in which the comparison was made. Error bars show SEMs. Ipsilaterally mediated suppression in A1 of monaurally deprived animals is increased in the hemisphere contralateral to the deprived ear **(E)**, but not in the corresponding hemisphere of the ICc **(F)**. Conversely, ipsilaterally mediated suppression is reduced in the ICc ipsilateral to the deprived ear **(F)**, but this effect is not apparent at the level of A1 **(E)**. These results suggest *(Continued)*

FIGURE 4 | Continued
that monaural deprivation induces persistent changes in the strength of ipsilateral input, which acts to weaken the representation of the deprived ear at the level of the ICc and strengthen the representation of the intact ear at the level of A1. In both cases, this increases the relative strength of the intact ear, and produces maladaptive shifts in ILD sensitivity. Modified with permission from Popescu and Polley (2010).

observed in the spatial response properties of IC neurons is often more extensive at higher levels of processing (Popescu and Polley, 2010). This suggests that additional changes may emerge either in the thalamus or the cortex (Popescu and Polley, 2010; Polley et al., 2013). Indeed, the involvement of multiple processing levels in adaptive plasticity has been demonstrated in adult ferrets. Thus, the ability of these animals to relearn to localize sound following a unilateral hearing loss depends on corticocollicular connections (Bajo et al., 2010) as well as the integrity of the cortex (Nodal et al., 2010). Similarly, plasticity induced by conditioning or by focal electrical stimulation in the tonotopic representation of the auditory cortex leads to changes in frequency tuning in the IC that depend on the relationship between activity in these two structures (Yan et al., 2005). There is therefore growing evidence that the effects of sensory experience on auditory perception may be mediated at the level of the cortex and then transmitted to subcortical sites via descending feedback connections (Bajo and King, 2013) (**Figure 1C**).

Whilst it is unclear whether similar principles apply to developing animals, these studies highlight the possibility that cue reweighting may be implemented by interactions between the midbrain and cortex. Consistent with this view, multisensory cue integration in the SC is thought to depend on descending input from "association" cortex, both during adulthood and development (Wallace and Stein, 1994; Jiang et al., 2006). However, since these results do not necessarily imply that cortical input influences unisensory integration at a subcortical level (Alvarado et al., 2007), a key step toward testing this model would be to determine whether IC neurons show evidence for cue reweighting.

INCOMPLETE AND MALADAPTIVE CHANGES IN SPATIAL PROCESSING

Although developmental plasticity can be beneficial, enabling an individual to adapt to a particular environment, these adaptive changes are often incomplete. For example, ferrets reared with an earplug in one ear localize sounds less well whilst wearing an earplug than controls with normal hearing (Keating et al., 2013a). Similarly, children who experience a unilateral hearing loss appear to be unable to fully adapt to the abnormal acoustical input available to them (Newton, 1983), and show clear deficits in sound localization (Viehweg and Campbell, 1960; Humes et al., 1980; Newton, 1983; Bess et al., 1986). In addition, whilst barn owls show very little residual bias in sound localization following adaptation to a unilateral hearing loss, the spatial precision of behavioral responses often remains slightly worse than controls (Knudsen et al., 1984a). Thus, despite clear differences between birds and mammals, an inability to fully compensate for the effects of asymmetric hearing loss is common to many different species. For tasks that are likely to require more complex processing, such as binaural unmasking in the presence of spatially discordant signals and noise, there is currently little evidence for any adaptation (Moore et al., 1999). The degree to which the developing auditory system can accommodate changes in input following hearing loss therefore depends on the nature of the task, and even where adaptation clearly occurs, such as in directional hearing tasks, this may not be enough to fully restore normal performance levels.

Perhaps more damagingly, however, any adaptive changes that do occur can become maladaptive if the environment is subsequently altered. This is particularly relevant to situations where a developmental hearing loss is resolved later in life, either spontaneously or through clinical intervention. In such cases, the auditory system may have altered the way in which spatial cues are processed, thereby compromising its ability to take full advantage of normal hearing when it becomes available.

Following a developmental hearing loss in one ear, for example, barn owls are, at least initially, unable to localize sounds correctly when normal hearing is restored (Knudsen et al., 1984b). This is because these animals have adapted to the imbalance in input between the two ears by remapping binaural spatial cues onto abnormal spatial locations. Although these mappings permit accurate localization when a hearing loss is experienced in one ear, they are not appropriate for localization under normal hearing conditions. The animals therefore exhibit systematic errors in sound localization when normal hearing becomes available, which can persist indefinitely if hearing is not restored early enough in development (Knudsen et al., 1984b). At a neural level, this is paralleled by persistent abnormalities in the tuning to binaural spatial cues (Keuroghlian and Knudsen, 2007) (**Figures 2B,C**).

Similarly, in mammals reared with a stable hearing loss in one ear, the neural representation of the developmentally occluded ear is typically [though not always (Moore and Irvine, 1981)] weakened, and does not immediately return to normal when the cause of the hearing loss is removed (Clopton and Silverman, 1977; Silverman and Clopton, 1977; Brugge et al., 1985; Popescu and Polley, 2010) (**Figure 4**), even when the period of monaural hearing loss is relatively brief (Polley et al., 2013). This is consistent with the cue reweighting mechanism of adaptation, which involves relying more on the input provided by the intact ear and less on the input from the occluded ear. Although this plasticity may help the auditory system to adapt to a hearing loss in one ear, it has been proposed that it may also be responsible for amblyaudia (Popescu and Polley, 2010; Whitton and Polley, 2011; Polley et al., 2013), a persistent condition in which the brain is unable to fully exploit the acoustical input provided to one ear. This is because the changes associated with asymmetric hearing loss can impair binaural processing of normal acoustical inputs, producing deficits in ILD sensitivity when normal hearing is restored (Moore and Irvine, 1981; Popescu and Polley, 2010; Polley et al., 2013).

In a recent study, for example, rats were reared with a conductive hearing loss in one ear and binaural interactions were quantified in the ICc and auditory cortex after the hearing loss was reversed (Popescu and Polley, 2010) (**Figures 4A,B**). In the ICc ipsilateral to the developmentally deprived ear, ipsilaterally-mediated suppression was weakened (**Figures 4D,F**), but this effect was not apparent at the level of A1 (**Figures 4C,E**). Conversely, ipsilaterally-mediated suppression in A1 of monaurally deprived animals was increased in the hemisphere contralateral to the deprived ear (**Figures 4C,E**), but not in the corresponding hemisphere of the ICc (**Figures 4D,F**). Together, these results show that binaural interactions may be altered by a developmental hearing loss in one ear, which can subsequently impair processing when normal hearing is restored.

Consistent with this view, humans and guinea pigs with a developmental history of asymmetric hearing loss tend to show persistent deficits in behavioral measures of binaural and spatial hearing even after normal hearing is restored (Clements and Kelly, 1978; Beggs and Foreman, 1980; Hall and Derlacki, 1988; Pillsbury et al., 1991; Wilmington et al., 1994; Moore et al., 1999; Gray et al., 2009). Since spatial hearing is important for listening in noisy and reverberant environments (Yost, 1997), this can affect performance in social and educational settings. In this way, deficits in spatial hearing may impair or delay linguistic, cognitive and social development (Moore et al., 2003; Tollin, 2010; Whitton and Polley, 2011).

Nevertheless, whilst long periods of unilateral hearing loss may weaken the neural representation of the deprived ear, this representation does not appear to be eliminated entirely. For example, ferrets reared with an earplug in one ear eventually show normal levels of binaural unmasking, although this can take up to approximately 2 years after the cause of the hearing loss has been removed (Moore et al., 1999). Consistent with these results, bilaterally deaf individuals who receive a unilateral cochlear implant typically retain some sensitivity to the non-implanted ear when a second implant is received in that ear later in life, despite experiencing a long period of unilateral stimulation (Kral et al., 2013). Although generally inferior to that associated with the first implant, this residual sensitivity might provide a neural basis for rehabilitation. A key goal for future research will therefore be to determine whether recovery from hearing loss during development can be enhanced or accelerated by specific training regimens, an approach that has been successfully used to treat deficits in language comprehension (Merzenich et al., 1996; Tallal et al., 1996). In this respect, it is critical to identify individuals who are particularly at risk and determine the developmental time point at which intervention is likely to be most successful.

EFFECTS OF ASYMMETRIC HEARING LOSS THROUGHOUT THE LIFESPAN

DIFFERENCES BETWEEN DEVELOPMENTAL AND ADULT PLASTICITY

One of the key findings to emerge from studies of spatial hearing following unilateral hearing loss is that the timing of hearing loss plays a critical role in mediating its effects. Early work in the barn owl, for example, emphasized the notion of sensitive or critical periods (Knudsen et al., 1984a,b), suggesting that auditory representations of space become relatively fixed at a particular stage of development. Initially, it was thought that the critical period for spatial hearing was determined by age rather than sensory experience (Knudsen and Knudsen, 1986). Subsequent work, however, suggested that critical periods for the visual recalibration of spatial hearing may be extended by environmental enrichment (Brainard and Knudsen, 1998). In a similar vein, the critical period for the effects of auditory experience on the organization of frequency maps in the auditory cortex (Zhang et al., 2001; De Villers-Sidani et al., 2007) can be extended by exposure to environmental noise (Chang and Merzenich, 2003).

A number of studies in which individuals have been exposed to altered auditory or visual experience have, however, demonstrated that spatial hearing remains plastic in adulthood [reviewed by Irvine and Wright (2005), Keuroghlian and Knudsen (2007); King (2009); King et al. (2011)]. In particular, adaptive changes in sound localization have been observed in adult ferrets (Kacelnik et al., 2006; Nodal et al., 2010; Irving et al., 2011) and humans (Kumpik et al., 2010; Irving and Moore, 2011; Strelnikov et al., 2011) after introducing an asymmetric hearing loss. While there are clear similarities with the experience-dependent changes that can take place during development, with adaptation in mammals likely to involve cue reweighting irrespective of age (Kacelnik et al., 2006; Kumpik et al., 2010; Keating et al., 2013a), this does not mean that the neurophysiological basis for this is necessarily the same. Indeed, plasticity in the young brain may differ from that in the adult in a number of important ways. Adult plasticity, for example, seems to depend to a greater extent on behavioral training (Bergan et al., 2005; Kacelnik et al., 2006), which may be mediated by increased focus and heightened arousal (Keuroghlian and Knudsen, 2007). In this respect, the plasticity of spatial hearing in adults parallels that of frequency and intensity processing (Polley et al., 2006).

Additional work, however, suggests that adult plasticity is possible even in the absence of behavioral training, with changes in frequency tuning induced by passive exposure to specific acoustic environments (Noreña et al., 2006; Zhou et al., 2008; Pienkowski and Eggermont, 2009, 2010; De Villers-Sidani and Merzenich, 2011; Pienkowski et al., 2011; Zhou et al., 2011; Pienkowski and Eggermont, 2012; Zheng, 2012; Zhou and Merzenich, 2012; Pienkowski et al., 2013). The results of one particular study, for example, suggest that it may be possible to reinstate more extensive plasticity in adults by exposure to moderate levels of acoustic noise (Zhou et al., 2011), a result that parallels findings of increased plasticity in visual cortex following a period of dark exposure (Duffy and Mitchell, 2013). This suggests that patterned sensory input may affect not only the development of neural processing but its subsequent maintenance later in life (Shepard et al., 2012).

On the other hand, the effects of attention and reward are not limited to adults, with developing circuits relevant to vocalization showing a similar susceptibility to these influences (Doupe and Kuhl, 1999). Together, these results question whether behavioral training plays a unique role in adult plasticity, and instead point toward the possibility that training enhances and accelerates plasticity throughout the lifespan. Indeed juvenile animals may be even more susceptible to the effects of auditory training than adults. For example, Sarro and Sanes (2011) found that behavioral training induced greater plasticity in juvenile gerbils than an equivalent amount of training in adulthood. The key difference between juveniles and adults may therefore lie in their susceptibility to change, with developing animals capable of more rapid and extensive changes. The reasons for this difference remain to be identified, but a variety of factors are thought to contribute, including differences in neuromodulatory influences (Shepard et al., 2012) as well as the relative balance of excitation and inhibition (Dorrn et al., 2010).

IMPORTANCE OF EARLY DEVELOPMENTAL EXPERIENCE

Although the auditory system can adapt to a unilateral hearing loss both during development and in adulthood, the consequences of this form of auditory deprivation have been shown to vary depending on the point in development at which hearing loss first occurs. Earlier developmental onsets result in a greater weakening of the neurophysiological (Clopton and Silverman, 1977; Popescu and Polley, 2010) and neuroanatomical (Blatchley et al., 1983; Webster, 1983b) representations corresponding to the affected ear. This suggests that neural circuits responsible for integrating inputs from the two ears may be particularly labile early in development.

If spatial hearing were particularly vulnerable to hearing loss early in development, we might expect clinical intervention to be more successful early in life. Consistent with this view, one recent study used hearing aids to restore balanced hearing to children who had previously been diagnosed with a sensorineural hearing loss in one ear (Johnstone et al., 2010). When tested more than 1 year later, children who received a hearing aid before the age of 5 showed improved sound localization performance under aided hearing conditions, but children who received a hearing aid later in life did not. Although the authors of this study noted that the two groups were tested at different ages, which could have influenced the outcome, these results are consistent with the notion that early developmental experience is particularly important. Further evidence for this view has been observed in studies of patients fitted with bone conduction devices following either congenital or acquired asymmetric hearing loss. In particular, patients with a congenital hearing loss benefit less from wearing a bone conduction device than patients who had normal hearing during early development (Agterberg et al., 2011).

Recipients of cochlear implants who are congenitally deaf also provide a unique opportunity to study this question. In recent work, for example, sequential implantation of the two ears was found to impair the ability to make use of the second implant if it was implanted much later in life than the first (Graham et al., 2009; Gordon et al., 2013; Illg et al., 2013), with the associated neural impairments persisting for at least 3–4 years following the onset of bilateral stimulation. Similarly, unilateral cochlear implantation in congenitally deaf cats leads to greater functional dominance of the implanted ear, but only if animals experience unilateral stimulation early in life (Kral et al., 2013). This suggests that the auditory system may be particularly vulnerable to early experience of unilateral stimulation, which has profound implications for rehabilitation strategies following asymmetric hearing loss.

More recent work, however, points toward a more complex situation, in which different aspects of binaural sensitivity are vulnerable to hearing loss at different stages of development (Polley et al., 2013) (**Figure 5**). In particular, this study showed that cortical neurons tend to preferentially respond to contralateral locations with short-latency spikes and ipsilateral locations with longer latency spikes (**Figures 5A–C**). Hearing loss at specific ages

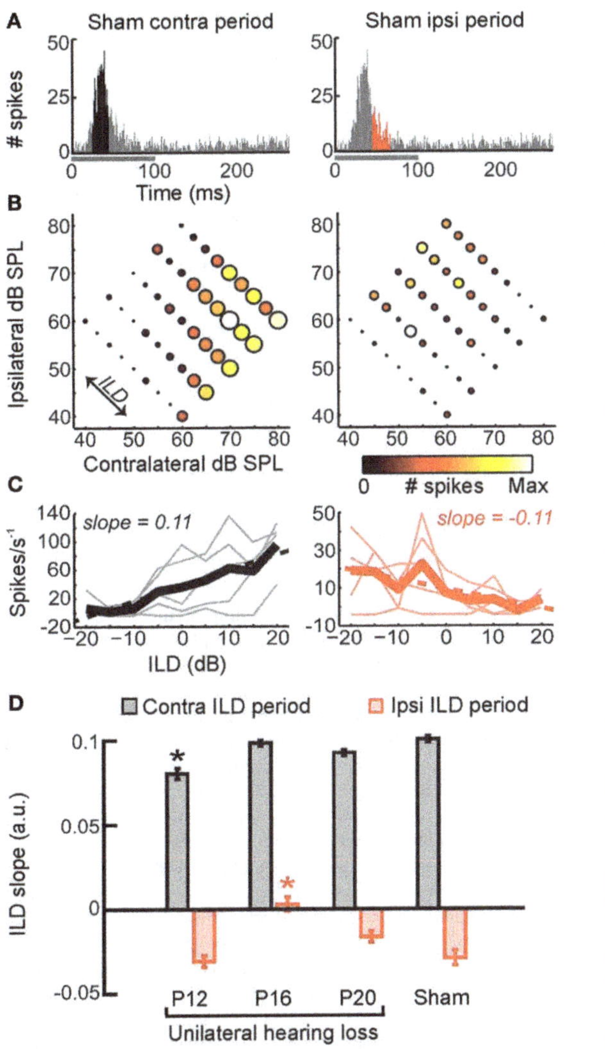

FIGURE 5 | Precise timing of unilateral hearing loss influences developmental outcome. (A) Poststimulus time histograms (PSTHs) of spikes recorded from neurons in the primary auditory cortex of the mouse can be divided into windows that show the strongest differential sensitivity to contralateral (black, left) and ipsilateral (red, right) ILDs. Greater contralateral ILD sensitivity is typically a feature of short-latency responses, whereas greater sensitivity to ipsilateral ILDs tends to be seen in longer latency responses. **(B)** Firing rate as a function of ILD at 5 different average binaural levels, with each plot corresponding to the response window shown immediately above. Heat map is scaled to the normalized firing rate within each time window, whereas circle diameter is normalized to the maximum firing rate across both time windows. **(C)** Faint lines show firing rates as a function of ILD for each of the average binaural levels shown in **(B)**. Thicker lines show the average of ILD functions obtained with different average binaural levels. **(D)** Slopes of linear fits were calculated for the thick lines in **(C)** and provide a measure of ILD sensitivity, with larger slope values indicating greater sensitivity. Mean slope values (±s.e.m.) are shown for sham operated controls as well as mice that experienced brief periods (1–2 weeks) of unilateral hearing loss beginning at different ages (either postnatal day 12, 16, or 20). Contralateral and ipsilateral ILD sensitivity are both reduced by asymmetric hearing loss, but these different aspects of spatial processing are vulnerable at different stages of development. Asterisk indicates significant differences relative to (sham-operated) controls (*post-hoc* tests following ANOVA, $P < 0.05$). Modified with permission from Polley et al. (2013).

can selectively impair one of these measures of binaural processing whilst leaving the other largely intact (**Figure 5D**). These results therefore point toward the possibility that vulnerability may be most pronounced when the neural circuits in question are maturing. Because different circuits are likely to mature at different times, this means that the consequences of hearing loss may depend on the precise developmental stage at which it is experienced.

EFFECTS OF A RECURRING ASYMMETRIC HEARING LOSS DURING DEVELOPMENT

INTERMITTENT PERIODS OF NORMAL EXPERIENCE MAY REVERSE AMBLYAUDIA

Although the timing and duration of hearing loss are likely to have a significant impact on spatial hearing, the temporal pattern of the impairment may also be a critical factor. In this respect, most research in this area has been restricted to studying a particular type of auditory deprivation, namely a single episode of unilateral hearing loss that remains stable over time (Clopton and Silverman, 1977; Silverman and Clopton, 1977; Clements and Kelly, 1978; Moore and Irvine, 1981; Blatchley et al., 1983; Webster, 1983b; Brugge et al., 1985; Popescu and Polley, 2010; Polley et al., 2013). It is much less clear, however, what would happen if the auditory system were exposed to a recurring hearing loss in one ear separated by periods of normal hearing. From a clinical perspective, this is important because recurring periods of hearing loss are extremely common during infancy (Hogan et al., 1997; Whitton and Polley, 2011). Otitis media with effusion, for example, is typically experienced in discrete episodes separated by periods of normal hearing (**Figure 6A**). It is therefore of considerable interest to determine the impact of intermittent hearing loss on auditory development.

On the one hand, we might expect that the effects of hearing loss would be reduced by periods of normal hearing. Studies of the visual system, for example, have shown that the negative effects of occluding one eye during development can be at least partially (Mitchell et al., 2003, 2006, 2011), albeit not necessarily completely (Mitchell et al., 2009), reversed by providing cats with brief intermittent periods of normal visual experience. If the same were true of the auditory system, then the symptoms associated with amblyaudia might be similarly ameliorated by providing intermittent experience of normal hearing throughout development.

Alternatively, intermittent periods of hearing loss might be damaging, producing an unstable acoustical environment in which the auditory system is unable to develop properly. In one early study, for example, barn owls were reared with unilateral earplugs that alternated between the two ears every second day (Knudsen and Knudsen, 1986). In contrast to the effects of chronic occlusion of one ear, these animals failed to adapt to a hearing loss in either ear and therefore made large localization errors, suggesting that inputs need to remain stable for a minimum period of time for adaptive changes in spatial cue processing to take place.

We addressed this issue in our recent study in which ferrets were reared with a unilateral hearing loss by providing brief intermittent periods of normal hearing throughout development

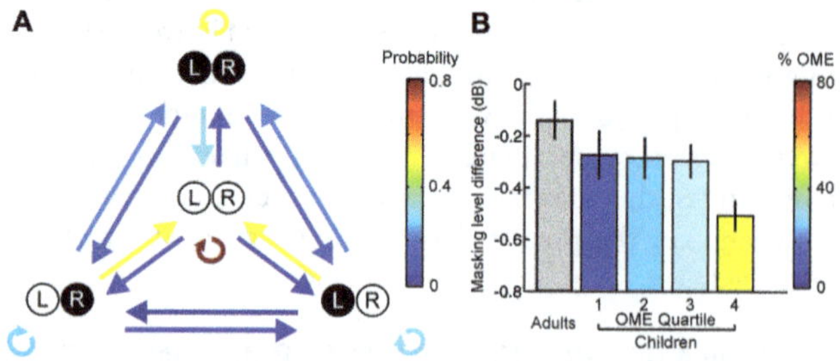

FIGURE 6 | Otitis media with effusion (OME) and its effects in humans. **(A)** State transition matrix for different effusion states, obtained via a prospective study among a group of 95 children aged 0–3 years. Arrow color shows the probability of transitioning from one effusion state to another. Effusion was either present (filled circles) or absent (open circles) in the left (L) and right (R) ears. Individuals often alternate between periods of normal and abnormal hearing. **(B)** Masking level difference, which provides a measure of spatial listening in noisy environments, is shown for adults as well as children with a history of OME (mean ± s.e.m.). Children are divided into quartiles depending on the amount of OME experienced during the first 5 years of life, with the colors indicating the mean prevalence of OME in each quartile. Adults with unknown OME experience are shown in gray. A deficit in masking level difference was observed in the upper quartile of children that experienced OME, corresponding to children that experienced OME at least 50% of the time. Based on Hogan et al. (1997) and Hogan and Moore (2003).

(Keating et al., 2013a). As shown in **Figure 3**, the sound localization behavior of these animals indicated that significant adaptation to the unilateral hearing loss had taken place. Instead of making systematic errors when normal inputs were provided in both ears, they were indistinguishable from controls in their ability to localize sounds (**Figure 7A**). Thus, although the animals showed clear evidence for experience-dependent changes in cue integration, these changes were selectively expressed, both behaviorally (**Figures 7B,C**) and neurophysiologically (**Figure 7D**), in the presence of a unilateral hearing loss, and disappeared whenever balanced binaural hearing was available (**Figures 7B–D**). These results contrast dramatically with the persistent changes observed following removal of the ear canal occlusion in animals reared with a stable hearing loss in one ear (Clopton and Silverman, 1977; Silverman and Clopton, 1977; Clements and Kelly, 1978; Moore and Irvine, 1981; Knudsen et al., 1984a; Brugge et al., 1985; Gold and Knudsen, 2000a; Popescu and Polley, 2010; Polley et al., 2013), which suggests that relatively brief periods of normal hearing may be able to preserve the ability to use binaural cues correctly.

This is consistent with clinical observations in humans, which show that the negative effects of a recurring hearing loss are reduced as the cumulative amount of abnormal hearing is decreased (Hogan and Moore, 2003) (**Figure 6B**). Together, these studies indicate that the symptoms of amblyaudia may be at least partially reversed by providing the developing auditory system with brief periods of normal hearing. Although it is currently unclear whether intermittent experience of normal hearing preserves the integrity of neuroanatomical pathways that are degraded by exposure to a stable unilateral hearing loss (Blatchley et al., 1983; Webster, 1983b), this is likely to be the case, and therefore remains an important question for future research.

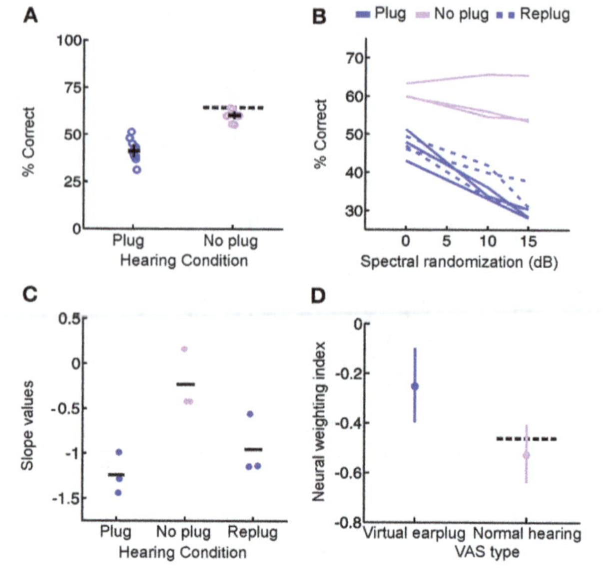

FIGURE 7 | Context-dependent reweighting of auditory spatial cues following a recurring developmental hearing loss in one ear. (A) Sound localization performance of ferrets reared with an earplug in one ear, either in the presence or absence of an earplug. Each symbol represents data from an individual animal. Although juvenile-plugged ferrets adapt to an earplug (see **Figure 3**), their performance improves when the earplug is removed, and approaches the mean performance level of controls under normal listening conditions (dotted black line). This means that juvenile-plugged ferrets adapt to an asymmetric hearing loss without compromising their ability to localize accurately when normal hearing becomes available. Error bars denote bootstrapped 95% confidence intervals, with solid black lines showing group means. **(B)** Context-specific reweighting of auditory spatial cues. Randomizing stimulus spectra across trials is known to degrade the usefulness of spectral cues, since it becomes unclear whether spectral features arise from the filtering effects of the head and ears or are instead properties of the stimulus itself. Whilst wearing an earplug, sound localization performance in juvenile-plugged ferrets declined as the amount of spectral randomization was increased, but this effect largely disappeared once the earplug was removed. Each line shows data for an individual animal, either with an earplug in place (solid, dark blue), following earplug removal (solid, pink), or after the reintroduction of an earplug (dotted, dark blue). **(C)** To quantify the effects of spectral randomization, slope values were calculated for the lines in **(B)** and are plotted for different hearing conditions. Each symbol shows data from an individual animal, with solid black lines indicating group means. Performance of juvenile-plugged ferrets was only impaired by randomization (negative slope values) when one ear was occluded. This means that the localization behavior of juvenile-plugged ferrets became more dependent on the spectral cues available to the contralateral ear whenever a unilateral earplug was present. The lack of effect of spectral randomization in the absence of the earplug suggests that the animals were relying on binaural cues when normal inputs were available. **(D)** Neural weighting index values are shown for neurons in the primary auditory cortex of juvenile-plugged ferrets, either in the presence or absence of a virtual earplug. Higher values indicate greater reliance on the spectral cues provided by the developmentally non-occluded ear. In juvenile-plugged ferrets, neural weighting index values change depending on whether a virtual earplug is present or not. Controls do not show the same effect, and are indistinguishable from juvenile-plugged ferrets under normal hearing conditions (dotted black line shows mean neural weighting index values for controls). This means that recurring monaural deprivation during development leads to cortical neurons weighting auditory spatial cues differently depending on whether a hearing loss is experienced, providing a possible neural basis for the cue reweighting observed behaviorally. Modified with permission from Keating et al. (2013a).

Another important issue, however, concerns the amount of normal sensory experience that is required to avoid the negative effects of hearing loss. In humans, deficits in spatial hearing are observed if the proportion of abnormal hearing exceeds 50% (Hogan and Moore, 2003) (**Figure 6B**). In ferrets, however, normal sound localization abilities can develop if the proportion of normal hearing is approximately 20% (Keating et al., 2013a). Although there are many factors that could explain this difference, it is likely that different tasks may be more or less sensitive to abnormal hearing during development. Consequently, whilst relatively simple tasks, such as localizing single sound sources in quiet environments (Keating et al., 2013a), may require very little experience of normal hearing, performance of tasks that involve more complex processing (Hogan and Moore, 2003) may require relatively more experience of normal hearing for these abilities to be preserved following a period of asymmetric hearing loss (Wilmington et al., 1994). An additional possibility is that it may be beneficial to have access to at least one set of cues that remains stable over time. If this were the case, then this would explain why subjects reared with entirely normal hearing in one ear (Keating et al., 2013a) appear to be less affected by hearing loss than individuals who intermittently experienced abnormal hearing in either ear (Knudsen and Knudsen, 1986; Hogan and Moore, 2003). Future work, however, will be necessary to resolve this issue.

CONTEXT-SPECIFICITY OF DEVELOPMENTAL PLASTICITY

Although studies of recurring hearing loss are directly relevant to otitis media with effusion and its treatment (Hogan et al., 1997; Whitton and Polley, 2011), they also have broader implications for our understanding of sensory processing in complex multi-context environments (Qian et al., 2012). In naturalistic situations, for example, the sensory environment may change dramatically over time. This variability, however, may not be entirely random, but may instead have specific statistical properties. The acoustical properties of a classroom, for example, may be very different from those experienced beside a busy road, although each may remain similar over time. The acoustical environment may therefore transition between distinct contexts, each of which is characterized by relatively stable statistical properties (Qian et al., 2012). By alternating between normal and abnormal acoustical contexts, recurring forms of hearing loss therefore provide an excellent experimental model for studying a much wider class of problem faced by the brain.

Our finding that juvenile ferrets can adapt to a recurring hearing loss in one ear by relying more on the monaural spectral cues provided to the intact ear when the hearing loss is present, whilst maintaining sensitivity to binaural cues under normal hearing conditions, suggests that the developing auditory system can process spatial cues in different ways depending on the specific environmental context in which they are experienced (Keating et al., 2013a) (**Figure 7**). Such context-dependent processing therefore enables the auditory system to adapt to a unilateral hearing loss without compromising its ability to use normal spatial cues. On the grounds that bilingual individuals can learn to interpret the same acoustic tokens in different ways depending on the linguistic context in which they occur (Werker, 2012; Buchweitz and Prat, 2013), we can think of this type of plasticity as "spatial bilingualism."

By showing that developmental plasticity enables context-dependent cue integration, this result ties together two distinct lines of research on cue integration. On the one hand, developmental studies have demonstrated that the emergence of cue integration depends on prior sensory experience (Wallace and Stein, 2007; Xu et al., 2012; Yu et al., 2013). On the other hand, numerous studies in adults have shown that cue weights can be rapidly updated to reflect their relative reliability (Ernst and Banks, 2002; Alais and Burr, 2004). In particular, behavioral experiments in adult humans have demonstrated that cue weights can be selectively updated for certain contexts or object classes, but not others (Jacobs and Fine, 1999; Atkins et al., 2001; Seydell et al., 2010). Very little is known, however, about the neural mechanisms that might enable the developing brain to learn to weight different cues (Fiser et al., 2010; Berkes et al., 2011).

Similarly, in the auditory system, there is accumulating neurophysiological evidence for various forms of context-dependent processing. Cortical activity, for example, shows rapid changes when individuals are required to perform specific tasks, with the nature of these changes being determined by the specific task requirements (Fritz et al., 2003, 2005; David et al., 2012; Mesgarani and Chang, 2012). Although these effects are thought to be mediated by attention, sensory context is also known to influence auditory processing, since the tuning properties of neurons can be modified by prior acoustical stimulation (Dean et al., 2008; Dahmen et al., 2010; Wen et al., 2012; Yaron et al., 2012; Nelken and De Cheveigne, 2013; Stange et al., 2013). Some studies have investigated the emergence of context-specific plasticity in the auditory system (Diamond and Weinberger, 1989; Cohen et al., 2011), but this work has tended to focus on the adult. Consequently, it is less clear how context-dependent processing emerges during development. In this respect, developmental studies of recurring hearing loss may therefore provide a useful tool for future work.

NEURAL TRACES OF CONTEXT-DEPENDENT PLASTICITY

In the specific case of spatial hearing, a key goal for future research will be to characterize the neural circuitry that enables developmental plasticity to be selectively expressed in specific contexts. One possibility is that the brain maintains neural circuits that are appropriate for different sensory contexts but functionally silences circuits that are not appropriate for the prevailing sensory conditions. Consistent with this view, studies in barn owls have shown that prism rearing results in the emergence of novel connections between the ICX and the optic tectum, which provide an anatomical basis for adaptive shifts in ITD tuning that realign the tectal maps of auditory and visual space. These abnormal connections persist following the removal of the prisms and coexist with connections that are appropriate to normal sensory experience, which likely accounts for the capacity of the owls to readapt in later life to the same audiovisual mismatch encountered during development (Linkenhoker and Knudsen, 2002; Linkenhoker et al., 2005).

Interestingly, only one set of connections between the ICX and optic tectum appears to be functionally expressed at any given time, with GABA-mediated inhibition implicated in the selection and stabilization of a particular set of connections (Zheng and Knudsen, 1999, 2001). Similarly, following temporary monocular occlusion during development, mice acquire novel anatomical specializations that persist long after normal vision is restored (Hofer et al., 2009). Although these changes have very little impact on neurophysiological response properties under conditions of normal vision, they nevertheless appear to facilitate more rapid and extensive changes in the visual cortex following a subsequent period of monocular occlusion later in life (Hofer et al., 2006, 2009).

In this way, prior experience can produce changes in neural circuitry that appear to be functionally silenced unless the brain is exposed to specific sensory conditions. Although sensory systems may require relatively long periods of time to switch on functionally silenced circuits, it is equally possible that the brain might learn to rapidly transition between using different circuits. This is likely to be particularly true in situations, such as a recurring hearing loss in one ear, where the auditory system has plenty of experience in switching between different acoustical conditions (Keating et al., 2013a).

However, whilst a recurring hearing loss can produce dramatic changes in auditory input, acoustical conditions can also vary, albeit to a lesser extent, in naturalistic environments. Context-dependent updating of spatial processing is therefore likely to be a general feature of the auditory system, even in individuals without a history of hearing loss. Consistent with this view, two recent studies have shown that the mature auditory system can undergo rapid changes in binaural spatial processing in response to prior acoustical stimulation. In one of these studies, shifts in ILD sensitivity were observed in the ICc as a function of prior stimulus statistics (Dahmen et al., 2010), whilst the other demonstrated $GABA_B$ receptor-mediated adaptation in the population code for ITDs found in the MSO (Stange et al., 2013). Although dynamic processing of binaural cues cannot account for the context-dependent plasticity induced by unilateral hearing loss in developing animals (Keating et al., 2013a), similar principles may be involved. Indeed, the adaptive mechanisms that have been observed in normally reared adults may themselves be plastic. In this way, adapting to a recurring hearing loss, either in development or adulthood, may utilize mechanisms that contribute to flexible processing of acoustical inputs under normal hearing conditions. Consequently, studies of recurring hearing loss may provide important insights into normal as well as abnormal adaptive processes in the brain.

CONCLUSIONS

Studies of asymmetric hearing loss have shown that the mechanisms underlying spatial hearing are remarkably plastic during development, with behavioral adaptation in response to altered sensory inputs reported in different species. The underlying basis for adaptation to asymmetric hearing loss appears, however, to vary across species. Thus, barn owls can learn with experience to use altered binaural spatial cues, whereas mammals appear to become more dependent on cues that remain intact and less on those that change in value as a result of the hearing loss. Further research is therefore needed to unravel the reasons for this difference. In addition, whilst the neural basis for behavioral plasticity has been well characterized in barn owls, corresponding studies in mammals are still at a comparatively early stage, highlighting the need for further work in this area.

Although this capacity for change enables the auditory system to adapt to abnormal acoustical inputs, it also represents a major source of developmental vulnerability. In many cases, prolonged periods of hearing loss may lead to amblyaudia, a condition in which the auditory system is unable to fully exploit acoustical input provided to the affected ear if normal hearing is subsequently restored. To the extent that binaural spatial hearing is important for speech comprehension in noisy, naturalistic environments, this may have secondary effects on linguistic, cognitive, social and educational development. It is therefore important to identify individuals who are particularly at risk and identify appropriate strategies for clinical intervention.

In this respect, a key finding to emerge from studies of asymmetric hearing loss is that spatial hearing may be particularly labile early in development. The timing and duration of hearing loss, as well as any necessary clinical intervention, are therefore of considerable importance. Although the stability of hearing loss is likely to play a similarly important role in determining whether intervention is necessary, as well as guiding how intervention might be successfully achieved, this issue has received much less attention in the experimental literature. Recent work, however, suggests that brief intermittent periods of normal hearing may play a protective role, reducing the longer term effects on auditory function when normal inputs become available. In this way, recurring forms of hearing loss may be less damaging than more stable deficits in hearing. Consequently, for individuals who experience a stable hearing loss in one ear, the provision of even relatively brief, intermittent periods of balanced hearing may help to protect against amblyaudia.

Investigation of how the auditory system responds to recurring hearing loss is likely to provide additional insight into a fundamental aspect of neural processing, namely the mechanisms that enable sensory inputs to be processed differently depending on the context in which they occur. In this respect, the context-dependent cue integration revealed by these studies may represent one of the mechanisms through which the auditory system maintains stable and efficient representations of auditory space in different acoustical environments.

To the extent that auditory processing and perception are influenced by sensory context, research in this field may also have important implications for rehabilitation strategies following hearing loss. It has been suggested, for example, that cochlear implants could make use of signal processing strategies that are optimized for specific acoustical contexts, and switch between those strategies depending on the prevailing acoustical conditions (Hu and Loizou, 2010). However, in addition to implementing context-dependence at the level of the device itself, stimulation and rehabilitation strategies might also be designed to exploit the ability of the auditory system to process identical inputs in different ways depending on the context in which they occur. In this way, it may be possible to leverage context-dependent processing for improving perceptual abilities following hearing loss.

ACKNOWLEDGMENTS

The authors' research is supported by the Wellcome Trust through a Principal Research Fellowship (WT076508AIA) to Andrew J. King and was previously supported by a Newton Abraham Studentship to Peter Keating.

REFERENCES

Agterberg, M. J., Hol, M. K., Cremers, C. W., Mylanus, E. A., Van Opstal, J., and Snik, A. F. (2011). Conductive hearing loss and bone conduction devices: restored binaural hearing? *Adv. Otorhinolaryngol.* 71, 84–91. doi: 10.1159/000323587

Agterberg, M. J., Snik, A. F., Hol, M. K., Van Wanrooij, M. M., and Van Opstal, A. J. (2012). Contribution of monaural and binaural cues to sound localization in listeners with acquired unilateral conductive hearing loss: improved directional hearing with a bone-conduction device. *Hear. Res.* 286, 9–18. doi: 10.1016/j.heares.2012.02.012

Alais, D., and Burr, D. (2004). The ventriloquist effect results from near-optimal bimodal integration. *Curr. Biol.* 14, 257–262. doi: 10.1016/S0960-9822(04)00043-0

Alais, D., Newell, F. N., and Mamassian, P. (2010). Multisensory processing in review: from physiology to behaviour. *Seeing Perceiving* 23, 3–38. doi: 10.1163/187847510X488603

Alvarado, J. C., Stanford, T. R., Vaughan, J. W., and Stein, B. E. (2007). Cortex mediates multisensory but not unisensory integration in superior colliculus. *J. Neurosci.* 27, 12775–12786. doi: 10.1523/JNEUROSCI.3524-07.2007

Atkins, J. E., Fiser, J., and Jacobs, R. A. (2001). Experience-dependent visual cue integration based on consistencies between visual and haptic percepts. *Vision Res.* 41, 449–461. doi: 10.1016/S0042-6989(00)00254-6

Bajo, V. M., and King, A. J. (2013). Cortical modulation of auditory processing in the midbrain. *Front. Neural Circuits* 6:114. doi: 10.3389/fncir.2012.00114

Bajo, V. M., Nodal, F. R., Moore, D. R., and King, A. J. (2010). The descending corticocollicular pathway mediates learning-induced auditory plasticity. *Nat. Neurosci.* 13, 253–260. doi: 10.1038/nn.2466

Beggs, W. D., and Foreman, D. L. (1980). Sound localization and early binaural experience in the deaf. *Br. J. Audiol.* 14, 41–48. doi: 10.3109/03005368009078899

Bergan, J. F., Ro, P., Ro, D., and Knudsen, E. I. (2005). Hunting increases adaptive auditory map plasticity in adult barn owls. *J. Neurosci.* 25, 9816–9820. doi: 10.1523/JNEUROSCI.2533-05.2005

Berkes, P., Orban, G., Lengyel, M., and Fiser, J. (2011). Spontaneous cortical activity reveals hallmarks of an optimal internal model of the environment. *Science* 331, 83–87. doi: 10.1126/science.1195870

Bernstein, L. R., and Trahiotis, C. (2002). Enhancing sensitivity to interaural delays at high frequencies by using "transposed stimuli." *J. Acoust. Soc. Am.* 112, 1026–1036. doi: 10.1121/1.1497620

Bess, F. H., Tharpe, A. M., and Gibler, A. M. (1986). Auditory performance of children with unilateral sensorineural hearing loss. *Ear Hear.* 7, 20–26. doi: 10.1097/00003446-198602000-00005

Blatchley, B. J., Williams, J. E., and Coleman, J. R. (1983). Age-dependent effects of acoustic deprivation on spherical cells of the rat anteroventral cochlear nucleus. *Exp. Neurol.* 80, 81–93. doi: 10.1016/0014-4886(83)90008-0

Blauert, J. (1997). *Spatial Hearing: The Psychophysics of Human Sound Localization.* Cambridge, MA; London: MIT Press.

Brainard, M. S., and Knudsen, E. I. (1998). Sensitive periods for visual calibration of the auditory space map in the barn owl optic tectum. *J. Neurosci.* 18, 3929–3942.

Brown, C. H., Beecher, M. D., Moody, D. B., and Stebbins, W. C. (1978). Localization of pure tones by old world monkeys. *J. Acoust. Soc. Am.* 63, 1484–1492. doi: 10.1121/1.381842

Brugge, J. F., Orman, S. S., Coleman, J. R., Chan, J. C., and Phillips, D. P. (1985). Binaural interactions in cortical area AI of cats reared with unilateral atresia of the external ear canal. *Hear. Res.* 20, 275–287. doi: 10.1016/0378-5955(85)90032-2

Brughera, A., Dunai, L., and Hartmann, W. M. (2013). Human interaural time difference thresholds for sine tones: the high-frequency limit. *J. Acoust. Soc. Am.* 133, 2839–2855. doi: 10.1121/1.4795778

Buchweitz, A., and Prat, C. (2013). The bilingual brain: flexibility and control in the human cortex. *Phys. Life Rev.* 10, 428–443. doi: 10.1016/j.plrev.2013.07.020

Carlile, S., Martin, R., and McAnally, K. (2005). Spectral information in sound localization. *Int. Rev. Neurobiol.* 70, 399–434. doi: 10.1016/S0074-7742(05)70012-X

Chang, E. F., and Merzenich, M. M. (2003). Environmental noise retards auditory cortical development. *Science* 300, 498–502. doi: 10.1126/science.1082163

Chase, S. M., and Young, E. D. (2005). Limited segregation of different types of sound localization information among classes of units in the inferior colliculus. *J. Neurosci.* 25, 7575–7585. doi: 10.1523/JNEUROSCI.0915-05.2005

Clayards, M., Tanenhaus, M. K., Aslin, R. N., and Jacobs, R. A. (2008). Perception of speech reflects optimal use of probabilistic speech cues. *Cognition* 108, 804–809. doi: 10.1016/j.cognition.2008.04.004

Clements, M., and Kelly, J. B. (1978). Auditory spatial responses of young guinea pigs (Cavia porcellus) during and after ear blocking. *J. Comp. Physiol. Psychol.* 92, 34–44. doi: 10.1037/h0077424

Clopton, B. M., and Silverman, M. S. (1977). Plasticity of binaural interaction. II. Critical period and changes in midline response. *J. Neurophysiol.* 40, 1275–1280.

Cohen, L., Rothschild, G., and Mizrahi, A. (2011). Multisensory integration of natural odors and sounds in the auditory cortex. *Neuron* 72, 357–369. doi: 10.1016/j.neuron.2011.08.019

Cohen, Y. E., and Knudsen, E. I. (1999). Maps versus clusters: different representations of auditory space in the midbrain and forebrain. *Trends Neurosci.* 22, 128–135. doi: 10.1016/S0166-2236(98)01295-8

Coleman, J. R., and O'Connor, P. (1979). Effects of monaural and binaural sound deprivation on cell development in the anteroventral cochlear nucleus of rats. *Exp. Neurol.* 64, 553–566. doi: 10.1016/0014-4886(79)90231-0

Dahmen, J. C., Keating, P., Nodal, F. R., Schulz, A. L., and King, A. J. (2010). Adaptation to stimulus statistics in the perception and neural representation of auditory space. *Neuron* 66, 937–948. doi: 10.1016/j.neuron.2010.05.018

David, S. V., Fritz, J. B., and Shamma, S. A. (2012). Task reward structure shapes rapid receptive field plasticity in auditory cortex. *Proc. Natl. Acad. Sci. U.S.A.* 109, 2144–2149. doi: 10.1073/pnas.1117717109

Daw, N. W. (2009). The foundations of development and deprivation in the visual system. *J. Physiol.* 587, 2769–2773. doi: 10.1113/jphysiol.2009.170001

Dean, I., Robinson, B. L., Harper, N. S., and McAlpine, D. (2008). Rapid neural adaptation to sound level statistics. *J. Neurosci.* 28, 6430–6438. doi: 10.1523/JNEUROSCI.0470-08.2008

De Villers-Sidani, E., Chang, E. F., Bao, S., and Merzenich, M. M. (2007). Critical period window for spectral tuning defined in the primary auditory cortex (A1) in the rat. *J. Neurosci.* 27, 180–189. doi: 10.1523/JNEUROSCI.3227-06.2007

De Villers-Sidani, E., and Merzenich, M. M. (2011). Lifelong plasticity in the rat auditory cortex: basic mechanisms and role of sensory experience. *Prog. Brain Res.* 191, 119–131. doi: 10.1016/B978-0-444-53752-2.00009-6

Diamond, D. M., and Weinberger, N. M. (1989). Role of context in the expression of learning-induced plasticity of single neurons in auditory cortex. *Behav. Neurosci.* 103, 471–494. doi: 10.1037/0735-7044.103.3.471

Dorrn, A. L., Yuan, K., Barker, A. J., Schreiner, C. E., and Froemke, R. C. (2010). Developmental sensory experience balances cortical excitation and inhibition. *Nature* 465, 932–936. doi: 10.1038/nature09119

Doupe, A. J., and Kuhl, P. K. (1999). Birdsong and human speech: common themes and mechanisms. *Annu. Rev. Neurosci.* 22, 567–631. doi: 10.1146/annurev.neuro.22.1.567

Duffy, K. R., and Mitchell, D. E. (2013). Darkness alters maturation of visual cortex and promotes fast recovery from monocular deprivation. *Curr. Biol.* 23, 382–386. doi: 10.1016/j.cub.2013.01.017

Engel, J., Anteunis, L., Volovics, A., Hendriks, J., and Marres, E. (1999). Prevalence rates of otitis media with effusion from 0 to 2 years of age: healthy-born versus high-risk-born infants. *Int. J. Pediatr. Otorhinolaryngol.* 47, 243–251. doi: 10.1016/S0165-5876(98)00185-2

Ernst, M. O., and Banks, M. S. (2002). Humans integrate visual and haptic information in a statistically optimal fashion. *Nature* 415, 429–433. doi: 10.1038/415429a

Fiser, J., Berkes, P., Orban, G., and Lengyel, M. (2010). Statistically optimal perception and learning: from behavior to neural representations. *Trends Cogn. Sci.* 14, 119–130. doi: 10.1016/j.tics.2010.01.003

Fritz, J. B., Elhilali, M., and Shamma, S. A. (2005). Differential dynamic plasticity of A1 receptive fields during multiple spectral tasks. *J. Neurosci.* 25, 7623–7635. doi: 10.1523/JNEUROSCI.1318-05.2005

Fritz, J., Shamma, S., Elhilali, M., and Klein, D. (2003). Rapid task-related plasticity of spectrotemporal receptive fields in primary auditory cortex. *Nat. Neurosci.* 6, 1216–1223. doi: 10.1038/nn1141

Gold, J. I., and Knudsen, E. I. (1999). Hearing impairment induces frequency-specific adjustments in auditory spatial tuning in the optic tectum of young owls. *J. Neurophysiol.* 82, 2197–2209.

Gold, J. I., and Knudsen, E. I. (2000a). Abnormal auditory experience induces frequency-specific adjustments in unit tuning for binaural localization cues in the optic tectum of juvenile owls. *J. Neurosci.* 20, 862–877.

Gold, J. I., and Knudsen, E. I. (2000b). A site of auditory experience-dependent plasticity in the neural representation of auditory space in the barn owl's inferior colliculus. *J. Neurosci.* 20, 3469–3486.

Gold, J. I., and Knudsen, E. I. (2001). Adaptive adjustment of connectivity in the inferior colliculus revealed by focal pharmacological inactivation. *J. Neurophysiol.* 85, 1575–1584.

Gordon, K. A., Wong, D. D., and Papsin, B. C. (2013). Bilateral input protects the cortex from unilaterally-driven reorganization in children who are deaf. *Brain* 136, 1609–1625. doi: 10.1093/brain/awt052

Graham, J., Vickers, D., Eyles, J., Brinton, J., Al Malky, G., Aleksy, W., et al. (2009). Bilateral sequential cochlear implantation in the congenitally deaf child: evidence to support the concept of a 'critical age' after which the second ear is less likely to provide an adequate level of speech perception on its own. *Cochlear Implants Int.* 10, 119–141. doi: 10.1002/cii.419

Gravel, J. S., and Wallace, I. F. (2000). Effects of otitis media with effusion on hearing in the first 3 years of life. *J. Speech Lang. Hear. Res.* 43, 631–644.

Gray, L., Kesser, B., and Cole, E. (2009). Understanding speech in noise after correction of congenital unilateral aural atresia: effects of age in the emergence of binaural squelch but not in use of head-shadow. *Int. J. Pediatr. Otorhinolaryngol.* 73, 1281–1287. doi: 10.1016/j.ijporl.2009.05.024

Grothe, B., Pecka, M., and McAlpine, D. (2010). Mechanisms of sound localization in mammals. *Physiol. Rev.* 90, 983–1012. doi: 10.1152/physrev.00026.2009

Hall, J. W. 3rd., and Derlacki, E. L. (1988). Binaural hearing after middle ear surgery. Masking-level difference for interaural time and amplitude cues. *Audiology* 27, 89–98. doi: 10.3109/00206098809081579

Harper, N. S., and McAlpine, D. (2004). Optimal neural population coding of an auditory spatial cue. *Nature* 430, 682–686. doi: 10.1038/nature02768

Hartley, D. E., and Moore, D. R. (2003). Effects of conductive hearing loss on temporal aspects of sound transmission through the ear. *Hear. Res.* 177, 53–60. doi: 10.1016/S0378-5955(02)00797-9

Hausmann, L., Von Campenhausen, M., Endler, F., Singheiser, M., and Wagner, H. (2009). Improvements of sound localization abilities by the facial ruff of the barn owl (Tyto alba) as demonstrated by virtual ruff removal. *PLoS ONE* 4:e7721. doi: 10.1371/journal.pone.0007721

Heffner, H. E., and Heffner, R. S. (1990). Effect of bilateral auditory cortex lesions on sound localization in Japanese macaques. *J. Neurophysiol.* 64, 915–931.

Henning, G. B. (1974). Detectability of interaural delay in high-frequency complex waveforms. *J. Acoust. Soc. Am.* 55, 84–90. doi: 10.1121/1.1928135

Hofer, S. B., Mrsic-Flogel, T. D., Bonhoeffer, T., and Hubener, M. (2006). Prior experience enhances plasticity in adult visual cortex. *Nat. Neurosci.* 9, 127–132. doi: 10.1038/nn1610

Hofer, S. B., Mrsic-Flogel, T. D., Bonhoeffer, T., and Hubener, M. (2009). Experience leaves a lasting structural trace in cortical circuits. *Nature* 457, 313–317. doi: 10.1038/nature07487

Hofman, P. M., and Van Opstal, A. J. (2002). Bayesian reconstruction of sound localization cues from responses to random spectra. *Biol. Cybern.* 86, 305–316. doi: 10.1007/s00422-001-0294-x

Hogan, S. C., and Moore, D. R. (2003). Impaired binaural hearing in children produced by a threshold level of middle ear disease. *J. Assoc. Res. Otolaryngol.* 4, 123–129. doi: 10.1007/s10162-002-3007-9

Hogan, S. C., Stratford, K. J., and Moore, D. R. (1997). Duration and recurrence of otitis media with effusion in children from birth to 3 years: prospective study using monthly otoscopy and tympanometry. *BMJ* 314, 350–353. doi: 10.1136/bmj.314.7077.350

Houben, D., and Gourevitch, G. (1979). Auditory lateralization in monkeys: an examination of two cues serving directional hearing. *J. Acoust. Soc. Am.* 66, 1057–1063. doi: 10.1121/1.383377

Hu, Y., and Loizou, P. C. (2010). Environment-specific noise suppression for improved speech intelligibility by cochlear implant users. *J. Acoust. Soc. Am.* 127, 3689–3695. doi: 10.1121/1.3365256

Humes, L. E., Allen, S. K., and Bess, F. H. (1980). Horizontal sound localization skills of unilaterally hearing-impaired children. *Audiology* 19, 508–518. doi: 10.3109/00206098009070082

Illg, A., Giourgas, A., Kral, A., Buchner, A., Lesinski-Schiedat, A., and Lenarz, T. (2013). Speech comprehension in children and adolescents after sequential bilateral cochlear implantation with long interimplant interval. *Otol. Neurotol.* 34, 682–689. doi: 10.1097/MAO.0b013e31828bb75e

Irvine, D. R., and Wright, B. A. (2005). Plasticity of spectral processing. *Int. Rev. Neurobiol.* 70, 435–472. doi: 10.1016/S0074-7742(05)70013-1

Irving, S., and Moore, D. R. (2011). Training sound localization in normal hearing listeners with and without a unilateral ear plug. *Hear. Res.* 280, 100–108. doi: 10.1016/j.heares.2011.04.020

Irving, S., Moore, D. R., Liberman, M. C., and Sumner, C. J. (2011). Olivocochlear efferent control in sound localization and experience-dependent learning. *J. Neurosci.* 31, 2493–2501. doi: 10.1523/JNEUROSCI.2679-10.2011

Jacobs, R. A. (1999). Optimal integration of texture and motion cues to depth. *Vision Res.* 39, 3621–3629. doi: 10.1016/S0042-6989(99)00088-7

Jacobs, R. A., and Fine, I. (1999). Experience-dependent integration of texture and motion cues to depth. *Vision Res.* 39, 4062–4075. doi: 10.1016/S0042-6989(99)00120-0

Javer, A. R., and Schwarz, D. W. (1995). Plasticity in human directional hearing. *J. Otolaryngol.* 24, 111–117.

Jiang, W., Jiang, H., and Stein, B. E. (2006). Neonatal cortical ablation disrupts multisensory development in superior colliculus. *J. Neurophysiol.* 95, 1380–1396. doi: 10.1152/jn.00880.2005

Johnstone, P. M., Nabelek, A. K., and Robertson, V. S. (2010). Sound localization acuity in children with unilateral hearing loss who wear a hearing aid in the impaired ear. *J. Am. Acad. Audiol.* 21, 522–534. doi: 10.3766/jaaa.21.8.4

Kacelnik, O., Nodal, F. R., Parsons, C. H., and King, A. J. (2006). Training-induced plasticity of auditory localization in adult mammals. *PLoS Biol.* 4, 627–638. doi: 10.1371/journal.pbio.0040071

Keating, P., Dahmen, J. C., and King, A. J. (2013a). Context-specific reweighting of auditory spatial cues following altered experience during development. *Curr. Biol.* 23, 1291–1299. doi: 10.1016/j.cub.2013.05.045

Keating, P., Nodal, F. R., and King, A. J. (2013b). Behavioral sensitivity to binaural spatial cues in ferrets: evidence for plasticity in the duplex theory of sound localization. *Eur. J. Neurosci.* doi: 10.1111/ejn.12402. [Epub ahead of print].

Keuroghlian, A. S., and Knudsen, E. I. (2007). Adaptive auditory plasticity in developing and adult animals. *Prog. Neurobiol.* 82, 109–121. doi: 10.1016/j.pneurobio.2007.03.005

Kidd, G. Jr., Arbogast, T. L., Mason, C. R., and Gallun, F. J. (2005). The advantage of knowing where to listen. *J. Acoust. Soc. Am.* 118, 3804–3815. doi: 10.1121/1.2109187

King, A. J. (2009). Visual influences on auditory spatial learning. *Philos. Trans. R. Soc. Lond. B Biol. Sci.* 364, 331–339. doi: 10.1098/rstb.2008.0230

King, A. J., Dahmen, J. C., Keating, P., Leach, N. D., Nodal, F. R., and Bajo, V. M. (2011). Neural circuits underlying adaptation and learning in the perception of auditory space. *Neurosci. Biobehav. Rev.* 35, 2129–2139. doi: 10.1016/j.neubiorev.2011.03.008

King, A. J., and Hutchings, M. E. (1987). Spatial response properties of acoustically responsive neurons in the superior colliculus of the ferret: a map of auditory space. *J. Neurophysiol.* 57, 596–624.

King, A. J., Schnupp, J. W., and Doubell, T. P. (2001). The shape of ears to come: dynamic coding of auditory space. *Trends Cogn. Sci.* 5, 261–270. doi: 10.1016/S1364-6613(00)01660-0

Knill, D. C., and Pouget, A. (2004). The Bayesian brain: the role of uncertainty in neural coding and computation. *Trends Neurosci.* 27, 712–719. doi: 10.1016/j.tins.2004.10.007

Knudsen, E. I. (1985). Experience alters the spatial tuning of auditory units in the optic tectum during a sensitive period in the barn owl. *J. Neurosci.* 5, 3094–3109.

Knudsen, E. I., Esterly, S. D., and Knudsen, P. F. (1984a). Monaural occlusion alters sound localization during a sensitive period in the barn owl. *J. Neurosci.* 4, 1001–1011.

Knudsen, E. I., Knudsen, P. F., and Esterly, S. D. (1984b). A critical period for the recovery of sound localization accuracy following monaural occlusion in the barn owl. *J. Neurosci.* 4, 1012–1020.

Knudsen, E. I., and Knudsen, P. F. (1986). The sensitive period for auditory localization in barn owls is limited by age, not by experience. *J. Neurosci.* 6, 1918–1924.

Kopčo, N., Huang, S., Belliveau, J. W., Raij, T., Tengshe, C., and Ahveninen, J. (2012). Neuronal representations of distance in human auditory cortex. *Proc. Natl. Acad. Sci. U.S.A.* 109, 11019–11024. doi: 10.1073/pnas.1119496109

Köppl, C. (1997). Phase locking to high frequencies in the auditory nerve and cochlear nucleus magnocellularis of the barn owl, Tyto alba. *J. Neurosci.* 17, 3312–3321.

Kral, A., Hubka, P., Heid, S., and Tillein, J. (2013). Single-sided deafness leads to unilateral aural preference within an early sensitive period. *Brain* 136, 180–193. doi: 10.1093/brain/aws305

Kumpik, D. P., Kacelnik, O., and King, A. J. (2010). Adaptive reweighting of auditory localization cues in response to chronic unilateral earplugging in humans. *J. Neurosci.* 30, 4883–4894. doi: 10.1523/JNEUROSCI.5488-09.2010

Linkenhoker, B. A., and Knudsen, E. I. (2002). Incremental training increases the plasticity of the auditory space map in adult barn owls. *Nature* 419, 293–296. doi: 10.1038/nature01002

Linkenhoker, B. A., Von Der Ohe, C. G., and Knudsen, E. I. (2005). Anatomical traces of juvenile learning in the auditory system of adult barn owls. *Nat. Neurosci.* 8, 93–98. doi: 10.1038/nn1367

Litovsky, R. Y., Jones, G. L., Agrawal, S., and Van Hoesel, R. (2010). Effect of age at onset of deafness on binaural sensitivity in electric hearing in humans. *J. Acoust. Soc. Am.* 127, 400–414. doi: 10.1121/1.3257546

Loftus, W. C., Bishop, D. C., and Oliver, D. L. (2010). Differential patterns of inputs create functional zones in central nucleus of inferior colliculus. *J. Neurosci.* 30, 13396–13408. doi: 10.1523/JNEUROSCI.0338-10.2010

Lupo, J. E., Koka, K., Thornton, J. L., and Tollin, D. J. (2010). The effects of experimentally induced conductive hearing loss on spectral and temporal aspects of sound transmission through the ear. *Hear. Res.* 272, 30–41. doi: 10.1016/j.heares.2010.11.003

Macpherson, E. A., and Middlebrooks, J. C. (2002). Listener weighting of cues for lateral angle: the duplex theory of sound localization revisited. *J. Acoust. Soc. Am.* 111, 2219–2236. doi: 10.1121/1.1471898

Malhotra, S., Hall, A. J., and Lomber, S. G. (2004). Cortical control of sound localization in the cat: unilateral cooling deactivation of 19 cerebral areas. *J. Neurophysiol.* 92, 1625–1643. doi: 10.1152/jn.01205.2003

Merzenich, M. M., Jenkins, W. M., Johnston, P., Schreiner, C., Miller, S. L., and Tallal, P. (1996). Temporal processing deficits of language-learning impaired children ameliorated by training. *Science* 271, 77–81. doi: 10.1126/science.271.5245.77

Mesgarani, N., and Chang, E. F. (2012). Selective cortical representation of attended speaker in multi-talker speech perception. *Nature* 485, 233–236. doi: 10.1038/nature11020

Middlebrooks, J. C., and Green, D. M. (1991). Sound localization by human listeners. *Annu. Rev. Psychol.* 42, 135–159. doi: 10.1146/annurev.ps.42.020191.001031

Miller, G. L., and Knudsen, E. I. (2001). Early auditory experience induces frequency-specific, adaptive plasticity in the forebrain gaze fields of the barn owl. *J. Neurophysiol.* 85, 2184–2194.

Miller, G. L., and Knudsen, E. I. (2003). Adaptive plasticity in the auditory thalamus of juvenile barn owls. *J. Neurosci.* 23, 1059–1065.

Mitchell, D. E., Kennie, J., Schwarzkopf, D. S., and Sengpiel, F. (2009). Daily mixed visual experience that prevents amblyopia in cats does not always allow the development of good binocular depth perception. *J. Vis.* 9:22. doi: 10.1167/9.5.22

Mitchell, D. E., Kind, P. C., Sengpiel, F., and Murphy, K. (2003). Brief daily periods of binocular vision prevent deprivation-induced acuity loss. *Curr. Biol.* 13, 1704–1708. doi: 10.1016/j.cub.2003.09.026

Mitchell, D. E., Kind, P. C., Sengpiel, F., and Murphy, K. (2006). Short periods of concordant binocular vision prevent the development of deprivation amblyopia. *Eur. J. Neurosci.* 23, 2458–2466. doi: 10.1111/j.1460-9568.2006.04755.x

Mitchell, D. E., Sengpiel, F., Hamilton, D. C., Schwarzkopf, D. S., and Kennie, J. (2011). Protection against deprivation amblyopia depends on relative not absolute daily binocular exposure. *J. Vis.* 11:13. doi: 10.1167/11.7.13

Mogdans, J., and Knudsen, E. I. (1992). Adaptive adjustment of unit tuning to sound localization cues in response to monaural occlusion in developing owl optic tectum. *J. Neurosci.* 12, 3473–3484.

Mogdans, J., and Knudsen, E. I. (1993). Early monaural occlusion alters the neural map of interaural level differences in the inferior colliculus of the barn owl. *Brain Res.* 619, 29–38. doi: 10.1016/0006-8993(93)91593-H

Mogdans, J., and Knudsen, E. I. (1994). Site of auditory plasticity in the brain stem (VLVp) of the owl revealed by early monaural occlusion. *J. Neurophysiol.* 72, 2875–2891.

Moiseff, A. (1989). Bi-coordinate sound localization by the barn owl. *J. Comp. Physiol. A* 164, 637–644. doi: 10.1007/BF00614506

Moiseff, A., and Konishi, M. (1981). Neuronal and behavioral sensitivity to binaural time differences in the owl. *J. Neurosci.* 1, 40–48.

Moore, D. R. (2002). Auditory development and the role of experience. *Br. Med. Bull.* 63, 171–181. doi: 10.1093/bmb/63.1.171

Moore, D. R., Hartley, D. E., and Hogan, S. C. (2003). Effects of otitis media with effusion (OME) on central auditory function. *Int. J. Pediatr. Otorhinolaryngol.* 67(Suppl. 1), S63–S67. doi: 10.1016/j.ijporl.2003.08.015

Moore, D. R., Hine, J. E., Jiang, Z. D., Matsuda, H., Parsons, C. H., and King, A. J. (1999). Conductive hearing loss produces a reversible binaural hearing impairment. *J. Neurosci.* 19, 8704–8711.

Moore, D. R., Hutchings, M. E., King, A. J., and Kowalchuk, N. E. (1989). Auditory brain stem of the ferret: some effects of rearing with a unilateral ear plug on the cochlea, cochlear nucleus, and projections to the inferior colliculus. *J. Neurosci.* 9, 1213–1222.

Moore, D. R., and Irvine, D. R. (1981). Plasticity of binaural interaction in the cat inferior colliculus. *Brain Res.* 208, 198–202. doi: 10.1016/0006-8993(81)90632-6

Moore, D. R., and King, A. J. (2004). "Plasticity of binaural systems," in *Plasticity of the Auditory System*, eds T. N. Parks, E. W. Rubel, and A. N. Popper (New York, NY: Springer), xii, 323 p.

Moore, D. R., and Kowalchuk, N. E. (1988). Auditory brainstem of the ferret: effects of unilateral cochlear lesions on cochlear nucleus volume and projections to the inferior colliculus. *J. Comp. Neurol.* 272, 503–515. doi: 10.1002/cne.902720405

Musicant, A. D., and Butler, R. A. (1984). The influence of pinnae-based spectral cues on sound localization. *J. Acoust. Soc. Am.* 75, 1195–1200. doi: 10.1121/1.390770

Musicant, A. D., Chan, J. C., and Hind, J. E. (1990). Direction-dependent spectral properties of cat external ear: new data and cross-species comparisons. *J. Acoust. Soc. Am.* 87, 757–781. doi: 10.1121/1.399545

Nelken, I., and De Cheveigne, A. (2013). An ear for statistics. *Nat. Neurosci.* 16, 381–382. doi: 10.1038/nn.3360

Newton, V. E. (1983). Sound localisation in children with a severe unilateral hearing loss. *Audiology* 22, 189–198. doi: 10.3109/00206098309072782

Nodal, F. R., Bajo, V. M., and King, A. J. (2012). Plasticity of spatial hearing: behavioural effects of cortical inactivation. *J. Physiol.* 590, 3965–3986. doi: 10.1113/jphysiol.2011.222828

Nodal, F. R., Kacelnik, O., Bajo, V. M., Bizley, J. K., Moore, D. R., and King, A. J. (2010). Lesions of the auditory cortex impair azimuthal sound localization and its recalibration in ferrets. *J. Neurophysiol.* 103, 1209–1225. doi: 10.1152/jn.00991.2009

Noreña, A. J., Gourevitch, B., Aizawa, N., and Eggermont, J. J. (2006). Spectrally enhanced acoustic environment disrupts frequency representation in cat auditory cortex. *Nat. Neurosci.* 9, 932–939. doi: 10.1038/nn1720

Palmer, A. R., and King, A. J. (1982). The representation of auditory space in the mammalian superior colliculus. *Nature* 299, 248–249. doi: 10.1038/299248a0

Parsons, C. H., Lanyon, R. G., Schnupp, J. W., and King, A. J. (1999). Effects of altering spectral cues in infancy on horizontal and vertical sound localization by adult ferrets. *J. Neurophysiol.* 82, 2294–2309.

Pienkowski, M., and Eggermont, J. J. (2009). Long-term, partially-reversible reorganization of frequency tuning in mature cat primary auditory cortex can be induced by passive exposure to moderate-level sounds. *Hear. Res.* 257, 24–40. doi: 10.1016/j.heares.2009.07.011

Pienkowski, M., and Eggermont, J. J. (2010). Intermittent exposure with moderate-level sound impairs central auditory function of mature animals without concomitant hearing loss. *Hear. Res.* 261, 30–35. doi: 10.1016/j.heares.2009.12.025

Pienkowski, M., and Eggermont, J. J. (2012). Reversible long-term changes in auditory processing in mature auditory cortex in the absence of hearing loss induced by passive, moderate-level sound exposure. *Ear Hear.* 33, 305–314. doi: 10.1097/AUD.0b013e318241e880

Pienkowski, M., Munguia, R., and Eggermont, J. J. (2011). Passive exposure of adult cats to bandlimited tone pip ensembles or noise leads to long-term response suppression in auditory cortex. *Hear. Res.* 277, 117–126. doi: 10.1016/j.heares.2011.02.002

Pienkowski, M., Munguia, R., and Eggermont, J. J. (2013). Effects of passive, moderate-level sound exposure on the mature auditory cortex: spectral edges, spectrotemporal density, and real-world noise. *Hear. Res.* 296, 121–130. doi: 10.1016/j.heares.2012.11.006

Pillsbury, H. C., Grose, J. H., and Hall, J. W. 3rd. (1991). Otitis media with effusion in children. Binaural hearing before and after corrective surgery. *Arch. Otolaryngol. Head Neck Surg.* 117, 718–723. doi: 10.1001/archotol.1991.01870190030008

Polley, D. B., Steinberg, E. E., and Merzenich, M. M. (2006). Perceptual learning directs auditory cortical map reorganization through top-down influences. *J. Neurosci.* 26, 4970–4982. doi: 10.1523/JNEUROSCI.3771-05.2006

Polley, D. B., Thompson, J. H., and Guo, W. (2013). Brief hearing loss disrupts binaural integration during two early critical periods of auditory cortex development. *Nat. Commun.* 4, 2547. doi: 10.1038/ncomms3547

Popescu, M. V., and Polley, D. B. (2010). Monaural deprivation disrupts development of binaural selectivity in auditory midbrain and cortex. *Neuron* 65, 718–731. doi: 10.1016/j.neuron.2010.02.019

Qian, T., Jaeger, T. F., and Aslin, R. N. (2012). Learning to represent a multi-context environment: more than detecting changes. *Front. Psychol.* 3:228. doi: 10.3389/fpsyg.2012.00228

Razak, K. A. (2011). Systematic representation of sound locations in the primary auditory cortex. *J. Neurosci.* 31, 13848–13859. doi: 10.1523/JNEUROSCI.1937-11.2011

Recanzone, G. H., and Sutter, M. L. (2008). The biological basis of audition. *Annu. Rev. Psychol.* 59, 119–142. doi: 10.1146/annurev.psych.59.103006.093544

Russell, F. A., and Moore, D. R. (1999). Effects of unilateral cochlear removal on dendrites in the gerbil medial superior olivary nucleus. *Eur. J. Neurosci.* 11, 1379–1390. doi: 10.1046/j.1460-9568.1999.00547.x

Sanes, D. H., Markowitz, S., Bernstein, J., and Wardlow, J. (1992). The influence of inhibitory afferents on the development of postsynaptic dendritic arbors. *J. Comp. Neurol.* 321, 637–644. doi: 10.1002/cne.903210410

Sarro, E. C., and Sanes, D. H. (2011). The cost and benefit of juvenile training on adult perceptual skill. *J. Neurosci.* 31, 5383–5391. doi: 10.1523/JNEUROSCI.6137-10.2011

Schnupp, J., Nelken, I., and King, A. (2011). *Auditory Neuroscience: Making Sense of Sound.* Cambridge, MA; London: MIT Press.

Schnupp, J. W., and King, A. J. (1997). Coding for auditory space in the nucleus of the brachium of the inferior colliculus in the ferret. *J. Neurophysiol.* 78, 2717–2731.

Seidl, A. H., and Grothe, B. (2005). Development of sound localization mechanisms in the mongolian gerbil is shaped by early acoustic experience. *J. Neurophysiol.* 94, 1028–1036. doi: 10.1152/jn.01143.2004

Seydell, A., Knill, D. C., and Trommershauser, J. (2010). Adapting internal statistical models for interpreting visual cues to depth. *J. Vis.* 10:1. doi: 10.1167/10.4.1.

Shepard, K. N., Kilgard, M. P., and Liu, R. C. (2012). "Experience-dependent plasticity and auditory cortex," in Neural *Correlates of Auditory Cognition*, ed Y. Cohen. (New York, NY: Springer), 293–327.

Shinn-Cunningham, B. G., Durlach, N. I., and Held, R. M. (1998). Adapting to supernormal auditory localization cues. I. Bias and resolution. *J. Acoust. Soc. Am.* 103, 3656–3666. doi: 10.1121/1.423088

Silverman, M. S., and Clopton, B. M. (1977). Plasticity of binaural interaction. I. Effect of early auditory deprivation. *J. Neurophysiol.* 40, 1266–1274.

Singheiser, M., Gutfreund, Y., and Wagner, H. (2012). The representation of sound localization cues in the barn owl's inferior colliculus. *Front. Neural. Circuits* 6:45. doi: 10.3389/fncir.2012.00045

Slattery, W. H. 3rd., and Middlebrooks, J. C. (1994). Monaural sound localization: acute versus chronic unilateral impairment. *Hear. Res.* 75, 38–46. doi: 10.1016/0378-5955(94)90053-1

Stange, A., Myoga, M. H., Lingner, A., Ford, M. C., Alexandrova, O., Felmy, F., et al. (2013). Adaptation in Sound localization: from GABA receptor-mediated synaptic modulation to perception. *Nat. Neurosci.* 16, 1840–1847. doi: 10.1038/nn.3548

Strelnikov, K., Rosito, M., and Barone, P. (2011). Effect of audiovisual training on monaural spatial hearing in horizontal plane. *PLoS ONE* 6:e18344. doi: 10.1371/journal.pone.0018344

Strutt, J. (1907). On our perception of sound direction. *Philos. Mag.* 13, 214–232. doi: 10.1080/14786440709463595

Sumner, C. J., and Palmer, A. R. (2012). Auditory nerve fibre responses in the ferret. *Eur. J. Neurosci.* 36, 2428–2439. doi: 10.1111/j.1460-9568.2012.08151.x

Tallal, P., Miller, S. L., Bedi, G., Byma, G., Wang, X., Nagarajan, S. S., et al. (1996). Language comprehension in language-learning impaired children improved with acoustically modified speech. *Science* 271, 81–84. doi: 10.1126/science.271.5245.81

Tollin, D. J. (2010). "Development of sound localization mechanisms," in *Oxford Handbook of Developmental Behavioral Neuroscience*, eds M. S. Blumberg, J. H. Freeman, and S. R. Robinson (New York, NY: Oxford University Press), 263–282.

Tollin, D. J., Ruhland, J. L., and Yin, T. C. (2013). The role of spectral composition of sounds on the localization of sound sources by cats. *J. Neurophysiol.* 109, 1658–1668. doi: 10.1152/jn.00358.2012

Tucci, D. L., Born, D. E., and Rubel, E. W. (1987). Changes in spontaneous activity and CNS morphology associated with conductive and sensorineural hearing loss in chickens. *Ann. Otol. Rhinol. Laryngol.* 96, 343–350.

Van Wanrooij, M. M., and Van Opstal, A. J. (2004). Contribution of head shadow and pinna cues to chronic monaural sound localization. *J. Neurosci.* 24, 4163–4171. doi: 10.1523/JNEUROSCI.0048-04.2004

Van Wanrooij, M. M., and Van Opstal, A. J. (2005). Relearning sound localization with a new ear. *J. Neurosci.* 25, 5413–5424. doi: 10.1523/JNEUROSCI.0850-05.2005

Van Wanrooij, M. M., and Van Opstal, A. J. (2007). Sound localization under perturbed binaural hearing. *J. Neurophysiol.* 97, 715–726. doi: 10.1152/jn.00260.2006

Viehweg, R., and Campbell, R. A. (1960). Localization difficulty in monaurally impaired listeners. *Ann. Otol. Rhinol. Laryngol.* 69, 622–634.

Wakeford, O. S., and Robinson, D. E. (1974). Lateralization of tonal stimuli by the cat. *J. Acoust. Soc. Am.* 55, 649–652. doi: 10.1121/1.1914577

Wallace, M. T., and Stein, B. E. (1994). Cross-modal synthesis in the midbrain depends on input from cortex. *J. Neurophysiol.* 71, 429–432.

Wallace, M. T., and Stein, B. E. (2007). Early experience determines how the senses will interact. *J. Neurophysiol.* 97, 921–926. doi: 10.1152/jn.00497.2006

Webster, D. B. (1983a). Auditory neuronal sizes after a unilateral conductive hearing loss. *Exp. Neurol.* 79, 130–140. doi: 10.1016/0014-4886(83)90384-9

Webster, D. B. (1983b). A critical period during postnatal auditory development of mice. *Int. J. Pediatr. Otorhinolaryngol.* 6, 107–118. doi: 10.1016/S0165-5876(83)80111-6

Webster, D. B., and Webster, M. (1979). Effects of neonatal conductive hearing loss on brain stem auditory nuclei. *Ann. Otol. Rhinol. Laryngol.* 88, 684–688.

Wen, B., Wang, G. I., Dean, I., and Delgutte, B. (2012). Time course of dynamic range adaptation in the auditory nerve. *J. Neurophysiol.* 108, 69–82. doi: 10.1152/jn.00055.2012

Werker, J. (2012). Perceptual foundations of bilingual acquisition in infancy. *Ann. N.Y. Acad. Sci.* 1251, 50–61. doi: 10.1111/j.1749-6632.2012.06484.x

Whitton, J. P., and Polley, D. B. (2011). Evaluating the perceptual and pathophysiological consequences of auditory deprivation in early postnatal life: a comparison of basic and clinical studies. *J. Assoc. Res. Otolaryngol.* 12, 535–547. doi: 10.1007/s10162-011-0271-6

Wightman, F. L., and Kistler, D. J. (1997). Monaural sound localization revisited. *J. Acoust. Soc. Am.* 101, 1050–1063. doi: 10.1121/1.418029

Wilmington, D., Gray, L., and Jahrsdoerfer, R. (1994). Binaural processing after corrected congenital unilateral conductive hearing loss. *Hear. Res.* 74, 99–114. doi: 10.1016/0378-5955(94)90179-1

Xu, J., Yu, L., Rowland, B. A., Stanford, T. R., and Stein, B. E. (2012). Incorporating cross-modal statistics in the development and maintenance of multisensory integration. *J. Neurosci.* 32, 2287–2298. doi: 10.1523/JNEUROSCI.4304-11.2012

Yan, J., Zhang, Y., and Ehret, G. (2005). Corticofugal shaping of frequency tuning curves in the central nucleus of the inferior colliculus of mice. *J. Neurophysiol.* 93, 71–83. doi: 10.1152/jn.00348.2004

Yaron, A., Hershenhoren, I., and Nelken, I. (2012). Sensitivity to complex statistical regularities in rat auditory cortex. *Neuron* 76, 603–615. doi: 10.1016/j.neuron.2012.08.025

Yin, T. C. T. (2002). "Neural mechanisms of encoding binaural localization cues in the auditory brainstem," in *Integrative Functions in the Mammalian Auditory Pathway*, eds D. Oertel, R. R. Fay, and A. N. Popper (New York, NY: Springer), 99–159.

Yost, W. A. (1997). "The cocktail party problem: forty years later," in *Binaural and Spatial Hearing in Real And Virtual Environments*, eds R. H. Gilkey and T. R. Anderson (Mahwah, NJ: Lawrence Erlbaum Associates), 329–347.

Young, E. D., Spirou, G. A., Rice, J. J., and Voigt, H. F. (1992). Neural organization and responses to complex stimuli in the dorsal cochlear nucleus. *Philos. Trans. R. Soc. Lond. B Biol. Sci.* 336, 407–413. doi: 10.1098/rstb.1992.0076

Yu, L., Xu, J., Rowland, B. A., and Stein, B. E. (2013). Development of cortical influences on superior colliculus multisensory neurons: effects of dark-rearing. *Eur. J. Neurosci.* 37, 1594–1601. doi: 10.1111/ejn.12182

Yu, X., Sanes, D. H., Aristizabal, O., Wadghiri, Y. Z., and Turnbull, D. H. (2007). Large-scale reorganization of the tonotopic map in mouse auditory midbrain revealed by MRI. *Proc. Natl. Acad. Sci. U.S.A.* 104, 12193–12198. doi: 10.1073/pnas.0700960104

Zahorik, P., Brungart, D. S., and Bronkhorst, A. W. (2005). Auditory distance perception in humans: a summary of past and present research. *Acta Acust. United Acust.* 91, 409–420.

Zhang, L. I., Bao, S., and Merzenich, M. M. (2001). Persistent and specific influences of early acoustic environments on primary auditory cortex. *Nat. Neurosci.* 4, 1123–1130. doi: 10.1038/nn745

Zheng, W. (2012). Auditory map reorganization and pitch discrimination in adult rats chronically exposed to low-level ambient noise. *Front. Syst. Neurosci.* 6:65. doi: 10.3389/fnsys.2012.00065

Zheng, W., and Knudsen, E. I. (1999). Functional selection of adaptive auditory space map by GABAA-mediated inhibition. *Science* 284, 962–965. doi: 10.1126/science.284.5416.962

Zheng, W., and Knudsen, E. I. (2001). Gabaergic inhibition antagonizes adaptive adjustment of the owl's auditory space map during the initial phase of plasticity. *J. Neurosci.* 21, 4356–4365.

Zhou, X., and Merzenich, M. M. (2012). Environmental noise exposure degrades normal listening processes. *Nat. Commun.* 3, 843. doi: 10.1038/ncomms1849

Zhou, X., Nagarajan, N., Mossop, B. J., and Merzenich, M. M. (2008). Influences of un-modulated acoustic inputs on functional maturation and critical-period plasticity of the primary auditory cortex. *Neuroscience* 154, 390–396. doi: 10.1016/j.neuroscience.2008.01.026

Zhou, X., Panizzutti, R., De Villers-Sidani, E., Madeira, C., and Merzenich, M. M. (2011). Natural restoration of critical period plasticity in the juvenile and adult primary auditory cortex. *J. Neurosci.* 31, 5625–5634. doi: 10.1523/JNEUROSCI.6470-10.2011

16

Is the auditory evoked P2 response a biomarker of learning?

Kelly L. Tremblay[1]*, Bernhard Ross[2,3], Kayo Inoue[1,4], Katrina McClannahan[1] and Gregory Collet[5,6]

[1] *Department of Speech and Hearing Sciences, University of Washington, Seattle, WA, USA*
[2] *Baycrest Centre, Rotman Research Institute, Toronto, ON, Canada*
[3] *Department of Medical Biophysics, University of Toronto, Toronto, ON, Canada*
[4] *Department of Radiology, Integrated Brian Imaging Center, University of Washington, Seattle, WA, USA*
[5] *Life Sciences Department, Royal Military Academy, Brussels, Belgium*
[6] *Unité de Recherche en Neurosciences Cognitives, Centre de Recherches en Cognition et Neurosciences Université Libre de Bruxelles, Brussels, Belgium*

Correspondence:
Kelly L. Tremblay, Department of Speech and Hearing Sciences, University of Washington, Eagleson Hall, 1417 NE 42nd St., Seattle WA 98105, USA
e-mail: tremblay@uw.edu

Even though auditory training exercises for humans have been shown to improve certain perceptual skills of individuals with and without hearing loss, there is a lack of knowledge pertaining to which aspects of training are responsible for the perceptual gains, and which aspects of perception are changed. To better define how auditory training impacts brain and behavior, electroencephalography (EEG) and magnetoencephalography (MEG) have been used to determine the time course and coincidence of cortical modulations associated with different types of training. Here we focus on P1-N1-P2 auditory evoked responses (AEP), as there are consistent reports of gains in P2 amplitude following various types of auditory training experiences; including music and speech-sound training. The purpose of this experiment was to determine if the auditory evoked P2 response is a biomarker of learning. To do this, we taught native English speakers to identify a new pre-voiced temporal cue that is not used phonemically in the English language so that coinciding changes in evoked neural activity could be characterized. To differentiate possible effects of repeated stimulus exposure and a button-pushing task from learning itself, we examined modulations in brain activity in a group of participants who learned to identify the pre-voicing contrast and compared it to participants, matched in time, and stimulus exposure, that did not. The main finding was that the amplitude of the P2 auditory evoked response increased across repeated EEG sessions for all groups, regardless of any change in perceptual performance. What's more, these effects are retained for months. Changes in P2 amplitude were attributed to changes in neural activity associated with the acquisition process and not the learned outcome itself. A further finding was the expression of a late negativity (LN) wave 600–900 ms post-stimulus onset, post-training exclusively for the group that learned to identify the pre-voiced contrast.

Keywords: auditory, training, ERP, P2, exposure, learning, rehabilitation, electrophysiology

INTRODUCTION

Long before the effects of auditory deprivation and stimulation on the brain were known, audiologists used auditory training exercises as a way to help people compensate for hearing loss (Carhart, 1960). The motivation for such exercises stemmed from the fact that adults and children with hearing loss often needed help in dealing with their speech perception deficits that remained after being fit with hearing aid amplification devices (Boothroyd, 2010). Some people reported training exercises to be helpful and others did not, so the use of auditory training exercises was questioned and slowly faded from clinical practice. By the year 2005, a mere 30% of audiology practices reported using auditory training type interventions in routine clinical practice (Kricos, 2006).

Advances in neuroscience reignited the interest in auditory training because of the plethora of research documenting the capacity of the human brain to change, depending on the type of sensory input or lack thereof. Here we focus on auditory perceptual training as a means of exploring the human capacity to learn so that brain plasticity can be optimized in ways that enhance the rehabilitation of people with hearing loss. Previous studies have shown that training-related changes in neural activity precede changes in auditory perception (Tremblay et al., 1998; Atienza et al., 2002) therefore, non-invasive physiological measures might provide an opportunity to monitor and optimize intervention efforts in people with different types of hearing loss.

Even though auditory training exercises in humans have been shown to improve certain perceptual skills of individuals with and without hearing loss (Boothroyd, 1997; Tremblay et al., 1997, 1998, 2001; Fu et al., 2004; Irvine and Wright, 2005; Sweetow and Sabes, 2006; Burk and Humes, 2007; Tremblay and Moore, 2012; Anderson et al., 2013; Chisolm et al., 2013; Sullivan et al., 2013), there is a lack of knowledge pertaining to which aspects of training are responsible for the perceptual gains, and which aspects of perception are changed (Amitay et al., 2006, 2013; Boothroyd, 2010; Henshaw and Ferguson, 2013; Jacoby and Ahissar, 2013). This lack of knowledge hinders the rehabilitation of people with hearing loss because individuals do not always respond as expected to the training program in which they participate. Even among normal hearing listeners, the effects of training can be highly heterogeneous. Without knowing which aspects of the training exercises are responsible for observed benefits, it is difficult to determine which components of the training paradigm are ineffective and what individual needs still require targeted intervention.

To better define how auditory training exercises impact brain and behavior, electroencephalography (EEG) and magnetoencephalography (MEG) have been used to determine the time course and coincidence of cortical and sub-cortical modulations in evoked activity associated with different types of auditory training (Tremblay et al., 1997, 2001, 2009, 2010; Brattico et al., 2003; Shahin et al., 2003; Bosnyak et al., 2004; Sheehan et al., 2005; Alain et al., 2010; Carcagno and Plack, 2011; Shahin, 2011; Anderson et al., 2013; Barrett et al., 2013). Here we focus on studies involving the P1-N1-P2 waves of the cortical auditory evoked response (AEP), as there are consistent reports of gains in P2 amplitude following various types of auditory training experiences; including music (Shahin et al., 2003; Kuriki et al., 2007; Seppänen et al., 2012; Kühnis et al., 2013) and speech-sound training. Despite converging evidence that increases in the amplitude of the P2 wave of the P1-N1-P2 complex coincides with improved perception, little is known about the functional meaning and neural generators of the auditory P2 response and whether or not it could serve as a biological marker of auditory learning. Our earlier studies show the center of activity for P2 to be in the anterior auditory cortex, but how this relates to learning is still unknown (Ross and Tremblay, 2009).

Speech sounds and acoustic elements thereof are represented in the neural activity patterns along the auditory pathway. One example is the representation of voice-onset time (VOT), as reflected through a sequence of onset responses recorded from primary auditory cortices in feline, primate, and human models (Eggermont, 1995; Steinschneider et al., 2005). Monotonic increases in VOT result in latency shifts and double onset responses involving the N1 peak of the P1-N1-P2 complex (Tremblay et al., 2003; Steinschneider et al., 2005). The N1 is often described to be an "exogenous" response, meaning that it is sensitive to physical characteristics of the sound used to evoke the response (see Picton, 2013 for a recent review). As an example, the N1 reflects the detection of acoustic changes; including, the onset of sound, and acoustic changes within an ongoing sound (such as a consonant-vowel transitions) (Ostroff et al., 1998; Wagner et al., 2013). The P1 wave is thought to reflect gating of auditory information to the auditory cortex (Alho et al., 1994) whereas the P2 may reflect auditory processing beyond sensation (Crowley and Colrain, 2004). It is for this reason; the P1-N1-P2 complex has been used to examine the neural representation of perceptually relevant temporal cues such as VOT.

In a series of past experiments, the effects of VOT training on the human P1-N1-P2 complex have also been studied (Tremblay et al., 2001, 2009, 2010; Sheehan et al., 2005; Alain et al., 2010). These experiments were used to determine if neural VOT codes could be altered through training. That is, could the perception of two within category VOT stimuli (e.g., identification and/or discrimination) that are perceived alike, and that evoke similar N1 peak latencies be altered with training? What's more, if perception changes, does the neural representation of VOT, marked by the latency of N1, change?

The VOT training studies described earlier did not reveal modifications in the latency of the N1 response. Instead, P2 amplitudes increased following VOT training. Training-related enhancements in P2 turned out not to be specific to VOT or VOT training. Enhanced P2 amplitudes appeared after various types of sound exposures (Tremblay and Ross, 2007; Tremblay et al., 2001, 2009; Atienza et al., 2002; Bosnyak et al., 2004; Sheehan et al., 2005) including identification or discrimination training; for different types of stimuli including tones and speech sounds; presented in different types of event-related potentials (ERPs) contexts (homogenous block or oddball paradigm, monaurally or binaurally); over different time courses (1 day vs. 1 year); using EEG or MEG. The P2 effect is robust, can be reliably seen in individuals, and is retained for months following initial exposure (Tremblay et al., 2010). This phenomenon is not limited to the laboratory either; enhanced P2 amplitudes appear to reflect life-long learning such as musical training (Kuriki et al., 2006; Shahin, 2011).

Even though P2 amplitude gains have been reported to be physiological correlates of auditory learning, it is important to challenge this notion by recognizing that contributions of stimulus exposure, executive function, cognitive tasks, and memory are inherent in any auditory training paradigm. Any one or combination of these components, rather than learning itself, could be influencing P2 changes reported in the literature. In fact, our previous studies (Ross and Tremblay, 2009; Tremblay et al., 2010), and others (Sheehan et al., 2005) suggest that mere stimulus exposure, during EEG and MEG recording sessions and behavioral baseline testing, in the absence of training or changes in perceptual performance, contribute to enhanced P2 amplitude.

Expanding this program of research by including different experimental designs, while involving the same stimuli, enables us to identify converging evidence across the studies. Therefore, the purpose of this study was to determine whether or not P2 amplitude changes represent biologic markers of auditory learning. To do so required examining modulations in brain activity in a group of participants who learned the task and comparing it to participants, matched in time, task, and stimulus exposure, that did not learn. Modulations in P2 amplitude could be viewed as a biomarker of auditory learning if P2 amplitudes increased only for the group that learned the VOT contrast, but not in the other groups.

We therefore recorded behavioral responses and brain activity, elicited by stimuli differing in VOT, from three groups of participants, who were tested within similar time windows (**Figure 1**). The first group served as a control group without intervening listening or training experience, so that quantifiable modulations in brain activity could be related solely to the passage of time. The remaining two experimental groups (Groups 2 and 3) participated in listening tasks during a 5 day intervening period between pre 2 and post sessions. Both groups heard the same number of stimulus sounds during these intervening days, but the two groups differed in the type of task and feedback they received. One facilitated learning whereas the other did not. For example, members of Group 2 were asked to click a mouse button (to proceed to the next sound) after hearing each sound without receiving any feedback to facilitate learning the VOT contrast. Group 3 members were instructed how to label each sound (the two-alternative force-choice task) by clicking a mouse button, feedback about their performance followed so to facilitate learning. In doing so, we were able to examine brain-related changes in activity among a group that did and did not learn the VOT contrast. We also looked beyond a typical P1-N1-P2 time window (<200 ms in latency), to determine if VOT training modulates more endogenous, higher-level, aspects of sound processing.

MATERIALS AND METHODS

PARTICIPANTS

Thirty normal-hearing native-English speakers (18–39 years) were randomly assigned to one of three groups (10 in each group). Normal hearing was defined as pure tone thresholds ≤25 dB HL across frequencies between 250 and 8000 Hz. All participants were right handed and provided their written informed consent prior to participation. The Research Ethics Board of the University of Washington approved the study. Data from ten of these subjects (Group 1) were previously described in a publication that

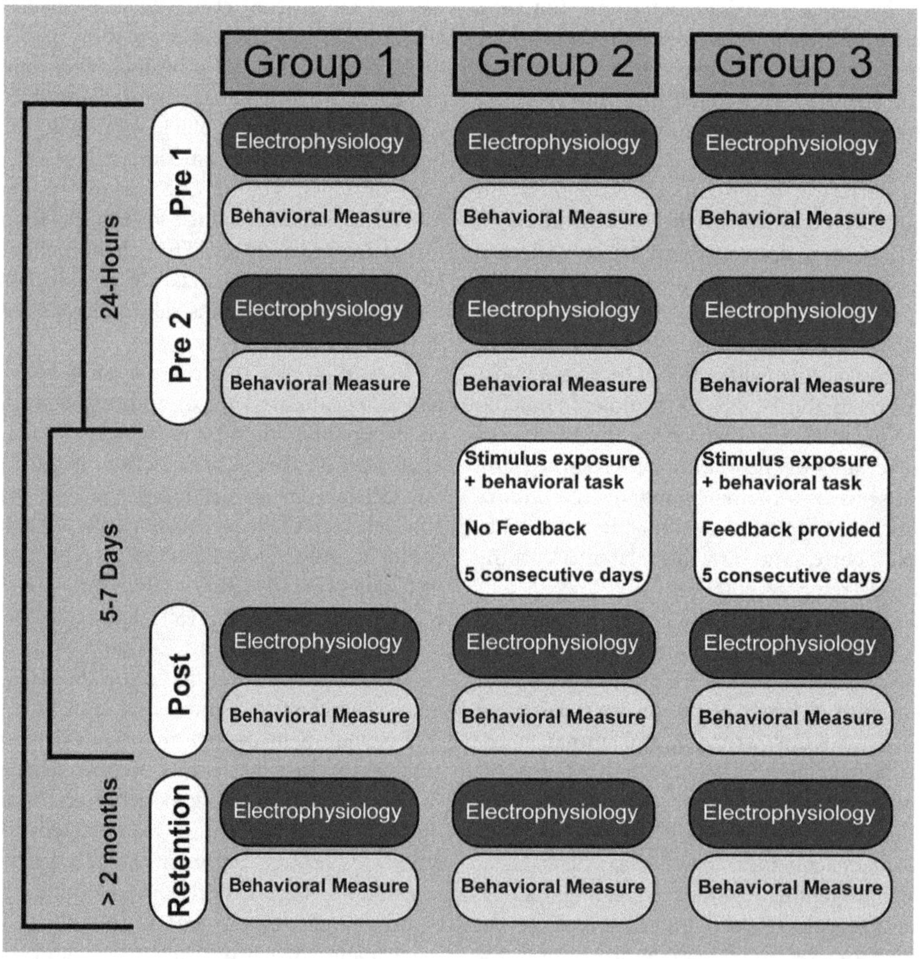

FIGURE 1 | Experiment design and time course. EEG recording and behavioral testing was performed at similar points in time, across four sessions, and involved three groups. EEG data were acquired separate from the behavioral sessions. Whereas participants in Groups 2 and 3 were exposed to, and interacted with, the stimuli over a 5 day period between test sessions, Group 1 did not. The number of stimuli (amount of stimulus exposure) was identical across Groups 2 and 3, and participants were required to perform a similar task (click the mouse to advance to the next stimulus), but what differed between the two groups was the instructions and feedback. Participants in Group 3 received instructions and response feedback intended to improve their ability to correctly identify each of the two pre-voiced stimuli, but participants in Group 2 did not.

reported only the effects of repeated stimulus exposure (Tremblay et al., 2010).

STIMULI

Two Klatt synthesized pre-voiced "ba" syllables, 180 ms in duration, were used in this experiment. They were the same stimuli used in a series of experiments designed to examine the neural encoding of VOT with training (see series of experiments by Tremblay et al., 1997 through 2010). Adult native English speakers consistently describe both pre-voiced stimuli as "ba" (McClaskey et al., 1983), but following training, they can learn to identify and label the −10 ms VOT stimulus as "ba" and the −20 ms VOT stimulus as "mba" (Tremblay et al., 1997).

BEHAVIORAL TESTS

The ability to correctly identify the two stimuli was tested in four sessions for all groups within the same time frame (**Figure 1**). The first two tests were performed on 2 subsequent days, termed pre 1 and 2, and provided baseline performance scores. A post-training test was administered 5–7 days later and a retention test more than 2 months later. All groups were involved in the identification task, which was the same for all sessions. Participants were presented with randomized trials of the "mba" and "ba" stimuli. Twenty-five of the "mba" and 25 "ba" stimuli were presented in each session binaurally at a level of 76 dB SPL using insert earphones (Etymotic Research ER3a). The test was self-paced and a response, entered via a computer mouse, triggered the presentation of the next sound. Feedback was not provided in any test. The instructions to all participants were: "*You will hear some sounds and I want you to label the sounds as you hear them using the left button on the computer mouse. You will label the sounds based on two choices that will be displayed on the computer monitor. There is no right or wrong answer; it is simply your perception of what you hear*". Two labels appeared on the computer screen as text: "mba" and "ba".

BEHAVIORAL TRAINING

Group 1 participated in the four-behavioral tests only and served as a control group for examining changes in perception and physiology, over the same time periods as Groups 2 and 3. Groups 2 and 3 participated in training sessions on 5 consecutive days, starting immediately following the pre 2 behavioral testing. Both groups heard four blocks of 50 randomized presentations of the "mba" and "ba" syllables, 25 of each on each day. Behavioral testing was self-paced and lasted approximately 20 min each day. Whereas the numbers of stimuli (amount of stimulus exposure) and the motor task of clicking the mouse were similar across the two groups, the instructions and feedback were different between groups. The task for Group 3 involved evaluating the stimulus they just heard, making a decision about what label they will assign to each sound, and then clicking the mouse to indicate which sound they heard. Group 3 also received feedback, which was intended to motivate participants to "correctly" label each sound.

Participants in Group 2 were instructed: "*You will hear some sounds. After each sound press the button on the screen to continue to the following sound*". A button labeled "NEXT" was displayed on the computer screen to advance the task following each stimulus presentation.

Group 3 participants were instructed: "*Now, we're going to help you label one sound /ba/ and one /mba/. You will be given feedback following each trial. If you select the correct label, it will turn green. If you do not select the correct label, the next trial will begin*". Two text labels, "mba" and "ba", were displayed on the computer screen.

ELECTROENCEPHALOGRAPHY (EEG) ACQUISITION

EEG recordings and behavioral testing were completed in a sound-attenuated booth on 2 consecutive days (Session pre 1 and 2) 1 week following initial testing (post-training session) and 2 months to 1+ year following initial testing (retention session). Retention tests were staggered in time so changes in brain and behavior could be tracked over a large time window.

Similar to our previous experiments, stimuli were delivered monaurally via insert earphones to the right ear at 76 dB SPL; the same intensity was used for the behavioral tests. A passive EEG paradigm was used, meaning participants watched closed-captioned movies and were instructed to stay alert but no particular attention to the stimuli was requested. No behavioral task took place during EEG recordings. Four hundred presentations of the same type stimuli ("ba" or "mba") were presented with an inter-stimulus interval of 1993 ms in a block. Following a 5 min break, a block of the other sound stimulus ("mba" or "ba") was recorded. Stimulus order was counter-balanced across groups and test sessions. This particular ISI was used because our previous studies have shown that younger and older adults are differentially sensitive to stimulus presentation rates faster than 2 s and in future studies we wish to compare these data to those of older adults (Tremblay et al., 2004).

Continuous EEG signals were recorded from 59 electrodes using an elastic cap (Electro-cap International, Inc.) and a PC-based Neuroscan system (SCAN, ver. 4.3.3) with SynAmps2 amplifiers. The electrode montage followed an extended 10–20 system, reported in more detail in Tremblay et al. (2010). Four additional electrodes were placed on the inferior and outer canthus of each eye to monitor eye blink activity. EEG signals were referenced to the Cz electrode, analog bandpass-filtered between 0.15 and 100 Hz (12 dB/octave roll off), amplified with a gain of 500, and digitized at a sampling rate of 1000 Hz.

For offline analysis, an artifact correction procedure using BESA (5.2) was applied to reduce the effects of contamination from eye-blinks and ocular movements. Eye-blink artifacts were identified by a threshold criterion and corresponding waveforms were averaged to obtain a template of ocular artifacts. A principal component analysis of these averaged recordings provided a set of components that best explained the eye movements. The scalp projections of these components were then removed from the EEG signal to minimize ocular contamination.

In BESA the continuous EEG signal was parsed into stimulus onset related epochs of 1200 ms length, including a 200 ms pre-stimulus interval, which was used for baseline-correction. The signals were averaged for each stimulus condition and re-referenced to the average across all electrodes. Waveforms were low pass filtered at 32 Hz. The peak amplitudes and latencies of the N1 and P2 waves were measured as the signal maxima at electrode Cz in the latency intervals of ±50 ms around 100 ms and 200 ms for each participant, each stimulus type and each session.

RESULTS

BEHAVIORAL DATA ANALYSIS

To assess perceptual performance across groups, *d*-prime (d') scores (Macmillan and Creelman, 1991) were computed for each participant from the rates of hits, misses, false alarms, and correct rejections for each behavioral test. A response was scored correct (hit) if the participant assigned the label "mba" to the −20 ms VOT stimulus. A correct rejection involved choosing the label "ba" for the −10 ms VOT stimulus. A split-plot 3 (fixed between groups; "Group") × 4 (fixed within groups; "Session") mixed model ANOVA was used to test the effects of "Group" and "Session" as well as their interaction on the d'-scores. *F*-statistics for the within-group effects and interactions were adjusted to control for Type I error due to significance of Mauchly's test of sphericity. Follow-up pairwise comparisons were made using the Dunn-Sidak multiple comparisons procedure to control for Type I error. **Figure 2A–C** summarize the behavioral results. Significant improvement in identification performance was seen for Group 3 only, and was retained for as long as 1 year for some individuals.

PERFORMANCE EVALUATION—PRE 1, PRE 2 AND POST SESSIONS

There was a significant main effect of "Session" on *d'-scores* ($F_{(2.33,53.50)} = 6.59$, $p < 0.01$, *partial* $\omega^2 = 0.13$); as well as a "Group" × "Session" interaction ($F_{(4.65,53.50)} = 7.17$, $p < 0.001$, partial $\omega^2 = 0.28$). Follow-up pairwise comparisons showed an increase in d' between baseline (Pre 2) and the post-test for

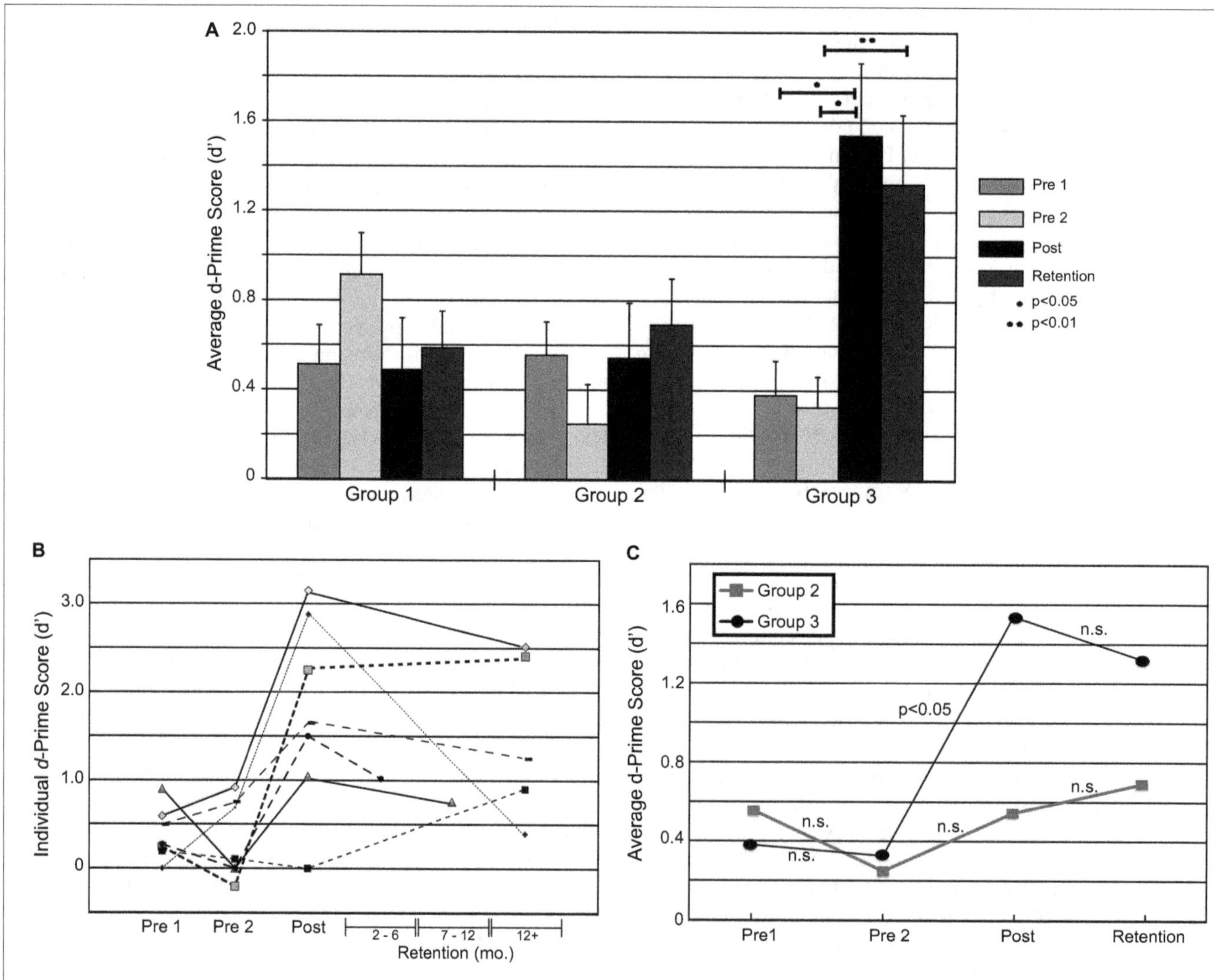

FIGURE 2 | Changes in behavioral performance over the time course of the experiment. (A) Significant increases in performance were seen only for Group 3. Members of Group 3 participated in the identification task and received feedback. **(B)** Changes in d' over time for 7 out of 10 individuals in Group 3 individuals who participated in the retention sessions. **(C)** A comparison in performance, over time, between Groups 2 and 3. Each group experienced the same number of trials and executed a button-pushing task, but Group 2 did not receive instructions or feedback designed to facilitate learning. No significant changes in performance were seen for Group 2.

Group 3 only i.e., for those participants in the training who received performance feedback (p-values < 0.05).

PERFORMANCE RETENTION

Figure 2B shows changes in d'-scores over time for Group 3. Three individuals were lost to attrition and were unavailable to return for retention testing. Analysis of d'-scores measured more than 2 months after the initial testing (Retention) revealed sustained improvements in performance for Group 3 (**Figure 2A**). Significant increases in d'-scores were seen between the baseline session (pre 2) and the post-training measures ($p = 0.033$), with significant differences between baseline and retention ($p = 0.009$) and no significant differences between post-training and retention measures ($p = 0.697$). An analysis of the d'-scores revealed that the improvements in performance, which was found between pre- and post-training measures persisted in the retention measure.

ELECTROENCEPHALOGRAPHY (EEG) ANALYSIS: AUDITORY EVOKED RESPONSES

To compare to our previously published studies, grand averaged evoked responses at electrode Cz are shown for the three groups and the four recording sessions in **Figures 3, 4**. All waveforms are in response to the −10 ms prevoiced "ba" stimulus and show prominent N1-P2 waves. The P1 wave is small. Although the response morphologies are quite different between groups as, for example, expressed in different ratios of the N1 and P2 amplitudes and variations at longer latencies beyond 300 ms, the effect of increasing P2 amplitudes between the first baseline recording and the post-training session is apparent in all three groups. Also, similar to our previous study (Tremblay et al., 2009), P2 amplitude measured across staggered retention sessions more than 2 months after the first recording, remained larger than the initially measured P2 amplitude. In contrast, changes in N1 amplitude over the time course of the experiment were small. Offset responses also appear to decrease over time, but we assume them to be driven by growth of P2.

The N1 amplitude showed smaller between-session changes than that of P2 (**Figure 4A**). N1 amplitude diminished over the time course of the first three recordings. A repeated measures ANOVA for the N1 amplitude revealed main effects of "Session" ($F_{(3,81)} = 4.67$, $p = 0.0046$) and "Stimulus" ($F_{(1,27)} = 5.32$, $p = 0.029$) and a "Session" × "Group" interaction ($F_{(6,81)} = 3.11$, $p = 0.0087$). When averaged across sessions, the stimulus effect appeared to be driven by the slightly larger "ba" amplitude for all three groups (mba: 1.63 μV and ba: 1.85 μV). The interaction diminished when considering the first three recordings only, suggesting it was mainly caused by the continuing N1 decrease in the retention session in Group 3 only. It should be kept in mind, that an N1 amplitude decrease means a positive voltage shift at the Cz electrode, which appeared in line with P2 amplitude increases, thus, a cross talk of the P2 changes has to be considered when interpreting the N1 changes. No significant changes in N1 latency were found for either stimulus, across sessions.

A repeated measures ANOVA on P2 amplitude with the between subjects factor "Group" (3 levels) and the within subjects factors "Session" (4 levels) and "Stimulus" (2 levels) revealed no main effect of "Group" ($F_{(2,27)} = 0.5$), but there were main effects of "Session" ($F_{(3,27)} = 62.7$, $p < 0.0001$) and of "Stimulus" ($F_{(2,27)} = 13.6$, $p = 0.001$). No "Group" × "Session" or "Group" × "Stimulus" interaction was significant. For the mean across groups, the P2 amplitude increased from 0.90 μV to 1.61 μV between the pre 1 and 2 baseline recordings, continued to increase to 2.59 μV in the post-training session, and decreased to 1.86 μV in the retention session. Compared to the first baseline recording, the P2 amplitude increased by 79% at the second

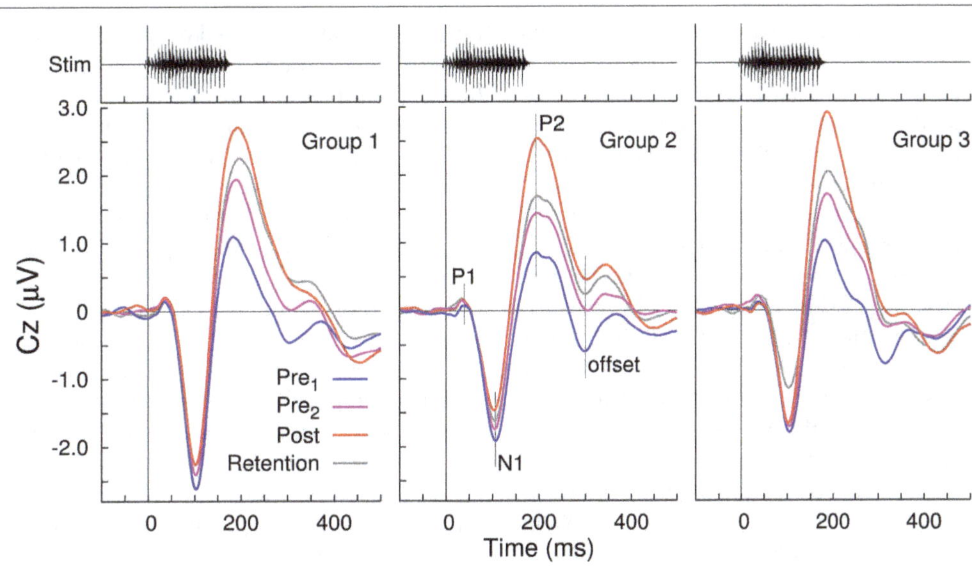

FIGURE 3 | Grand averaged voltages at the vertex electrode Cz in response to the −10 ms VOT stimulus "ba". Prominent N1 and P2 waves are visible in all time-series as well as the gradual increase in the P2 amplitude across the three sessions. Offset responses decrease across sessions, presumably due to the P2 amplitude growth.

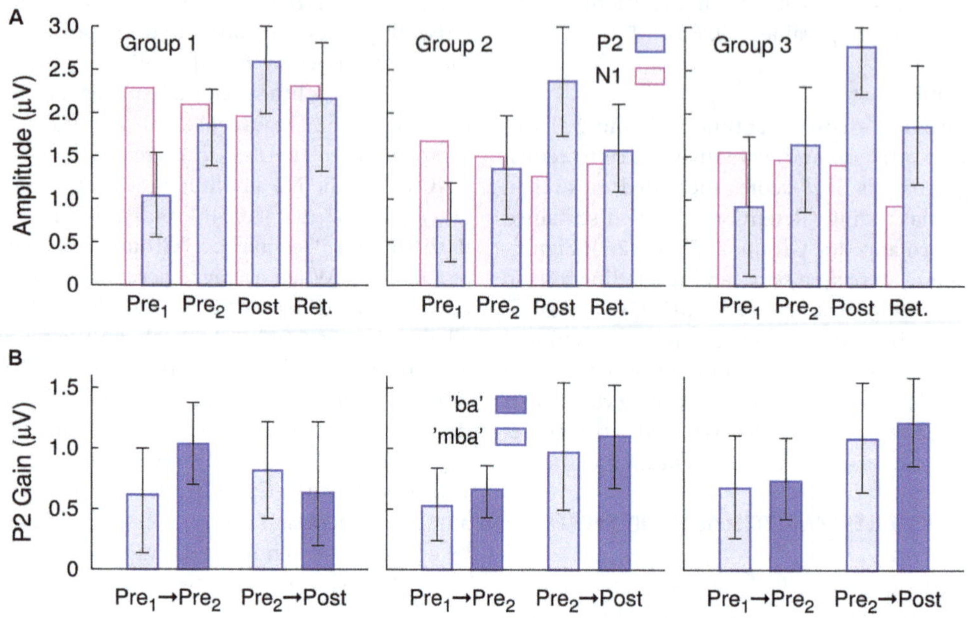

FIGURE 4 | Changes in the group mean P2 amplitudes, measured at electrode Cz. (A) In all three groups, P2 amplitude gains were seen for the Pre 2, post-training, and even during the retention sessions. P2 amplitudes were still larger in the retention session than in the first session. By comparison, changes in the N1 amplitude were small. The error bars indicate the 95% confidence intervals for each group mean. **(B)** Gain in the P2 amplitudes between Pre 1 and Pre 2 sessions and between the Pre 2 and post-training sessions

baseline recording, by 187% at the post-training session, and retained larger than twice the initial amplitude after more than 2 months.

Gains in P2 amplitude between the pre-training sessions and between pre- and post-training sessions are illustrated in **Figure 4B**. An ANOVA revealed a main effect of "Session" ($F_{(1,27)} = 4.9$, $p = 0.035$) and a "Session" × "Group" interaction ($F_{(2,27)} = 5.2$, $p = 0.030$) because the P2 gain between pre- and post-training was larger than the P2 increase between the baseline sessions in Group 2 ($t_{(19)} = 2.21$, $p = 0.040$) and in Group 3 ($t_{(19)} = 2.31$, $p = 0.035$) but not in Group 1 ($t_{(19)} = 0.3$). There were no differences in the amount of P2 gain between Groups 2 and 3.

Results of a spatio-temporal principal component analysis on the evoked response waveforms observed in Group 3 are summarized in **Figure 5** with the topographic distributions of the five largest components, which explain in total 98.4% of the variance, and the corresponding waveforms separately for the two baseline sessions and the post-training session. Overlaid are the responses to the "ba" and the "mba" stimuli. The aim of this analysis was to explore whether learning to identify the two stimuli would result in a different responses to "ba" and "mba". Recognizing there are spatial precision limitations with EEG, we report the largest component, characterized by the N1-P2 waves, as being maximal at frontal midline electrodes, and the second largest component was predominant above the posterior parietal region. Smaller components were localized to left and right temporal and inferior frontal regions. Although the smallest component explained only 2.2% of the signal variance, the corresponding time series were clearly reproduced between sessions. Most importantly, no clear distinction between "ba" and "mba" responses became obvious. Accordingly, a formal multivariate test using PLS analysis showed a main effect of "Session" but no "Session" × "Stimulus" interaction. So far, the current data do not suggest that learning results in different cortical representation of the learned stimulus item beyond the statistical power of our analysis.

LATE NEGATIVITY

Changes in evoked neural activity, in the 600–900 ms latency interval, were also observed during post- training and retention-sessions in the trained Group 3. Therefore, the mean amplitude in the 600–900 ms latency interval was measured and compared between groups and recording sessions. The repeated measures ANOVA for this late negativity (LN) revealed only a tendency toward significance for "Group" ($F_{(2,27)} = 2.71$, $p = 0.085$); however, a main effect of the within-subject factor "Session" ($F_{(2,54)} = 6.92$, $p = 0.0021$) and the "Session" × "Group" interaction ($F_{(4,54)} = 3.47$, $p = 0.0135$) was observed. Pairwise comparisons help to explain the interaction because between-session differences in the LN were significant in Group 3 only (**Figure 6**). In Group 3, the LN was larger after the training compared to the pre 1 session ($t_{(19)} = 4.18$, $p < 0.0001$) and compared to the pre 2 session ($t_{(19)} = 3.62$, $p = 0.0018$). Despite the significant training-related changes in the LN latency range for Group 3, the magnitude of perceptual change did not correlate with the amount of amplitude LN change ($R^2 = 0.07$, $F = 0.61$, $p = 0.46$). Also, even though a visible LN can be seen in the retention data, the between subject variability was large (likely because of the staggered test times) and thus the retention effect was not significant.

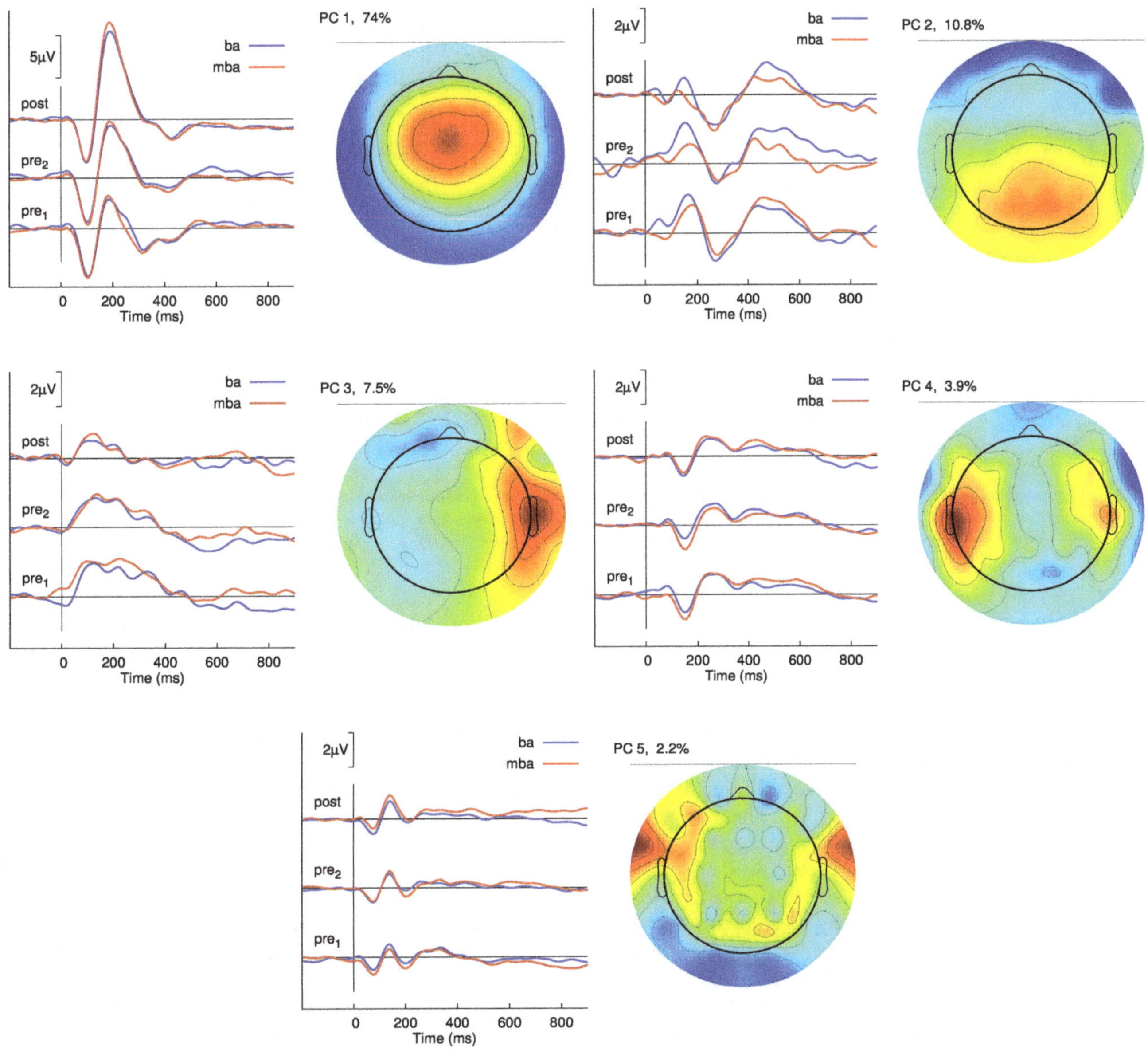

FIGURE 5 | Principal component analysis of the group averaged responses in the training group with feedback (Group 3). The graphs show the time series of the five largest principal components (PC) for the two pre-training and the post-training recordings. The responses to the "ba" and "mba" stimuli are overlaid for comparison. The topographic map of the potential distribution across the head is shown right to the graphs of time series. The first PC explains 74% of the signal variance and shows the typical fronto-central maximum corresponding to two tangential dipole sources in left and right auditory cortices.

DISCUSSION

There is a long history of using auditory training exercises as a part of auditory rehabilitation programs for people with and without hearing loss. One assumption is that listening training modifies the way sound is encoded and processed in the central auditory system, another is that listening exercises permit the person to make better use of existing neural codes. We still do not know what aspects of auditory training are responsible for perceptual gains (Boothroyd, 2010) and how coincident changes in neural activity relate to the auditory cue being trained. To address this issue, we compared training-related changes in perception and physiology, evoked by the same VOT stimuli, so brain and behavior relationships could be made. N1 and P2 latencies are consistently reported to be important neural correlates of VOT (Wagner et al., 2013); however, when people are trained to alter the perception of VOT, P2 amplitude, rather than N1 or P2 latencies are observed. Therefore, the purpose of this experiment was to determine

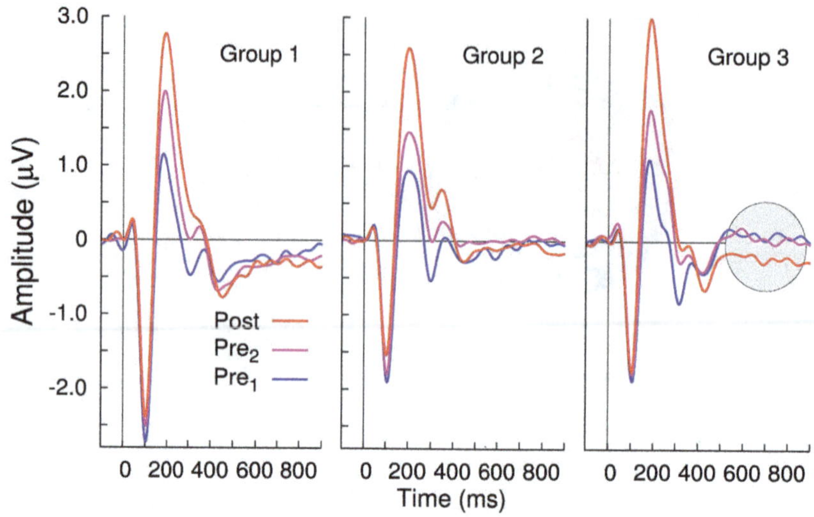

FIGURE 6 | Group averaged time series of the largest principal component of the evoked responses. Whereas no between-session changes in the 600–900 ms latency interval are noticeable in Groups 1 and 2; in Group 3, there is an increased negativity following training.

if the auditory evoked P2 response is a biomarker of VOT learning.

IS P2 A BIOMARKER OF LEARNING?

The main finding was that P2 amplitude growths were observed for people who did and did not learn the novel VOT contrast. Based on these data, the most obvious conclusion is that P2 amplitude is not a biomarker of learning. This conclusion is reinforced by the growing body of evidence suggesting it is the elements of training (exposure, task execution) that contribute to P2 enhancements, and not the learned product of a goal-directed act. It would also explain why no study has been able to establish a one-to-one relationship between the magnitude of P2 change and the magnitude of perceptual change (Tremblay et al., 2001; Sheehan et al., 2005) and why enhancements appear to generalize to other stimuli exposed to but not necessarily learned (Tremblay et al., 2009). However, it is also possible that the large training related changes in P2 might overlay and obscure smaller effects of learning; or reflect other related processes not measured here. Therefore, to entirely dismiss a relationship between P2 and auditory learning would be to ignore converging evidence, from multiple laboratories, linking enhanced neuroplastic P2 activity to multiple forms of learned behaviors. When learning to discriminate the rate of frequency modulation in tones, for example, differences in performance gain related to different learning strategies, and were reported be reflected in P2 amplitude increases (Orduña et al., 2012). In a study of pitch discrimination training, absolute P2 amplitude correlated with reaction time (Tong et al., 2009). Also, long-term experience in musicianship and effects of auditory training in musicians were expressed in larger P2 amplitudes and amplitude increments compared to non-musicians (Seppänen et al., 2012). Collectively, there is a growing body of literature linking enhanced P2 amplitudes to auditory learning that it makes it difficult to entirely reject some type of brain-behavior relationship. We therefore put forth an alternative hypothesis; changes in P2 amplitude reflect neural activity associated with the acquisition process, but not the learned outcome itself. What neural mechanisms are associated with the process, and driving modulations in P2 activity, still need to be defined.

Based on source modeling we can assume some degree of auditory cortex involvement. Ross and Tremblay (2009) showed N1 and P2 to originate from different anatomical structures that likely serve different functions. N1 sources lay in the posterior part of auditory cortex, the planum temporale, whereas the center of activity for P2 lay in anterior auditory cortex, the lateral part of Heschl's gyrus. P2 sources have also been identified in planum temporale, Brodmann's area 22, and auditory association cortices (Crowley and Colrain, 2004). Whereas the P2 increase exhibits a neuroplastic nature, with enhanced activity becoming evident only after a period of sleep (Atienza et al., 2002; Ross and Tremblay, 2009; Zhu, 2010) and persisting for months; decreases in N1 amplitude occur within an experimental session and return to baseline in subsequent recordings (Ross and Tremblay, 2009). This type of N1 behavior pattern is more in line with habituation and less so with the types of learning-related N1 changes exhibited during active EEG recordings where modulations in brain activity are recorded while the participant is attending and executing the training task (Alain et al., 2010). Then again, habituation is sometimes termed "non-associative learning" and may be facilitating the P2 effects reported here (Rankin et al., 2009). N1 suppression mechanisms may also help consolidation, resulting in an increase of P2 between sessions.

The stimuli and passive recording paradigms used in our original VOT studies were designed to determine if neural codes reflecting VOT, and reflected by the N1, could be altered through training. If so, these far-field AEP recordings could be used clinically to assess the temporal resolution and rehabilitation of populations with suspected temporal processing disorders. The passive EEG recording paradigm is ideal for difficult to test populations and avoids potential confounds that can interfere with perceptual performance. Moreover, the stimulus block design was designed with future clinical applications in mind as these types of recording paradigms are within the capacity, and similar to electrophysiological procedures, used in audiology clinics today. However, to date, using this approach, no evidence of significant N1 latency shifts, reflecting perceptual changes in VOT, over time, have been reported. One possibility is that N1 latencies do not reflect subtle differences in *pre*-voicing. Another is that mechanisms underlying N1 are resistant to training (Wagner et al., 2013), or changes in synchronous activity are so modest that they cannot be detected using far-field recordings in humans. However, there is some evidence that N1 (and some subcomponents) can be modified with training but these were all observed as amplitude rather than latency changes (Menning et al., 2000; Brattico et al., 2003; Bosnyak et al., 2004). An exception is Reinke et al. (2003) who reported decreased N1 and P2 latencies, as well as enhanced P2 amplitudes following training, but these latency changes were recorded using an active EEG task while listeners partook in a vowel segregation-training task. This means, attention, auditory and visual sensory processing, memory and executive function could have contributed to the observed latency changes. Thus, it is difficult to differentiate sensory vs. cognitive (top-down) contributions to learning, as well as the various types of top-down contributors.

The P1-N1-P2 responses recorded here were acquired in a passive way and as such are described as being mainly exogenous in nature, meaning they are highly dependent on the physical properties of the stimulus used to evoke it. However, these AEPs can be endogenous, and modulated by attention in certain circumstances (Hillyard et al., 1973; Woldorff and Hillyard, 1991; Woods, 1995). This point is important when considering potential contributors to enhanced P2 activity. In our design, participants heard stimuli during the AEP sessions and during each perceptual training and testing task. They saw visual instructions and text response options. In all instances, auditory and visual input tapped into memory sources because sessions were repeated on different days. So, as described by Tremblay et al. (2001) and others, it is possible that some of the training-related physiological changes reported here might reflect other top-down modulatory influences that are activated during AEP recordings as well as focused listening tasks. What's more, the P2 effects might not even be auditory specific. Similar to the auditory evoked P2, the visually evoked P2 is modulated by attention, language context information, and memory and repetition effects. It is also considered to be part of cognitive matching system that compares sensory inputs with stored memory (Luck and Hillyard, 1994; Freunberger et al., 2007). Therefore, although our source modeling studies (Ross and Tremblay, 2009) showed involvement of primary and association cortical areas, we have not yet ruled out multisensory interactions from contributing to our results. Until future experiments are designed to disentangle the various multi-sensory top-down contributing components such as: attention, memory, and executive function, we are left to speculate about neural mechanisms, and their contributions to the results reported here.

One possibility worth exploring in future studies is the concept of object representation (Näätänen and Winkler, 1999; Ross et al., 2013). If we view N1 and P2 as reflecting synchronous evoked auditory involved in the early stages of perceptual learning, where the neural representation of the sensory input takes place, we could speculate that the P2 indicates memory updating, and consolidation, where the two similar sounding ("ba" and "mba") stimuli, are stored in a buffer. This phase could be passive, not requiring engagement of the participants, which would explain enhanced P2 activity from session to session in the absence of training. With directions and feedback, it would become possible to separate this sensory information into two objects "mba" and "ba". Within this framework, we suggest that P2 plays a role in stimulus familiarization and auditory object representation; critical processes for successful perception. The second phase of learning is likely mediated by top-down processes and probably involves many interactive aspects involving attention, motivation, reinforcement etc. Whereas the first stage applies to the neural detection of sound, the second stage reflects how the brain makes use of the sound. To better understand later stages in sound processing, we expanded our prior analyses to determine if auditory training, and its components, result in recordable modulations in brain activity—later in time. As seen in previous studies (Tremblay et al., 2009) there might be experience-related changes occurring outside the P2 latency region that are visible in different scalp locations.

LATE NEGATIVITY (LN)

A previously unreported finding was the presence of the LN in the post-training session, for the group that learned to identify the pre-voiced contrast. It appears to a lesser degree in the retention data as well, but brain-and-behavior scores do not correlate with each other. Like the P2, the magnitude of LN change does not predict a person's perceptual change score. So what does the LN reflect?

It is well established that distinct forms of cognitive control are associated with unique patterns of activation over a distributed network of regions. These networks can include the dorsolateral prefrontal cortex (DLPFC), ventrolateral prefrontal cortex (VLPFC), supplementary and pre-supplementary motor areas, the anterior cingulate cortex (ACC), superior and inferior aspects of the posterior parietal cortex (Corbetta and Shulman, 2002; Cole and Schneider, 2007). What's more, many aspects of cognitive control have been shown to manifest themselves as negativities in ERP recordings (e.g., N2, Nd, MMN, N400, Late Difference Negativity (LDN) and Error Related Negativity (ERN)). However, these types of negativities are typically recorded when the task involved attention switching, or other complex stimulus paradigms like an oddball paradigm, or often require active participation during the EEG recording. In the present experiment, participants were not engaged in a purposeful attention task and the stimuli were presented as a homogenous train of equiprobable events with no salient deviant stimuli. Thus, our use of the term LN is descriptive and does not neatly fit a well-characterized ERP profile. If left to speculate, we hypothesize that members of Group 3 learned to identify subtle acoustic cues that separated the two pre-voiced stimuli prior to the final ERP session. It is possible then that the training sessions drew greater attention to the stimuli as being separate objects. At the time of post-training EEG sessions, these two stimuli were automatically recognized as two separate auditory objects, but members of Group 3 were the only ones who were taught to attach each object to a perceptual label.

SUMMARY AND CONCLUSIONS

The purpose of this study was to determine if enhanced auditory evoked P2 activity is a biomarker of learning. The question is relevant to the study of auditory rehabilitation in that neurophysiological correlates of auditory training are needed to better understand the mechanisms of action presumed to be involved when using training as an intervention approach for people with and without hearing loss. This study showed increases in P2 AEP amplitude following exposure to auditory stimuli as well as the participation in tasks (with and without feedback). Enhanced P2 amplitudes were seen regardless of any change in perceptual performance and therefore not interpreted to be a biomarker of learning. Instead, modulations in P2 amplitude were attributed to changes in neural activity associated with the acquisition process and not the learned outcome itself. A process that is robust enough to be retained for months. A further finding was the expression of a LN wave 600–900 ms post-stimulus onset, in the post-training session, exclusively for the group that learned to identify the pre-voiced contrast. Collectively, we conclude that being exposed to and interacting with sound, alters the way those sounds are represented in the brain and these changes in neural activity are part of the learning process. Consistent with our earlier findings (Tremblay et al., 1998, 2009), changes in neural activity appear to precede changes in auditory perception and are retained for months. The application of this information to the assessment and rehabilitation of people with hearing loss and other communication-based disorders will depend on future studies aimed at disentangling multi modal bottom-up and top-down neural mechanisms contributing to changes in the N1, P2 and LN. However, a final take home point is that research directed at identifying neural mechanisms related to training and learning should take into consideration the contribution of repeated stimulus exposure as well as other possible coincident contributors to reported physiological changes.

AUTHOR CONTRIBUTIONS

All authors contributed substantially to the concept/design of the work; the interpretation of data; draft reviews including revisions, and approved the final version to be published. Collectively we are accountable for all aspects of the work, including accuracy and integrity. Additionally, Katrina McClannahan and Gregory Collet contributed to data collection.

ACKNOWLEDGMENTS

This work was supported by the National Institutes of Health (R01-DC007705; R01DC012769), (P30-DC04661), (F30-DC010297), and the Fonds National de Recherche Scientifique (FRS-FNRS), Brussels, Belgium. Funding from the American Academy of Audiology awarded to Katrina McClannahan is also acknowledged. The authors would also like to thank Dr. Chris Bishop for his review of earlier drafts and Yu He for her assistance with data processing.

REFERENCES

Alain, C., Campeanu, S., and Tremblay, K. (2010). Changes in sensory evoked responses coincide with rapid improvement in speech identification performance. *J. Cogn. Neurosci.* 22, 392–403. doi: 10.1162/jocn.2009.21279

Alain, C., Snyder, J. S., He, Y., and Reinke, K. S. (2007). Changes in auditory cortex parallel rapid perceptual learning. *Cereb. Cortex* 17, 1074–1084. doi: 10.1093/cercor/bhl018

Alho, K., Teder, W., Lavikainen, J., and Näätänen, R. (1994). Strongly focused attention and auditory event-related potentials. *Biol. Psychol.* 38, 73–90. doi: 10.1016/0301-0511(94)90050-7

Amitay, S., Irwin, A., and Moore, D. R. (2006). Discrimination learning induced by training with identical stimuli. *Nat. Neurosci.* 9, 1446–1448. doi: 10.1038/nn1787

Amitay, S., Zhang, Y. X., Jones, P. R., and Moore, D. R. (2013). Perceptual learning: top to bottom. *Vision Res.* doi: 10.1016/j.visres.2013.11.006. [Epub ahead of print].

Anderson, S., White-Schwoch, T., Parbery-Clark, A., and Kraus, N. (2013). A dynamic auditory-cognitive system supports speech-in-noise perception in older adults. *Hear. Res.* 300, 18–32. doi: 10.1016/j.heares.2013.03.006

Atienza, M., Cantero, J. L., and Dominguez-Marin, E. (2002). The time course of neural changes underlying auditory perceptual learning. *Learn. Mem.* 9, 138–150. doi: 10.1101/lm.46502

Barrett, K. C., Ashley, R., Strait, D. L., and Kraus, N. (2013). Art and science: how musical training shapes the brain. *Front. Psychol.* 4:713. doi: 10.3389/fpsyg.2013.00713

Boothroyd, A. (1997). Auditory development of the hearing child. *Scand. Audiol. Suppl.* 46, 9–16.

Boothroyd, A. (2010). Adapting to changed hearing: the potential role of formal training. *J. Am. Acad. Audiol.* 21, 601–611. doi: 10.3766/jaaa.21.9.6

Bosnyak, D. J., Eaton, R. A., and Roberts, L. E. (2004). Distributed auditory cortical representations are modified when non-musicians are trained at pitch discrimination with 40 Hz amplitude modulated tones. *Cereb. Cortex* 14, 1088–1099. doi: 10.1093/cercor/bhh068

Brattico, E., Tervaniemi, M., and Picton, T. W. (2003). Effects of brief discrimination-training on the auditory N1 wave. *Neuroreport* 14, 2489–2492. doi: 10.1097/00001756-200312190-00039

Burk, M. H., and Humes, L. E. (2007). Effects of training on speech recognition performance in noise using lexically hard words. *J. Speech Lang. Hear. Res.* 50, 25–40. doi: 10.1044/1092-4388(2007/003)

Carcagno, S., and Plack, C. J. (2011). Subcortical plasticity following perceptual learning in a pitch discrimination task. *J. Assoc. Res. Otolaryngol.* 12, 89–100. doi: 10.1007/s10162-010-0236-1

Carhart, R. (1960). Assessment of sensorineural response in otosclerotics. *AMA Arch. Otolaryngol.* 71, 141–149. doi: 10.1001/archotol.1960.03770020013004

Chisolm, T. H., Saunders, G. H., Frederick, M. T., McArdle, R. A., Smith, S. L., and Wilson, R. H. (2013). Learning to listen again: the role of compliance in auditory training for adults with hearing loss. *Am. J. Audiol.* doi: 10.1044/1059-0889(2013/12-0081). [Epub ahead of print].

Cole, M. W., and Schneider, W. (2007). The cognitive control network: integrated cortical regions with dissociable functions. *Neuroimage* 37, 343–360. doi: 10.1016/j.neuroimage.2007.03.071

Corbetta, M., and Shulman, G. L. (2002). Control of goal-directed and stimulus-driven attention in the brain. *Nat. Rev. Neurosci.* 3, 201–215. doi: 10.1038/nrn755

Crowley, K. E., and Colrain, I. M. (2004). A review of the evidence for P2 being an independent component process: age, sleep and modality. *Clin. Neurophysiol.* 115, 732–744. doi: 10.1016/j.clinph.2003.11.021

Eggermont, J. J. (1995). Representation of a voice onset time continuum in primary auditory cortex of the cat. *J. Acoust. Soc. Am.* 98, 911–920. doi: 10.1121/1.413517

Freunberger, R., Klimiesch, W., Doppelmayr, M., and Holler, Y. (2007). Visual P2 component is related to theta phase-locking. *Neurosci. Lett.* 426, 181–186. doi: 10.1016/j.neulet.2007.08.062

Fu, Q. J., Galvin, J., Wang, X., and Nogaki, G. (2004). Effects of auditory training on adult cochlear implant patients: a preliminary report. *Cochlear Implants Int.* 5(Suppl. 1), 84–90. doi: 10.1002/cii.181

Henshaw, H., and Ferguson, M. A. (2013). Efficacy of individual computer-based auditory training for people with hearing loss: a systematic review of the evidence. *PLoS One* 8:e62836. doi: 10.1371/journal.pone.0062836

Hillyard, S. A., Hink, R. F., Schwent, V. L., and Picton, T. W. (1973). Electrical signs of selective attention in the human brain. *Science* 182, 177–180. doi: 10.1126/science.182.4108.177

Irvine, D. R., and Wright, B. A. (2005). Plasticity of spectral processing. *Int. Rev. Neurobiol.* 70, 435–472. doi: 10.1016/s0074-7742(05)70013-1

Jacoby, N., and Ahissar, M. (2013). What does it take to show that a cognitive training procedure is useful? A critical evaluation. *Prog. Brain Res.* 207, 121–140. doi: 10.1016/B978-0-444-63327-9.00004-7

Kricos, P. B. (2006). Audiologic management of older adults with hearing loss and compromised cognitive/psychoacoustic auditory processing capabilities. *Trends Amplif.* 10, 1–28. doi: 10.1177/108471380601000102

Kühnis, J., Elmer, S., Meyer, M., and Jäncke, L. (2013). Musicianship boosts perceptual learning of pseudoword-chimeras: an electrophysiological approach. *Brain Topogr.* 26, 110–125. doi: 10.1007/s10548-012-0237-y

Kuriki, S., Kanda, S., and Hirata, Y. (2006). Effects of musical experience on different components of MEG responses elicited by sequential piano-tones and chords. *J. Neurosci.* 26, 4046–4053. doi: 10.1523/jneurosci.3907-05.2006

Kuriki, S., Ohta, K., and Koyama, S. (2007). Persistent responsiveness of long-latency auditory cortical activities in response to repeated stimuli of musical timbre and vowel sounds. *Cereb. Cortex* 17, 2725–2732. doi: 10.1093/cercor/bhl182

Luck, S. J., and Hillyard, S. A. (1994). Electrophysiological correlates of feature analysis during visual search. *Psychophysiology* 31, 291–308. doi: 10.1111/j.1469-8986.1994.tb02218.x

Macmillan, N. A., and Creelman, C. D. (1991). *Detection Theory: A User's Guide.* Mahwah, NJ: Lawrence Erlbaum Association.

McClaskey, C. L., Pisoni, D. B., and Carrell, T. D. (1983). Transfer of training of a new linguistic contrast in voicing. *Percept. Psychophys.* 34, 323–330. doi: 10.3758/bf03203044

Menning, H., Roberts, L. E., and Pantev, C. (2000). Plastic changes in the auditory cortex induced by intensive frequency discrimination training. *Neuroreport* 11, 817–822. doi: 10.1097/00001756-200003200-00032

Näätänen, R., and Winkler, I. (1999). The concept of auditory stimulus representation in cognitive neuroscience. *Psychol. Bull.* 125, 826–859. doi: 10.1037/0033-2909.125.6.826

Orduña, I., Liu, E. H., Church, B. A., Eddins, A. C., and Mercado, E. (2012). Evoked-potential changes following discrimination learning involving complex sounds. *Clin. Neurophysiol.* 123, 711–719. doi: 10.1016/j.clinph.2011.08.019

Ostroff, J. M., Martin, B. A., and Boothroyd, A. (1998). Cortical evoked response to acoustic change within a syllable. *Ear Hear.* 19, 290–297. doi: 10.1097/00003446-199808000-00004

Picton, T. (2013). Hearing in time: evoked potential studies of temporal processing. *Ear Hear.* 34, 385–401. doi: 10.1097/aud.0b013e31827ada02

Rankin, H. A., Abrams, T., Barry, R. J., Bhatnagar, S., Clayton, D. F., Colombo, J., et al. (2009). Habituation revisited: an updated and revised description of the behavioral characteristics of habituation. *Neurobiol. Learn. Mem.* 92, 135–138. doi: 10.1016/j.nlm.2008.09.012

Reinke, K. S., He, Y., Wang, C., and Alain, C. (2003). Perceptual learning modulates sensory evoked response during vowel segregation. *Brain Res. Cogn. Brain Res.* 17, 781–791. doi: 10.1016/s0926-6410(03)00202-7

Ross, B., Jamali, S., and Tremblay, K. L. (2013). Plasticity in neuromagnetic cortical responses suggests enhanced auditory object representation. *BMC Neurosci.* 14:151. doi: 10.1186/1471-2202-14-151

Ross, B., and Tremblay, K. (2009). Stimulus experience modifies auditory neuromagnetic responses in young and older listeners. *Hear. Res.* 248, 48–59. doi: 10.1016/j.heares.2008.11.012

Seppänen, M., Hämäläinen, J., Pesonen, A. K., and Tervaniemi, M. (2012). Music training enhances rapid neural plasticity of N1 and P2 source activation for unattended sounds. *Front. Hum. Neurosci.* 6:43. doi: 10.3389/fnhum.2012.00043

Shahin, A. J. (2011). Neurophysiological influence of musical training on speech perception. *Front. Psychol.* 2:126. doi: 10.3389/fpsyg.2011.00126

Shahin, A., Bosnyak, D. J., Trainor, L. J., and Roberts, L. E. (2003). Enhancement of neuroplastic P2 and N1c auditory evoked potentials in musicians. *J. Neurosci.* 23, 5545–5552.

Sheehan, K. A., Mcarthur, G. M., and Bishop, D. V. (2005). Is discrimination training necessary to cause changes in the P2 auditory event-related brain potential to speech sounds? *Brain Res. Cogn. Brain Res.* 25, 547–553. doi: 10.1016/j.cogbrainres.2005.08.007

Steinschneider, M., Volkov, I. O., Fishman, Y. I., Oya, H., Arezzo, J. C., and Howard, M. A. 3rd. (2005). Intracortical responses in human and monkey primary auditory cortex support a temporal processing mechanism for encoding of the voice onset time phonetic parameter. *Cereb. Cortex* 15, 170–186. doi: 10.1093/cercor/bhh120

Sullivan, J. R., Thibodeau, L. M., and Assmann, P. F. (2013). Auditory training of speech recognition with interrupted and continuous noise maskers by children with hearing impairment. *J. Acoust. Soc. Am.* 133, 495–501. doi: 10.1121/1.4770247

Sweetow, R. W., and Sabes, J. H. (2006). The need for and development of an adaptive listening and communication enhancement (LACE™) program. *J. Am. Acad. Audiol.* 17, 538–558. doi: 10.3766/jaaa.17.8.2

Tong, Y., Melara, R. D., and Rao, A. (2009). P2 enhancement from auditory discrimination training is associated with improved reaction times. *Brain Res.* 1297, 80–88. doi: 10.1016/j.brainres.2009.07.089

Tremblay, K. L., Billings, C., and Rohila, N. (2004). Speech evoked cortical potentials: effects of age and stimulus presentation rate. *J. Am. Acad. Audiol.* 15, 226–237. doi: 10.3766/jaaa.15.3.5

Tremblay, K. L., Inoue, K., Mcclannahan, K., and Ross, B. (2010). Repeated stimulus exposure alters the way sound is encoded in the human brain. *PLoS One* 5:e10283. doi: 10.1371/journal.pone.0010283

Tremblay, K., Kraus, N., Carrell, T. D., and Mcgee, T. (1997). Central auditory system plasticity: generalization to novel stimuli following listening training. *J. Acoust. Soc. Am.* 102, 3762–3773. doi: 10.1121/1.420139

Tremblay, K., Kraus, N., and Mcgee, T. (1998). The time course of auditory perceptual learning: neurophysiological changes during speech-sound training. *Neuroreport* 9, 3557–3560. doi: 10.1097/00001756-199811160-00003

Tremblay, K., Kraus, N., Mcgee, T., Ponton, C., and Otis, B. (2001). Central auditory plasticity: changes in the N1-P2 complex after speech-sound training. *Ear Hear.* 22, 79–90. doi: 10.1097/00003446-200104000-00001

Tremblay, K., and Moore, D. R. (2012). Current issues in auditory plasticity and auditory training. *Transl. Perspect. Aud. Neurosci.* BOOK 3, 165–189.

Tremblay, K. L., Piskosz, M., and Souza, P. (2003). Effects of age and age-related hearing loss on the neural representation of speech cues. *Clin. Neurophysiol.* 114, 1332–1343. doi: 10.1016/s1388-2457(03)00114-7

Tremblay, K. L., and Ross, B. (2007). Auditory rehabilitation and the aging brain. *ASHA Lead.* 12, 12–13.

Tremblay, K. L., Shahin, A. J., Picton, T., and Ross, B. (2009). Auditory training alters the physiological detection of stimulus-specific cues in humans. *Clin. Neurophysiol.* 120, 128–135. doi: 10.1016/j.clinph.2008.10.005

Van Veen, V., and Carter, C. S. (2002). The timing of action-monitoring processing in the anterior cingulate cortex. *J. Cogn. Neurosci.* 14, 593–602.

Wagner, M., Shafer, V. L., Martin, B., and Steinschneider, M. (2013). The effect of native-language experience on the sensory-obligatory components, the P1-N1-P2 and the T-complex. *Brain Res.* 1522, 31–37. doi: 10.1016/j.brainres.2013.04.045

Woldorff, M. G., and Hillyard, S. A. (1991). Modulation of early auditory processing during selective listening to rapidly presented tones. *Electroencephalogr. Clin. Neurophysiol.* 79, 170–191. doi: 10.1016/0013-4694(91)90136-r

Woods, D. L. (1995). The component structure of the N1 wave of the human auditory evoked potential. *Electroencephalogr. Clin. Neurophysiol. Suppl.* 44, 102–109.

Zhu, Kuang Da. (2010). Neuroplastic changes during auditory perceptual learning over multiple practice sessions within and between days. *Master of Arts Degree.* Department of Psychology, University of Toronto. https://tspace.library.utoronto.ca/bitstream/1807/24291/3/Zhu_KuangDa_20103_MA_thesis.pdf

17

Effects of age-related hearing loss and background noise on neuromagnetic activity from auditory cortex

Claude Alain[1,2,3]*, Anja Roye[1] and Claire Salloum[1]

[1] Rotman Research Institute, Baycrest Centre for Geriatric Care, Toronto, ON, Canada
[2] Department of Psychology, University of Toronto, Toronto, ON, Canada
[3] Institute of Medical Sciences, University of Toronto, Toronto, ON, Canada

***Correspondence:**
Claude Alain, Rotman Research Institute, Baycrest Centre for Geriatric Care, 3560 Bathurst Street, Toronto, ON M6A 2E1, Canada
e-mail: calain@research.baycrest.org

Aging is often accompanied by hearing loss, which impacts how sounds are processed and represented along the ascending auditory pathways and within the auditory cortices. Here, we assess the impact of mild binaural hearing loss on the older adults' ability to both process complex sounds embedded in noise and to segregate a mistuned harmonic in an otherwise periodic stimulus. We measured auditory evoked fields (AEFs) using magnetoencephalography while participants were presented with complex tones that had either all harmonics in tune or had the third harmonic mistuned by 4 or 16% of its original value. The tones (75 dB sound pressure level, SPL) were presented without, with low (45 dBA SPL), or with moderate (65 dBA SPL) Gaussian noise. For each participant, we modeled the AEFs with a pair of dipoles in the superior temporal plane. We then examined the effects of hearing loss and noise on the amplitude and latency of the resulting source waveforms. In the present study, results revealed that similar noise-induced increases in N1m were present in older adults with and without hearing loss. Our results also showed that the P1m amplitude was larger in the hearing impaired than in the normal-hearing adults. In addition, the object-related negativity (ORN) elicited by the mistuned harmonic was larger in hearing impaired listeners. The enhanced P1m and ORN amplitude in the hearing impaired older adults suggests that hearing loss increased neural excitability in auditory cortices, which could be related to deficits in inhibitory control.

Keywords: aging, MEG, hearing loss, auditory cortex, inhibition (psychology)

INTRODUCTION

Hearing abilities diminish with age largely due to changes that take place in the cochlea. However, there is increasing evidence suggesting that changes in the peripheral system alone cannot adequately account for all hearing problems encountered by older adults. Rather deficits in central auditory processing are also likely playing an important role (Martin and Jerger, 2005; Humes et al., 2012). Scalp recordings of auditory evoked potentials (AEPs) and auditory evoked fields (AEFs, the magnetic counterpart of AEPs) may be useful for differentiating an "aging" from a "hearing loss" basis for the auditory deficits observed in older adults. Furthermore, it may also help identify brain areas that are more susceptible to hearing loss and/or the aging process.

In healthy normal hearing adults, AEPs are usually composed of a positive, a negative, and then a positive wave that peak at about 50 (P1), 100 (N1), and 180 ms (P2) after sound onset, respectively. Converging evidence from lesion studies in humans (e.g., Woods et al., 1987; Alain et al., 1998), magnetoencephaplography (MEG) (e.g., Hari et al., 1980; Hari, 1991; Reite et al., 1994), and brain source modeling (e.g., Scherg and Von Cramon, 1986; Picton et al., 1999) are consistent with generators located in or near Heschl's gyrus. The P1, N1, and P2 waves are mainly stimulus-driven (i.e., exogenous) responses thought to index signal detection (Hillyard et al., 1971). The amplitude and latency of these responses are influenced by the signal-to-noise ratio (Martin et al., 1997, 1999; Whiting et al., 1998; Martin and Stapells, 2005). Martin and colleagues, for example, examined the effects of competing signals by presenting speech signals embedded in noise (Martin et al., 1997; Martin and Stapells, 2005). They found that speech identification abilities decreased when exposed to poorer signal-to-noise ratios with the performance decrement paralleled by both increased N1 latencies and decreased N1 amplitudes. More importantly, the latency and amplitude of the N1 significantly correlated with behavioral assessments of signal detectability (Martin et al., 1997) with electrophysiological thresholds closely approximating behavioral thresholds (Lightfoot and Kennedy, 2006). These findings suggest that AEPs provide a sensitive measure of signal audibility, which may prove useful at evaluating the effects of age-related hearing loss on central auditory processing.

The effects of normal aging on AEPs and AEFs have been examined in numerous reports using a variety of paradigms and stimuli. In many studies, the P1 wave has been found to be larger in older adults than in younger adults. (e.g., Smith et al., 1980; Pekkonen et al., 1995; Bertoli et al., 2005; Kovacevic et al., 2005;

Fabiani et al., 2006; Alain and Snyder, 2008; Ross and Tremblay, 2009; Soros et al., 2009; Ross et al., 2010; Lister et al., 2011; Alain et al., 2012) Similar age-related increases in the N1 amplitude have been reported (e.g., Anderer et al., 1996; Chao and Knight, 1997; Alain and Woods, 1999; Amenedo and Diaz, 1999; Harkrider et al., 2006; Ross and Tremblay, 2009; Soros et al., 2009), albeit with less consistency (for a failure to find age difference see, Pfefferbaum et al., 1980; Smith et al., 1980; Picton et al., 1984; Barrett et al., 1987; Iragui et al., 1993; Bertoli et al., 2002; Tremblay et al., 2004; Kovacevic et al., 2005; Lister et al., 2011). The effect of age on the P2 amplitude is more equivocal with some studies reporting no age difference (Ford et al., 1979; Picton et al., 1984; Barrett et al., 1987; Iragui et al., 1993; Tremblay et al., 2004) while others observing smaller (Goodin et al., 1978; Smith et al., 1980; Ross and Tremblay, 2009) or larger (Pfefferbaum et al., 1980; Ford and Pfefferbaum, 1991; Fabiani et al., 2006; Alain and Snyder, 2008) amplitudes in older adults. However, the effects of age on the P2 latency are more consistent, with most studies reporting an age-related increase in P2 latency (e.g., Goodin et al., 1978; Iragui et al., 1993; Tremblay et al., 2004; Alain and McDonald, 2007). Together these findings are often taken as evidence for an age-related change in central auditory processing. The implicit assumption is that the changes are specific to age rather than to other factors such as hearing loss. However, in most studies, the young and older adults do not only differ in terms of age, they often also differ in hearing thresholds. This potential confound is acknowledged in many studies and there have been some attempts to control for it, for example, by adjusting sound intensity using the mean audiometric thresholds (e.g., Ross et al., 2007) or by using hearing thresholds as a covariate (e.g., Alain and McDonald, 2007).

Another approach to separate the contribution of age and hearing loss on central auditory processing consists of comparing older normal-hearing adults with those who have mild or severe hearing loss. The few studies published so far using this approach have yielded unexpected and surprising results. For instance, Harkrider et al. (2006) compared young adults, older normal-hearing adults, and older adults with mild to moderate hearing loss. They found that the speech-evoked N1 wave was larger in hearing impaired than in normal-hearing older adults. Tremblay et al. (2003) also report a larger N1 in older adults with hearing impairment but only for a subset of speech sounds with voice onset time greater than 40 ms. Conversely, Bertoli et al. (2005) tested young adults, normal-hearing older adults, and hearing-impaired older adults. They found reduced N1 amplitudes to pure tone stimuli in hearing-impaired older adults compared to older normal hearing adults. Hence, it remains unclear whether hearing loss contributes to the age-related difference in N1 amplitude. The results for the P2 are slightly more consistent, with studies reporting no difference in P2 amplitude between normal-hearing and hearing-impaired older adults (Bertoli et al., 2005; Harkrider et al., 2006). In older adults, there is little evidence that hearing loss per se affects the P1, N1, or P2 latency (Tremblay et al., 2003; Bertoli et al., 2005; Harkrider et al., 2006).

The present study aims to further investigate the effect of hearing loss on central auditory processing using MEG. This study is an extension of an earlier study that examined the effects of age and background noise on listeners' ability to process a mistuned harmonic in an otherwise harmonic complex tone (Alain et al., 2012). The use of harmonic complex sounds with and without a mistuned harmonic provide the means to assess age-related differences related to processing sound onset as well as neural activity associated with encoding frequency periodicity. The study from Alain et al. (2012) revealed an age-related increase in P1m (magnetic counterpart of the P1 wave from EEG) as well as a delayed P2m compared to young adults. The mistuned harmonic generated an object-related negativity (ORN), which was comparable in amplitude between young and older adults. The ORN is a relatively new event-related potential (ERP) component that has been associated with the perception of concurrent sound objects induced by the mistuning of a low tonal element of a harmonic complex tone (e.g., Alain et al., 2001, 2002; Hautus and Johnson, 2005). It is usually illustrated by subtracting the ERPs elicited by tuned from those elicited by mistuned stimuli. The ORN provides a metric to assess whether age and/or hearing loss impaired listeners' ability to segregate concurrent sounds based on periodicity cues, which is important for understanding speech in noisy situations. If hearing loss plays an important role in the age-related difference in central auditory processing, as previously reported, then we should observe a group difference in neuromagnetic brain activity elicited by sound onset and mistuning between older adults with normal-hearing and those who are hearing-impaired.

MATERIALS AND METHODS

PARTICIPANTS

A total of 36 older adults were recruited for the study. Based on their hearing status (pure tone thresholds, see below), they were categorized into one of two groups, normal hearing vs. mildly hearing impaired. All were screened to exclude health or mental problems and/or medications that might affect cognitive function or brain activity.

Participants were recruited from the local community and provided informed consent in accordance with the guidelines established by the University of Toronto and Baycrest Centre. Two participants were excluded due to excessive head motion during the MEG recording (one from each group). A final sample of 17 hearing impaired adults (range: 62–82; mean age = 70.6, standard deviation (s.d.) = 6.3; 8 men) were compared with a sample of 17 normal hearing adults (range: 63–76; mean age = 67.8, s.d. = 3.6; 9 men). The two groups did not differ in their mean age ($t_{(32)}$ = 1.60; P = 0.12). All but one participant in each group were right handed.

HEARING ASSESSMENT

Our criteria for mild hearing loss were pure-tone thresholds greater than 25 decibel (dB) and hearing level (HL) for octave frequencies from 250 to 2000 Hz in both ears. Participants with pure-tone thresholds less than or equal to 25 dB hearing level were included in the normal hearing group. All participants completed a speech-in-noise (SIN) test. Four lists of six sentences were used from the Quick SIN (Etymotic Research, 2001; Killion et al., 2004) test. All sentences were spoken by a female in a background of four-talker "babble" at 70 dB sound pressure level

(SPL). The babble in each list of sentences was increased in 5 dB steps in order to vary the signal-to-noise ratio (SNR) from 0 dB to +25 dB. Participants repeated back the target sentence. Each sentence included five "keywords". A point was awarded for each key word of a possible total of five points per sentence. The SNR loss was determined by subtracting the total number of correct words from 25.5. This number represents the SNR required to correctly identify 50% of the sentences (Killion et al., 2004).

All hearing impaired participants filled in a brief hearing checklist (self-report questionnaire) that was based on the Revised American Academy of Otolaryngology-Head & Neck Surgery's 5 min hearing test (Koike et al., 1994), to compare the amount of hearing loss with the hearing loss of other older adults.

STIMULI AND TASK

The stimuli used during the recording of neuromagnetic activity consisted of complex sounds created by combining ten pure tones of equal intensity (i.e., 200, 400, 600, 800, 1000, 1200, 1400, 1600, 1800, and 2000 Hz). The fundamental frequency (f_0) was 200 Hz and the third partial could either be tuned (i.e., 0% mistuning at 600 Hz) or mistuned upwards from its original value by 4% (to 624 Hz) or 16% (to 696 Hz). Stimuli were digitally generated at a sampling rate of 24,414 Hz using a System 3 Real-Time Processor (Tucker Davis Technologies, Alachua, FL) and presented binaurally via an OB 822 Clinical Audiometer using ER-3A transducers (Etymotic Research, Elk Grove, IL, USA) and reflectionless 2.5-m plastic tubes. All three stimulus types (0%, 4%, and 16% mistuning) had durations of 200 ms and rise/fall times of 5 ms. They were equiprobable and presented in random order with an inter-stimulus interval (ISI) that varied randomly between 800 and 1200 ms in 100 ms steps (rectangular distribution). All participants, regardless of their hearing status, were presented with stimuli at a fixed 75 dB SPL. There were three listening conditions corresponding to the background against which the stimuli were presented within a block of trials. That is, within the entire block of trials, the stimuli were either presented without background noise, or against a continuous low (45 dBA), or against a continuous moderate (65 dBA) level broadband Gaussian white noise. For each noise condition, participants were presented with a total of 300 trials (100 of each stimulus type: 0%, 4%, and 16% mistuning), for a grand total of 900 stimuli during the course of the experiment. The order of noise conditions was counterbalanced between participants. The intensity of the stimuli and the intensity of the noise were measured using a Larson-Davis SPL meter (Model 824, Provo, Utah). The plastic tubes from the ER-3A transducers were attached to a 2 cc coupler on an artificial ear (Model AEC100l) connected to the SPL meter. Separate measurements were taken for left and right ear channels.

All participants completed a behavioral task that was performed after the MEG recording in a double-walled sound attenuated chamber (IAC model 1204A, Electromedical Instruments, Mississauga, ON). The same stimuli were presented over Eartone ER-3A insert earphones using a System 3 Real Time Processor and a GSI 61 Clinical Audiometer. Following the presentation of each stimulus, participants were asked to indicate if they heard one sound (i.e., a buzz) or two sounds (i.e., a buzz plus another sound with a pure tone quality) by pressing two different buttons label as "1" or "2", respectively. These responses (i.e., 1 or 2) reflected participants' perceptions based on the mistuning manipulation. Responses were registered using a multi-button response box and the next stimulus was presented 1500 ms following the previous response. Participants did not receive feedback on their performance. Prior to the behavioral experiment, participants were presented with a sample of stimuli to familiarize themselves with the task and the response box. After this familiarization phase, participants completed six blocks of trials. For each noise condition, two blocks of 150 trials were presented for a total of 300 trials (100 of each stimulus type: 0%, 4%, and 16% mistuning). For each participant, we calculated the proportion of trials in which participants reported hearing two sounds as well as dprime (d') and beta (β) values. For the calculation of d' and β, trials whereby participants were presented with 0% mistuning and responded "2" were treated as "false alarms", and trials whereby participants were presented with mistuned stimuli and responded "2" were treated as "hits" (Moore et al., 1986; Alain et al., 2012).

NEUROMAGNETIC RECORDING AND ANALYSIS

The MEG recording took place in a magnetically shielded room using a helmet shaped 151-channel whole cortex neuromagnetometer (OMEGA, CTF Systems, VSM Medtech Inc., Vancouver, Canada). AEFs were recorded in a passive listening session as participants watched a muted, subtitled movie of their choice. This design allowed us to examine the impact of noise on cortical activity elicited by stimuli while minimizing the influence of top-down processes on AEF amplitude. The use of muted subtitled movies has been shown to effectively capture attention without interfering with auditory processing (Pettigrew et al., 2004). To minimize movement, participants laid down throughout the recording.

The neuromagnetic activity was recorded continuously with a sampling rate of 625 Hz and an on-line, low-pass filter with a cutoff frequency of 200 Hz. The analysis epoch included 200 ms of pre-stimulus activity and 600 ms of post-stimulus activity. The epochs were scanned for artifacts using Brain Electrical Source Analysis (BESA) software (version 5.2). To account for individual differences in the amplitude of neuromagnetic brain activity, the maximum intensity for accepting single epochs of the MEG signals was adjusted for each participant and ranged from 1515 to 6607 fT/cm. AEFs were averaged separately for each stimulus type and noise condition (i.e., block of trials). For normal hearing adults, the number of trials included in the single-subject grand average (i.e., all stimulus type and noise condition combined) ranged from 587 to 697 while for hearing impaired adults it ranged from 587 to 752. For each participant and for each noise condition, we computed the grand average of AEFs that comprised all stimulus types. This average was used to generate a dipole source model of the scalp recorded AEFs. The source waveforms for each experimental condition were computed from the resulting source model.

We used BESA software (version 5.2) for dipole source modeling. The analysis used the spherical head model of Sarvas (1987).

Before dipole source modeling, the averaged data were low-pass filtered at 20 Hz (12 dB/octave; zero phase). First, we seeded a left and a right dipole in the temporal lobe near Heschl's gyrus using a magnetic resonance imaging template from BESA. Then, we fitted the location and orientation of each dipole to account for a 40 ms interval centered on the peak of the N1m wave. We chose to model the N1m wave because it was the largest and most reliable deflection from the AEF elicited by the harmonic complex tones. The analysis was performed on the grand average across stimulus types to enhance signal-to-noise ratio and because the differences in source location between the N1m elicited by tuned and mistuned stimuli were expected to be small (Arnott et al., 2011). Peak amplitude and latency were determined as the largest positivity (P) or negativity (N) in the individual source waveforms during a specific interval. The measurement intervals were 30–90 ms (P1m), 70–160 ms (N1m), 150–260 ms (P2m), and 120–220 ms (ORN). AEF amplitude and latency were analyzed using a mixed model repeated measures ANOVA with hearing status (normal, impaired) as the between-groups factor and mistuning (0%, 4%, 16%), noise condition (no, low, moderate), and hemisphere (left, right) as the within-group factors. When appropriate, the degrees of freedom were adjusted with the Greenhouse-Geisser epsilon (ϵ) and all reported probability estimates are based on the reduced degrees of freedom, although the original degrees of freedom are reported. Bonferroni corrections were applied for all posthoc, pairwise comparisons. For the behavioral data, we performed mixed model repeated measures ANOVA with hearing status (normal, impaired) as the between-groups factor and mistuning (0%, 4%, 16%), and noise condition (no, low, moderate) as the within-group factors.

RESULTS

BEHAVIORAL DATA

Pure tone thresholds

The two experimental groups significantly differed in pure tone thresholds (**Figure 1**) with normal hearing adults having lower average thresholds (M = 12.7 dB HL) than hearing impaired adults (M = 32.3 dB HL), $F_{(1,32)} = 75.64$, $P < 0.001$, $\eta^2 = 0.70$) for 250–2000 Hz. Despite the difference, both normal hearing and hearing impaired groups showed typical age-related decline in pure tone thresholds, most prominent in the higher frequencies, $F_{(3,96)} = 11.62$, $P < 0.001$, $\eta^2 = 0.27$. This decline was even more prominent in the hearing impaired group (interaction group × tone frequency, $F_{(3,96)} = 3.62$, $P = 0.002$, $\eta^2 = 0.01$). There were no differences in hearing thresholds between the left and the right ear in either the normal hearing group or hearing impaired group (hemisphere $F < 1$; group × hemisphere $F < 1$; hemisphere × tone frequency, $F_{(3,96)} = 1.48$, $P = 0.23$).

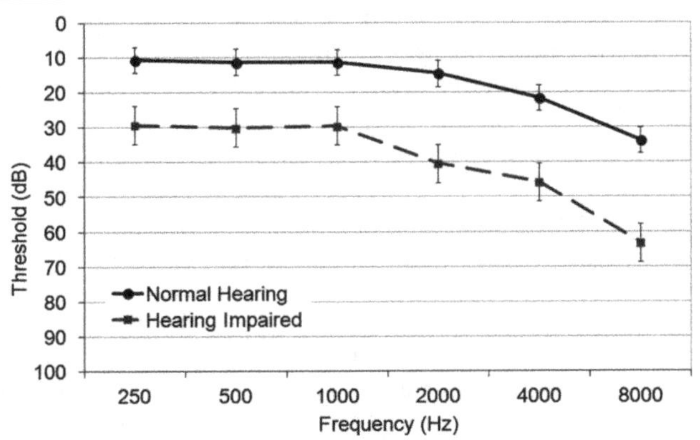

FIGURE 1 | Group mean audiometric thresholds in normal hearing and hearing impaired older adults for octave frequencies between 250 and 8000 Hz. The error bars indicate standard error of the mean.

Quick hearing check

According to the quick hearing check, all participants classified as hearing impaired reached scores that were within the lower 10 to 35% of other older adults classified as hearing impaired (Koike et al., 1994). Furthermore, the hearing impaired group performed worse in the Quick SIN test as revealed by a higher SNR loss (M = 4.21, *s.e.* = 0.72) compared to the normal hearing group (M = 1.90, *s.e.* = 0.64; $t_{(32)} = -2.40$, $P = 0.02$).

Behavioral task

Within the hearing impaired group, 5 of 17 participants did not finish the behavioral task and hence only 12 hearing impaired participants were included in the final analysis of the behavioral data. Overall, results showed that the proportion whereby participants indicated hearing two concurrent sounds increased with mistuning, $F_{(2,56)} = 64.33$, $P < 0.001$, $\eta^2 = 0.70$, with the steepest slope for the low noise condition (interaction mistuning × noise, $F_{(4,112)} = 2.23$, $P = 0.07$, $\eta^2 = 0.07$; **Figure 2**). The main effect of hearing status and noise was not significant, nor was the interaction between hearing status and noise. The three-way interaction between hearing status, noise and mistuning was not significant.

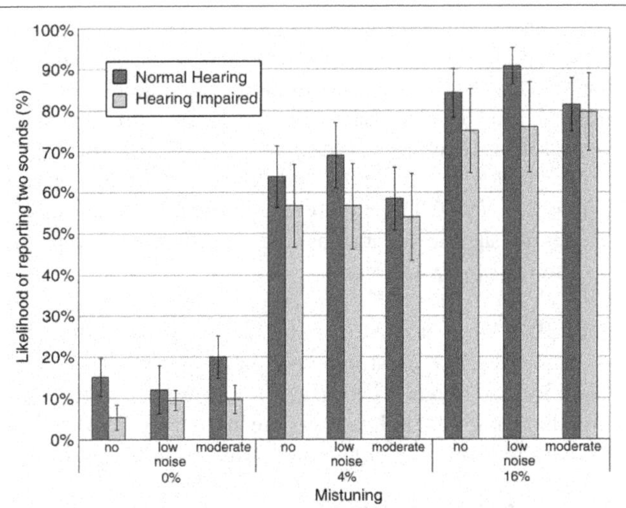

FIGURE 2 | Group mean likelyhood of reporting hearing two concurrent sounds as a function of mistuning and background noise. The error bars indicate ±1 standard error of the mean. Normal hearing: darker gray bar; Hearing impaired: lighter gray bar.

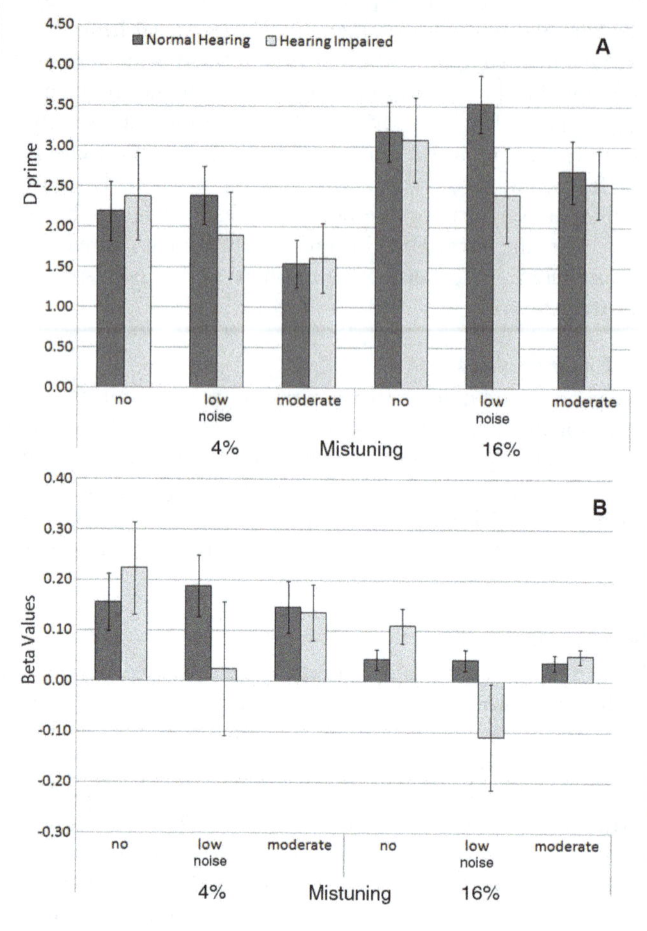

FIGURE 3 | (A) Group mean sensitivity (d') and **(B)** response bias (β) for each background noise condition for the 4% and for the 16% mistuned harmonics in normal hearing and in hearing impaired older adults. The error bars indicate ±1 standard error of the mean.

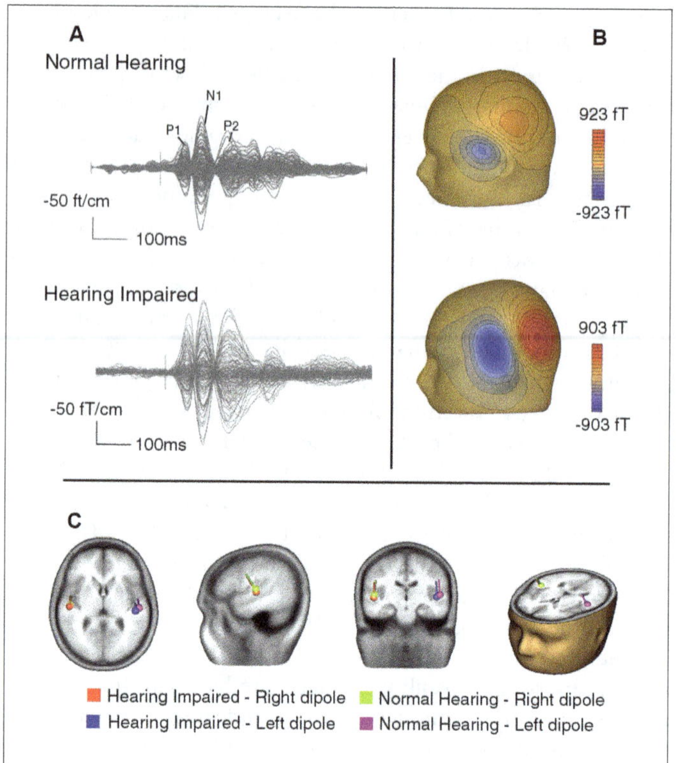

FIGURE 4 | (A) Butterfly plot showing AEFs from a representative normal hearing older adult (top) and a hearing impaired older adult (bottom) averaged over all stimulus types from all sensors. **(B)** The contour maps for the N1m for these two participants indicate the direction of the magnetic flux (i.e., blue = negative, red = positive). **(C)** The group mean dipole location for the N1m from the normal and hearing impaired older adults overlaid on a magnetic resonance imaging template from BESA (5.3).

Figure 3 shows the group mean sensitivity (i.e., d') and response bias (i.e., β) in hearing impaired older adults compared to normal hearing older adults in the three noise conditions. There was an increase in d' with mistuning (**Figure 3A**; $F_{(1,27)} = 14.23$, $P = 0.001$, $\eta^2 = 0.34$), but a decrease with increasing noise ($F_{(2,54)} = 5.27$, $P = 0.008$, $\eta^2 = 0.16$). The main effect of hearing status was not significant, nor was the interaction between hearing status and mistuning or noise.

Overall, the response bias varied as a function of mistuning (**Figure 3B**), $F_{(1,27)} = 5.03$, $P = 0.03$, $\eta^2 = 0.16$, with smaller β values for the 16% mistuning condition. However, there was no significant difference between normal hearing and hearing impaired older adults in β, nor was the interaction between hearing status and mistuning or hearing status and noise significant.

AUDITORY EVOKED FIELDS AND DIPOLE SOURCE LOCATION

Figure 4 overlays the time course of the AEFs recorded with all MEG sensors averaged over the three noise conditions. The AEFs comprise an initial P1m peak at 68 ms followed by the larger N1m and P2m responses at 125 and 220 ms, respectively. The magnetic field topography at the latency of N1m for two representative participants is consistent with bilateral sources in the auditory cortices along the superior temporal gyrus.

The group mean locations for the N1m are also shown in **Figure 4**. The effects of hearing status and noise on N1m source locations were examined by comparing source coordinates (x, y, and z coordinates) separately. For the lateral-medial axis, the main effects of hearing status, noise, and hemisphere were not significant nor was the interaction between any of the factors. For the anterior-posterior axis, there was the typical main effect of hemisphere, $F_{(1,32)} = 18.25$, $P < 0.001$, $\eta^2 = 0.36$), indicating that the source in the right hemisphere was more anterior than the one in the left hemisphere. The main effect of hearing status was also significant ($F_{(1,32)} = 4.80$, $P = 0.04$, $\eta^2 = 0.13$), with more posterior N1 source locations for the hearing impaired group. There was also a main effect of noise ($F_{(2,64)} = 6.84$, $P = 0.002$, $\eta^2 = 0.18$). Pairwise comparisons revealed that the N1m source location was more anterior under moderate noise conditions compared to no and low noise conditions ($P < 0.05$ in both cases). There was no difference in source location between the no and low noise conditions ($P = 0.50$).

For the inferior-superior axis, the hearing impaired group showed more inferior N1m source locations than the normal

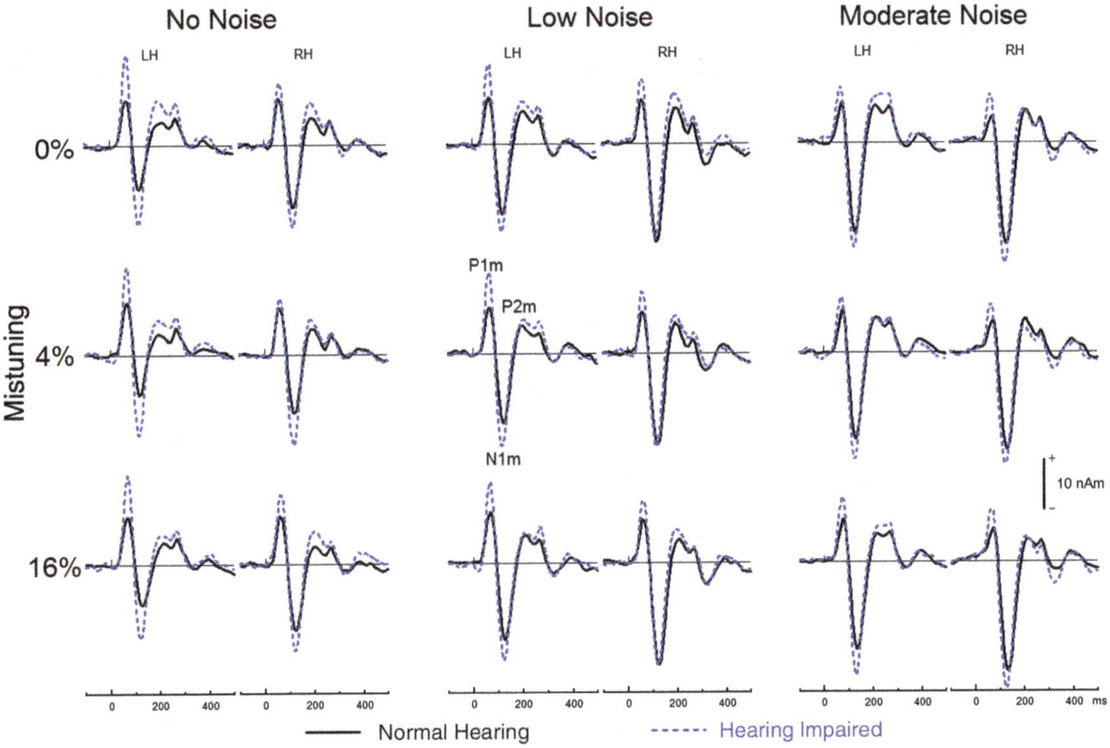

FIGURE 5 | Group mean source waveform from the left hemisphere (LH) and the right hemisphere (RH) for tuned (top) and mistuned stimuli.

hearing group ($F_{(1,32)} = 4.89$, $P = 0.03$, $\eta^2 = 0.13$). Furthermore, the N1m source was located more superior in the left hemisphere compared to the right hemisphere ($F_{(1,32)} = 4.20$, $P = 0.049$, $\eta^2 = 0.11$). No other effect reached statistical significance.

SOURCE WAVEFORMS

Figure 5 shows the group mean source waveforms in each hemisphere for hearing impaired and normal hearing older adults as well as for each stimulus type as a function of background noise. In both groups, the source waveforms comprised a P1m, N1m, and P2m peaking at about 68 ms, 125 ms, and 220 ms after sound onset.

Effects of hearing status, mistuning, and noise on auditory evoked field (AEF) latency

Analysis revealed no main effect of hearing status on P1m latency ($F < 1$). For both groups the P1m peaked earlier in the right ($M = 66.00$, *s.e.* = 1.47 ms) than in the left ($M = 71.45$, *s.e.* = 1.47 ms) hemisphere, $F_{(1,32)} = 43.05$, $P < 0.001$, $\eta^2 = 0.57$. There was a main effect of noise such that stimuli embedded in moderate noise levels generated longer P1m latency compared to lower or no noise conditions, $F_{(2,64)} = 8.75$, $P < 0.005$, $\eta^2 = 0.21$ (**Table 1**). The interaction between hearing status and noise conditions was significant ($F_{(2,64)} = 4.36$, $P = 0.03$, $\eta^2 = 0.15$). P1m latency increased with noise only in normal hearing older adults ($F_{(2,32)} = 13.03$, $P < 0.001$). In hearing impaired older adults, the main effect of noise on P1m latency was not significant ($F < 1$). The main effect of mistuning was significant, $F_{(2,64)} = 5.50$, $P = 0.007$, $\eta^2 = 0.15$. The 16% mistuned stimuli generated a longer P1m latency than the tuned or 4% mistuned stimuli ($P < 0.05$ in both cases). There was no difference in latency between the tuned and

Table 1 | Group mean P1m latency and amplitude.

Group	Noise	Tuning	Latency (ms)	Std. Error	Amplitude (nAm)	Std. Error
Normal Hearing	No	0%	68.141	2.35	11.048	1.837
		4%	67.906	2.158	8.05	1.058
		16%	68.188	2.323	11.536	1.93
	Low	0%	65.976	2.097	10.405	1.621
		4%	66.165	2.256	10.095	1.51
		16%	66.824	2.361	10.882	1.624
	Moderate	0%	73.741	2.699	8.051	1.358
		4%	75.153	2.498	8.448	1.342
		16%	76.376	2.429	8.544	1.388
Hearing Impaired	No	0%	66.871	2.35	17.094	1.837
		4%	66.024	2.158	9.926	1.058
		16%	69.412	2.323	17.71	1.93
	Low	0%	66.447	2.097	15.972	1.621
		4%	66.400	2.256	16.136	1.51
		16%	67.906	2.361	16.199	1.624
	Moderate	0%	67.812	2.699	12.203	1.358
		4%	68.471	2.498	11.714	1.342
		16%	69.224	2.429	13.09	1.388

Table 2 | Group mean N1m latency and amplitude.

Group	Noise	Tuning	Latency (ms)	Std. Error	Amplitude (nAm)	Std. Error
Normal Hearing	No	0%	119.012	3.231	−12.564	2.776
		4%	118.494	3.157	−11.901	2.759
		16%	126.871	3.627	−12.786	2.759
	Low	0%	124.376	2.77	−18.623	3.423
		4%	124.329	3.008	−18.144	3.543
		16%	125.412	2.878	−19.56	3.564
	Moderate	0%	130.494	2.311	−20.521	2.821
		4%	131.859	2.226	−19.569	2.732
		16%	133.506	2.246	−21.065	2.791
Hearing Impaired	No	0%	117.647	3.231	−18.658	2.776
		4%	118.306	3.157	−19.197	2.759
		16%	123.718	3.627	−18.992	2.759
	Low	0%	117.459	2.77	−20.929	3.423
		4%	117.459	3.008	−21.279	3.543
		16%	122.306	2.878	−23.043	3.564
	Moderate	0%	123.153	2.311	−24.8	2.821
		4%	124.518	2.226	−24.351	2.732
		16%	126.588	2.246	−26.587	2.791

Table 3 | Group mean P2m latency and amplitude.

Group	Noise	Tuning	Latency (ms)	Std. Error	Amplitude (nAm)	Std. Error
Normal Hearing	No	0%	213.176	7.239	7.335	1.294
		4%	203.247	6.706	6.914	1.292
		16%	216.424	6.755	6.121	1.411
	Low	0%	208.047	6.213	8.665	1.42
		4%	209.129	7.005	7.895	1.474
		16%	214.918	6.459	7.006	1.36
	Moderate	0%	220.329	5.321	8.317	1.363
		4%	219.859	5.402	8.151	1.337
		16%	229.412	5.612	6.642	1.263
Hearing Impaired	No	0%	209.176	7.239	11.469	1.294
		4%	215.388	6.706	10.014	1.292
		16%	214.306	6.755	9.659	1.411
	Low	0%	207.812	6.213	11.59	1.42
		4%	218.588	7.005	10.123	1.474
		16%	217.976	6.459	9.955	1.36
	Moderate	0%	224.141	5.321	11.116	1.363
		4%	218.588	5.402	8.793	1.337
		16%	224.518	5.612	8.987	1.263

4% mistuned stimuli nor did mistuning interact with any other factors.

As with P1m, there was no main effect of hearing status on N1m peak latency, $F_{(1,32)} = 1.78$, $P = 0.19$, (**Table 2**) and the N1m peaked earlier in the right ($M = 122.32$, *s.e.* = 1.92 ms) than in the left ($M = 124.96$, *s.e.* = 1.84 ms) hemisphere, $F_{(1,32)} = 6.13$, $P = 0.02$, $\eta^2 = 0.16$. N1m latency increased with increasing background noise levels, $F_{(2,64)} = 28.62$, $P < 0.001$, $\eta^2 = 0.47$, and this effect of noise was more pronounced for normal hearing adults (noise × group interaction, $F_{(2,64)} = 3.55$, $P = 0.04$, $\eta^2 = 0.10$). Furthermore, the effect of noise on the N1m latency was more pronounced in the left than in the right hemisphere (noise × hemisphere interaction, $F_{(2,64)} = 3.59$, $P = 0.04$, $\eta^2 = 0.10$). The main effect of mistuning was significant, $F_{(2,64)} = 2.36$, $P < 0.001$, $\eta^2 = 0.13$ such that the 16% mistuned stimuli generated a longer latency than the tuned or 4% mistuned stimuli ($P < 0.001$, in both cases). There was no difference between the tuned and 4% mistuned stimuli ($P = 0.63$).

The effects of hearing status and experimental condition on the P2m latency are summarized in **Table 3**. As with the P1m and N1m, the P2m peak latency was unaffected by hearing status ($F < 1$). The P2m peaked earlier in the right ($M = 210$, *s.e.* = 4.3 ms) than in the left ($M = 221$, *s.e.* = 4.0 ms) hemisphere, $F_{(1,32)} = 9.47$, $P = 0.004$, $\eta^2 = 0.23$. The main effect of noise level was significant, $F_{(2,64)} = 11.86$, $P < 0.001$, $\eta^2 = 0.27$. Stimuli embedded in a moderate level of noise generated a longer P2m latency than those in the no noise or low noise condition ($P < 0.001$, in both cases). There was no difference in P2m latency between the no noise and the low noise conditions ($P = 0.99$). The main effect of mistuning was significant, $F_{(2,64)} = 3.82$, $P < 0.03$, $\eta^2 = 0.11$. The 16% mistuned stimuli generated a longer latency than the tuned stimuli ($P = 0.03$). There was no significant difference between the 16% and the 4% mistuned stimuli ($P = 0.11$), nor was the difference between tuned and 4% mistuned stimuli significant ($P = 0.99$).

To sum it up, the latency of the P1m, N1m, and P2m was little affected by hearing loss. The source waveforms elicited by harmonic complex tones peaked earlier in the right than in the left hemisphere. Background noise and mistuning increased the latency of source activity from the auditory cortex. This effect of background noise on the latency of source waveforms was greater in normal hearing older adults than hearing impaired older adults. The effect of mistuning on the latency of source waveforms was comparable in both groups.

Effects of hearing impairment and noise on auditory evoked field (AEF) amplitude

The main effect of hearing status on P1m amplitude was significant ($F_{(1,32)} = 5.76$, $P = 0.02$, $\eta^2 = 0.15$), with hearing impaired older adults generating a larger P1m response ($M = 14.45$, *s.e.* = 1.41) than normal hearing older adults ($M = 9.67$, *s.e.* = 1.41). The main effect of noise was also significant, $F_{(2,64)} = 15.55$, $P < 0.001$, $\eta^2 = 0.33$). The P1m amplitude was smaller in the moderate noise condition than in the no noise or low noise conditions ($P < 0.005$, in both cases). There was no difference in P1m amplitude between the no noise and the low noise condition ($P = 0.63$). The interaction between hearing status and noise condition was not significant ($F_{(2,64)} = 1.14$, $P = 0.32$). There was a main effect of mistuning, $F_{(2,64)} = 25.23$, $P < 0.001$, $\eta^2 = 0.44$ as well as a significant interaction between hearing status and mistuning ($F_{(2,64)} = 3.71$, $P = 0.04$, $\eta^2 = 0.10$). Overall, the P1m was smaller for the 4% mistuned stimuli than for the tuned or the 16% mistuned stimuli ($P < 0.001$ in both cases) whereas the P1m generated by the 16% mistuned harmonic was larger than the one elicited by the tuned stimuli ($P = 0.024$). The interaction between hearing status and mistuning was due to greater changes in P1m as a function of harmonicity in older adults with mild hearing loss than older adults with normal hearing.

The ANOVA on the P1m amplitude also revealed a significant interaction between mistuning and noise ($F_{(4,128)} = 22.09$, $P < 0.001$, $\eta^2 = 0.41$) and between hearing status, mistuning and noise ($F_{(4,128)} = 3.96$, $P = 0.005$, $\eta^2 = 0.11$). Post hoc testing revealed that the effect of mistuning on P1m amplitude was actually present only in the no noise condition and that this effect was bigger for the hearing impaired group (no noise, main effect mistuning $F_{(2,64)} = 34.83$, $P < 0.001$; no noise, hearing status × mistuning $F_{(2,64)} = 5.39$, $P = 0.007$; no noise, effect of mistuning for hearing impaired $F_{(2,32)} = 24.25$, $P < 0.001$; no noise, effect of mistuning for normal hearing $F_{(2,32)} = 10.61$, $P = 0.002$; no significant effect of mistuning for low noise and moderate noise). Further, the interactions of noise by hemisphere ($F_{(2,62)} = 7.59$, $P = 0.002$, $\eta^2 = 0.19$), mistuning by hemisphere ($F_{(2,64)} = 18.51$, $P < 0.001$, $\eta^2 = 0.37$), and mistuning by noise by hemisphere ($F_{(4,128)} = 12.42$, $P < 0.001$, $\eta^2 = 0.28$) were significant.

The N1m amplitude was not significantly affected by hearing status ($F_{(1,32)} = 1.46$, $P = 0.24$). However, there was a main effect of noise ($F_{(2,64)} = 14.84$, $P < 0.001$, $\eta^2 = 0.32$). The N1m was larger when stimuli were embedded in low or moderate background noise than when there was no background noise ($P = 0.01$ in both cases). There was no difference between the low and moderate noise condition ($P = 0.27$). The main effect of mistuning was also significant, ($F_{(2,64)} = 6.74$, $P = 0.005$, $\eta^2 = 0.17$), and this effect is likely due to the ORN superimposed on the N1m thereby increasing its amplitude (see below). The interaction between hearing status and noise was not significant ($F < 1$) nor was the interaction between hearing status and mistuning ($F < 1$). The three-way interaction between hearing status, noise, and mistuning was not significant ($F < 1$). Lastly, the N1m amplitude was larger in the right than in the left hemisphere, $F_{(1,32)} = 5.06$, $P = 0.03$, $\eta^2 = 0.14$.

For the P2m peak amplitude, the main effect of hearing loss was not significant ($F_{(1,32)} = 2.61$, $P = 0.12$) nor was the main effect of noise ($F < 1$), or the interaction between hearing status and noise ($F < 1$). The main effect of mistuning was significant ($F_{(2,64)} = 17.29$, $P < 0.001$, $\eta^2 = 0.35$), with the P2m amplitude decreasing with the presence of mistuning. Pairwise comparison revealed smaller P2m for the 4% and 16% mistuned stimuli relative to tuned stimuli ($P < 0.001$, in both cases). The difference between 4% and 16% was not significant ($P = 0.28$). Further, the interaction between noise and hemisphere was significant ($F_{(2,64)} = 6.15$, $P = 0.004$, $\eta^2 = 0.16$). However, none of the pairwise comparisons reached statistical significance. No other main effects or interactions reached significance.

Object-related negativity (ORN)

The effects of hearing status and noise on concurrent sound segregation are best illustrated in the difference waves between source waveforms for the tuned stimuli and for the 4% and the 16% mistuned stimuli (cf. Alain et al., 2001). For both groups, this difference wave showed an ORN that peaked at about 170 ms after sound onset (**Figure 6**).

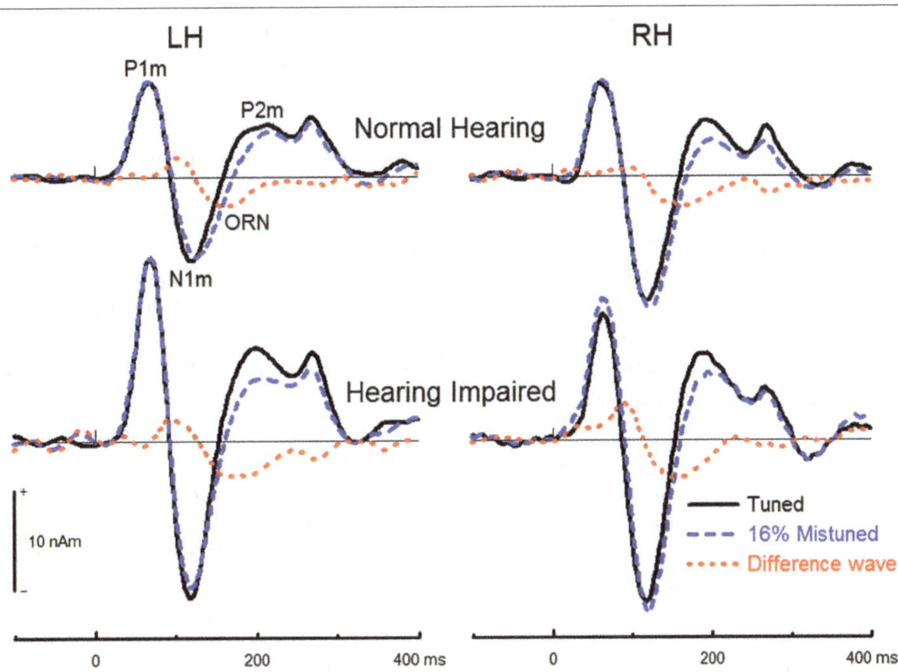

FIGURE 6 | Group mean source waveform for the tuned and the 16%mistuned stimuli and the corresponding difference in source waveforms. The ORN peaked earlier when the harmonic was mistuned by 16% ($M = 165$, *s.e.* = 1.7 ms) than when it was mistuned by 4% ($M = 175$, *s.e.* = 1.7 ms), $F_{(1,32)} = 18.71$, $P < 0.001$, $\eta^2 = 0.37$. The effect of hearing status was not significant ($F_{(1,32)} = 2.10$, $P = 0.16$) nor was the effect of noise ($F < 1$) or hemisphere ($F_{(1,32)} = 2.70$, $P = 0.11$). The interaction between hearing status and mistuning was not significant ($F_{(1,32)} = 2.01$, $P = 0.17$) nor was the interaction between hearing status and noise ($F < 1$).

The 16% mistuned harmonic stimuli generated a larger ORN amplitude than the 4% mistuned stimuli, $F_{(1,32)} = 65.66$, $P < 0.001$, $\eta^2 = 0.67$. The effect of hearing status on the ORN peak amplitude was significant ($F_{(1,32)} = 9.70$, $P = 0.004$, $\eta^2 = 0.23$), with hearing impaired older adults generating larger ORN than normal hearing older adults. The interaction between hearing status and mistuning was not significant ($F < 1$), nor was the three way interaction between group, mistuning and hemisphere ($F < 1$). No further main effects or interactions reached statistical significance.

DISCUSSION

The primary aim of this study was to assess the impact of mild hearing loss on cortical evoked responses in an effort to clarify age-related changes in auditory evoked responses. Specifically, this study examines whether these previously reported changes in the literature reflect age per se or whether they are partly due to age-related hearing loss. In the present study, there was a difference in pure tone thresholds of about 20 dB HL between older adults with normal hearing and those included in the mild hearing loss group. Moreover, older adults with mild hearing loss, as defined by pure tone thresholds, showed elevated thresholds for understanding speech in noise. Surprisingly, there was no significant difference between the two groups in the proportion of trials for which participants indicated hearing two concurrent sounds as a function of mistuning. That is, the likelihood of hearing the mistuned harmonic as a separate sound was little affected by mild hearing loss. Although this may appear surprising, the lack of differences between groups might be due to the drop out of bad performers during the behavioral part of the experiment in the hearing impaired group only. The lack of group difference could also be related to the forced choice procedure, which involved a subjective component and did not capture participants' thresholds in detecting mistuning or parsing the mistuned harmonic as a separate tone.

EFFECT OF MILD HEARING LOSS ON AUDITORY EVOKED FIELDS (AEFs)

In both groups, the source waveforms derived from modeling the N1m wave with bilateral dipoles in or near Heschl's gyrus comprised a P1m, N1m, and P2m deflection. The N1m source location was more anterior and more inferior in the right than in the left hemisphere, and this is consistent with prior MEG studies (e.g., Pantev et al., 1998; Ross et al., 2010). These differences between left and right N1m sources map onto the anatomical asymmetry that showed a more anterior auditory cortex in the right than in the left hemisphere (Penhune et al., 1996; Leonard et al., 1998; Rademacher et al., 2001). The N1m source location was more posterior and more inferior in older adults with hearing impairment than without. This group difference was unexpected and may reflect neuroplastic changes in auditory cortices associated with peripheral hearing loss. For example, the changes in N1m source location could reflect the recruitment of cortical neurons that have lost their afferent input due to peripheral hearing loss (Dietrich et al., 2001). The recruitment of de-afferented neurons could also contribute to the increased amplitude of neuromagnetic responses.

The P1m amplitude was larger in older adults with mild hearing loss than in older adults with normal hearing, which suggests that aging is not the sole contributor to increased sensory evoked response amplitude. Hearing loss, therefore, plays an important role in modulating cortical evoked response amplitude. Furthermore, since stimuli and noise SPL levels were identical for all participants, sound intensity cannot account for increased P1m amplitude between the two groups. However, identical sound intensity may not have yielded the same loudness and it is possible that older adults with hearing impairment experienced greater loudness recruitment than older adults with normal hearing. Loudness recruitment refers to the perceptual phenomenon of sounds becoming rapidly louder with increasing sound levels and has been proposed to contribute to increased N1m amplitude in patients with hearing impairment (Morita et al., 2003).

Prior research examining the effect of hearing impairment on auditory evoked responses have observed larger N1 amplitudes in hearing impaired than in normal hearing adults (Morita et al., 2003; Tremblay et al., 2003; Harkrider et al., 2006). In the present study, the main effect of hearing status on N1m amplitude was not significant, despite the N1m source waveforms appearing slightly larger in the hearing impaired. The difference between the present study and prior work could be related to the material used. Prior research used speech sounds (Tremblay et al., 2003; Harkrider et al., 2006) or pure tones (Morita et al., 2003) with relatively long rise/fall times whereas we used complex sounds that had a well-defined and abrupt rise time. Consequently, our stimuli were more optimal to generate P1m and N1m responses whereas the material used in prior studies only generated a clear N1 response. Thus, our finding coupled with those of prior research provides converging evidence for increased neural excitability in primary and associative auditory cortices following sensory-neural hearing loss. Future experiments that manipulate the stimulus envelope is, however, needed to better understand the origin of these differences in the latency of the effect of hearing loss on cortical evoked responses.

In aging research, the enhanced amplitude of sensory evoked responses (i.e., P1 and N1 deflections) is often thought to index listeners' difficulty in filtering out task-irrelevant information (Chao and Knight, 1997; Alain and Woods, 1999; West and Alain, 2000; Gazzaley et al., 2005), which has been related to a decline in prefrontal function (West, 1996; Chao and Knight, 1997; Alain and Woods, 1999). This account emphasizes the role of top-down control processes mediated by higher brain functions and assumes deficits in descending auditory pathways. Empirical support for this proposal includes studies in humans that showed increased amplitudes of middle latency auditory evoked responses following lesions to the dorsolateral prefrontal cortex (Knight et al., 1989; Alho et al., 1994). An alternative of this top-down account focuses on impaired inhibitory functions along the ascending auditory pathways as well as a loss of frequency selectivity. Evidence from animal studies has revealed a relationship between sensory-neural hearing loss and increased neural excitability within the ascending auditory pathway (Willott and Lu, 1982) and primary auditory cortex (Kotak et al., 2005), which likely reflects deficits in inhibition (Willott and Lu, 1982; Caspary et al., 1995, 2005; Kotak et al., 2005). It is worth noting that we observed effects of mild hearing loss primarily on early exogenous evoked responses. This suggests that sensory-neural hearing loss impacts early cortical registration of acoustic information and further research is needed to determine whether even earlier stages of cortical processing would be impacted by hearing loss and how this relates to auditory perception and attention.

As in our previous aging study, we also found that the ORN amplitude increased with increasing mistuning. Interestingly, the effect of mistuning on perception was comparable in older adults with or without mild hearing loss. However, the ORN elicited by the mistuned harmonic was enhanced in older adults with mild hearing loss compared to normal hearing older adults. The enhanced ORN amplitude in mildly hearing impaired older adults was unexpected and could be due to loudness recruitment and/or increased cortical reactivity. The effect of mild hearing loss on both transient onset responses and ORN provides converging evidence for a general decline in inhibitory processes along the ascending auditory pathway, which likely contributes to increased time-locked cortical activity.

EFFECTS OF HEARING LOSS AND NOISE ON THE SPEED OF AUDITORY PROCESSING

The peak latency of AEFs indicates the amount of time taken to generate the neuromagnetic response after sound onset and provides a means for assessing speed of auditory processing. In the present study, the P1m latency was comparable for the two groups. This suggests that conduction time in the ascending auditory pathways may be little affected by mild hearing loss. The N1m and P2m latencies were also comparable in older adults with and without mild hearing loss. Our findings are consistent with those of earlier EEG studies using speech sounds (Tremblay et al., 2003; Harkrider et al., 2006), which also found that mild hearing loss had little impact on the latencies of the N1 and P2 waves. This is important as it suggests that mild hearing loss does not impact the speed of processing. In a prior study using the same stimuli and listening conditions (Alain et al., 2012), we found age-related increases in N1m and P2m latencies, which was consistent with earlier research (e.g.,Tremblay et al., 2002; Matilainen et al., 2010). The age-related increase in latency of auditory evoked responses may reflect a slowing in auditory processing and/or a broadening of the temporal integration window (Emmer et al., 2006; Gleich et al., 2007; Huang et al., 2009) with older adults reaching a saturation in the auditory evoked responses at a longer latency than young adults. The fact that the ORN latency was comparable between older adults with and without hearing loss suggests that mild hearing loss does not significantly delay the early computation needed to segregate the mistuned harmonic as a separate sound object.

Presenting auditory stimuli against moderate background noise increased latencies of P1m, N1m, and P2m deflections. The noise-related increase in latencies of exogenous components is consistent with prior studies using speech sounds (Whiting et al., 1998; Parbery-Clark et al., 2011). In the present study, the noise-related increase in P1m and N1m latencies was only present for the normal hearing group, suggesting that mild hearing loss and background noise do not independently affect central auditory processing. Further research is needed to characterize in more detail the impact of hearing loss on speed of processing and how it interacts with age.

NOISE-INDUCED INCREASE IN N1m AMPLITUDE

Another goal of the present study was to assess whether the noise-induced increase in N1m amplitude previously reported for young adults would also be observed in older adults with mild hearing loss. For both groups, the N1m amplitude was larger when stimuli were embedded in low and moderate background noise than when there was no background noise. As such, this finding replicates and extends those of earlier studies (Alain et al., 2009, 2012) to older adults with mild hearing loss. This noise-induced increase in sensory evoked responses is not limited to harmonic complexes, but has also been observed for speech sounds in young adults (Shtyrov et al., 1999; Parbery-Clark et al., 2011) and children (Anderson et al., 2010). The increased N1 amplitude may be related to efferent feedback connections between the auditory cortex and the thalamus, inferior colliculus, and/or auditory brainstem nuclei, whose role would be to enhance the SNR in adverse listening situations (Alain et al., 2009). Such a proposal is supported by a positive correlation between the N1 amplitude for stimuli embedded in noise and the performance in a speech-in-noise task (Parbery-Clark et al., 2011). Another possibility is that low and moderate levels of background noise enhance states of arousal, which then similarly enhance the amplitude of sensory evoked responses to improve performance in working memory tasks (Han et al., 2013).

CONCLUDING REMARKS

The present study aimed to clarify the role of age-related hearing loss in the enhancement of cortical evoked responses previously reported in the literature. We found increased cortical evoked responses in older adults with mild hearing loss compared to age-matched controls that have clinically normal hearing. Our findings suggest that age-related decline in hearing sensitivity plays an important role in modulating the amplitude of auditory evoked responses. More importantly, our findings highlight the importance to control for age-related difference in hearing sensitivity while investigating the impact of aging on central auditory processing.

ACKNOWLEDGMENTS

This research was supported by grants from the Canadian Institutes of Health Research (MOP 106619) and the Natural Sciences and Engineering Research Council of Canada. We wish to thank Jeffrey Wong for his help in preparing the illustrations and for his helpful comments and suggestions regarding the manuscript.

REFERENCES

Alain, C., Arnott, S. R., and Picton, T. W. (2001). Bottom-up and top-down influences on auditory scene analysis: evidence from event-related brain potentials. *J. Exp. Psychol. Hum. Percept. Perform.* 27, 1072–1089. doi: 10.1037/0096-1523.27.5.1072

Alain, C., and McDonald, K. L. (2007). Age-related differences in neuromagnetic brain activity underlying concurrent sound perception. *J. Neurosci.* 27, 1308–1314. doi: 10.1523/jneurosci.5433-06.2007

Alain, C., McDonald, K., and Van Roon, P. (2012). Effects of age and background noise on processing a mistuned harmonic in an otherwise periodic complex sound. *Hear. Res.* 283, 126–135. doi: 10.1016/j.heares.2011.10.007

Alain, C., Quan, J., McDonald, K., and Van Roon, P. (2009). Noise-induced increase in human auditory evoked neuromagnetic fields. *Eur. J. Neurosci.* 30, 132–142. doi: 10.1111/j.1460-9568.2009.06792.x

Alain, C., Schuler, B. M., and McDonald, K. L. (2002). Neural activity associated with distinguishing concurrent auditory objects. *J. Acoust. Soc. Am.* 111, 990–995. doi: 10.1121/1.1434942

Alain, C., and Snyder, J. S. (2008). Age-related differences in auditory evoked responses during rapid perceptual learning. *Clin. Neurophysiol.* 119, 356–366. doi: 10.1016/j.clinph.2007.10.024

Alain, C., and Woods, D. L. (1999). Age-related changes in processing auditory stimuli during visual attention: evidence for deficits in inhibitory control and sensory memory. *Psychol. Aging* 14, 507–519. doi: 10.1037/0882-7974.14.3.507

Alain, C., Woods, D. L., and Knight, R. T. (1998). A distributed cortical network for auditory sensory memory in humans. *Brain Res.* 812, 23–37. doi: 10.1016/s0006-8993(98)00851-8

Alho, K., Woods, D. L., Algazi, A., Knight, R. T., and Naatanen, R. (1994). Lesions of frontal cortex diminish the auditory mismatch negativity. *Electroencephalogr. Clin. Neurophysiol.* 91, 353–362. doi: 10.1016/0013-4694(94)00173-1

Amenedo, E., and Diaz, F. (1999). Ageing-related changes in the processing of attended and unattended standard stimuli. *Neuroreport* 10, 2383–2388. doi: 10.1097/00001756-199908020-00030

Anderer, P., Semlitsch, H. V., and Saletu, B. (1996). Multichannel auditory event-related brain potentials: effects of normal aging on the scalp distribution of N1, P2, N2 and P300 latencies and amplitudes. *Electroencephalogr. Clin. Neurophysiol.* 99, 458–472. doi: 10.1016/s0013-4694(96)96518-9

Anderson, S., Chandrasekaran, B., Yi, H. G., and Kraus, N. (2010). Cortical-evoked potentials reflect speech-in-noise perception in children. *Eur. J. Neurosci.* 32, 1407–1413. doi: 10.1111/j.1460-9568.2010.07409.x

Arnott, S. R., Bardouille, T., Ross, B., and Alain, C. (2011). Neural generators underlying concurrent sound segregation. *Brain Res.* 1387, 116–124. doi: 10.1016/j.brainres.2011.02.062

Barrett, G., Neshige, R., and Shibasaki, H. (1987). Human auditory and somatosensory event-related potentials: effects of response condition and age. *Electroencephalogr. Clin. Neurophysiol.* 66, 409–419. doi: 10.1016/0013-4694(87)90210-0

Bertoli, S., Smurzynski, J., and Probst, R. (2002). Temporal resolution in young and elderly subjects as measured by mismatch negativity and a psychoacoustic gap detection task. *Clin. Neurophysiol.* 113, 396–406. doi: 10.1016/s1388-2457(02)00013-5

Bertoli, S., Smurzynski, J., and Probst, R. (2005). Effects of age, age-related hearing loss, and contralateral cafeteria noise on the discrimination of small frequency changes: psychoacoustic and electrophysiological measures. *J. Assoc. Res. Otolaryngol.* 6, 207–222. doi: 10.1007/s10162-005-5029-6

Caspary, D. M., Milbrandt, J. C., and Helfert, R. H. (1995). Central auditory aging: GABA changes in the inferior colliculus. *Exp. Gerontol.* 30, 349–360. doi: 10.1016/0531-5565(94)00052-5

Caspary, D. M., Schatteman, T. A., and Hughes, L. F. (2005). Age-related changes in the inhibitory response properties of dorsal cochlear nucleus output neurons: role of inhibitory inputs. *J. Neurosci.* 25, 10952–10959. doi: 10.1523/jneurosci.2451-05.2005

Chao, L. L., and Knight, R. T. (1997). Prefrontal deficits in attention and inhibitory control with aging. *Cereb. Cortex* 7, 63–69. doi: 10.1093/cercor/7.1.63

Dietrich, V., Nieschalk, M., Stoll, W., Rajan, R., and Pantev, C. (2001). Cortical reorganization in patients with high frequency cochlear hearing loss. *Hear. Res.* 158, 95–101. doi: 10.1016/s0378-5955(01)00282-9

Emmer, M. B., Silman, S., Silverman, C. A., and Levitt, H. (2006). Temporal integration of the contralateral acoustic-reflex threshold and its age-related changes. *J. Acoust. Soc. Am.* 120, 1467–1473. doi: 10.1121/1.2221415

Etymotic Research. (2001). "QuickSIN Speech-in-Noise Test, Version 1.3." (Compact Disk) 61 Martin Lane, Elk Grove Village, IL 60007.

Fabiani, M., Low, K. A., Wee, E., Sable, J. J., and Gratton, G. (2006). Reduced suppression or labile memory? Mechanisms of inefficient filtering of irrelevant information in older adults. *J. Cogn. Neurosci.* 18, 637–650. doi: 10.1162/jocn.2006.18.4.637

Ford, J. M., and Pfefferbaum, A. (1991). Event-related potentials and eyeblink responses in automatic and controlled processing: effects of age. *Electroencephalogr. Clin. Neurophysiol.* 78, 361–377. doi: 10.1016/0013-4694(91)90098-o

Ford, J. M., Roth, W. T., Mohs, R. C., Hopkins, W. F. 3rd, and Kopell, B. S. (1979). Event-related potentials recorded from young and old adults during a memory retrieval task. *Electroencephalogr. Clin. Neurophysiol.* 47, 450–459. doi: 10.1016/0013-4694(79)90161-5

Gazzaley, A., Cooney, J. W., Rissman, J., and D'Esposito, M. (2005). Top-down suppression deficit underlies working memory impairment in normal aging. *Nat. Neurosci.* 8, 1298–1300. doi: 10.1038/nn1543

Gleich, O., Kittel, M. C., Klump, G. M., and Strutz, J. (2007). Temporal integration in the gerbil: the effects of age, hearing loss and temporally unmodulated and modulated speech-like masker noises. *Hear. Res.* 224, 101–114. doi: 10.1016/j.heares.2006.12.002

Goodin, D. S., Squires, K. C., Henderson, B. H., and Starr, A. (1978). Age-related variations in evoked potentials to auditory stimuli in normal human subjects. *Electroencephalogr. Clin. Neurophysiol.* 44, 447–458. doi: 10.1016/0013-4694(78)90029-9

Han, L., Liu, Y., Zhang, D., Jin, Y., and Luo, Y. (2013). Low-arousal speech noise improves performance in N-Back task: an ERP study. *PLoS One* 8:e76261. doi: 10.1371/journal.pone.0076261

Hari, R. (1991). Activation of the human auditory cortex by speech sounds. *Acta Otolaryngol. Suppl.* 491, 132–137; discussion 138. doi: 10.3109/00016489109136790

Hari, R., Aittoniemi, K., Jarvinen, M. L., Katila, T., and Varpula, T. (1980). Auditory evoked transient and sustained magnetic fields of the human brain. Localization of neural generators. *Exp. Brain Res.* 40, 237–240. doi: 10.1007/bf00237543

Harkrider, A. W., Plyler, P. N., and Hedrick, M. S. (2006). Effects of hearing loss and spectral shaping on identification and neural response patterns of stop-consonant stimuli. *J. Acoust. Soc. Am.* 120, 915–925. doi: 10.1121/1.2204588

Hautus, M. J., and Johnson, B. W. (2005). Object-related brain potentials associated with the perceptual segregation of a dichotically embedded pitch. *J. Acoust. Soc. Am.* 117, 275–280. doi: 10.1121/1.1828499

Hillyard, S. A., Squires, K. C., Bauer, J. W., and Lindsay, P. H. (1971). Evoked potential correlates of auditory signal detection. *Science* 172, 1357–1360. doi: 10.1126/science.172.3990.1357

Huang, Y., Huang, Q., Chen, X., Wu, X., and Li, L. (2009). Transient auditory storage of acoustic details is associated with release of speech from informational masking in reverberant conditions. *J. Exp. Psychol. Hum. Percept. Perform.* 35, 1618–1628. doi: 10.1037/a0015791

Humes, L. E., Dubno, J. R., Gordon-Salant, S., Lister, J. J., Cacace, A. T., Cruickshanks, K. J., et al. (2012). Central presbycusis: a review and evaluation of the evidence. *J. Am. Acad. Audiol.* 23, 635–666. doi: 10.3766/jaaa.23.8.5

Iragui, V. J., Kutas, M., Mitchiner, M. R., and Hillyard, S. A. (1993). Effects of aging on event-related brain potentials and reaction times in an auditory oddball task. *Psychophysiology* 30, 10–22. doi: 10.1111/j.1469-8986.1993.tb03200.x

Killion, M. C., Niquette, P. A., Gudmundsen, G. I., Revit, L. J., and Banerjee, S. (2004). Development of a quick speech-in-noise test for measuring signal-to-noise ratio loss in normal-hearing and hearing-impaired listeners. *J. Acoust. Soc. Am.* 116, 2395–2405. doi: 10.1121/1.2166610

Knight, R. T., Scabini, D., and Woods, D. L. (1989). Prefrontal cortex gating of auditory transmission in humans. *Brain Res.* 504, 338–342. doi: 10.1016/0006-8993(89)91381-4

Koike, K. J., Hurst, M. K., and Wetmore, S. J. (1994). Correlation between the American Academy of Otolaryngology-Head and Neck Surgery five-minute hearing test and standard audiologic data. *Otolaryngol. Head Neck Surg.* 111, 625–632. doi: 10.1016/s0194-5998(94)70531-3

Kotak, V. C., Fujisawa, S., Lee, F. A., Karthikeyan, O., Aoki, C., and Sanes, D. H. (2005). Hearing loss raises excitability in the auditory cortex. *J. Neurosci.* 25, 3908–3918. doi: 10.1523/JNEUROSCI.5169-04.2005

Kovacevic, S., Qualls, C., Adair, J. C., Hudson, D., Woodruff, C. C., Knoefel, J., et al. (2005). Age-related effects on superior temporal gyrus activity during an auditory oddball task. *Neuroreport* 16, 1075–1079. doi: 10.1097/00001756-200507130-00009

Leonard, C. M., Puranik, C., Kuldau, J. M., and Lombardino, L. J. (1998). Normal variation in the frequency and location of human auditory cortex landmarks. Heschl's gyrus: where is it? *Cereb. Cortex* 8, 397–406. doi: 10.1093/cercor/8.5.397

Lightfoot, G., and Kennedy, V. (2006). Cortical electric response audiometry hearing threshold estimation: accuracy, speed and the effects of stimulus presentation features. *Ear Hear.* 27, 443–456. doi: 10.1097/01.aud.0000233902.53432.48

Lister, J. J., Maxfield, N. D., Pitt, G. J., and Gonzalez, V. B. (2011). Auditory evoked response to gaps in noise: older adults. *Int. J. Audiol.* 50, 211–225. doi: 10.3109/14992027.2010.526967

Martin, B. A., Kurtzberg, D., and Stapells, D. R. (1999). The effects of decreased audibility produced by high-pass noise masking on N1 and the mismatch negativity to speech sounds /ba/and/da. *J. Speech Lang. Hear. Res.* 42, 271–286.

Martin, B. A., Sigal, A., Kurtzberg, D., and Stapells, D. R. (1997). The effects of decreased audibility produced by high-pass noise masking on cortical event-related potentials to speech sounds/ba/and/da. *J. Acoust. Soc. Am.* 101, 1585–1599. doi: 10.1121/1.418146

Martin, B. A., and Stapells, D. R. (2005). Effects of low-pass noise masking on auditory event-related potentials to speech. *Ear Hear.* 26, 195–213. doi: 10.1097/00003446-200504000-00007

Martin, J. S., and Jerger, J. F. (2005). Some effects of aging on central auditory processing. *J. Rehabil. Res. Dev.* 42, 25–44. doi: 10.1682/jrrd.2004.12.0164

Matilainen, L. E., Talvitie, S. S., Pekkonen, E., Alku, P., May, P. J., and Tiitinen, H. (2010). The effects of healthy aging on auditory processing in humans as indexed by transient brain responses. *Clin. Neurophysiol.* 121, 902–911. doi: 10.1016/j.clinph.2010.01.007

Moore, B. C., Glasberg, B. R., and Peters, R. W. (1986). Thresholds for hearing mistuned partials as separate tones in harmonic complexes. *J. Acoust. Soc. Am.* 80, 479–483. doi: 10.1121/1.394043

Morita, T., Naito, Y., Nagamine, T., Fujiki, N., Shibasaki, H., and Ito, J. (2003). Enhanced activation of the auditory cortex in patients with inner-ear hearing impairment: a magnetoencephalographic study. *Clin. Neurophysiol.* 114, 851–859. doi: 10.1016/s1388-2457(03)00033-6

Pantev, C., Ross, B., Berg, P., Elbert, T., and Rockstroh, B. (1998). Study of the human auditory cortices using a whole-head magnetometer: left vs. right hemisphere and ipsilateral vs. contralateral stimulation. *Audiol. Neurootol.* 3, 183–190. doi: 10.1159/000013789

Parbery-Clark, A., Marmel, F., Bair, J., and Kraus, N. (2011). What subcortical-cortical relationships tell us about processing speech in noise. *Eur. J. Neurosci.* 33, 549–557. doi: 10.1111/j.1460-9568.2010.07546.x

Pekkonen, E., Huotilainen, M., Virtanen, J., Sinkkonen, J., Rinne, T., Ilmoniemi, R. J., et al. (1995). Age-related functional differences between auditory cortices: a whole-head MEG study. *Neuroreport* 6, 1803–1806. doi: 10.1097/00001756-199509000-00023

Penhune, V. B., Zatorre, R. J., MacDonald, J. D., and Evans, A. C. (1996). Interhemispheric anatomical differences in human primary auditory cortex: probabilistic mapping and volume measurement from magnetic resonance scans. *Cereb. Cortex* 6, 661–672. doi: 10.1093/cercor/6.5.661

Pettigrew, C. M., Murdoch, B. E., Ponton, C. W., Kei, J., Chenery, H. J., and Alku, P. (2004). Subtitled videos and mismatch negativity (MMN) investigations of spoken word processing. *J. Am. Acad. Audiol.* 15, 469–485. doi: 10.3766/jaaa.15.7.2

Pfefferbaum, A., Ford, J. M., Roth, W. T., and Kopell, B. S. (1980). Age-related changes in auditory event-related potentials. *Electroencephalogr. Clin. Neurophysiol.* 49, 266–276.

Picton, T. W., Alain, C., Woods, D. L., John, M. S., Scherg, M., Valdes-Sosa, P., et al. (1999). Intracerebral sources of human auditory-evoked potentials. *Audiol. Neurootol.* 4, 64–79. doi: 10.1159/000013823

Picton, T. W., Stuss, D. T., Champagne, S. C., and Nelson, R. F. (1984). The effects of age on human event-related potentials. *Psychophysiology* 21, 312–325. doi: 10.1111/j.1469-8986.1984.tb02941.x

Rademacher, J., Morosan, P., Schormann, T., Schleicher, A., Werner, C., Freund, H. J., et al. (2001). Probabilistic mapping and volume measurement of human primary auditory cortex. *Neuroimage* 13, 669–683. doi: 10.1006/nimg.2000.0714

Reite, M., Adams, M., Simon, J., Teale, P., Sheeder, J., Richardson, D., et al. (1994). Auditory M100 component 1: relationship to Heschl's gyri. *Brain Res. Cogn. Brain Res.* 2, 13–20. doi: 10.1016/0926-6410(94)90016-7

Ross, B., Fujioka, T., Tremblay, K. L., and Picton, T. W. (2007). Aging in binaural hearing begins in mid-life: evidence from cortical auditory-evoked responses to changes in interaural phase. *J. Neurosci.* 27, 11172–11178. doi: 10.1523/jneurosci.1813-07.2007

Ross, B., Schneider, B., Snyder, J. S., and Alain, C. (2010). Biological markers of auditory gap detection in young, middle-aged and older adults. *PLoS One* 5:e10101. doi: 10.1371/journal.pone.0010101

Ross, B., and Tremblay, K. (2009). Stimulus experience modifies auditory neuromagnetic responses in young and older listeners. *Hear. Res.* 248, 48–59. doi: 10.1016/j.heares.2008.11.012

Sarvas, J. (1987). Basic mathematical and electromagnetic concepts of the biomagnetic inverse problem. *Phys. Med. Biol.* 32, 11–22. doi: 10.1088/0031-9155/32/1/004

Scherg, M., and Von Cramon, D. (1986). Evoked dipole source potentials of the human auditory cortex. *Electroencephalogr. Clin. Neurophysiol.* 65, 344–360. doi: 10.1016/0168-5597(86)90014-6

Shtyrov, Y., Kujala, T., Ilmoniemi, R. J., and Naatanen, R. (1999). Noise affects speech-signal processing differently in the cerebral hemispheres. *Neuroreport* 10, 2189–2192. doi: 10.1097/00001756-199907130-00034

Smith, D. B., Michalewski, H. J., Brent, G. A., and Thompson, L. W. (1980). Auditory averaged evoked potentials and aging: factors of stimulus, task and topography. *Biol. Psychol.* 11, 135–151. doi: 10.1016/0301-0511(80)90048-4

Soros, P., Teismann, I. K., Manemann, E., and Lutkenhoner, B. (2009). Auditory temporal processing in healthy aging: a magnetoencephalographic study. *BMC Neurosci.* 10:34. doi: 10.1186/1471-2202-10-34

Tremblay, K. L., Billings, C., and Rohila, N. (2004). Speech evoked cortical potentials: effects of age and stimulus presentation rate. *J. Am. Acad. Audiol.* 15, 226–237; quiz 264. doi: 10.3766/jaaa.15.3.5

Tremblay, K. L., Piskosz, M., and Souza, P. (2002). Aging alters the neural representation of speech cues. *Neuroreport* 13, 1865–1870. doi: 10.1097/00001756-200210280-00007

Tremblay, K. L., Piskosz, M., and Souza, P. (2003). Effects of age and age-related hearing loss on the neural representation of speech cues. *Clin. Neurophysiol.* 114, 1332–1343. doi: 10.1016/s1388-2457(03)00114-7

West, R., and Alain, C. (2000). Age-related decline in inhibitory control contributes to the increased Stroop effect observed in older adults. *Psychophysiology* 37, 179–189. doi: 10.1111/1469-8986.3720179

West, R. L. (1996). An application of prefrontal cortex function theory to cognitive aging. *Psychol. Bull.* 120, 272–292. doi: 10.1037//0033-2909.120.2.272

Whiting, K. A., Martin, B. A., and Stapells, D. R. (1998). The effects of broadband noise masking on cortical event-related potentials to speech sounds /ba/ and /da. *Ear Hear.* 19, 218–231. doi: 10.1097/00003446-199806000-00005

Willott, J. F., and Lu, S. M. (1982). Noise-induced hearing loss can alter neural coding and increase excitability in the central nervous system. *Science* 216, 1331–1334. doi: 10.1126/science.7079767

Woods, D. L., Clayworth, C. C., Knight, R. T., Simpson, G. V., and Naeser, M. A. (1987). Generators of middle- and long-latency auditory evoked potentials: implications from studies of patients with bitemporal lesions. *Electroencephalogr. Clin. Neurophysiol.* 68, 132–148. doi: 10.1016/0168-5597(87)90040-2

18

Developmental hearing loss impairs signal detection in noise: putative central mechanisms

Jennifer D. Gay*[1,2]*, Sergiy V. Voytenko*[1]*, Alexander V. Galazyuk*[1] *and Merri J. Rosen*[1]*

[1] *Department of Anatomy and Neurobiology, Northeast Ohio Medical University, Rootstown, OH, USA*
[2] *Biomedical Sciences Program, Kent State University, Kent, OH, USA*

***Correspondence:**
Merri J. Rosen, Department of Anatomy and Neurobiology, Northeast Ohio Medical University, P.O. Box 95, 4209 State Route 44, Rootstown, OH 44272, USA
e-mail: mrosen@neomed.edu

Listeners with hearing loss have difficulty processing sounds in noisy environments. This is most noticeable for speech perception, but is reflected in a basic auditory processing task: detecting a tonal signal in a noise background, i.e., simultaneous masking. It is unresolved whether the mechanisms underlying simultaneous masking arise from the auditory periphery or from the central auditory system. Poor detection in listeners with sensorineural hearing loss (SNHL) is attributed to cochlear hair cell damage. However, hearing loss alters neural processing in the central auditory system. Additionally, both psychophysical and neurophysiological data from normally hearing and impaired listeners suggest that there are additional contributions to simultaneous masking that arise centrally. With SNHL, it is difficult to separate peripheral from central contributions to signal detection deficits. We have thus excluded peripheral contributions by using an animal model of early conductive hearing loss (CHL) that provides auditory deprivation but does not induce cochlear damage. When tested as adults, animals raised with CHL had increased thresholds for detecting tones in simultaneous noise. Furthermore, intracellular *in vivo* recordings in control animals revealed a cortical correlate of simultaneous masking: local cortical processing reduced tone-evoked responses in the presence of noise. This raises the possibility that altered cortical responses which occur with early CHL can influence even simple signal detection in noise.

Keywords: conductive hearing loss, masking, noise, signal detection, auditory cortex, intracellular, electrophysiology, gerbil

INTRODUCTION

Listeners with hearing loss often struggle to understand speech in noisy environments. This difficulty is reflected in increased thresholds for detecting a simple signal in noise, i.e., simultaneous masking. Sensorineural hearing loss (SNHL) affects both the peripheral (cochlear) and central auditory system (cochlear nucleus and above), making it challenging to determine the mechanisms underlying impaired signal detection. We thus use a model of conductive hearing loss (CHL) that leaves the cochlea intact, allowing us to determine whether and how central auditory changes induced by hearing loss affect signal processing in noise.

CHL has effects on the central auditory system. In children, chronic middle ear infections (otitis media) produce a fluctuating CHL that can overlap with critical periods of neural development. Auditory deprivation during these periods alters intrinsic cellular and synaptic properties throughout the central auditory system (Vale and Sanes, 2000, 2002; Leao et al., 2004; Youssoufian et al., 2005; Leão et al., 2006). Developmental CHL is correlated with persistent perceptual problems that are presumably linked to changes in the central auditory system (Whitton and Polley, 2011). Support for this idea arises from animal developmental studies (Knudsen et al., 1984; King et al., 2000; Popescu and Polley, 2010). For example, binaural CHL leads to increased perceptual detection thresholds for slow amplitude modulations, and these behavioral deficits match the magnitude of neural shifts in auditory cortex (ACx; Rosen et al., 2012).

Acoustically demanding conditions, such as noisy environments, are particularly challenging for children who experience CHL. In multiple studies, children with a history of CHL have greater difficulty correctly identifying words or understanding speech in background noise than controls, requiring higher signal-to-noise ratios (SNRs) to attain equivalent performance (Gravel and Wallace, 1992; Schilder et al., 1994; Hall et al., 2003; Eapen et al., 2008; Hsieh et al., 2009; Keogh et al., 2010). These speech processing difficulties are likely due to changes in the central auditory system that arise from auditory deprivation (Sanes and Bao, 2009).

Detection of simple signals in noise should also be susceptible to CHL-induced central auditory system changes. Auditory percepts that reach mature performance levels gradually are susceptible to central changes that can arise due to hearing loss-induced deprivation (Moore, 2002). In particular, for the detection of brief signals in noise (simultaneous masking), thresholds do not reach adult levels until 10 years of age or later in humans (Hartley et al., 2000; Huyck, personal communication).

Neural elements that are affected by early hearing loss may contribute to these deficits. In auditory cortex, many hearing loss-induced effects are considered to involve modifications in local inhibitory networks (Calford et al., 1993; Kral et al., 2000; Chang et al., 2005; Razak et al., 2008; Takesian et al., 2010, 2012). Importantly, at least some of these changes persist into adulthood (Takesian et al., 2012). Thus, cortical neural changes during development as a result of hearing loss may contribute to signal detection problems that persist into maturity.

Deficits in simultaneous masking are also seen in SNHL listeners, but are usually attributed to peripheral mechanisms. In SNHL listeners, elevated simultaneous masking thresholds are ascribed to broadened filters and abnormal intensity perception that arise from cochlear damage, particularly of outer hair cells (Moore and Glasberg, 1986; Glasberg et al., 1987; Florentine, 1992; Kidd et al., 2002; Oxenham and Bacon, 2003). In normal listeners, psychophysical models attribute signal-in-noise detection thresholds to processing within the cochlea (Dai et al., 1991; Schlauch and Hafter, 1991; Moore, 2012). However, both psychophysical and neurophysiological data indicate that the central auditory system contributes to simultaneous masking performance.

Several psychophysical phenomena and auditory cortical responses implicate the central auditory system in simultaneous masking. One is overshoot, when a signal presented in the middle of a noise masker is more detectable than a signal presented at or near the noise onset (Elliott, 1965; Zwicker, 1965). Peripheral mechanisms cannot explain this phenomena (Smith and Zwislocki, 1975; Moore et al., 1987; Bacon and Smith, 1991), but neurons in primary ACx have response properties consistent with overshoot: signals presented at a delay relative to a background sound elicited more action potentials than those presented close to background sound onset, and this was directly attributable to inhibition from local cortical circuits (Volkov and Galazyuk, 1992). Another compelling indicator of central involvement is that a subject's expectation influences performance. In the presence of a continuous noise, detection of a tone can drop nearly to chance when the tone occurs at an unexpected frequency or duration (Scharf et al., 1987; Dai et al., 1991; Schlauch and Hafter, 1991; Wright and Dai, 1994). This susceptibility to stimulus variability has no peripheral correlate and implicates higher processing elements such as sensory memory and attention. A central correlate may exist in neurons from auditory cortical areas, which modulate their discharge rates in response to sound elements that deviate from expected values (Ulanovsky et al., 2003; Gill et al., 2008; Buran et al., 2014a).

Although it is difficult to pinpoint mechanisms underlying perceptual deficits, CHL, which does not result in hair cell damage, can disambiguate the contributions of peripheral and central elements to perception (Tucci et al., 1999; Lee et al., 2013). Early CHL induces central synaptic and cellular changes across the auditory neuraxis (Webster, 1983; Stuermer and Scheich, 2000; Tucci et al., 2001; Sumner et al., 2005; Xu et al., 2007; Takesian et al., 2010, 2012). Thus perceptual deficits resulting from CHL are presumably due to central contributions. Here we use an animal model of early CHL to demonstrate the effects of hearing loss on basic auditory perception, and to examine putative neural correlates in the central auditory system. Mongolian gerbils underwent surgery prior to the onset of hearing to induce a permanent moderate CHL. Animals with this permanent loss were then tested in adulthood compared with normal-hearing controls. Performance on an operant conditioning task demonstrated that early CHL impaired the perception of tones in simultaneous noise maskers. Then in normal-hearing animals, we used intracellular recordings to reveal a cortical correlate of simultaneous masking: local cortical processing reduced tone-evoked responses in the presence of noise. This raises the possibility that altered cortical responses affect simultaneous masking thresholds in animals with hearing loss.

METHODS

ANIMALS

All procedures relating to the maintenance and use of animals were approved by the Institutional Animal Care and Use Committee at the Northeast Ohio Medical University. Adult Mongolian gerbils (*Meriones unguiculatus*) ranging between postnatal (P) day 54–125 were tested in one of two procedures. Cortical responses to signals in noise were measured with intracellular recordings from a group of control (CTR) animals ($n = 7$). Perceptual detection thresholds were obtained from separate groups using an operant conditioning procedure. Control animals ($n = 8$) received normal auditory experience during development and were compared to animals with developmental CHL ($n = 10$). All animals were weaned at P30 and housed with litter mates in a 12 h light/12 h dark cycle. Groups were comprised of animals from multiple litters and included both males and females.

CONDUCTIVE HEARING LOSS INDUCTION AND MEASUREMENT

Malleus removal

Bilateral CHL was induced at P10–11 prior to the onset of hearing by tympanic membrane puncture and malleus extirpation (Tucci et al., 1999). Pups were anesthetized with methoxyflurane (Metofane, Ivesco Holdings) and the malleus was removed bilaterally through perforations in each tympanic membrane. At the conclusion of the study, hearing thresholds were measured via auditory brainstem responses (ABRs) from all animals. In addition, CHL animals were sacrificed and both ears examined to confirm malleus removal and to verify that the cochlea was not damaged by visual inspection of the bony labyrinth.

Auditory brainstem response (ABR)

After behavioral testing, ABRs from a subset of animals were measured to assess neural hearing thresholds. Tucker Davis Technologies (TDT) software and hardware were used to generate and present sounds (SigGen, BioSigRZ, RZ6), and to digitize and record neural responses (RZ6, RA4PA). Animals were anesthetized with ketamine and chloral hydrate and presented with auditory stimuli from a free-field calibrated speaker (TDT MF-1) positioned 6 cm in front of the animal. Responses were measured using stainless steel needle electrodes inserted subdermally at the dorsal midline between the eyes (non inverting), posterior to each pinna (inverting), and base of the tail (common ground). Auditory stimuli were 3 ms pure tones with 1 ms rise/fall times, repeated at 15/s. Sound level was adjusted in 5 dB steps to obtain a threshold response (i.e., a visually detectable N1 potential).

BEHAVIORAL TRAINING AND TESTING

Experimental environment

Gerbils were placed in a custom built test cage in a double-walled room (ETS Lindgren Acoustic Systems) lined with echo-attenuating material, and were observed via closed circuit monitor. The test cage contained a stainless steel drinking spout and metal floor plate. Gerbil contact with both plate and spout completed a circuit that initiated water delivery via a syringe pump (New Era). A personal computer connected to a digital I/O interface TDT measured animal contact and controlled the timing of acoustic stimuli, water delivery (0.2–0.25 ml/min), and a small aversive current delivered at the end of warning trials. Auditory stimuli were generated by the TDT system and delivered via a calibrated custom speaker (Madisound) centered ~ 60 cm in front of the lick spout. Sound level at the test cage was measured with a spectrum analyzer (Bruel and Kjaer 2690-OF2) via a 1/4 inch free-field condenser microphone (Bruel and Kjaer 4939) positioned at the location of the animal head when in contact with the spout. Noise levels are in dB SPL, converted from RMS measurements.

Auditory stimuli and operant conditioning task

During training and testing, animals heard continuous repeated bursts of a 300 ms noise masker (30% BW noise centered linearly at 4 kHz) with 700 ms inter-burst intervals. Within this repeated background were intermittent SAFE and WARN trials (**Figure 1A**). SAFE trials contained only the noise masker, while WARN trials contained the masker and signal (4 kHz pure tone, 40 ms duration, 2 ms rise/fall; **Figure 1A**). Contact with the spout was monitored immediately prior to each trial and the trial only proceeded if the animal was in contact with the spout for 75% of the 50 ms pre-check window. The warning stimulus was followed by an aversive unconditioned stimulus (300 ms electrical current via the lick spout) delivered 300 ms after the end of the 40 ms signal. To determine if the animal detected the signal, contact with the spout was monitored during the 50 ms prior to delivery of the shock. Contact for ≤75% of this window was scored as a hit. For the same window during SAFE trials a contact time of ≤75% was scored as a false alarm (FA). WARN trials always occurred at the end of a block of 2–4 SAFE trials, randomized to avoid temporal conditioning.

Sound levels

Control and CHL animals were tested at approximately equivalent sensation levels based on previous measures of hearing loss induced by malleus removal. This procedure typically produces an attenuation of ~45 dB as assessed by ABR (Tucci et al., 1999; Rosen et al., 2012), and of ~30 dB at 4 kHz as assessed by behavioral testing (Buran et al., 2014b; see Section Results for more detail). Sound levels were presented 35 dB louder for CHLs (85 dB SPL masker) than CTRs (50 dB SPL masker). The signal levels began at 23 dB SPL above the masker level and were reduced to determine detection threshold. We determined that the stimulus was not distorted at the loudest levels presented.

Procedural training

Behavioral training and testing involved a conditioned avoidance procedure (Heffner and Heffner, 1995; Kelly et al., 2006). Animals were water deprived for 48 h prior to training and remained on controlled water access for the duration of the training and testing. Animals were introduced to the behavioral cage and trained to initiate water delivery via contact with the metal spout, during repeated presentations of gated noise maskers (**Figure 1A**). Animals learned to withdraw from the spout when an acoustic cue

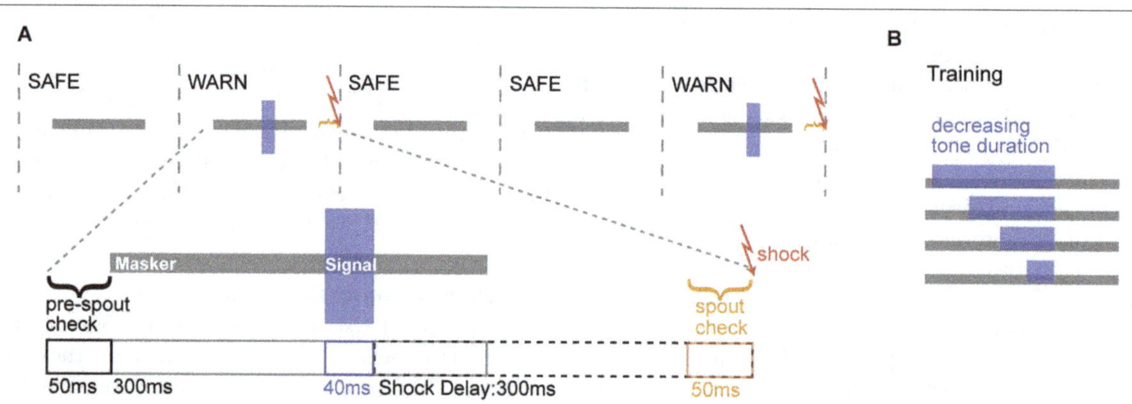

FIGURE 1 | Operant conditioning schematic. (A) *Top*: Trial structure for the simultaneous masking task, where 300 ms noise maskers were presented either with (WARN trial) or without (SAFE trial) overlapping tonal signals. Warn trials were followed by an aversive shock. *Bottom*: The timeline of a single warn trial is illustrated, with the masker (*gray*) and signal (*blue*) just above. For the trial to be initiated, the animal needed to maintain contact with the spout for >75% of the pre-spout check period. WARN trials contained a 300 ms masker and a 40 ms signal. A mild shock was delivered 300 ms after the offset of the signal. During the 50 ms prior to the shock, a spout check determined whether the animal was correctly off the spout (Hit) or incorrectly on the spout (Miss). For SAFE trials (not illustrated), neither the signal nor shock were presented, but the spout check determined whether the animal was correctly on the spout (Correct Rejection) or incorrectly off the spout (False Alarm). **(B)** During training, the duration of the signal was progressively decreased as animals reached criterion performance at each duration. The shock always occurred 300 ms after signal offset, regardless of signal duration.

(tonal signal) was presented within the noise, in order to avoid a low AC current (0.25–2.5 mA, 300 ms, Coulbourn) delivered through the lick spout. Since animals display large between-subject variability in pain sensitivity (Mogil, 1999; Wasner and Brock, 2008; Nielsen et al., 2009), the shock level was adjusted continuously for each animal to produce reliable withdrawal from the spout without dissuading the animal from returning to the spout. For initial training, a long (200 ms) signal was presented and shortened in 20–30 ms steps until animals reliably detected the target duration of 40 ms (**Figure 1B**). To establish criterion performance at the target duration, warning trials were presented until performance reached 70% correct over 10 consecutive trials.

Perceptual testing

Once animals reached criterion on the conditioned avoidance procedure, they were tested with decreasing signal levels using the method of constant limits: five signal levels separated by 3 dB presented in decreasing order. Each day of testing used a range of sound levels that bracketed the previous day's threshold (Sarro and Sanes, 2010). Animals were tested for 4–5 days with increasing difficulty in order to determine thresholds for detecting the signal in noise (signal-to-noise ratio, SNR, quantified as the signal in dB minus the noise in dB). Pilot data indicated that this duration of testing produced reliable performance, while longer testing resulted in poorer performance, as the difficulty of the task induced animals to adopt strategies that resulted in increased thresholds (e.g., high FA rates or long lapses of attention). SNRs for the best day along with the best 3 days of performance were taken as perceptual thresholds.

Data analysis

A performance value, $d' = z(\text{hits}) - z(\text{false alarms})$, was obtained for z-scores that corresponded to right-tail p-values (Swets, 1973; Yanz, 1984), and was calculated for each signal level. Thresholds were defined as the signal level at which performance reached $d' = 1$; only sessions in which animals performed on a minimum of 25 WARN trials were included in the analysis. Psychometric functions of d' across signal level were constructed for each day of testing. Performance during the best 3 days of testing served as the assessment of practiced detection thresholds. Performance across groups was compared with two-sided Wilcoxon rank sum tests for unpaired data. All values are given as mean ± standard error (SEM).

Inclusion criteria

All animals that performed behavioral testing were included in the analysis. In order to compare the effects of treatment group, no animals were excluded for poor performance, as is common in behavioral studies examining best performance capability. Animals that did not reach criteria after 10 days of training with the long-duration signal were excluded. This removed three controls and six CHL animals from the study.

INTRACELLULAR RECORDINGS

Surgical preparation

Mongolian gerbils ($n = 7$) were anesthetized through isoflurane inhalation (1.5–2.5% in oxygen) and held secure in a stereotaxic apparatus. A headpost was cemented to the skull using dental acrylic, and a small craniotomy was made over left auditory cortex, leaving the dura intact. Following this brief surgical procedure, animals were anesthetized with ketamine (30 mg/kg) and chloral hydrate (350 mg/kg) in preparation for recordings, and were maintained as necessary with supplemental doses.

Acoustic stimuli

Stimuli were generated using TDT software (SigGen) and hardware (RP 2.1) and delivered via a calibrated custom built speaker. The signal was a 40 ms FM downsweep with a 10 kHz bandwidth, extending through a range chosen to encompass the cell's best frequency (BF). This range was based on an initial extracellular recording that determined the general BF of cells within the region. The masker was a 200 ms broadband noise, with onset 100 ms before the FM signal. Signal and masker were presented at equal amplitudes.

Electrophysiology

Intracellular recordings were made using techniques described previously (Voytenko and Galazyuk, 2008). Animals were placed inside a single-walled acoustic chamber (Industrial Acoustics), and positioned on an air table 7″ from a freefield speaker. Sharp microelectrodes were pulled from 1.2-mm-diameter quartz glass (Sutter Instruments) on a Flaming-Brown micropipette puller and filled with 3M potassium acetate. Impedance ranged between 40 and 90 MΩ. After placement on the dorsal surface of the brain, the exposure was filled with 4% agar and the electrode was advanced in 3-μm steps using a precision microdrive (Kopf, Model 660). Intracellular responses were amplified (Cygnus Technologies NeuroData IR183A), monitored with Pulse software (v. 8.65) and digitized using a data acquisition system (Heka model EPC-10) at a sampling rate of 100 kHz.

Analysis

Responses to masked and unmasked signals were compared within cells. 10–20 repetitions were presented for each stimulus, and mean traces calculated from membrane potentials (V_m) after truncating spikes. Hyperpolarization within a given time window was measured from mean traces as the area under the curve in relation to baseline V_m. For each cell, the time window in which a specific response occurred (either a hyperpolarization or rebound action potentials) was determined from the mean V_m trace elicited by the signal alone. This time window was used to measure response magnitudes with and without a masker present; these were compared with two-sided Wilcoxon signed rank tests for paired data. All values are given as mean ± SEM.

RESULTS

DEVELOPMENTAL CONDUCTIVE HEARING LOSS DEGRADES SIGNAL DETECTION IN NOISE

Behavioral thresholds for signal detection in noise were obtained from two groups of adult gerbils: animals reared with CHL prior to hearing onset, and age-matched controls (CTR). Animals were trained to detect a brief 4 kHz signal embedded in a longer noise masker (30% bandwidth centered around the signal frequency). Once animals were reliably performing the task, they received several days of procedural testing to determine threshold (defined as the quietest tone level that could be reliably detected in the presence of the masker, reported here as SNR in dB). Thresholds were compared across groups for each animal's best day (**Figure 2A**) and mean across the best 3 days (**Figure 2B**). CTR animals displayed significantly lower detection thresholds compared to CHLs (Best day: $p < 0.001$; Best 3 days: $p = 0.01$, Wilcoxon rank-sum). Differences in thresholds were not due to differences in training or performance on the task. Groups received a comparable number of procedural training trials (**Figure 2C**: $p = 0.97$, Wilcoxon rank sum) and learned the task at a similar rate (days of training: CTR 5.6 ± 0.9 vs. CHL 5.8 ± 0.6, $p = 0.69$, Wilcoxon rank-sum). Furthermore, the amount of procedural training on the task was not correlated to threshold for either group (**Figure 2D**: CTR: $R^2 = 0.192$, $p = 0.28$, CHL: $R^2 = 0.021$, $p = 0.69$).

One might expect that early hearing loss would affect learning or improvement on perceptual tasks. For this simple simultaneous masking task that was not the case. In addition to equivalent time-courses of training, both groups improved but did so equivalently across testing days (**Figure 2E**; First day minus last day threshold (dB SNR): CTR 7.8 ± 2.7 vs. CHL 4.7 ± 4.6, $p = 0.15$, Wilcoxon rank-sum). Furthermore, the rate of learning did not differ between groups, as animals reached best performance over an equivalent number of testing days (number of testing days to reach threshold (dB SNR): CTR 4.6 ± 0.2 vs. CHL 3.7 ± 0.4, $p = 0.19$, Wilcoxon rank-sum).

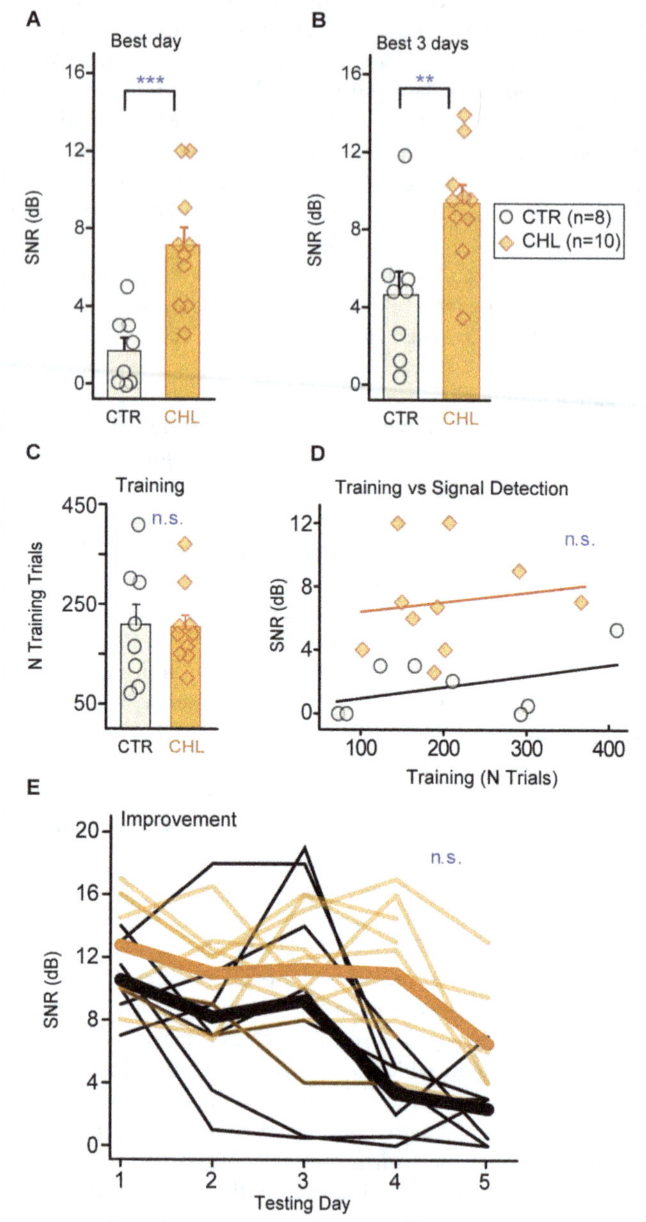

FIGURE 2 | Early CHL increases behavioral detection thresholds for simultaneously masked signals. Detection thresholds (quantified as SNR; see Section Methods) were significantly higher for conductive hearing loss (CHL; *shaded orange*) compared with control (CTR; *cream-filled black*) animals, as measured by **(A)** the best performance day and **(B)** the mean across the best 3 performance days. Thresholds from individual animals are depicted as *circles* or *diamonds* atop each bar. **(C)** Groups required similar numbers of training trials to reach criterion performance. **(D)** The amount of training did not predict final detection thresholds. *Lines* show non-significant linear fits. **(E)** Detection thresholds across testing days indicate gradual improvement which did not differ across groups. *Thin lines* are thresholds from individual animals, and *thick lines* are means. Abbreviations: CTR: controls, CHL: conductive hearing loss, n.s.: not significant, **: $p < 0.01$, ***: $p = 0.001$.

PERFORMANCE VARIABLES DO NOT ACCOUNT FOR THE EFFECT OF EARLY HEARING LOSS

Higher thresholds for the CHL animals did not appear to be due to poorer attention to the task. Poor attention can be indicated by high FA rates, measured here as withdrawal from the spout during SAFE trials (which minimizes the chance of receiving a shock during poor attention to the signal). CTR and CHL animals did not differ in their FA rates (**Figure 3A**: $p = 0.26$, Wilcoxon rank-sum) and this measure of attention did not predict threshold for either group (**Figure 3B**: CTR: $R^2 = 0.172$, $p = 0.31$, CHL: $R^2 = 0.159$, $p = 0.25$).

Attention can also be indicated by licking consistency. During testing, animals ideally maintain constant contact with the spout, and withdraw only upon detecting a signal. Another strategy is to drink continuously but make poor contact with the spout, with continuous micro-withdrawals to minimize the magnitude of shock received. This hesitant contact can be an indicator of poor attention or performance anxiety and can be quantified as the number of times an animal breaks contact with the spout between WARNs. CTR animals displayed significantly more breaks in contact between WARNs compared to CHLs (**Figure 3C**: $p < 0.01$, Wilcoxon rank-sum) indicating group differences in overall performance strategy. However, this was independent of signal detection thresholds (**Figure 3D**: CTR: $R^2 = 0.06$, $p = 0.57$, CHL: $R^2 = 0.001$, $p = 0.93$). Notably, this performance strategy would be likely to increase the false alarm rate in CTR animals, thus increasing their thresholds as calculated by the d' measure. Despite this, CTR thresholds were significantly lower than those of CHLs, suggesting that, if anything, the threshold differences measured here may underestimate perceptual differences across groups.

Task proficiency and performance consistency can also affect behavioral thresholds. As an indicator of task proficiency, we measured performance at the easiest level on the best testing

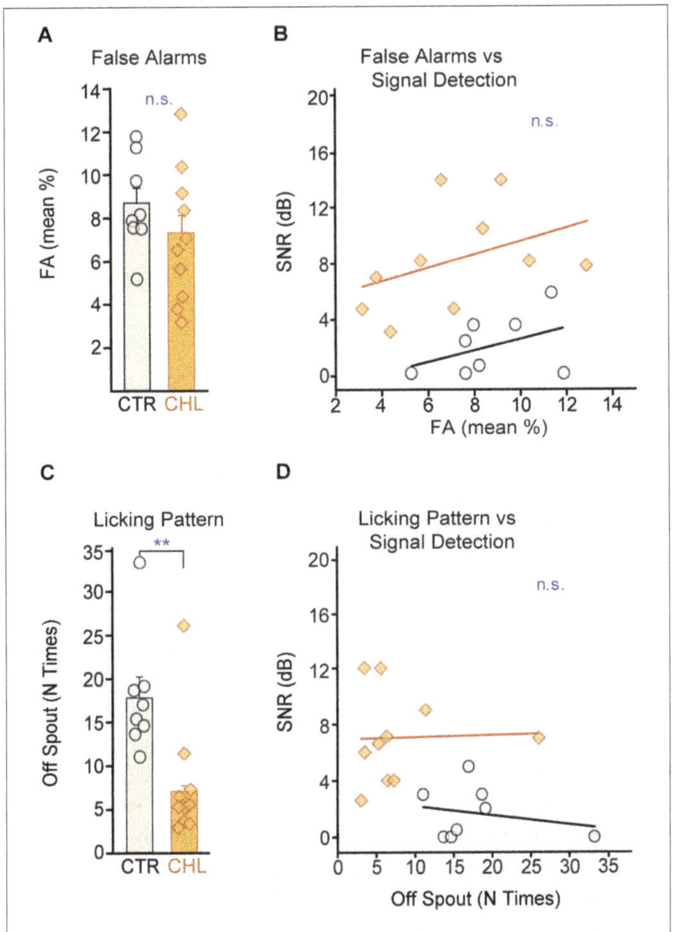

FIGURE 3 | Performance strategies do not account for differences in behavioral detection thresholds. **(A)** False alarm (FA) rates, a measure of attention, did not differ across CTR (*open black*) and CHL (*shaded orange*) animals. FA rates from individual animals are depicted as *circles* or *diamonds* atop each bar. **(B)** FA rates did not correlate with behavioral detection thresholds for either group (*lines* show non-significant linear fits). **(C)** CTR animals adopted a less consistent licking strategy than CHL animals (quantified as the number of breaks with the water spout between WARNs: N times off spout). **(D)** Despite a difference in licking stragegy, the number of breaks did not correlate with final detection thresholds for either group (*lines* show non-significant linear fits). Abbreviations as in **Figure 2**.

day (**Figure 4A**). As an indicator of performance consistency we measured the range of d' scores for the easiest level presented across days; a wider range indicates increased variability in performance (**Figure 4B**). Neither the d' score for the easiest level on the best performance day (CTR: $R^2 = 0.35, p = 0.12$, CHL: $R^2 = 0.11, p = 0.34$) nor the range of d' scores at the easiest level (CTR: $R^2 = 0.17, p = 0.30$, CHL: $R^2 = 0.42, p = 0.57$) correlated with behavioral threshold for either group. Thus perceptual deficits in CHL animals are independent from their ability to perform the task.

SENSATION LEVEL ALONE DOES NOT ACCOUNT FOR THE EFFECT OF EARLY HEARING LOSS

In order to attribute deficits in masked thresholds to central changes, it is essential to demonstrate that the attenuation provided by CHL is not sufficient to explain these deficits. It is possible that increased signal detection thresholds for CHL animals could be attributed to the stimuli not being presented at sensation levels equivalent to CTRs. To account for this, the two groups were tested with stimuli that differed by 35 dB (for both masker and signal). This level difference was based on behaviorally-measured level thresholds for separate groups of CHL animals in two tasks: AM detection (Rosen et al., 2012) and tone-detection (Buran et al., 2014b), which indicated 35 and 30 dB shifts respectively. We then tested to ensure that the amount of hearing loss at 4 kHz did not predict detection thresholds for our 4 kHz masked tones. **Figure 4C** shows that hearing levels for a 4 kHz tone, as measured by ABRs for each animal, did not correlate with behavioral thresholds in either CTRs ($R^2 = 0.01$, $p = 0.84$) or CHLs ($R^2 = 0.10$, $p = 0.55$). As there was no differential difficulty in hearing the signal, non-equivalent sensation levels could not account for the increased masked thresholds seen in CHL animals. That is, the characteristics of the perceptual deficit are not what would be predicted based solely on the amount of signal attenuation caused by the CHL.

AUDITORY CORTEX CONTRIBUTES TO REDUCED RESPONSES DURING SIMULTANEOUS MASKING

Since the mechanisms by which central areas contribute to simultaneous masking are not resolved, intracellular responses to noise-masked signals were measured via sharp electrode recordings in auditory cortex. We focused on signal-evoked hyperpolarizations, as these are of cortical origin and reflect central processing (Somogyi et al., 1983; DeFelipe and Jones, 1985; Matsubara, 1988; Albus et al., 1991; Albus and Wahle, 1994; Tomioka et al., 2005; Higo et al., 2007). The spikes that occurred when hyperpolarizations returned to baseline were examined because they were likely to be generated by post-inhibitory rebound. Such spikes can be attributed to local cortical processes.

The subset of cells ($n = 16$) that exhibited hyperpolarization in response to the signal were examined. For each cell, the response to the signal alone was compared with the response to the masked signal. An example of overlaid traces in **Figure 5A** (top) shows a FM signal-evoked spiking onset response followed by a hyperpolarization, with rebound spikes upon return to baseline. The bottom trace shows a reduced hyperpolarization with no clear rebound spikes in response to the FM signal during a masker. For the sample of cells tested, the magnitude of the signal-evoked hyperpolarization (measured as the area under the curve relative to the membrane resting potential) was significantly reduced during presentation of the masker (**Figure 5B**; Wilcoxon signed rank, $p = 0.049$). Furthermore, those cells that spiked on rebound from the FM signal-evoked hyperpolarization fired significantly fewer rebound spikes during masker presentation (**Figure 5C**; Wilcoxon signed rank, $p = 0.008$). A reduced firing response to a masked signal is one measure of a neural correlate of perceptual masking. As this signal-evoked hyperpolarization must arise locally, from intrinsic cortical cellular mechanisms or local inhibitory circuitry, these data are evidence for a cortical contribution to simultaneous masking.

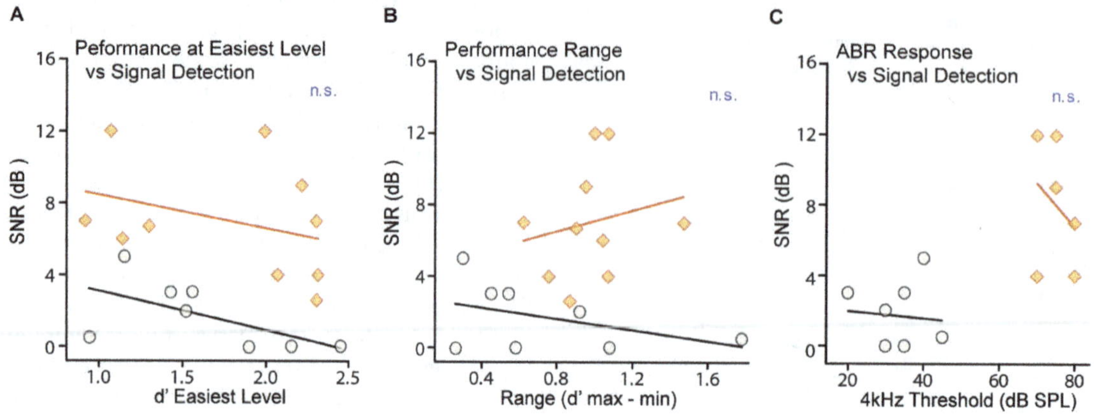

FIGURE 4 | Neither task proficiency nor hearing ability account for differences in detection thresholds. Detection thresholds were not correlated with either **(A)** *d′* performance for the easiest signal levels or **(B)** the variability of *d′* performance for the easiest signal level across testing days, for either CTR (*shaded orange*) or CHL (*open black*) groups. Thresholds from individual animals are depicted as *circles* or *diamonds*, and *lines* are non-significant linear fits. **(C)** Neural ABR thresholds measured across frequency were predictably increased in CHL animals by ~40 dB. There was no correlation in either CTRs or CHLs between neural hearing thresholds and signal detection thresholds. Abbreviations as in **Figure 2**.

DISCUSSION

This study demonstrates that simultaneous masking involves the central auditory system and is impaired by early CHL. Developmental auditory deprivation induces anatomical and physiological changes in the central auditory system that persist into adulthood in animals (Harrison et al., 1993; Chang and Merzenich, 2003; Kral et al., 2005; Sanes and Bao, 2009). Perceptions that involve the central auditory system should be affected. We thus asked whether animals with early CHL had increased detection thresholds for simple signals in noise. When tested with a conditioned avoidance procedure, adult animals reared with CHL displayed significantly poorer detection thresholds than CTRs for a brief tone embedded in a simultaneous noise masker, despite equivalent training (**Figure 2**). These masked threshold increases could not be attributed to the amount of attenuation induced by the hearing loss. Furthermore, they were not due to task proficiency, strategy, or attention, as these did not differ across groups (**Figures 3, 4**). This type of developmental CHL maintains cochlear integrity and is known to alter intrinsic and synaptic properties in the central auditory system, particularly in ACx (Xu et al., 2007; Takesian et al., 2010, 2012). For such alterations to affect thresholds for simultaneous masking in deprived animals, neural areas central to the periphery should directly contribute to the responses to these signals, rather than merely inheriting responses from the auditory periphery. We therefore made intracellular *in vivo* recordings from ACx in control animals, and demonstrated a cortical contribution to simultaneous masking. This can be attributed to local sources, either intrinsic neural properties or local inhibitory synaptic inputs (**Figure 5;** Somogyi et al., 1983; DeFelipe and Jones, 1985; Matsubara, 1988; Albus et al., 1991; Albus and Wahle, 1994; Tomioka et al., 2005; Higo et al., 2007).

TECHNICAL CONSIDERATIONS OF THE DEVELOPMENTAL CHL MODEL

The CHL induced here, via malleus removal, attenuates sound transmission to the inner ear but leaves the cochlea intact: ossicle removal does not alter hair cell counts on the basilar membrane, and bone conduction thresholds are normal (Tucci and Rubel, 1985). Here, visual postmortem analyses excluded the possibility of accidental cochlear damage. In SNHL listeners, reduced cochlear nonlinearities are often used to explain raised thresholds for simultaneous masked signals (Moore and Glasberg, 1986; Oxenham and Bacon, 2003), but this should not be the source of the raised thresholds seen here. The possibility exists that the permanent CHL induced compensatory changes at the periphery, perhaps via efferent alterations of the middle ear reflex (Munro and Blount, 2009). However, signal detection thresholds were not correlated with hearing thresholds at the same frequency (**Figure 4C**). Another possible peripheral contribution would be the induction of a hearing loss that was not consistent across the frequency range used in the behavioral masking task. Hearing loss with malleus removal is relatively flat across the frequency spectrum (Rosen et al., 2012), mimicking the flat CHL that occurs during otitis media in children (Kokko, 1974; Anteby et al., 1986; Hunter et al., 1994). Here, signals of 4 kHz were masked with a noise spanning 3.4–4.6 kHz, which approximates the gerbil critical band at that center frequency (~1 kHz; Kittel et al., 2002). Finally, it is worth noting that CHL induced via malleus removal is not the best mimic of otitis media, but is well-suited to examine central contributions to hearing loss deficits. Our CHL is permanent, whereas early otitis media typically produces a fluctuating CHL that resolves after childhood. Our model does not reproduce the effusion viscosity that occurs with otitis media, which alters sound transmission delays (Hartley and Moore, 2003). It therefore avoids introducing an element of altered peripheral processing that may affect temporal processing in listeners with otitis media.

CORTICAL CONTRIBUTIONS TO SIMULTANEOUS MASKING

Our evidence in combination with previous work indicates that responses to simultaneous masked signals evolve from the periphery to central regions. In the periphery, simultaneous

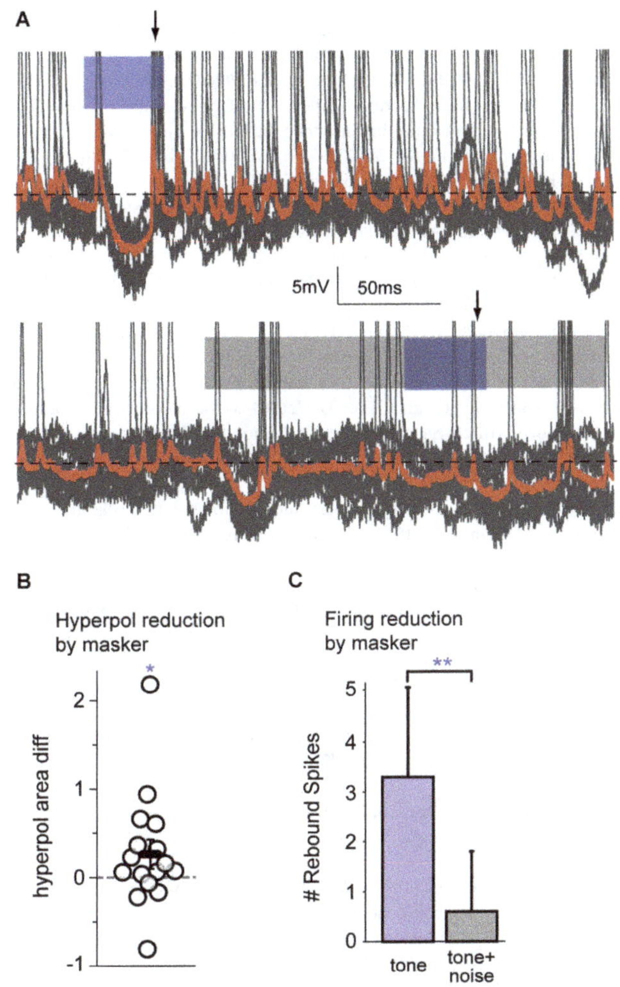

FIGURE 5 | Auditory cortex alters firing responses to simultaneous masked signals. (A) An example of overlaid traces (*gray traces* with mean in *red*) from a cortical neuron in response to 10 presentations of a FM tone (*top; blue bar*) or a FM tone occurring during a broadband noise (*bottom; blue bar within gray bar*). The traces show changes in voltage over time. *Top*: This neuron has an onset spiking response to the FM tone followed by a hyperpolarization, with rebound spikes (*arrow*) upon return to baseline (*black dotted line*). *Bottom*: When a simultaneous masker is presented, there is a reduced hyperpolarization and no clear rebound spikes (*arrow*) in response to the masked FM signal. **(B)** During masker presentation compared with tone alone, there was a significant reduction in the magnitude of signal-evoked hyperpolarizations. **(C)** When a simultaneous masker was present (*gray bar*), there were significantly fewer spikes immediately following hyperpolarizations, as compared with the tone presented alone (*blue bar*). Since hyperpolarizations arise within cortex and indicate central processing, a reduction in their magnitude, and a reduction of the number of post-inhibitory rebound spikes, are attributable to central mechanisms. **: $p < 0.01$, *: $p < 0.05$.

masking functions in auditory nerve fibers are based upon cochlear nonlinearities. For example, with a continuous broadband noise masker, auditory nerve fiber responses to tones shift in a manner consistent with two-tone suppression (the reduction of the response to one tone by simultaneous presentation of another tone) (Costalupes et al., 1984; Ruggero et al., 1992). This suppression is attributable to outer hair cell interactions with the basilar membrane (Robles and Ruggero, 2001). SNHL reduces those nonlinearities, which affects simultaneous masked thresholds (Oxenham and Bacon, 2003). In comparison, CHL, which does not alter cochlear nonlinearities, also affects simultaneous masked thresholds, and this is presumably due to central processes.

Our intracellular data reveal a cortical correlate of simultaneous masking. In neurons that exhibited signal-evoked hyperpolarization, the responses to FM tones showed a reduced hyperpolarization and fewer subsequent spikes in the presence of a noise masker (**Figures 5B,C**). The action potentials that immediately follow the hyperpolarization are likely to be rebound spikes, resulting from intrinsic cellular properties and thus of cortical origin. Cortical inhibition is known to arise locally, via intrinsic horizontal, intralaminar, and some long-range projections (Somogyi et al., 1983; DeFelipe and Jones, 1985; Matsubara, 1988; Albus et al., 1991; Albus and Wahle, 1994; Tomioka et al., 2005; Higo et al., 2007). As the hyperpolarizations seen here arise locally, our data are an example of the cortex modifying inherited subcortical information. The two possible sources of this hyperpolarization are either inhibition from local interneurons, or intrinsic cellular properties that generate afterhyperpolarizations. Intracellular *in vivo* recordings of ACx pyramidal neurons show responses similar to those seen here: signal-evoked depolarization often followed by hyperpolarization. The hyperpolarization has characteristics of a chloride-mediated IPSP that is likely mediated by $GABA_A$ receptors (De Ribaupierre et al., 1972; Ojima and Murakami, 2002). Here, the hyperpolarization time courses were similar to those previously described. Therefore they are likely to arise from local inhibition rather than intrinsic hyperpolarizing currents activated by depolarization. If the hyperpolarization indeed arises from local cortical interneurons, the reduced hyperpolarization seen during masking may arise from reduced excitatory input onto those interneurons. Reduced neural responses are seen in subcortical regions during simultaneous masking, and may be a source of these excitatory feedforward inputs (Costalupes et al., 1984; Rees and Palmer, 1988; May and Sachs, 1992).

To our knowledge, the only other direct demonstration of inhibitory reduction of spiking during simultaneous masking in ACx is by Volkov and Galazyuk (1992), where a background sound evoked a local inhibitory current that reduced the response to an overlaid signal. However, they did not directly compare unmasked and masked conditions and only tested binaural interactions. Previous neurophysiological analyses of ACx and inferior colliculus have provided some evidence for central contributions to simultaneous masking involving local inhibition. In the inferior colliculus, tone-evoked responses were shifted during simultaneous noise in a manner consistent with local inhibition, providing responses that differed from auditory nerve fibers (Rees and Palmer, 1988). In primary ACx, monotonic cells (those whose discharge rate increases with sound level) responded like auditory nerve fibers, dominated by whichever sound (signal or masker) elicited a stronger response alone. In contrast, nonmonotonic cells (those with more complex level-sensitivity) were suppressed by a noise masker, suggestive of inhibitory influences (Phillips and Cynader, 1985; Phillips and Kelly, 1992). Consistent with this idea, nonmonotonic response profiles do not reflect inputs inherited from lower hierarchical areas. Instead, they arise from local excitatory and inhibitory interactions (Wu et al., 2006). Thus our result is expected: local cortical inhibition shapes responses to signals masked by simultaneous noise. We did not explicitly test for monotonicity, but would predict that the neurons analyzed here were nonmonotonic.

NEURAL CORRELATES OF SIGNAL DETECTION

A challenging element is connecting changes in neural discharge with altered auditory perception. The reduced spiking shown in this study indicates a reduced output to a masked signal and would be expected to increase signal detection thresholds. This idea is supported by recordings of cortical auditory evoked potentials (CAEPs) in humans, which show a correlate for the detection of masked signals in the P1/N1/P2 waveform. The amplitude of CAEP peaks is correlated with detectability of signals in noise (Martin et al., 1997). Since the CAEP primarily reflects synchronous activity arising from ACx (Näätänen and Picton, 1987; Eggermont, 2007), the reduction in ACx spiking seen here during the presence of a masker could manifest as reduced CAEP amplitude, and may thus contribute to poor perception in noise.

Cortical changes known to occur with hearing loss suggest a simple mechanism for impaired signal detection. Early CHL directly affects the central auditory system, generally reducing inhibition relative to excitation in order to maintain homeostasis (Sanes, 2013). For example, animals raised with early CHL have reduced IPSC amplitude, decreased firing rates in fast-spiking interneurons, and facilitating rather than the normal depressing short-term plasticity (Takesian et al., 2010, 2012). Inhibition is known to sharpen neural tuning curves at the level of cortex (Ojima, 2011). In normal listeners, inhibition would reduce the magnitude of noise-evoked responses. With reduced cortical inhibition seen from early hearing loss, the frequency components of a noise surrounding a neuron's BF would *increase* the response magnitude to noise. At the same time, early CHL reduces the magnitude of ACx firing to tones (Rosen et al., 2012). Concurrently, these effects would reduce the SNR of tones presented in a noise masker. In this manner, changes to the cortical network may subserve the impaired simultaneous masked thresholds seen in this study. This prediction can be directly tested in our animal model. Future experiments that measure neural activity during perceptual detection tasks in CHL animals can connect changes in central auditory regions with perceptual impairments arising from developmental deprivation.

ACKNOWLEDGMENTS

This work was supported by R01DC013314 to Merri J. Rosen and R01DC011330 to Alexander V. Galazyuk. We thank Julia Huyck, Kyle Nakamoto, and Sharad Shanbhag for helpful ideas, discussions, and comments on the manuscript.

REFERENCES

Albus, K., and Wahle, P. (1994). The topography of tangential inhibitory connections in the postnatally developing and mature striate cortex of the cat. *Eur. J. Neurosci.* 6, 779–792. doi: 10.1111/j.1460-9568.1994.tb00989.x

Albus, K., Wahle, P., Lubke, J., and Matute, C. (1991). The contribution of GABA-ergic neurons to horizontal intrinsic connections in upper layers of the cat's striate cortex. *Exp. Brain Res.* 85, 235–239. doi: 10.1007/bf00230006

Anteby, I., Hafner, H., Pratt, H., and Uri, N. (1986). Auditory brainstem evoked potentials in evaluating the central effects of middle ear effusion. *Int. J. Pediatr. Otorhinolaryngol.* 12, 1–11. doi: 10.1016/s0165-5876(86)80051-9

Bacon, S. P., and Smith, M. A. (1991). Spectral, intensive and temporal factors influencing overshoot. *Q. J. Exp. Psychol. A* 43, 373–399. doi: 10.1080/14640749108400978

Buran, B. N., Sarro, E. C., Manno, F. A., Kang, R., Caras, M. L., and Sanes, D. H. (2014b). A sensitive period for the impact of hearing loss on auditory perception. *J. Neurosci.* 34, 2276–2284. doi: 10.1523/JNEUROSCI.0647-13.2014

Buran, B. N., von Trapp, G., and Sanes, D. H. (2014a). Behaviorally gated reduction of spontaneous discharge can improve detection thresholds in auditory cortex. *J. Neurosci.* 34, 4076–4081. doi: 10.1523/JNEUROSCI.4825-13.2014

Calford, M. B., Rajan, R., and Irvine, D. R. (1993). Rapid changes in the frequency tuning of neurons in cat auditory cortex resulting from pure-tone-induced temporary threshold shift. *Neuroscience* 55, 953–964. doi: 10.1016/0306-4522(93)90310-c

Chang, E. F., Bao, S., Imaizumi, K., Schreiner, C. E., and Merzenich, M. M. (2005). Development of spectral and temporal response selectivity in the auditory cortex. *Proc. Natl. Acad. Sci. U S A* 102, 16460–16465. doi: 10.1073/pnas.0508239102

Chang, E. F., and Merzenich, M. M. (2003). Environmental noise retards auditory cortical development. *Science* 300, 498–502. doi: 10.1126/science.1082163

Costalupes, J. A., Young, E. D., and Gibson, D. J. (1984). Effects of continuous noise backgrounds on rate response of auditory nerve fibers in cat. *J. Neurophysiol.* 51, 1326–1344.

Dai, H. P., Scharf, B., and Buus, S. (1991). Effective attenuation of signals in noise under focused attention. *J. Acoust. Soc. Am.* 89, 2837–2842. doi: 10.1121/1.400721

DeFelipe, J., and Jones, E. G. (1985). Vertical organization of gamma-aminobutyric acid-accumulating intrinsic neuronal systems in monkey cerebral cortex. *J. Neurosci.* 5, 3246–3260.

De Ribaupierre, F., Goldstein, M. H. Jr., and Yeni-Komshian, G. (1972). Intracellular study of the cat's primary auditory cortex. *Brain Res.* 48, 185–204. doi: 10.1016/0006-8993(72)90178-3

Eapen, R. J., Buss, E., Grose, J. H., Drake, A. F., Dev, M., and Hall, J. W. (2008). The development of frequency weighting for speech in children with a history of otitis media with effusion. *Ear Hear.* 29, 718–724. doi: 10.1097/AUD.0b013e31817a98cb

Eggermont, J. J. (2007). "Electric and magnetic fields of synchronous neural activity," in *Auditory Evoked Potentials*, eds R. F. Burkard, M. Don and J. J. Eggermont (Philadelphia: Lippincott Williams and Wilkins), 3–21.

Elliott, L. L. (1965). Changes in the simultaneous masked threshold of brief tones. *J. Acoust. Soc. Am.* 38, 738–746. doi: 10.1121/1.1909798

Florentine, M. (1992). Effects of cochlear impairment and equivalent-threshold masking on psychoacoustic tuning curves. *Audiology* 31, 241–253. doi: 10.3109/00206099209072913

Gill, P., Woolley, S. M., Fremouw, T., and Theunissen, F. E. (2008). What's that sound? Auditory area CLM encodes stimulus surprise, not intensity or intensity changes. *J. Neurophysiol.* 99, 2809–2820. doi: 10.1152/jn.01270.2007

Glasberg, B. R., Moore, B. C., and Bacon, S. P. (1987). Gap detection and masking in hearing-impaired and normal-hearing subjects. *J. Acoust. Soc. Am.* 81, 1546–1556. doi: 10.1121/1.394507

Gravel, J. S., and Wallace, I. F. (1992). Listening and language at 4 years of age: effects of early otitis media. *J. Speech Hear. Res.* 35, 588–595. doi: 10.1044/jshr.3503.588

Hall, J. W., Grose, J. H., Buss, E., Dev, M. B., Drake, A. F., and Pillsbury, H. C. (2003). The effect of otitis media with effusion on perceptual masking. *Arch. Otolaryngol. Head Neck Surg.* 129, 1056–1062. doi: 10.1001/archotol.129.10.1056

Harrison, R. V., Stanton, S. G., Ibrahim, D., Nagasawa, A., and Mount, R. J. (1993). Neonatal cochlear hearing loss results in developmental abnormalities of the central auditory pathways. *Acta Otolaryngol.* 113, 296–302. doi: 10.3109/00016489309135812

Hartley, D. E., and Moore, D. R. (2003). Effects of conductive hearing loss on temporal aspects of sound transmission through the ear. *Hear. Res.* 177, 53–60. doi: 10.1016/s0378-5955(02)00797-9

Hartley, D. E., Wright, B. A., Hogan, S. C., and Moore, D. R. (2000). Age-related improvements in auditory backward and simultaneous masking in 6- to 10-year-old children. *J. Speech Lang. Hear. Res.* 43, 1402–1415. doi: 10.1044/jslhr.4306.1402

Heffner, H. E., and Heffner, R. S. (1995). "Conditioned avoidance," in *Methods in Comparative Psychoacoustics*, eds G. M. Klump, R. J. Dooling, R. R. Fay and W. C. Stebbins (Basel, Switzerland: Birkhauser Verlag), 79–93.

Higo, S., Udaka, N., and Tamamaki, N. (2007). Long-range GABAergic projection neurons in the cat neocortex. *J. Comp. Neurol.* 503, 421–431. doi: 10.1002/cne.21395

Hsieh, D. L., Lin, K. N., Ho, J. H., and Liu, T. C. (2009). Hearing in noise test in subjects with conductive hearing loss. *J. Formos. Med. Assoc.* 108, 937–942. doi: 10.1016/S0929-6646(10)60006-X

Hunter, L. L., Margolis, R. H., and Giebink, G. S. (1994). Identification of hearing loss in children with otitis media. *Ann. Otol. Rhinol. Laryngol. Suppl.* 163, 59–61.

Kelly, J. B., Cooke, J. E., Gilbride, P. C., Mitchell, C., and Zhang, H. (2006). Behavioral limits of auditory temporal resolution in the rat: amplitude modulation and duration discrimination. *J. Comp. Psychol.* 120, 98–105. doi: 10.1037/0735-7036.120.2.98

Keogh, T., Kei, J., Driscoll, C., and Khan, A. (2010). Children with minimal conductive hearing impairment: speech comprehension in noise. *Audiol. Neurootol.* 15, 27–35. doi: 10.1159/000218360

Kidd, G. Jr., Arbogast, T. L., Mason, C. R., and Walsh, M. (2002). Informational masking in listeners with sensorineural hearing loss. *J. Assoc. Res. Otolaryngol.* 3, 107–119. doi: 10.1007/s101620010095

King, A. J., Parsons, C. H., and Moore, D. R. (2000). Plasticity in the neural coding of auditory space in the mammalian brain. *Proc. Natl. Acad. Sci. U S A* 97, 11821–11828. doi: 10.1073/pnas.97.22.11821

Kittel, M., Wagner, E., and Klump, G. M. (2002). An estimate of the auditory-filter bandwidth in the Mongolian gerbil. *Hear. Res.* 164, 69–76. doi: 10.1016/s0378-5955(01)00411-7

Knudsen, E. I., Esterly, S. D., and Knudsen, P. F. (1984). Monaural occlusion alters sound localization during a sensitive period in the barn owl. *J. Neurosci.* 4, 1001–1011.

Kokko, E. (1974). Chronic secretory otitis media in children. A clinical study. *Acta Otolaryngol. Suppl.* 327, 1–44.

Kral, A., Hartmann, R., Tillein, J., Heid, S., and Klinke, R. (2000). Congenital auditory deprivation reduces synaptic activity within the auditory cortex in a layer-specific manner. *Cereb. Cortex* 10, 714–726. doi: 10.1093/cercor/10.7.714

Kral, A., Tillein, J., Heid, S., Hartmann, R., and Klinke, R. (2005). Postnatal cortical development in congenital auditory deprivation. *Cereb. Cortex* 15, 552–562. doi: 10.1093/cercor/bhh156

Leao, R. N., Berntson, A., Forsythe, I. D., and Walmsley, B. (2004). Reduced low-voltage activated K+ conductances and enhanced central excitability in a congenitally deaf (dn/dn) mouse. *J. Physiol.* 559, 25–33. doi: 10.1113/jphysiol.2004.067421

Leão, R. N., Naves, M. M., Leão, K. E., and Walmsley, B. (2006). Altered sodium currents in auditory neurons of congenitally deaf mice. *Eur. J. Neurosci.* 24, 1137–1146. doi: 10.1111/j.1460-9568.2006.04982.x

Lee, H., Kim, J., and Nguyen, V. (2013). Ear infections: otitis externa and otitis media. *Prim. Care* 40, 671–686. doi: 10.1016/j.pop.2013.05.005

Martin, B. A., Sigal, A., Kurtzberg, D., and Stapells, D. R. (1997). The effects of decreased audibility produced by high-pass noise masking on cortical event-related potentials to speech sounds/ba/and/da. *J. Acoust. Soc. Am.* 101, 1585–1599. doi: 10.1121/1.418146

Matsubara, J. A. (1988). Local, horizontal connections within area 18 of the cat. *Prog. Brain Res.* 75, 163–172. doi: 10.1016/s0079-6123(08)60475-6

May, B. J., and Sachs, M. B. (1992). Dynamic range of neural rate responses in the ventral cochlear nucleus of awake cats. *J. Neurophysiol.* 68, 1589–1602.

Mogil, J. S. (1999). The genetic mediation of individual differences in sensitivity to pain and its inhibition. *Proc. Natl. Acad. Sci. U S A* 96, 7744–7751. doi: 10.1073/pnas.96.14.7744

Moore, D. R. (2002). Auditory development and the role of experience. *Br. Med. Bull.* 63, 171–181. doi: 10.1093/bmb/63.1.171

Moore, B. C. (2012). *An Introduction to the Psychology of Hearing.* Bingley, UK: Emerald Group Publishing.

Moore, B. C., and Glasberg, B. R. (1986). Comparisons of frequency selectivity in simultaneous and forward masking for subjects with unilateral cochlear impairments. *J. Acoust. Soc. Am.* 80, 93–107. doi: 10.1121/1.394087

Moore, B. C., Poon, P. W., Bacon, S. P., and Glasberg, B. R. (1987). The temporal course of masking and the auditory filter shape. *J. Acoust. Soc. Am.* 81, 1873–1880. doi: 10.1121/1.394751

Munro, K. J., and Blount, J. (2009). Adaptive plasticity in brainstem of adult listeners following earplug-induced deprivation. *J. Acoust. Soc. Am.* 126, 568–571. doi: 10.1121/1.3161829

Näätänen, R., and Picton, T. (1987). The N1 wave of the human electric and magnetic response to sound: a review and an analysis of the component structure. *Psychophysiology* 24, 375–425. doi: 10.1111/j.1469-8986.1987.tb00311.x

Nielsen, C. S., Staud, R., and Price, D. D. (2009). Individual differences in pain sensitivity: measurement, causation and consequences. *J. Pain* 10, 231–237. doi: 10.1016/j.jpain.2008.09.010

Ojima, H. (2011). Interplay of excitation and inhibition elicited by tonal stimulation in pyramidal neurons of primary auditory cortex. *Neurosci. Biobehav. Rev.* 35, 2084–2093. doi: 10.1016/j.neubiorev.2010.11.009

Ojima, H., and Murakami, K. (2002). Intracellular characterization of suppressive responses in supragranular pyramidal neurons of cat primary auditory cortex in vivo. *Cereb. Cortex* 12, 1079–1091. doi: 10.1093/cercor/12.10.1079

Oxenham, A. J., and Bacon, S. P. (2003). Cochlear compression: perceptual measures and implications for normal and impaired hearing. *Ear Hear.* 24, 352–366. doi: 10.1097/01.aud.0000090470.73934.78

Phillips, D. P., and Cynader, M. S. (1985). Some neural mechanisms in the cat's auditory cortex underlying sensitivity to combined tone and wide-spectrum noise stimuli. *Hear. Res.* 18, 87–102. doi: 10.1016/0378-5955(85)90112-1

Phillips, D. P., and Kelly, J. B. (1992). Effects of continuous noise maskers on tone-evoked potentials in cat primary auditory cortex. *Cereb. Cortex* 2, 134–140. doi: 10.1093/cercor/2.2.134

Popescu, M. V., and Polley, D. B. (2010). Monaural deprivation disrupts development of binaural selectivity in auditory midbrain and cortex. *Neuron* 65, 718–731. doi: 10.1016/j.neuron.2010.02.019

Razak, K. A., Richardson, M. D., and Fuzessery, Z. M. (2008). Experience is required for the maintenance and refinement of FM sweep selectivity in the developing auditory cortex. *Proc. Natl. Acad. Sci. U S A* 105, 4465–4470. doi: 10.1073/pnas.0709504105

Rees, A., and Palmer, A. R. (1988). Rate-intensity functions and their modification by broadband noise for neurons in the guinea pig inferior colliculus. *J. Acoust. Soc. Am.* 83, 1488–1498. doi: 10.1121/1.395904

Robles, L., and Ruggero, M. A. (2001). Mechanics of the mammalian cochlea. *Physiol. Rev.* 81, 1305–1352.

Rosen, M. J., Sarro, E. C., Kelly, J. B., and Sanes, D. H. (2012). Diminished behavioral and neural sensitivity to sound modulation is associated with moderate developmental hearing loss. *PLoS One* 7:e41514. doi: 10.1371/journal.pone.0041514

Ruggero, M. A., Robles, L., and Rich, N. C. (1992). Two-tone suppression in the basilar membrane of the cochlea: mechanical basis of auditory-nerve rate suppression. *J. Neurophysiol.* 68, 1087–1099.

Sanes, D. (2013). "Synaptic and cellular consequences of hearing loss," in *Springer Handbook of Auditory Research: Deafness*, eds A. Kral, A. N. Popper and R. R. Fay (New York: Springer-Verlag), 129–150.

Sanes, D. H., and Bao, S. (2009). Tuning up the developing auditory CNS. *Curr. Opin. Neurobiol.* 19, 188–199. doi: 10.1016/j.conb.2009.05.014

Sarro, E. C., and Sanes, D. H. (2010). Prolonged maturation of auditory perception and learning in gerbils. *Dev. Neurobiol.* 70, 636–648. doi: 10.1002/dneu.20801

Scharf, B., Quigley, S., Aoki, C., Peachey, N., and Reeves, A. (1987). Focused auditory attention and frequency selectivity. *Percept. Psychophys.* 42, 215–223. doi: 10.3758/bf03203073

Schilder, A. G., Snik, A. F., Straatman, H., and van den Broek, P. (1994). The effect of otitis media with effusion at preschool age on some aspects of auditory perception at school age. *Ear Hear.* 15, 224–231. doi: 10.1097/00003446-199406000-00003

Schlauch, R. S., and Hafter, E. R. (1991). Listening bandwidths and frequency uncertainty in pure-tone signal detection. *J. Acoust. Soc. Am.* 90, 1332–1339. doi: 10.1121/1.401925

Smith, R. L., and Zwislocki, J. J. (1975). Short-term adaptation and incremental responses of single auditory-nerve fibers. *Biol. Cybern.* 17, 169–182. doi: 10.1007/bf00364166

Somogyi, P., Cowey, A., Kisvarday, Z. F., Freund, T. F., and Szentagothai, J. (1983). Retrograde transport of gamma-amino[3H]butyric acid reveals specific interlaminar connections in the striate cortex of monkey. *Proc. Natl. Acad. Sci. U S A* 80, 2385–2389. doi: 10.1073/pnas.80.8.2385

Stuermer, I. W., and Scheich, H. (2000). Early unilateral auditory deprivation increases 2-deoxyglucose uptake in contralateral auditory cortex of juvenile Mongolian gerbils. *Hear. Res.* 146, 185–199. doi: 10.1016/s0378-5955(00)00113-1

Sumner, C. J., Tucci, D. L., and Shore, S. E. (2005). Responses of ventral cochlear nucleus neurons to contralateral sound after conductive hearing loss. *J. Neurophysiol.* 94, 4234–4243. doi: 10.1152/jn.00401.2005

Swets, J. A. (1973). The relative operating characteristic in psychology: a technique for isolating effects of response bias finds wide use in the study of perception and cognition. *Science* 182, 990–1000. doi: 10.1126/science.182.4116.990

Takesian, A. E., Kotak, V. C., and Sanes, D. H. (2010). Presynaptic GABA(B) receptors regulate experience-dependent development of inhibitory short-term plasticity. *J. Neurosci.* 30, 2716–2727. doi: 10.1523/JNEUROSCI.3903-09.2010

Takesian, A. E., Kotak, V. C., and Sanes, D. H. (2012). Age-dependent effect of hearing loss on cortical inhibitory synapse function. *J. Neurophysiol.* 107, 937–947. doi: 10.1152/jn.00515.2011

Tomioka, R., Okamoto, K., Furuta, T., Fujiyama, F., Iwasato, T., Yanagawa, Y., et al. (2005). Demonstration of long-range GABAergic connections distributed throughout the mouse neocortex. *Eur. J. Neurosci.* 21, 1587–1600. doi: 10.1111/j.1460-9568.2005.03989.x

Tucci, D. L., Cant, N. B., and Durham, D. (1999). Conductive hearing loss results in a decrease in central auditory system activity in the young gerbil. *Laryngoscope* 109, 1359–1371. doi: 10.1097/00005537-199909000-00001

Tucci, D. L., Cant, N. B., and Durham, A. (2001). Conductive hearing loss results in changes in cytochrome oxidase activity in gerbil gentral auditory system. *J. Assoc. Res. Otolaryngol.* 3, 89–106. doi: 10.1007/s101620010091

Tucci, D. L., and Rubel, E. W. (1985). Afferent influences on brain stem auditory nuclei of the chicken: effects of conductive and sensorineural hearing loss on n. magnocellularis. *J. Comp. Neurol.* 238, 371–381. doi: 10.1002/cne.902380402

Ulanovsky, N., Las, L., and Nelken, I. (2003). Processing of low-probability sounds by cortical neurons. *Nat. Neurosci.* 6, 391–398. doi: 10.1038/nn1032

Vale, C., and Sanes, D. H. (2000). Afferent regulation of inhibitory synaptic transmission in the developing auditory midbrain. *J. Neurosci.* 20, 1912–1921.

Vale, C., and Sanes, D. H. (2002). The effect of bilateral deafness on excitatory and inhibitory synaptic strength in the inferior colliculus. *Eur. J. Neurosci.* 16, 2394–2404. doi: 10.1046/j.1460-9568.2002.02302.x

Volkov, I. O., and Galazyuk, A. V. (1992). Peculiarities of inhibition in cat auditory cortex neurons evoked by tonal stimuli of various durations. *Exp. Brain Res.* 91, 115–120. doi: 10.1007/bf00230019

Voytenko, S. V., and Galazyuk, A. V. (2008). Timing of sound-evoked potentials and spike responses in the inferior colliculus of awake bats. *Neuroscience* 155, 923–936. doi: 10.1016/j.neuroscience.2008.06.031

Wasner, G. L., and Brock, J. A. (2008). Determinants of thermal pain thresholds in normal subjects. *Clin. Neurophysiol.* 119, 2389–2395. doi: 10.1016/j.clinph.2008.07.223

Webster, D. B. (1983). Auditory neuronal sizes after a unilateral conductive hearing loss. *Exp. Neurol.* 79, 130–140. doi: 10.1016/0014-4886(83)90384-9

Whitton, J. P., and Polley, D. B. (2011). Evaluating the perceptual and pathophysiological consequences of auditory deprivation in early postnatal life: a comparison of basic and clinical studies. *J. Assoc. Res. Otolaryngol.* 12, 535–547. doi: 10.1007/s10162-011-0271-6

Wright, B. A., and Dai, H. (1994). Detection of unexpected tones with short and long durations. *J. Acoust. Soc. Am.* 95, 931–938. doi: 10.1121/1.410010

Wu, G. K., Li, P., Tao, H. W., and Zhang, L. I. (2006). Nonmonotonic synaptic excitation and imbalanced inhibition underlying cortical intensity tuning. *Neuron* 52, 705–715. doi: 10.1016/j.neuron.2006.10.009

Xu, H., Kotak, V. C., and Sanes, D. H. (2007). Conductive hearing loss disrupts synaptic and spike adaptation in developing auditory cortex. *J. Neurosci.* 27, 9417–9426. doi: 10.1523/jneurosci.1992-07.2007

Yanz, J. L. (1984). The application of the theory of signal detection to the assessment of speech perception. *Ear Hear.* 5, 64–71. doi: 10.1097/00003446-198403000-00002

Youssoufian, M., Oleskevich, S., and Walmsley, B. (2005). Development of a robust central auditory synapse in congenital deafness. *J. Neurophysiol.* 94, 3168–3180. doi: 10.1152/jn.00342.2005

Zwicker, E. (1965). Temporal effects in simultaneous masking by white-noise bursts. *J. Acoust. Soc. Am.* 37, 653–663. doi: 10.1121/1.1909389

19

Auditory training during development mitigates a hearing loss-induced perceptual deficit

Ramanjot Kang[1], Emma C. Sarro[1] and Dan H. Sanes[1,2]*

[1] _Center for Neural Science, New York University, New York, NY, USA_
[2] _Department of Biology, New York University, New York, NY, USA_

***Correspondence:**
Dan H. Sanes, Center for Neural Science, New York University, 4 Washington Place, New York, NY 10003, USA
e-mail: dhs1@nyu.edu

Sensory experience during early development can shape the central nervous system and this is thought to influence adult perceptual skills. In the auditory system, early induction of conductive hearing loss (CHL) leads to deficits in central auditory coding properties in adult animals, and this is accompanied by diminished perceptual thresholds. In contrast, a brief regimen of auditory training during development can enhance the perceptual skills of animals when tested in adulthood. Here, we asked whether a brief period of training during development could compensate for the perceptual deficits displayed by adult animals reared with CHL. Juvenile gerbils with CHL, and age-matched controls, were trained on a frequency modulation (FM) detection task for 4 or 10 days. The performance of each group was subsequently assessed in adulthood, and compared to adults with normal hearing (NH) or adults raised with CHL that did not receive juvenile training. We show that as juveniles, both CHL and NH animals display similar FM detection thresholds that are not immediately impacted by the perceptual training. However, as adults, detection thresholds and psychometric function slopes of these animals were significantly improved. Importantly, CHL adults with juvenile training displayed thresholds that approached NH adults. Additionally, we found that hearing impaired animals trained for 10 days displayed adult thresholds closer to untrained adults than those trained for 4 days. Thus, a relatively brief period of auditory training may compensate for the deleterious impact of hearing deprivation on auditory perception on the trained task.

Keywords: conductive hearing loss, plasticity, auditory training, frequency modulation, development, perceptual learning

INTRODUCTION

The developmental sensory environment can initiate life long modifications to central nervous system computations and has been demonstrated for a broad range of sensory systems (for review see (visual) Hubel, 1978; Wiesel, 1982; Hooks and Chen, 2007; (somatosensory) Feldman and Brecht, 2005; (auditory) Keuroghlian and Knudsen, 2007; Sanes and Bao, 2009). In the auditory system, these neural deficits are closely associated with impaired perceptual skills. For example, developmental auditory deprivation leads to diminished behavioral performance on frequency discrimination, amplitude modulation detection, and sound localization (Clements and Kelly, 1978; Kerr et al., 1979; Knudsen et al., 1984; Moore et al., 1999; Rosen et al., 2012). Consistent with this, developmental hearing loss in humans can lead to persistent deficiencies in sound localization and signal detection, as well as impairments in the acquisition of speech and language (Hall and Grose, 1994; Wilmington et al., 1994; Hall et al., 1995; Kidd et al., 2002; Halliday and Bishop, 2005, 2006). Even transient periods of conductive hearing loss (CHL), due to chronic otitis media with effusion, may cause perceptual deficits (Whitton and Polley, 2011).

In contrast to the detrimental impact of developmental hearing loss, a brief period of auditory training during development can enhance performance on the trained task when animals are tested in adulthood (Sarro and Sanes, 2011). The long-term effect, as assessed in adulthood, is similar to the impact of adult perceptual training (Wright et al., 1997; Wright and Fitzgerald, 2001; Wright and Sabin, 2007). However, the short term effect of training during development can be surprisingly limited (Sarro and Sanes, 2010; Huyck and Wright, 2011). These findings suggest that developmental auditory training could counteract the long-term perceptual deficits induced by early sound deprivation. Here, we asked whether the diminished performance skills of adult animals reared with CHL could be rescued with a brief period of auditory perceptual training during juvenile development.

In the present study, we examined the performance of gerbils on a frequency modulation (FM) detection task. Adults reared with CHL display much poorer performance on this task than adults reared with normal hearing (NH; Buran et al., 2014). Therefore, we provided both CHL and NH juveniles with a brief period of auditory training on the FM detection task, and reassessed their detection thresholds in adulthood. Juvenile training permitted animals with hearing loss to display superior FM detection thresholds and decreased variance (as measured with psychometric function slope) as compared to CHL animals without juvenile training. These results suggest that training induces a long-term compensation for the perceptual deficits on the trained task caused by early hearing loss.

MATERIALS AND METHODS

ANIMALS

Gerbil (*Meriones unguiculatus*) pups were weaned from commercial breeding pairs (Charles River) at postnatal days (P) 23–30. Males and females were caged separately and maintained in a 12 h light/dark cycle. All procedures related to the maintenance and uses of animals were in accordance with the "Institutional Animal & Use Committee Handbook" and approved by the University Animal Welfare Committee (UAWC) at New York University.

DEVELOPMENTAL HEARING LOSS

Bilateral CHL was induced via surgical removal of a middle ear bone, the malleus, prior to the onset of hearing at P10. At postnatal day 10 (P10), pups were anesthetized with the halogenated ethyl methyl ether, methoxyflurane. Anesthetic induction occurred within 10 min and produced complete elimination of responses to nociceptive stimuli. CHL was induced by tympanic membrane puncture and malleus extirpation (Tucci et al., 1999). A postauricular skin incision was made, and the tympanic membrane was visualized and punctured with a forceps. The malleus was then removed through this opening. The postauricular wound was closed with cyanoacrylate glue, and procedure repeated on the other side. After surgery, animals were warmed on a heating pad and returned to the litter when respiration and motor activity had recovered. The age of surgery was chosen based on the finding that anteroventral cochlear nucleus cell number is unaffected by cochlear ablation after P9 in gerbils (Tierney and Moore, 1997). This manipulation induces an attenuation of ≈55 dB at 4 kHz, as assessed by auditory brainstem response (Tucci et al., 1999; Rosen et al., 2012), but behavioral measures indicate an attenuation of ≈40 dB at 4 kHz (Buran et al., 2014). We did not use sham controls for this study, however previous work from our lab has published findings that show similar effects of CHL when compared to sham controls or non-sham controls (Takesian et al., 2012; Kotak et al., 2013), demonstrating the neurophysiological effects of CHL were not due to the anesthesia or surgery procedures.

EXPERIMENTAL GROUPS

FM depth detection thresholds were obtained from gerbils as both juveniles and adults. Data from adults reared with NH, and adults reared with CHL were collected previously for a study on the critical period of vulnerability to hearing loss (Buran et al., 2014). Both of these groups received procedural training and 10 days of perceptual training (described below) on an FM detection task from ~P70–P90. The new data collected in this study was obtained from the following groups: (1) Juvenile trained NH animals (n = 11 (2f, 9m)) received procedural training and 4 or 10 days of perceptual training on an FM detection task beginning on ~P23, the earliest age at which animals could be weaned and placed on controlled water access; (2) Juvenile trained CHL gerbils (n = 13 (7f, 6m)) also received procedural training and 4 or 10 days of perceptual training on an FM detection task beginning at ~P23. As adults (~P70–P90), after the age at which gerbils reach sexual maturity (Field and Sibold, 1999) these animals were retested on the FM detection task; (3) Adult trained NH gerbils (n = 6 (6m)) received procedural training and 10 days of perceptual training on an FM detection task beginning at ~P70. As older adults (~P120–150) these animals were retested on the FM detection task. These animals were not exposed to handling or the testing context prior to adult testing; (4) An additional group (n = 6 (2f, 4m)) of adults reared with NH were obtained, and added to the data obtained previously and re-shown here (Buran et al., 2014). These animals were not exposed to handling or the testing context prior to adult testing.

BEHAVIORAL TESTING APPARATUS

Gerbils were placed in a testing cage of approximated 1 ft^2 that was housed within a sound isolation booth (Gretch-Ken Industries), and observed from a separate room via a closed circuit monitor. When the animal contacted both a metal footplate and lick spout, they completed a circuit that initiated water delivery via a syringe pump (Yale Apparatus). A personal computer, connected to a digital interface (Tucker-Davis Technologies, TDT RZ6), generated the acoustic stimuli, timed the water delivery (0.3 ml/min), and controlled a small current that was delivered through the metal lick spout. Auditory stimuli were delivered via a calibrated tweeter (KEF Electronics) positioned 1 m in front of the test cage at 0° elevation. Sound level was calibrated with a spectrum analyzer (Bruel and Kjaer 3550) via a 1/4″ free-field condenser microphone positioned at the head location when in contact with the lick spout.

PROCEDURAL TRAINING

All training used a conditioned avoidance Go-Nogo procedure to measure detection of FM stimuli (Heffner and Heffner, 1995; Kelly et al., 2006; Sarro and Sanes, 2010, 2011). Animals were placed on controlled water access and, upon introduction to the experimental cage, learned to obtain water from the metal lick spout. This training occurred in the presence of a continuous unmodulated 4 kHz tone. Sound level was set to 45 dB SPL for NH animals, and 95 dB SPL for animals with CHL to compensate for the elevated thresholds. These values were identical to those used in a published report on FM detection (Buran et al., 2014). Additionally, we previously found that sensation level was not correlated with FM detection threshold (Buran et al., 2014). Animals were then trained to withdraw from the spout when a FM stimulus was presented. To train the withdrawal response, a low AC current (0.5–1.0 mA, 300 ms; Lafayette Instruments) was delivered through the lick spout immediately after each FM stimulus. Since animals display between-subject variability in pain sensitivity (Mogil, 1999; Wasner and Brock, 2008; Nielsen et al., 2009) the strength of the shock was adjusted for each animal to reliably produce withdrawal from the spout, but not so great as to dissuade an animal from approaching the spout on subsequent trials (Sarro and Sanes, 2010). To train animals on the procedure, go trials (4 kHz center frequency; 5 Hz modulation rate; 500 Hz modulation depth) were presented until performance reached a criterion of ≥70% correct over 10 consecutive trials. All animals received procedural training to establish criterion performance when they were first introduced to the task as juveniles, and again when they were reintroduced to the task for assessment in adulthood.

PERCEPTUAL TRAINING AND ASSESSMENT OF FM DETECTION THRESHOLDS

Once this criterion was reached, we tested animals on a range of at least 5 FM depths within each session, presented in descending order from largest to smallest. On each subsequent day of perceptual training, an animal's performance on the previous day determined the range of depths that were presented; these depths always bracketed the previous day's detection threshold. This protocol was used for all treatment groups. For juvenile perceptual training, animals were trained for either 4 or 10 days. This choice was chosen to remain consistent with the number of juvenile training days used in a prior study (Sarro and Sanes, 2011). Subsequently, we found that adults approach their best detection thresholds on the FM detection task when using at least 10 days of detection training (Buran et al., 2014). Adult animals were tested until their performance stabilized (i.e., did not improve for 3 consecutive days).

TRIAL STRUCTURE

Each trial was 1000 ms long, either containing the FM stimulus (go trials) or not containing a modulation of the 4 kHz center frequency (nogo trials). To determine if the animal detected the FM stimulus, contact with the spout was monitored during the final 100 ms of each go trial. A contact time of <50 ms was scored as a correct response (i.e., a hit), and a contact time of >50 ms was scored as a miss. For nogo trials, a contact time of <50 ms was scored as a false alarm, and a contact time of >50 ms was scored as a correct rejection. Go trials always occurred after a block of 3–5 nogo trials, randomized to avoid temporal conditioning.

DATA ANALYSIS

Behavioral sensitivity, $d' = z(\text{false alarm}) - z(\text{hit})$, was obtained for z-scores that corresponded to the right-tail p-values (Swets, 1973), and was calculated for each FM depth. Only sessions in which an animal performed a minimum of 5 trials per stimulus value were included in the analysis. Performance functions from sessions consisting of at least five presentations of five different depths were fitted using the open-source package psignifit as described in Buran et al. (2014). To ensure fits were of sufficient quality we discarded fits where the deviance of the fit to the original dataset exceeded the 95th percentile of the deviance of the fit to 1,000 simulated datasets (see Fründ et al., 2011 for details). Threshold was defined as the FM depth at which performance reached a $d' = 1$, and slope was also calculated at a d' of 1, as obtained from fitted psychometric functions (see examples shown in **Figures 1, 2**). Average threshold for each treatment group was determined by averaging the threshold for the best 3 days of testing for each animal.

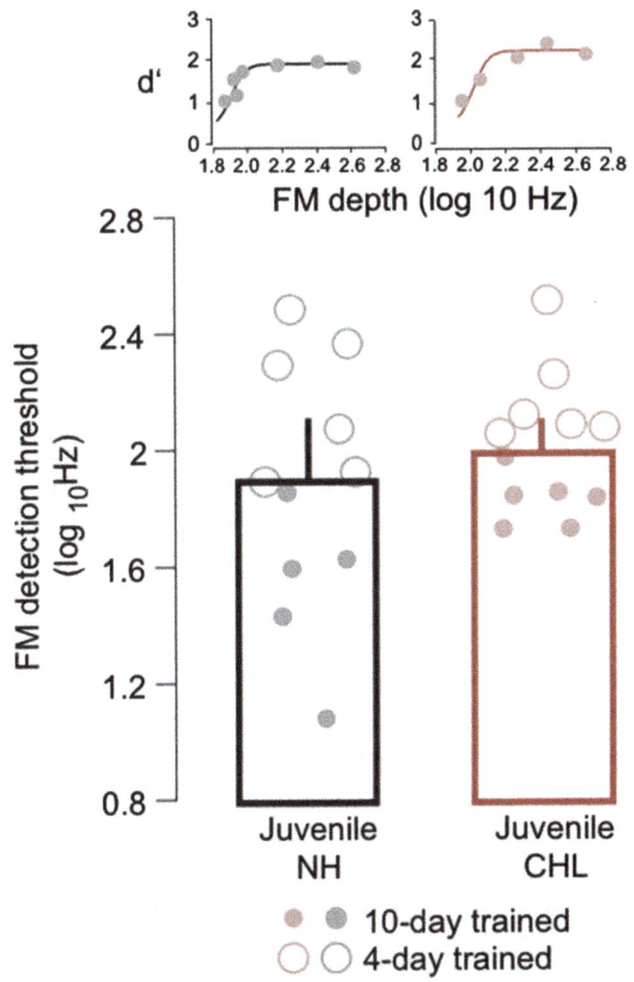

FIGURE 1 | Normal hearing (NH) and conductive hearing loss (CHL) juveniles display similar frequency modulation (FM) detection thresholds. Average FM detection thresholds ($\log_{10}$Hz; mean ± SEM) are plotted for NH juveniles (black bar, gray circles) and CHL juveniles (red bar; light red circles). Data points from individual animals are the average of the best 3 days of performance. Open circles indicate 4 days of perceptual training, and closed circles indicate 10 days of perceptual training. Insets: Example psychometric function fits from one NH juvenile and one CHL juvenile, taken from a single day of testing.

Statistical tests were first performed to determine whether the dependent variable was normally distributed for each treatment group (NH, CHL, juvenile-trained CHL), using a Shapiro-Wilk normality test. We found two departures from normality (slope of psychometric function for NH adults, $p = 0.02$ and Juvenile-trained CHL adults, $p = 0.007$) and used Levene's test for equal variance (using the median value as an estimate of each group's center) since it is more robust when samples deviate from a normal distribution. Two of the dependent variables displayed unequal variance (Adult FM thresholds, $df = 2$, $F = 4.6$, $p = 0.02$; and slope of psychometric function, $df = 2$, $F = 33.6$, $p < 0.001$). For all multiple comparison tests, we used the non-parametric Kruskal-Wallis test followed by pairwise comparisons using a two-sided Wilcoxon test with Holm-corrected p-values.

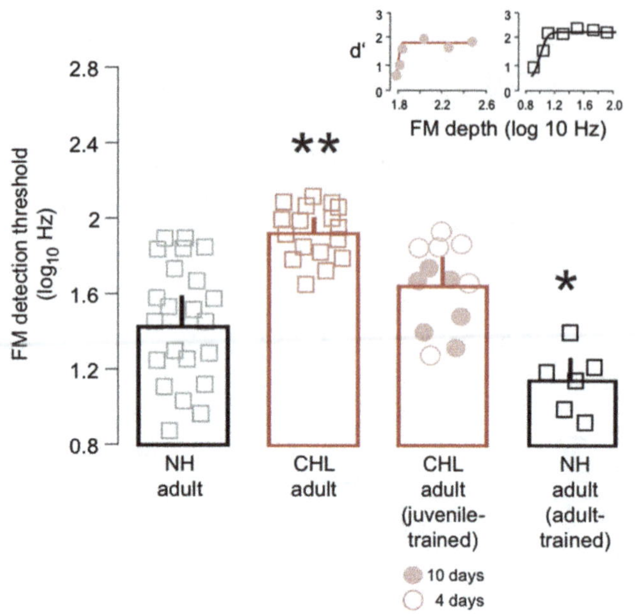

FIGURE 2 | Training on FM detection as a juvenile improved detection thresholds assessed in adulthood. Average FM detection thresholds ($\log_{10}$Hz; mean ± SEM) are plotted for NH adult (black bar, gray squares), CHL adult (red bar; red squares), CHL adult animals trained on the FM task as juveniles (red bar; red circles), and NH adult animals trained on the FM task as adults and retested at a later time (black bar, black squares). For the juvenile trained animals, open circles indicate 4 days of perceptual training, and closed circles indicate 10 days of perceptual training. Data points from individual animals are the average of the best 3 days of performance. Significant differences for between-group comparisons are presented in the text and indicated here by asterisks (** significantly greater than all other groups; * significantly smaller than all other groups). Insets: Example psychometric function fits from CHL adult animals trained on the FM task as juveniles (red circles, red line) and the NH adult animals trained on the FM task as adults and retested at a later time (black bar, black squares), taken from a single day of testing. Examples from the same set of NH adults and CHL adults are provided in a previous published report (Buran et al., 2014).

For normally distributed depended variables (Juvenile FM detection thresholds), we used a one-way ANOVA as a way to compare the groups.

RESULTS

FM DETECTION ABILITY FOR NH AND CHL GERBILS IS SIMILAR DURING DEVELOPMENT

To address whether developmental CHL influenced perception during the juvenile period, we obtained FM detection thresholds from NH and CHL animals at P23–P40. **Figure 1** plots the mean FM detection thresholds, and the performance of individual animals, with days of training indicated by the symbol type. An ANOVA reported a main effect of training duration ($F = 35.0$, $df = 1$, $p < 0.0001$), but there was neither an effect of hearing status ($F = 3.3$, $df = 1$, $p = 0.08$) nor an interaction between hearing status and training duration ($F = 2.8$, $df = 1$, $p = 0.11$). Therefore, it appears that CHL does not immediately diminish FM detection thresholds.

ADULT FM DETECTION IS IMPROVED BY JUVENILE TRAINING

We have previously shown that developmental CHL leads to degraded FM detection thresholds in adulthood (Buran et al., 2014). Here, we tested whether training on the FM detection task during juvenile development could rescue this perceptual skill in adulthood. NH and CHL animals were trained on the FM detection task from P23–P40, and retested as adults. **Figure 2** illustrates a main effect of treatment group on FM detection thresholds (Kruskal-Wallis: $\chi^2 = 31.03$, $df = 3$, $p < 0.0001$). The average FM detection threshold for NH adults (1.44 ± 0.05 $\log_{10}$Hz) was significantly lower than for CHL adults (1.93 ± 0.06 $\log_{10}$Hz) (Wilcoxon test: $\chi^2 = 19.8$, $df = 1$, $p < 0.0001$). Notably, the average FM detection threshold for juvenile trained CHL-reared animals (1.64 ± 0.07 $\log_{10}$Hz) was significantly better than CHL adults (Wilcoxon test: $\chi^2 = 10.73$, $df = 1$, $p < 0.001$), and only slightly worse than the detection thresholds of NH animals (Wilcoxon test: $\chi^2 = 3.4$, $df = 1$, $p = 0.07$). However, the CHL animals that had been trained for 10 days (**Figure 2**, closed red circles; 1.54 ± 0.09 $\log_{10}$Hz) generally displayed better detection thresholds than those animals trained for only 4 days (**Figure 2**, open circles; 1.74 ± 0.09 $\log_{10}$Hz). This suggests that developmental training on FM detection rescued adult abilities for animals raised with moderate hearing loss.

Finally, we asked whether training on the FM detection task in adulthood could improve performance of NH animals when subsequently tested again. NH adults with prior adult training on the FM detection task displayed better detection thresholds (1.14 ± 0.12 $\log_{10}$Hz) than NH adults (Wilcoxon test: $\chi^2 = 4.77$, $df = 1, p < 0.05$), untrained CHL adults (Wilcoxon test: $\chi^2 = 12.8$, $df = 1, p < 0.001$), and the juvenile trained CHL adults (Wilcoxon test: $\chi^2 = 10.1$, $df = 1$, $p < 0.01$). Therefore, the effect of juvenile training on animals with CHL did not restore the highest level of performance that was observed in NH animals.

To determine whether developmental training modifies the variance of performance, the psychometric function slopes were obtained at $d' = 1$ for the three best sessions. **Figure 3** shows a main effect of treatment group (Kruskal-Wallis: $\chi^2 = 34.3$, $df = 2$, $p < 0.0001$). The average slope for NH adults (0.06 ± 0.01 $d'/\log_{10}$Hz) was significantly steeper than found in CHL adults (0.02 ± 0.007 $\log_{10}$Hz) (Wilcoxon test: $\chi^2 = 18.65$, $df = 1$, $p < 0.0001$). However, the average slope for juvenile trained CHL-reared animals (0.17 ± 0.02 $d'/\log_{10}$Hz) was significantly steeper than CHL adults (Wilcoxon test: $\chi^2 = 20.4$, $df = 1$, $p < 0.0001$), and also significantly steeper from NH animals (Wilcoxon test: $\chi^2 = 15.9$, $df = 1$, $p < 0.001$). The CHL animals that had been trained for 10 days (**Figure 3**, closed red circles; 0.2 ± 0.03 $d'/\log_{10}$Hz) generally displayed steeper slopes than those animals trained for only 4 days (**Figure 3**, open circles; 0.13 ± 0.03 $d'/\log_{10}$Hz). This suggests that developmental training on FM detection decreases performance variability for animals raised with hearing loss.

DISCUSSION

Auditory deprivation during development can induce long-term changes to the central nervous system, and these are associated with perceptual deficits in adulthood (Sanes and Bao, 2009; Sanes and Woolley, 2011). For example, CHL that is induced prior to

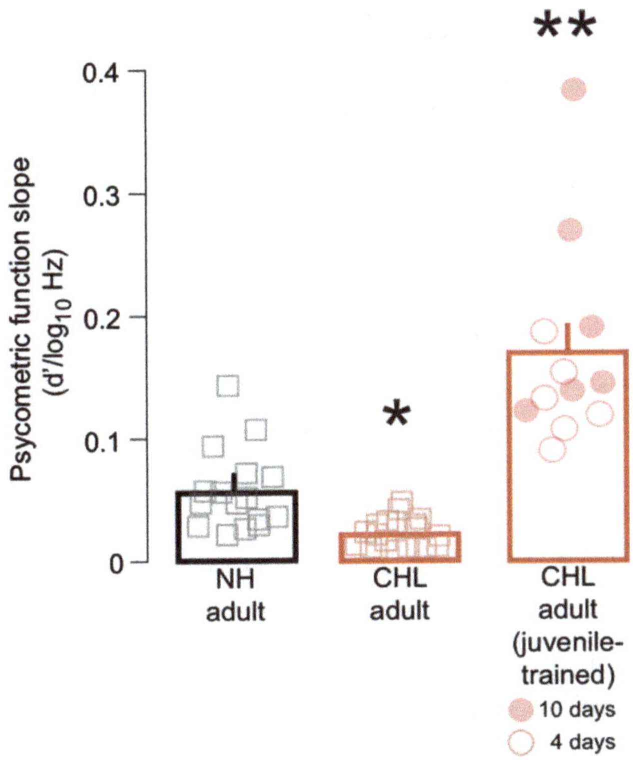

FIGURE 3 | Training on FM detection as a juvenile improved psychometric function slopes in adulthood. Average slope of fitted psychometric functions ($d'/\log_{10}$Hz; mean ± SEM) are plotted for NH adult (black bar, gray squares), CHL adult (red bar; red squares), and CHL adult animals trained on the FM task as juveniles (red bar; red circles). Data points from individual animals are the average of the best 3 days of performance. For the trained animals, open circles indicate 4 days of perceptual training, and closed circles indicate 10 days of perceptual training. Significant differences for between-group comparisons are presented in the text and indicated here by asterisks (** significantly greater than all other groups; * significantly smaller than all other groups).

hearing onset results in poorer performance on both frequency and amplitude modulation detection tasks, even when audibility is compensated (Rosen et al., 2012; Buran et al., 2014), where our lab's prior work on FM detection in animals with hearing loss tested the theory that there is a critical period for hearing loss on adult perception (Buran et al., 2014). However, the developmental period also provides an opportune time to train animals on perceptual tasks. A brief period of auditory perceptual training during the juvenile period results in a long-term benefit to adult performance on the trained task (Sarro and Sanes, 2011). This current study was a logical extension of this because it led us to explore whether long-term deficits on auditory perceptual skills on FM detection could be rescued with a brief period of training during development. Here, we trained juvenile gerbils with CHL on a FM detection task, and found that their performance on this task in adulthood was better than untrained CHL animals.

The performance of CHL animals was initially assessed immediately at the termination of the training period while animals were still juveniles. At this time, the FM detection thresholds of CHL animals were similar to those displayed by NH juvenile animals (**Figure 1**). This suggests that the deficits in performance, as measured in adults (Buran et al., 2014), emerge gradually as the duration of deprivation accumulates. Because of inadequate sensory input, the animals with CHL may not display a normal trajectory of improvement. A similar phenomenon is found in children with language based learning disorders who display slower auditory perceptual maturation, and do not attain adult levels of performance (Wright and Zecker, 2004). Consistent with this, children with hearing impairments display immature measures of cortical function when compared to NH children that is only partially restored by cochlear implants, suggesting a delay in the developmental process that does not resolve following an extended duration of hearing (Ponton and Eggermont, 2001).

The results from the present study demonstrate that a brief period of FM detection training during this period is sufficient to improve adult detection FM thresholds in animals with CHL, and thus possibly impede the accumulation of the deficit as a function of age. The two training regimens, 4 or 10 days, were not sufficient to restore a normal level of performance (**Figure 2**). However, our results indicate that the amount of developmental training can impact adult performance. Thus, those adults that had received 10 days of developmental training had slightly better adult detection thresholds than those with only 4 days of training (**Figure 2**). The impact of juvenile training on psychometric function slopes (**Figure 3**) suggests that the limited amount of training given to the juveniles with CHL allowed these animals to become more consistent within a narrower range of FM depths. It is possible that, with more training on the FM detection task during development, these animals may have become more confident across a broader range of FM depths and eventually approached NH adult thresholds, while also modifying the slope closer to NH adults. Taken together, these findings suggest that perceptual learning that occurs during development can provide long-term benefits on perceptual abilities and may, in fact, be able to rescue deficits in perception.

The long-term enhancements to performance were the result of only a brief period of developmental training. Each daily session during development occurred over a period of about 10–15 min in duration and only for a total or either 4 or 10 sessions. Following this training period, animals were not exposed to the training stimuli until reaching adulthood. This suggests that the practice required to improve performance may be small, at least for this task. In fact, the amount of perceptual training required to induce learning does differ, depending on the specific percept being trained (Wright and Fitzgerald, 2001; Wright and Sabin, 2007; Fitzgerald and Wright, 2011). For example, in adult humans, the number of sessions required to show dramatic improvement can be as low as one session for tasks such as amplitude modulation detection and interaural time difference detection, but as high as three sessions for interaural level difference detection (Wright and Fitzgerald, 2001; Fitzgerald and Wright, 2011). In the present study, the amount of training had an impact on the degree of improvement in adulthood (**Figure 2**), indicating that a further increase of practice could lead to even greater improvements (Hussain et al., 2009), and possibly full recovery of normal adult perception.

DEVELOPMENTAL TRAINING MAY COMPENSATE FOR CENTRAL IMPAIRMENTS

One basis for the ameliorative influence of juvenile training is that central impairments caused by CHL (Xu et al., 2007, 2010; Takesian et al., 2010, 2012, 2013) were either corrected or compensated for by learning learning-associated plasticity. Prior studies demonstrate that primary auditory cortex displays induced modifications for both frequency representation and cortical temporal processing (Recanzone et al., 1993; Weinberger and Bakin, 1998; Beitel et al., 2003; Bao et al., 2004). Moreover, behavioral training has been shown to restore impaired cortical processing in animals with developmentally induced hearing loss. For example, in prelingually deafened cats, behaviorally relevant training leads to enhanced temporal processing in auditory cortex that is close to normal levels (Beitel et al., 2011; Vollmer and Beitel, 2011). Consistent with this, congenitally deaf humans who receive cochlear prostheses early in life display improvements in speech perception and language skills, suggesting a long-term effect of exposure and use of auditory input (Busby et al., 1991; Dawson et al., 1992; Svirsky et al., 2004). Thus, modifications and improvements to an impairment of cortical function may accompany the behavioral improvements displayed by the CHL animals with developmental training.

ACKNOWLEDGMENTS

This work was supported by DC009237 (Dan H. Sanes). We thank Antje Ihlefeld and Brad Buran for help with data analysis.

REFERENCES

Bao, S., Chang, E. F., Woods, J., and Merzenich, M. M. (2004). Temporal plasticity in the primary auditory cortex induced by operant perceptual learning. *Nat. Neurosci.* 7, 974–981. doi: 10.1038/nn1293

Beitel, R. E., Schreiner, C. E., Cheung, S. W., Wang, X., and Merzenich, M. M. (2003). Reward-dependent plasticity in the primary auditory cortex of adult monkeys trained to discriminate temporally modulated signals. *Proc. Natl. Acad. Sci. U S A* 100, 11070–11075. doi: 10.1073/pnas.1334187100

Beitel, R. E., Vollmer, M., Raggio, M. W., and Schreiner, C. E. (2011). Behavioral training enhances cortical temporal processing in neonatally deafened juvenile cats. *J. Neurophysiol.* 106, 944–959. doi: 10.1152/jn.00731.2010

Buran, B. N., Sarro, E. C., Manno, F. A., Kang, R., Caras, M. L., and Sanes, D. H. (2014). A sensitive period for the impact of hearing loss on auditory perception. *J. Neurosci.* 34, 2276–2284. doi: 10.1523/JNEUROSCI.0647-13.2014

Busby, P. A., Roberts, S. A., Tong, Y. C., and Clark, G. M. (1991). Results of speech perception and speech production training for three prelingually deaf patients using a multiple-electrode cochlear implant. *Br. J. Audiol.* 25, 291–302. doi: 10.3109/03005369109076601

Clements, M., and Kelly, J. B. (1978). Auditory spatial responses of young guinea pigs (Cavia porcellus) during and after ear blocking. *J. Comp. Physiol. Psychol.* 92, 34–44. doi: 10.1037/h0077424

Dawson, P. W., Blamey, P. J., Rowland, L. C., Dettman, S. J., Clark, G. M., Busby, P. A., et al. (1992). Cochlear implants in children, adolescents, and prelinguistically deafened adults: speech perception. *J. Speech Hear. Res.* 35, 401–417.

Feldman, D. E., and Brecht, M. (2005). Map plasticity in somatosensory cortex. *Science* 310, 810–815. doi: 10.1126/science.1115807

Field, K. J., and Sibold, A. L. (1999). "Husbandry, breeding," in *The Laboratory Hamster and Gerbil*, ed M. A. Suckow (Boca Raton, FL: CRC Press LLC), 43–46.

Fitzgerald, M. B., and Wright, B. A. (2011). Perceptual learning and generalization resulting from training on an auditory amplitude-modulation detection task. *J. Acoust. Soc. Am.* 129, 898–906. doi: 10.1121/1.3531841

Fründ, I., Haenel, N. V., and Wichmann, F. A. (2011). Inference for psychometric functions in the presence of nonstationary behavior. *J. Vis.* 11:16. doi: 10.1167/11.6.16

Hall, J. W., and Grose, J. H. (1994). The effect of otitis media with effusion on comodulation masking release in children. *J. Speech Hear. Res.* 37, 1441–1449.

Hall, J. W., Grose, J. H., and Pillsbury, H. C. (1995). Long-term effects of chronic otitis media on binaural hearing in children. *Arch. Otolaryngol. Head Neck Surg.* 121, 847–852. doi: 10.1001/archotol.1995.01890080017003

Halliday, L. F., and Bishop, D. V. M. (2005). Frequency discrimination and literacy skills in children with mild to moderate sensorineural hearing loss. *J. Speech Lang. Hear. Res.* 48, 1187–1203. doi: 10.1044/1092-4388(2005/083)

Halliday, L. F., and Bishop, D. V. (2006). Is poor frequency modulation detection linked to literacy problems? A comparison of specific reading disability and mild to moderate sensorineural hearing loss. *Brain Lang.* 97, 200–213. doi: 10.1016/j.bandl.2005.10.007

Heffner, H. E., and Heffner, R. S. (1995). "Conditioned avoidance," in *Methods in Comparative Psychoacoustics*, eds G. M. Klump, R. J. Dooling, R. R. Fay and W. C. Stebbins (Basel, Switzerland: Birkhauser Verlag), 79–93.

Hooks, B. M., and Chen, C. (2007). Critical periods in the visual system: changing views for a model of experience-dependent plasticity. *Neuron* 56, 312–326. doi: 10.1016/j.neuron.2007.10.003

Hubel, D. H. (1978). Effects of deprivation on the visual cortex of cat and monkey. *Harvey Lect.* 72, 1–51.

Hussain, Z., Sekuler, A. B., and Bennett, P. J. (2009). How much practice is needed to produce perceptual learning? *Vision Res.* 49, 2624–2634. doi: 10.1016/j.visres.2009.08.022

Huyck, J. J., and Wright, B. A. (2011). Late maturation of auditory perceptual learning. *Dev. Sci.* 14, 614–621. doi: 10.1111/j.1467-7687.2010.01009.x

Kelly, J. B., Cooke, J. E., Gilbride, P. C., Mitchell, C., and Zhang, H. (2006). Behavioral limits of auditory temporal resolution in the rat: amplitude modulation and duration discrimination. *J. Comp. Psychol.* 120, 98–105. doi: 10.1037/0735-7036.120.2.98

Kerr, L. M., Ostapoff, E. M., and Rubel, E. W. (1979). Influence of acoustic experience on the ontogeny of frequency generalization gradients in the chicken. *J. Exp. Psychol. Anim. Behav. Process.* 5, 97–115. doi: 10.1037/0097-7403.5.2.97

Keuroghlian, A. S., and Knudsen, E. I. (2007). Adaptive auditory plasticity in developing and adult animals. *Prog. Neurobiol.* 82, 109–121. doi: 10.1016/j.pneurobio.2007.03.005

Kidd, G. Jr., Arbogast, T. L., Mason, C. R., and Walsh, M. (2002). Informational masking in listeners with sensorineural hearing loss. *J. Assoc. Res. Otolaryngol.* 3, 107–119. doi: 10.1007/s101620010095

Knudsen, E. I., Esterly, S. D., and Knudsen, P. F. (1984). Monaural occlusion alters sound localization during a sensitive period in the barn owl. *J. Neurosci.* 4, 1001–1011.

Kotak, V. C., Takesian, A. E., MacKenzie, P. C., and Sanes, D. H. (2013). Rescue of inhibitory synapse strength following developmental hearing loss. *PLoS One* 8:e53438. doi: 10.1371/journal.pone.0053438

Mogil, J. S. (1999). The genetic mediation of individual differences in sensitivity to pain and its inhibition. *Proc. Natl. Acad. Sci. U S A* 96, 7744–7751. doi: 10.1073/pnas.96.14.7744

Moore, D. R., Hine, J. E., Jiang, Z. D., Matsuda, H., Parsons, C. H., and King, A. J. (1999). Conductive hearing loss produces a reversible binaural hearing impairment. *J. Neurosci.* 19, 8704–8711.

Mossbridge, J. A., Fitzgerald, M. B., O'Connor, E. S., and Wright, B. A. (2006). Perceptual-learning evidence for separate processing of asynchrony and order tasks. *J. Neurosci.* 26, 12708–12716. doi: 10.1523/jneurosci.2254-06.2006

Nielsen, C. S., Staud, R., and Price, D. D. (2009). Individual differences in pain sensitivity: measurement, causation, and consequences. *J. Pain* 10, 231–237. doi: 10.1016/j.jpain.2008.09.010

Ponton, C. W., and Eggermont, J. J. (2001). Of kittens and kids: altered cortical maturation following profound deafness and cochlear implant use. *Audiol. Neurootol.* 6, 363–380. doi: 10.1159/000046846

Recanzone, G. H., Schreiner, C. E., and Merzenich, M. M. (1993). Plasticity in the frequency representation of primary auditory cortex following discrimination training in adult owl monkeys. *J. Neurosci.* 13, 87–103.

Rosen, M. J., Sarro, E. C., Kelly, J. B., and Sanes, D. H. (2012). Diminished behavioral and neural sensitivity to sound modulation is associated with moderate developmental hearing loss. *PLoS One* 7:e41514. doi: 10.1371/journal.pone.0041514

Sanes, D. H., and Bao, S. (2009). Tuning up the developing auditory CNS. *Curr. Opin. Neurobiol.* 19, 188–199. doi: 10.1016/j.conb.2009.05.014

Sanes, D. H., and Woolley, S. M. N. (2011). A behavioral framework to guide research on central auditory development and plasticity. *Neuron* 72, 912–929. doi: 10.1016/j.neuron.2011.12.005

Sarro, E. C., and Sanes, D. H. (2010). Prolonged maturation of auditory perception and learning in gerbils. *Dev. Neurobiol.* 70, 636–648. doi: 10.1002/dneu.20801

Sarro, E. C., and Sanes, D. H. (2011). The cost and benefit of juvenile training on adult perceptual skill. *J. Neurosci.* 31, 5383–5391. doi: 10.1523/JNEUROSCI.6137-10.2011

Svirsky, M. A., Teoh, S. W., and Neuburger, H. (2004). Development of language and speech perception in congenitally, profoundly deaf children as a function of age at cochlear implantation. *Audiol. Neurootol.* 9, 224–233. doi: 10.1159/000078392

Swets, J. A. (1973). The relative operating characteristic in psychology. *Science* 182, 990–1000. doi: 10.1126/science.182.4116.990

Takesian, A. E., Kotak, V. C., and Sanes, D. H. (2010). Presynaptic GABA(B) receptors regulate experience-dependent development of inhibitory short-term plasticity. *J. Neurosci.* 30, 2716–2727. doi: 10.1523/JNEUROSCI.3903-09.2010

Takesian, A. E., Kotak, V. C., and Sanes, D. H. (2012). Age-dependent effect of hearing loss on cortical inhibitory synapse function. *J. Neurophysiol.* 107, 937–947. doi: 10.1152/jn.00515.2011

Takesian, A. E., Kotak, V. C., Sharma, N., and Sanes, D. H. (2013). Hearing loss differentially disrupts thalamic drive to two cortical interneurons. *J. Neurophysiol.* 110, 999–1008. doi: 10.1152/jn.00182.2013

Tierney, T. S., and Moore, D. R. (1997). Naturally occurring neuron death during postnatal development of the gerbil ventral cochlear nucleus begins at the onset of hearing. *J. Comp. Neurol.* 387, 421–429. doi: 10.1002/(sici)1096-9861(19971027)387:3<421::aid-cne7>3.0.co;2-2

Tucci, D. L., Cant, N. B., and Durham, D. (1999). Conductive hearing loss results in a decrease in central auditory system activity in the young gerbil. *Laryngoscope* 109, 1359–1371. doi: 10.1097/00005537-199909000-00001

Vollmer, M., and Beitel, R. E. (2011). Behavioral training restores temporal processing in auditory cortex of long-deaf cats. *J. Neurophysiol.* 106, 2423–2436. doi: 10.1152/jn.00565.2011

Wasner, G. L., and Brock, J. A. (2008). Determinants of thermal pain thresholds in normal subjects. *Clin. Neurophysiol.* 119, 2389–2395. doi: 10.1016/j.clinph.2008.07.223

Weinberger, N. M., and Bakin, J. S. (1998). Learning-induced physiological memory in adult primary auditory cortex: receptive field plasticity, model, and mechanisms. *Audiol. Neurootol.* 3, 145–167. doi: 10.1159/000013787

Whitton, J. P., and Polley, D. B. (2011). Evaluating the perceptual and pathophysiological consequences of auditory deprivation in early postnatal life: a comparison of basic and clinical studies. *J. Assoc. Res. Otolaryngol.* 12, 535–547. doi: 10.1007/s10162-011-0271-6

Wiesel, T. N. (1982). Postnatal development of the visual cortex and the influence of the environment. *Nature* 299, 583–591. doi: 10.1038/299583a0

Wilmington, D., Gray, L., and Jahrsdoerfer, R. (1994). Binaural processing after corrected congenital unilateral conductive hearing loss. *Hear. Res.* 74, 99–114. doi: 10.1016/0378-5955(94)90179-1

Wright, B. A., Buonomano, D. V., Mahncke, H. W., and Merzenich, M. M. (1997). Learning and generalization of auditory temporal-interval discrimination in humans. *J. Neurosci.* 17, 3956–3963.

Wright, B. A., and Fitzgerald, M. B. (2001). Different patterns of human discrimination learning for two interaural cues to sound-source location. *Proc. Natl. Acad. Sci. U S A* 98, 12307–12312. doi: 10.1073/pnas.211220498

Wright, B. A., and Sabin, A. T. (2007). Perceptual learning: how much daily training is enough? *Exp. Brain Res.* 180, 727–736. doi: 10.1007/s00221-007-0898-z

Wright, B. A., and Zecker, S. G. (2004). Learning problems, delayed development, and puberty. *Proc. Natl. Acad. Sci. U S A* 101, 9942–9946. doi: 10.1073/pnas.0401825101

Xu, H., Kotak, V. C., and Sanes, D. H. (2007). Conductive hearing loss disrupts synaptic and spike adaptation in developing auditory cortex. *J. Neurosci.* 27, 9417–9426. doi: 10.1523/jneurosci.1992-07.2007

Xu, H., Kotak, V. C., and Sanes, D. H. (2010). Normal hearing is required for the emergence of long-lasting inhibitory potentiation in cortex. *J. Neurosci.* 30, 331–341. doi: 10.1523/JNEUROSCI.4554-09.2010

Permissions

All chapters in this book were first published by Frontiers; hereby published with permission under the Creative Commons Attribution License or equivalent. Every chapter published in this book has been scrutinized by our experts. Their significance has been extensively debated. The topics covered herein carry significant findings which will fuel the growth of the discipline. They may even be implemented as practical applications or may be referred to as a beginning point for another development.

The contributors of this book come from diverse backgrounds, making this book a truly international effort. This book will bring forth new frontiers with its revolutionizing research information and detailed analysis of the nascent developments around the world.

We would like to thank all the contributing authors for lending their expertise to make the book truly unique. They have played a crucial role in the development of this book. Without their invaluable contributions this book wouldn't have been possible. They have made vital efforts to compile up to date information on the varied aspects of this subject to make this book a valuable addition to the collection of many professionals and students.

This book was conceptualized with the vision of imparting up-to-date information and advanced data in this field. To ensure the same, a matchless editorial board was set up. Every individual on the board went through rigorous rounds of assessment to prove their worth. After which they invested a large part of their time researching and compiling the most relevant data for our readers.

The editorial board has been involved in producing this book since its inception. They have spent rigorous hours researching and exploring the diverse topics which have resulted in the successful publishing of this book. They have passed on their knowledge of decades through this book. To expedite this challenging task, the publisher supported the team at every step. A small team of assistant editors was also appointed to further simplify the editing procedure and attain best results for the readers.

Apart from the editorial board, the designing team has also invested a significant amount of their time in understanding the subject and creating the most relevant covers. They scrutinized every image to scout for the most suitable representation of the subject and create an appropriate cover for the book.

The publishing team has been an ardent support to the editorial, designing and production team. Their endless efforts to recruit the best for this project, has resulted in the accomplishment of this book. They are a veteran in the field of academics and their pool of knowledge is as vast as their experience in printing. Their expertise and guidance has proved useful at every step. Their uncompromising quality standards have made this book an exceptional effort. Their encouragement from time to time has been an inspiration for everyone.

The publisher and the editorial board hope that this book will prove to be a valuable piece of knowledge for researchers, students, practitioners and scholars across the globe.

List of Contributors

Andrej Kral and Peter Hubka
Cluster of Excellence, Department of Experimental Otology, Institute of Audioneurotechnology, ENT Clinics, Hannover Medical School, Hannover, Germany

Silvia Heid and Jochen Tillein
Cluster of Excellence, Department of Experimental Otology, Institute of Audioneurotechnology, ENT Clinics, Hannover Medical School, Hannover, Germany
Department of Physiology and Otolaryngology, J. W. Goethe University, Frankfurt am Main, Germany

Samira Anderson, Travis White-Schwoch and Hee Jae Choi
Auditory Neuroscience Laboratory, Department of Communication Sciences and Disorders, Northwestern University, Evanston, IL, USA
Department of Communication Sciences, Northwestern University, Evanston, IL, USA

Nina Kraus
Auditory Neuroscience Laboratory, Department of Communication Sciences and Disorders, Northwestern University, Evanston, IL, USA
Department of Communication Sciences, Northwestern University, Evanston, IL, USA
Institute for Neuroscience, Northwestern University, Evanston, IL, USA
Department of Neurobiology and Physiology, Northwestern University, Evanston, IL, USA
Department of Otolaryngology, Northwestern University, Evanston, IL, USA

Alan Kan and Ruth Y. Litovsky
Waisman Center, University of Wisconsin, Madison, WI, USA

Antje Ihlefeld
Waisman Center, University of Wisconsin, Madison, WI, USA
Center for Neural Science, New York University, New York, NY, USA

Carolyn McGettigan
Department of Psychology, Royal Holloway, University of London, Egham, UK
Institute of Cognitive Neuroscience, University College London, London, UK

Sophie K. Scott
Institute of Cognitive Neuroscience, University College London, London, UK

Stuart Rosen
Department of Speech, Hearing and Phonetic Sciences, University College London, London, UK

Meital Avivi-Reich, Meredyth Daneman and Bruce A. Schneider
Human Communication Laboratory, Department of Psychology, University of Toronto Mississauga, Mississauga, ON, Canada

Julia Erb and Jonas Obleser
Max Planck Research Group "Auditory Cognition", Max Planck Institute for Human Cognitive and Brain Sciences, Leipzig, Germany

Tara Rachakonda and Judith E. C. Lieu
Department of Otolaryngology-Head and Neck Surgery, Washington University School of Medicine, St. Louis, MO, USA

Joshua S. Shimony and Rebecca S. Coalson
Department of Radiology, Mallinckrodt Institute of Radiology, Washington University School of Medicine, St. Louis, MO, USA

Sushmit Mishra, Jerker Rönnberg and Mary Rudner Stefan Stenfelt
Linnaeus Centre HEAD, Swedish Institute for Disability Research, Department of Behavioural Sciences and Learning, Linköping University, Linköping, Sweden
Department of Clinical and Experimental Medicine, Linköping University, Linköping, Sweden

Thomas Lunner
Linnaeus Centre HEAD, Swedish Institute for Disability Research, Department of Behavioural Sciences and Learning, Linköping University, Linköping, Sweden
Department of Clinical and Experimental Medicine, Linköping University, Linköping, Sweden
Eriksholm Research Centre, Oticon A/S, Snekkersten, Denmark

Jill B. Firszt, Ruth M. Reeder and Timothy A. Holden
Department of Otolaryngology-Head and Neck Surgery, Washington University School of Medicine, St. Louis, MO, USA

Harold Burton
Department of Anatomy and Neurobiology, Washington University School of Medicine, St. Louis, MO, USA
Department of Radiology, Washington University School of Medicine, St. Louis, MO, USA

Richard A. Chole
Department of Otolaryngology-Head and Neck Surgery, Washington University School of Medicine, St. Louis, MO, USA
Department of Developmental Biology, Washington University School of Medicine, St. Louis, MO, USA

Fatima T. Husain
Department of Speech and Hearing Science, University of Illinois at Urbana-Champaign, Champaign, IL, USA
The Neuroscience Program, University of Illinois at Urbana-Champaign, Champaign, IL, USA
Beckman Institute for Advanced Science and Technology, University of Illinois at Urbana-Champaign, Champaign, IL, USA

Jake R. Carpenter-Thompson and Sara A. Schmidt
The Neuroscience Program, University of Illinois at Urbana-Champaign, Champaign, IL, USA
Beckman Institute for Advanced Science and Technology, University of Illinois at Urbana-Champaign, Champaign, IL, USA

Hari M. Bharadwaj and Barbara G. Shinn-Cunningham
Center for Computational Neuroscience and Neural Technology, Boston University, Boston, MA, USA
Department of Biomedical Engineering, Boston University, Boston, MA, USA

Sarah Verhulst
Center for Computational Neuroscience and Neural Technology, Boston University, Boston, MA, USA
Department of Otology and Laryngology, Harvard Medical School, Boston, MA, USA

Luke Shaheen
Eaton-Peabody Laboratories, Massachusetts Eye and Ear Infirmary, Boston, MA, USA
Harvard-MIT Division of Health Sciences and Technology, Speech and Hearing Bioscience and Technology Program, Cambridge, MA, USA

M. Charles Liberman
Department of Otology and Laryngology, Harvard Medical School, Boston, MA, USA
Eaton-Peabody Laboratories, Massachusetts Eye and Ear Infirmary, Boston, MA, USA
Harvard-MIT Division of Health Sciences and Technology, Speech and Hearing Bioscience and Technology Program, Cambridge, MA, USA

Robert Becker and Christoph M. Michel
Functional Brain Mapping Lab, Department of Fundamental Neuroscience, University of Geneva, Geneva, Switzerland

Maria Pefkou and Alexis G. Hervais-Adelman
Brain and Language Lab, Department of Clinical Neuroscience, University of Geneva, Geneva, Switzerland

Kenneth S. Henry
Department of Speech, Language, and Hearing Sciences, Purdue University, West Lafayette, IN, USA

Sushrut Kale
Weldon School of Biomedical Engineering, Purdue University, West Lafayette, IN, USA

Michael G. Heinz
Department of Speech, Language, and Hearing Sciences, Purdue University, West Lafayette, IN, USA
Weldon School of Biomedical Engineering, Purdue University, West Lafayette, IN, USA

Chloé Huetz, Maud Guedin and Jean-Marc Edeline
Centre de Neurosciences Paris-Sud, CNRS, UMR 8195, Université Paris-Sud, Orsay, France

Peter Keating and Andrew J. King
Department of Physiology, Anatomy and Genetics, University of Oxford, Oxford, UK

Kelly L. Tremblay and Katrina McClannahan
Department of Speech and Hearing Sciences, University of Washington, Seattle, WA, USA

Bernhard Ross
Baycrest Centre, Rotman Research Institute, Toronto, ON, Canada
Department of Medical Biophysics, University of Toronto, Toronto, ON, Canada

Kayo Inoue
Department of Speech and Hearing Sciences, University of Washington, Seattle, WA, USA
Department of Radiology, Integrated Brian Imaging Center, University of Washington, Seattle, WA, USA

Gregory Collet
Life Sciences Department, Royal Military Academy, Brussels, Belgium
Unité de Recherche en Neurosciences Cognitives, Centre de Recherches en Cognition et Neurosciences Université Libre de Bruxelles, Brussels, Belgium

Anja Roye and Claire Salloum
Rotman Research Institute, Baycrest Centre for Geriatric Care, Toronto, ON, Canada

Ramanjot Kang and Emma C. Sarro
Center for Neural Science, New York University, New York, NY, USA

Claude Alain
Rotman Research Institute, Baycrest Centre for Geriatric Care, Toronto, ON, Canada
Department of Psychology, University of Toronto, Toronto, ON, Canada
Institute of Medical Sciences, University of Toronto, Toronto, ON, Canada

Sergiy V. Voytenko, Alexander V. Galazyuk and Merri J. Rosen
Department of Anatomy and Neurobiology, Northeast Ohio Medical University, Rootstown, OH, USA

Jennifer D. Gay
Department of Anatomy and Neurobiology, Northeast Ohio Medical University, Rootstown, OH, USA
Biomedical Sciences Program, Kent State University, Kent, OH, USA

Dan H. Sanes
Center for Neural Science, New York University, New York, NY, USA
Department of Biology, New York University, New York, NY, USA

Index

www.ingramcontent.com/pod-product-compliance
Lightning Source LLC
LaVergne TN
LVHW082149200926
848484LV00008B/2127

* 9 7 9 8 8 8 7 4 0 1 7 3 7 *